Wear of orthopaedic implants and artificial joints

Related titles:

Joint replacement technology
(ISBN 978-1-84569-245-2)
Increasing numbers of joint revision and replacement operations drive the demand for improved prostheses. This book comprehensively reviews developments in joint replacement technology, covering the most pertinent materials science and engineering issues, specific joints, clinical trial results and sterilisation techniques. Part I discusses biomechanics, tribology, the chemical environment of the body and an overview of materials and engineering of joint replacement. The second part of the book reviews specific materials, bearing surfaces and bone cements, in addition to the failure mechanisms and lifetime prediction of joints. Part III discusses the biological environment and interaction of replacement joints. Specific joints are analysed in detail in Part IV.

Bone repair biomaterials
(ISBN 978-1-84569-385-5)
Bone repair is a fundamental part of the rapidly expanding medical care sector and has benefited from many recent technological developments. This unique book provides a comprehensive review of the materials science, engineering principles and recent advances in this important area. The first part of the book reviews the fundamentals of bone repair and regeneration. Further chapters discuss the science and properties of biomaterials used for bone repair such as metals and biocomposites. The final set of chapters analyses device considerations such as implant lifetime, failure, applications and ethics of bone repair biomaterials.

Orthopaedic bone cements
(ISBN 978-1-84569-376-3)
Bone cements are widely used in orthopaedic applications to bond an implant to existing bone and in remodelling following bone loss. *Orthopaedic bone cements* is an authoritative review of research that focuses on improving the mechanical and biological performance of bone cements. The first part of the book discusses the use of bone cements in medicine in addition to commercial aspects and delivery systems. Bone cement materials are reviewed in Part II, followed by their mechanical properties in Part III. Techniques to enhance bone cements, such as antibiotic loading and bioactive cements, are discussed in the final part.

Details of these and other Woodhead Publishing materials books can be obtained by

- visiting our web site at www.woodheadpublishing.com
- contacting Customer Services (e-mail: sales@woodheadpublishing.com; fax: +44 (0) 1223 832819; tel.: +44 (0) 1223 499140 ext. 130; address: Woodhead Publishing Limited, 80 High Street, Sawston, Cambridge CB22 3HJ, UK)
- contacting our US office (e-mail: usmarketing@woodheadpublishing.com; tel.: (215) 928 9112; address: Woodhead Publishing, 1518 Walnut Street, Suite 1100, Philadelphia, PA 19102-3406, USA)

If you would like e-versions of our content, please visit our online platform: www.woodheadpublishing.com. Please recommend it to your librarian so that everyone in your institution can benefit from the wealth of content on the site.

Wear of orthopaedic implants and artificial joints

Edited by
Saverio Affatato

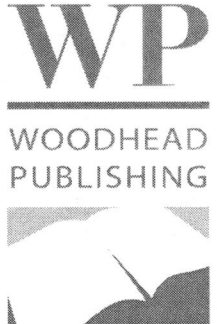

Oxford   Cambridge   Philadelphia   New Delhi

Published by Woodhead Publishing Limited,
80 High Street, Sawston, Cambridge CB22 3HJ, UK
www.woodheadpublishing.com
www.woodheadpublishingonline.com

Woodhead Publishing, 1518 Walnut Street, Suite 1100, Philadelphia, PA 19102-3406, USA

Woodhead Publishing India Private Limited, G-2, Vardaan House, 7/28 Ansari Road, Daryaganj, New Delhi – 110002, India
www.woodheadpublishingindia.com

First published 2012, Woodhead Publishing Limited
© Woodhead Publishing Limited, 2012
The authors have asserted their moral rights.

This book contains information obtained from authentic and highly regarded sources. Reprinted material is quoted with permission, and sources are indicated. Reasonable efforts have been made to publish reliable data and information, but the authors and the publishers cannot assume responsibility for the validity of all materials. Neither the authors nor the publishers, nor anyone else associated with this publication, shall be liable for any loss, damage or liability directly or indirectly caused or alleged to be caused by this book.

Neither this book nor any part may be reproduced or transmitted in any form or by any means, electronic or mechanical, including photocopying, microfilming and recording, or by any information storage or retrieval system, without permission in writing from Woodhead Publishing Limited.

The consent of Woodhead Publishing Limited does not extend to copying for general distribution, for promotion, for creating new works, or for resale. Specific permission must be obtained in writing from Woodhead Publishing Limited for such copying.

Trademark notice: Product or corporate names may be trademarks or registered trademarks, and are used only for identification and explanation, without intent to infringe.

British Library Cataloguing in Publication Data
A catalogue record for this book is available from the British Library.

Library of Congress Control Number: 2012932629

ISBN 978-0-85709-128-4 (print)
ISBN 978-0-85709-612-8 (online)

The publisher's policy is to use permanent paper from mills that operate a sustainable forestry policy, and which has been manufactured from pulp which is processed using acid-free and elemental chlorine-free practices. Furthermore, the publisher ensures that the text paper and cover board used have met acceptable environmental accreditation standards.

Typeset by Data Standards Ltd, Frome, Somerset, UK
Printed by TJ Digital, Padstow, Cornwall, UK

Contents

	Contributor contact details	xi
	Acknowledgements	xv
Part I	**Fundamentals of implant wear**	1
1	**Introduction to wear phenomena of orthopaedic implants**	3
	S. AFFATATO and D. BRANDO, Istituto Ortopedico Rizzoli, Italy	
1.1	History of wear	3
1.2	Wear mechanisms	5
1.3	Importance of wear mechanisms and their evaluation	17
1.4	*In vivo* wear measurements	18
1.5	*In vitro* wear measurements	19
1.6	Socio-economic wear impact	21
1.7	Future trends	22
1.8	References	22
2	**Biology of implant wear**	27
	G. CIAPETTI, Istituto Ortopedico Rizzoli, Italy	
2.1	Introduction	27
2.2	Inflammatory reaction to particulate materials	28
2.3	Cellular/molecular response to wear	32
2.4	Conclusion and therapeutic targets	40
2.5	References	48
3	**Biomechanics of the hip and knee: implant wear**	56
	F. E. KENNEDY, Dartmouth College, USA	
3.1	Introduction	56
3.2	Kinematics of hip and knee joints	57
3.3	Kinetics and joint forces	64

3.4	Lubrication and contact conditions in hip and knee implants	71
3.5	Implications for implant wear	80
3.6	Future trends in biomechanics of hip and knee joints	86
3.7	Sources of further information	87
3.8	References	87
4	**Anatomy of the hip and suitable prostheses**	**93**

F. TRAINA, M. DE FINE and S. AFFATATO, Istituto Ortopedico Rizzoli, Italy

4.1	Anatomy of the hip	93
4.2	Kinematics of the hip	98
4.3	Biomechanics of the hip	101
4.4	History and indications for total hip replacement	104
4.5	Prosthetic designs and bearing surfaces	105
4.6	Future trends	109
4.7	Acknowledgments	110
4.8	References	111
5	**Anatomy of the knee and suitable prostheses**	**115**

F. TRAINA, M. DE FINE and S. AFFATATO, Istituto Ortopedico Rizzoli, Italy

5.1	Bones and ligaments	115
5.2	Kinematics	120
5.3	Biomechanics	123
5.4	History and indications for total knee replacement	124
5.5	Prosthetic designs and bearing surfaces	126
5.6	Future trends	129
5.7	Acknowledgment	129
5.8	References	130
6	**Orthopaedic implant materials and design**	**133**

D. TIGANI, Santa Maria alle Scotte Hospital, Italy, M. FOSCO, R. BEN AYAD and R. FANTASIA, Istituto Ortopedico Rizzoli, Italy

6.1	Introduction	133
6.2	Materials in knee and hip arthroplasty	134
6.3	Evolution of total knee arthroplasty	147
6.4	History of total hip arthroplasty	151
6.5	Future trends	168
6.6	Sources of further information and advice	169
6.7	Acknowledgments	169
6.8	References	170

| 7 | Materials used for hip and knee implants | 178 |

E. KAIVOSOJA, Helsinki University Central Hospital, Finland, V.-M. TIAINEN, Orton Orthopaedic Hospital of the Invalid Foundation, Finland, Y. TAKAKUBO, Helsinki University Central Hospital, Finland and Yamagata University School of Medicine, Japan, B. RAJCHEL, Polish Academy of Sciences, Poland, J. SOBIECKI, Warsaw University of Technology, Poland, Y. T. KONTTINEN, Helsinki University Central Hospital, Finland, Orton Orthopaedic Hospital of the Invalid Foundation, Finland and COXA Hospital for Joint Replacement, Finland and M. TAKAGI, Yamagata University School of Medicine, Japan

7.1	Introduction	178
7.2	Polymer evolution and internal/surface treatments	179
7.3	Metal evolution and internal/surface treatments to use *in vivo*	187
7.4	Ceramic evolution and internal/surface treatments to use *in vivo*	196
7.5	Conclusion	206
7.6	References	206

Part II	Wear phenomena	219

| 8 | Wear phenomena of ultra-high molecular weight polyethylene (UHMWPE) joints | 221 |

C. CHO, The University of Kitakyushu, Japan, T. MURAKAMI and Y. SAWAE, Kyushu University, Japan

8.1	Introduction	221
8.2	Wear phenomena of UHMWPE knee joints	227
8.3	Concluding remarks	242
8.4	Acknowledgments	242
8.5	References	243

| 9 | Wear phenomena of metal joints | 246 |

N. DIOMIDIS, Ecole Polytechnique Fédérale de Lausanne, Switzerland

9.1	Alloys for orthopaedic implants	246
9.2	Electrochemical aspects of corrosion	249
9.3	Passivity and corrosion of implant alloys	253
9.4	Surface phenomena in biotribocorrosion	257
9.5	Tribocorrosion at the articulating interface	262

9.6	Fretting corrosion	267
9.7	Conclusions	272
9.8	References	272
10	**Wear phenomena of ceramic joints**	**278**

S. AFFATATO, Istituto Ortopedico Rizzoli, Italy and P. TADDEI, Università di Bologna, Italy

10.1	Introduction	278
10.2	Developments in ceramic technology	280
10.3	Wear of ceramic components	288
10.4	References	293
11	**The influence of surgical techniques on implant wear**	**298**

X. FLECHER, S. PARRATTE, J.-M. AUBANIAC and J.-N. ARGENSON, Institut du Mouvement et de l'Appareil Locomoteur, France

11.1	Introduction	298
11.2	Hip arthroplasty	299
11.3	Knee arthroplasty	303
11.4	Conclusion	305
11.5	References	305
12	**Factors contributing to orthopaedic implant wear**	**310**

L. C. JONES, Johns Hopkins University School of Medicine, USA, A. K. TSAO, Sun Valley Orthopedic Surgeons, USA and L. D. T. TOPOLESKI, University of Maryland, Baltimore County, USA

12.1	Introduction	310
12.2	Implant-specific factors – materials and design	318
12.3	Surgical factors	327
12.4	Patient factors	330
12.5	Interactions between different factors	333
12.6	Conclusion	334
12.7	References	334
13	**Diagnosis and surveillance of orthopaedic implants**	**351**

S. AFFATATO, D. BRANDO, Istituto Ortopedico Rizzoli, Italy and D. TIGANI, Santa Maria alle Scotte Hospital, Italy

13.1	The importance of a correct diagnosis	351
13.2	Predictive and detection methods	364
13.3	Choice of prosthesis	366

13.4	Patient education	369
13.5	Surveillance	370
13.6	References	372
14	**Failure analysis of orthopaedic implants**	**377**
	D. W. VAN CITTERS, Dartmouth College, USA	
14.1	Introduction	377
14.2	Implant retrieval laboratories	378
14.3	Failure modes	379
14.4	Analysis techniques	391
14.5	Importance of validation	394
14.6	Conclusion	395
14.7	References	395
15	**Wear prediction of orthopaedic implants**	**403**
	F. LIU, J. FISHER, University of Leeds, UK and Z. JIN, University of Leeds, UK and Xi'an Jiatong University, People's Republic of China	
15.1	Introduction	403
15.2	Overall wear modelling	404
15.3	Wear models	405
15.4	Determination of wear factors and coefficients	407
15.5	Contact models	409
15.6	Numerical calculation of wear	409
15.7	Applications	410
15.8	Future trends	414
15.9	Further information	416
15.10	Acknowledgments	416
15.11	References	417
	Index	*419*

Contributor contact details

(* = main contact)

Editor and chapters 1, 4, 5, 10 and 13

Saverio Affatato
Laboratorio di Tecnologia Medica
Istituto Ortopedico Rizzoli
Via di Barbiano, 1/10
40136 Bologna
Italy
E-mail: affatato@tecno.ior.it

Chapter 1

Saverio Affatato*
E-mail: affatato@tecno.ior.it

Dorina Brando
Laboratorio di Tecnologia Medica
Istituto Ortopedico Rizzoli
Via di Barbiano, 1/10
40136 Bologna
Italy

Chapter 2

Gabriela Ciapetti
Lab for Orthopaedic
  Pathophysiology and
  Regenerative Medicine
Istituto Ortopedico Rizzoli
Via di Barbiano, 1/10
40136 Bologna
Italy
E-mail: gabriela.ciapetti@ior.it

Chapter 3

Francis E. Kennedy
Thayer School of Engineering
Dartmouth College
Hanover
NH 03755
USA
E-mail: Francis.kennedy@
  dartmouth.edu

Chapters 4 and 5

Francesco Traina
Laboratorio di Tecnologia Medica
Istituto Ortopedico Rizzoli
Bologna
Italy

Marcello De Fine
Traumatologia e Chirurgia
  Protesica e dei Reimpianti di
  Anca e di Ginocchio
Istituto Ortopedico Rizzoli
Bologna
Italy

Saverio Affatato*
E-mail: affatato@tecno.ior.it

Chapter 6

Domenico Tigani*
Department of Orthopaedic Surgery
Santa Maria alle Scotte Hospital
Viale Bracci, 1
53100 Siena
Italy
E-mail: domenico.tigani@fast webnet.it

Matteo Fosco, Rida Ben Ayad and Rossana Fantasia
First Ward of Orthopaedic Surgery
Istituto Ortopedico Rizzoli
Bologna
Italy

Chapter 7

E. Kaivosoja
Department of Medicine
Helsinki University Central Hospital, Haartmaninkatu 8
FI-00029 HUS
Helsinki
Finland

V.-M. Tiainen
Orton Orthopaedic Hospital of the Invalid Foundation
Tenholantie 10
00280, Helsinki
Finland

Y. Takakubo
Department of Medicine
Helsinki University Central Hospital
Helsinki
Finland

and

Department of Orthopaedic Surgery
Yamagata University School of Medicine, 2-2-2 Iida-Nishi
Yamagata, 990-9585
Japan

B. Rajchel
Institute of Nuclear Physics
Polish Academy of Sciences
ul. Radzikowskiego 152
31-342, Kraków
Poland

J. Sobiecki
Faculty of Materials Science and Engineering
Warsaw University of Technology
Narbutta 85
02-524, Warsaw
Poland

Y. T. Konttinen*
Department of Medicine
Helsinki University Central Hospital, Haartmaninkatu 8
FI-00029 HUS
Helsinki
Finland
E-mail: yrjo.konttinen@helsinki.fi

and

Orton Orthopaedic Hospital of the Invalid Foundation
Tenholantie 10
00280, Helsinki
Finland

and

COXA Hospital for Joint
   Replacement
Biokatu 6B
33520, Tampere
Finland

M. Takagi
Department of Orthopaedic Surgery
Yamagata University School of
   Medicine, 2-2-2 Iida-Nishi
Yamagata, 990-9585
Japan

Chapter 8

Changhee Cho*
Department of Mechanical Systems
   Engineering
Faculty of Environmental
   Engineering
The University of Kitakyushu
1–1 Hibikino, Wakamatsu-ku,
   Kitakyushu
Fukuoka 808–0135
Japan
E-mail: cho@kitakyu-u.ac.jp

Teruo Murakami and Yoshinori
   Sawae
Department of Mechanical
   Engineering
Faculty of Engineering
Kyushu University
744 Motooka
Nishi-ku
Fukuoka 819–0395
Japan

Chapter 9

Nikitas Diomidis
Tribology and Interfacial Chemistry
   Group
Ecole Polytechnique Fédérale de
   Lausanne
MXC231, Station 12
CH-1015 Lausanne
Switzerland
E-mail: nikitas.diomidis@epfl.ch

Chapter 10

Saverio Affatato*
E-mail: affatato@tecno.ior.it

P. Taddei
Dipartimento di Biochimica "G.
   Moruzzi"
Sezione di Chimica e Propedeutica
   Biochimica
Via Belmeloro, 8/2
Università di Bologna
Bologna
Italy

Chapter 11

Xavier Flecher*, Sebastien Parratte,
   Jean-Mannel Aubaniac and Jean-
   Noël Argenson
Institut du Mouvement et de
   l'Appareil Locomoteur
Assistance Publique des Hôpitaux
   de Marseille
Université de la Méditerranée
270, Bd Sainte Marguerite
Marseille 13009
France
E-mail: Xavier.flecher@ap-hm.fr

Chapter 12

Lynne C. Jones*
Department of Orthopaedic Surgery
Johns Hopkins University School of
   Medicine

JHU Orthopaedics @ Good
  Samaritan Hospital
Suite 201 Smyth Bldg.
5601 Loch Raven Blvd.
Baltimore
MD 21239
USA
E-mail: ljones3@jhmi.edu

Audrey K. Tsao
Sun Valley Orthopedic Surgeons
Surprise
Arizona
USA

L. D. Timmie Topoleski
Department of Mechanical
  Engineering
University of Maryland
Baltimore County
Baltimore
Maryland
USA

Chapter 13

Saverio Affatato*
E-mail: affatato@tecno.ior.it

Dorina Brando
Laboratorio di Tecnologia Medica
Istituto Ortopedico Rizzoli
Via di Barbiano, 1/10
40136 Bologna
Italy

Domenico Tigani
Department of Orthopaedic Surgery
Santa Maria alle Scotte Hospital
Viale Bracci, 1
53100 Siena
Italy

Chapter 14

Douglas W. Van Citters
Thayer School of Engineering
Dartmouth College
8000 Cummings Hall
Hanover
NH 03755
USA
E-mail: dvancitters@dartmouth.edu

Chapter 15

Feng Liu and John Fisher
Institute of Medical and Biological
  Engineering
School of Mechanical Engineering
University of Leeds
LS2 9JT
UK

Zhongmin Jin*
Institute of Medical and Biological
  Engineering
School of Mechanical Engineering
University of Leeds
LS2 9JT
UK
E-mail: z.jin@leeds.ac.uk;
  menfl@leeds.ac.uk

and

Institute of Advanced
  Manufacturing Technology
School of Manufacturing
  Engineering
Xi'an Jiatong University
No. 99 Yanxiang Rd
Yanta District
Xi'an City
Shaanxi Province, 710054
People's Republic of China

Acknowledgements

The Editor would like to thank all people that contributed, directly or indirectly, to this book. The primary source is the team of Laboratorio di Tecnologia Medica of the Istituto Ortopedico Rizzoli in Bologna. Many thanks are owed to all the Editor's colleagues for their precious contributions to this book. Thanks are given to Woodhead Publishing for this opportunity and for their enthusiastic and professional support. Particular thanks are also owed to Laura Overend and Lucy Beg for their efforts. Luigi Lena prepared most of the original illustrations in this book.

The book is dedicated to Susanna and Stefania.

Part I
Fundamentals of implant wear

1
Introduction to wear phenomena of orthopaedic implants

S. AFFATATO and D. BRANDO, Istituto Ortopedico Rizzoli, Italy

Abstract: The term 'wear' could be defined as an undesirable progressive loss of material from one or both surfaces in relative motion between them. Wear is not a basic material property, but is a system response of the material; because of this, the mechanism can have a variegate nature. The mechanism of wear is very complex and there are two broad approaches to the classification of wear: the first is descriptive of the results of wear, while the second is based on the physical nature of the underlying processes. It is, however, the second form of classification that is most useful. According to this approach, five wear processes have been clearly recognized: abrasion, adhesion, fatigue, erosion and corrosion. It has been agreed that wear cannot be totally prevented, but most of these mechanisms can be attenuated and, in some cases, can be avoided. It is very important for a designer to know the amount a component can wear before it must be replaced. Since manufacturers must recommend replacement or overhaul times for the equipment they supply, they must be able to ascertain, for each component, when sufficient wear has occurred so that the component is no longer usable.

Key words: wear, wear mechanism, *in vivo* wear measurements, *in vitro* wear measurements, socio-economic wear impact.

1.1 History of wear

Wear is a phenomenon that occurs between two bodies that are in contact. The term 'wear' could be defined as an undesirable progressive loss of material from one or both of the surfaces during relative motion between them (Bhushan, 1999; Schmalzried and Callaghan, 1999). An ancient observation that gave a good description of wear phenomena was made by Lucretius in *De rerum natura*, I (95–55 BC) (Dowson, 1998a):

... a ring is worn thin next to the finger with continual rubbing. Dripping water hollows a stone, a curved ploughshare, iron though it is, dwindles imperceptibly in the furrow. We see the cobblestones of the highway worn be the feet of many wayfarers. The bronze statues by the city gates show their right hands worn thin by the touch of all travellers who have greeted them in passing. We see that all these are being diminished since they are worn away. But to perceive what particles drop off at any particular time is a power grudged us by our ungenerous sense of sight.

More recently, it was Ragnar Holm, working first in the Siemens-Konzern laboratories in Berlin and later with the Stackpole Carbon Company of St Marys, Pennsylvania, who made one of the earliest substantial contributions to the study of wear (Dowson, 1998b; Holm, 1946). Initially, Holm considered wear to be a uniform atomic transfer process taking place at asperity contacts. He later introduced the concept of a uniform layer of transferred material having a thickness equal to an integral number of molecules, mainly to establish a physical appreciation of the wear process (Holm, 1946).

Wear is probably the most important aspect of tribology, yet it has remained largely unexplored until recent times. The recent overflow of publications is difficult to appreciate in historical terms, partly because of the sheer volume of material, but also because we must wait awhile before some of the basic and intrinsic concepts can be confirmed by experiment and practice as valid signposts on the road of truth.

Wear can result from a variety of different processes triggered by the sliding contact between two surfaces and can cause different effects depending upon the component in question and its functional requirements. Wear is not a basic material property, but a system response of the material so that this mechanism can have a variegate nature (Bayer, 1994).

There is no simple relationship between wear and any other materials property and the wear phenomenon can be split into two majority categories: wear dominated by the mechanical behavior of materials and wear dominated by the chemical behavior of materials (McKellop et al., 1995; Peterson, 1980). Both these effects produce changes in the appearance (the morphological features) of the bearing surfaces. During the wear process, worn material is expelled from the contact between two surfaces in the form of debris and these wear products can cause adverse reactions leading to massive bone loss around the implant and consequently loosening of the fixation (Brown and Clarke, 2006; McGee et al., 2000).

The mechanism of wear is very complex; it should also be understood that the real area of contact between two solid surfaces compared with the apparent area of contact is invariably very small, being limited to points of contact between surface asperities. The load applied to the surfaces will be transferred through these points of contact and the localized forces can be very large. The material intrinsic surface properties such as hardness, strength, ductility, work hardening, etc. are very important factors for wear resistance, but other factors such as surface finish, lubrication, load, speed, corrosion, temperature and properties of the opposing surface are equally important.

1.2 Wear mechanisms

There are two broad approaches to the classification of wear. The first is descriptive of the results of wear and the second is based on the physical nature of the underlying processes (Dowson, 1998b; Peterson, 1980). It is, however, the second form of classification that is the most useful.

A wear mechanism is the fundamental microscopic process by which material is removed from a surface (Scherge et al., 2003). Wear can also be defined as a process in which interaction of the surfaces or bounding faces of a solid with its working environment results in dimensional loss of the solid, with or without loss of material. According to this approach, five wear processes have been clearly recognized: abrasion, adhesion, fatigue, erosion and corrosion (Archard, 1980; Callaghan et al., 1995; Peterson, 1980; Schmalzried and Callaghan, 1999). These general classifications of wear were well established by the early 1970s, but much of the work supporting these views was undertaken on metals under dry rubbing conditions (Dowson, 1998b).

Both polymers and ceramics have assumed important positions in the spectrum of tribological materials in recent decades. Polymers now occupy a major position in the bearings field, while the inertness, hardness and excellent surface finish of ceramics make them particularly attractive in both monolithic and coating forms (Lawn, 2002; Martorana et al., 2009). As interest moved away from the 'severe' end of the wear scale, a major step forward was recorded by Suh in 1973 when he introduced the concept of delamination wear (Suh, 1973). Quinn et al. (1980) also attacked the problem of chemical or oxidative wear. The different wear modes are now explained in more detail.

1.2.1 Abrasive wear

Abrasive wear occurs when a hard rough surface slides across a softer surface; in this case, wear is defined as a damage to a solid surface that generally involves progressive loss of material and is due to relative motion between that surface and a contacting substance or substances (ASM, 1998; ASTM, 1987). Abrasive wear is commonly classified according to the type of contact and the contact environment; the type of contact determines the mode of abrasive wear (ASM, 1998). The two modes of abrasive wear are

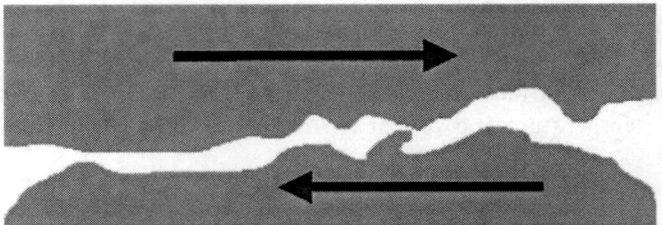

1.1 Schematization of the abrasive wear mechanism.

known as two-body and three-body abrasive wear. Two-body abrasive wear occurs when one surface (usually harder than the other) cuts material away from the other surface; this mechanism very often changes to three-body abrasion as the wear debris then acts as an abrasive between the two surfaces. Three-body wear occurs when particles are not constrained, but are free to roll and slide down a surface (ASM, 1998; Peterson, 1980). A schematic illustration of the phenomenon is shown in Fig. 1.1.

The most common mechanisms of abrasive wear are plowing, cutting and fragmentation. Plowing is the mechanism by which, during the formation of grooves, material is not directly removed but is displaced to the side, resulting in ridges adjacent to grooves, which may be removed by subsequent passage of abrasive particles. During cutting, material is taken away from the surface as primary debris, in the same way as machining. Fragmentation is a type of wear typical for brittle materials due to indentation followed by crack propagation (ASM, 1998). Rabinowicz (1965) described one of the most important models to better define this wear phenomenon. He considered that if a conical asperity with diameter D and angle θ penetrates a softer surface under a load L, the equilibrium condition will be described by:

$$L = \frac{H\pi D^2}{4} \qquad [1.1]$$

The groove section in the plane perpendicular to the wear surface will be:

$$A_s = \frac{D^2 \tan\theta}{4} = \frac{L \tan\theta}{\pi H} \qquad [1.2]$$

When the cone moves a distance S, the removed volume because of wear is:

$$W = \frac{LS \tan\theta}{\pi H} = k\frac{LS}{H} \qquad [1.3]$$

where $k = (\tan\theta)/\pi$ is the wear coefficient.

In orthopaedic implants, abrasive third-body wear occurs in polyethylene, metals and ceramics because of bone cement particles that can produce

Introduction to wear phenomena of orthopaedic implants

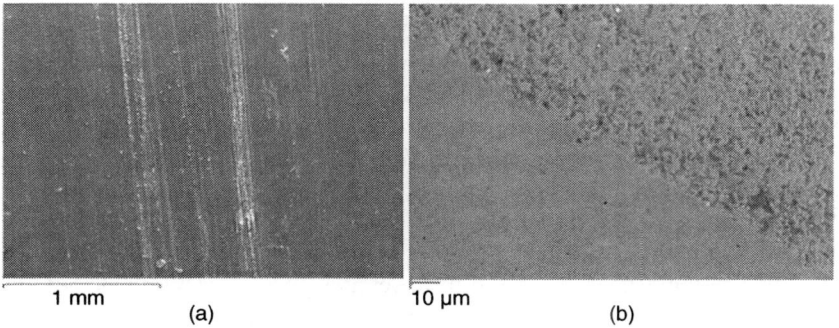

1.2 Examples of abrasive wear in retrieved hip implants: (a) scanning electron microscopy (SEM) image of a metal femoral head; (b) SEM image of a ceramic femoral head.

damage in the surface materials, removing material during their movement. The dimension of abrasive wear in these materials depends on the roughness surface and the presence of third-body particles (Santavirta *et al.*, 1999). Two examples of abrasive wear in hip implants are shown in Fig. 1.2.

1.2.2 Adhesive wear

Adhesive wear is generated by the sliding of one solid surface along another surface (Peterson, 1980). This kind of wear mode occurs when the asperities on mutually opposing surfaces become fused together and are then subsequently ruptured because of their relative motion. In other words, when two bodies slide over each other; or are pressed into another one, which promotes material transfer between the two surfaces, this is called adhesive wear. It is necessary for the surfaces to be in intimate contact with each other; in surfaces that are held apart by lubricating films, oxide films, etc., the tendency for adhesion to occur is reduced. The phenomenon is illustrated schematically in Fig. 1.3.

Adhesive wear can be described as plastic deformation of very small fragments within the surface layer when two surfaces slide against each

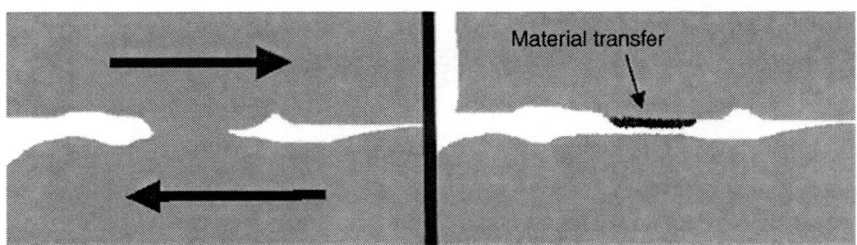

1.3 Schematization of the adhesive wear mechanism.

other. The asperities (i.e. microscopic high points) found on the mating surfaces will penetrate the opposing surface and develop a plastic zone around the penetrating asperity (ASM, 1998; Bhushan, 2001; Dowson, 1998b). In these areas that are strictly in contact (order of atomic distances), adhesive micro-junctions can be formed by two distinct processes – micro-welding and adhesion. During micro-welding, a sort of welding occurs with interdiffusion of one material into the second and re-crystallization associated with the variation in grain size. In micro-welding, the localized interfacial temperature, called the flash temperature, is of the order of the material melting temperature. The occurrence of micro-welding can be due to the plastic stage of the material during the interaction between asperities, allowing melting of the material at a temperature lower than the relative melting temperature. During adhesion, superficial interatomic forces associated with the interfacial energy of the junction surface are the most important elements. There is no interdiffusion between the two materials or recrystallization and the junction occurs between the separation line of the two surfaces (Sin et al., 1979).

During the relative motion of sliding, micro-junctions undergo a shear stress and the brake can occur in two different positions: on the line of junction, when the junction is weak; or at the bases of the asperities at the lower shear straight, if the junction is strong enough (ASM, 1998; ASTM, 1987; Peterson, 1980). In the first case, surface plastic deformations occur and the interacting surfaces will be subjected to plowing, with no creation of wear particles. In the second case, there is a transfer of particles from one body to the other with the trigger of micro-seizure, which may extend to different levels of intensity. Adhesive wear is the most common form of wear and is commonly encountered in conjunction with lubricant failures. In engineering science, some aspects of adhesive wear are commonly referred to as welding wear due to the exhibited surface characteristics; the tribology process is usually referred to as galling and is a common fault factor in sheet metal forming (SMF) and other industrial applications.

Adhesive wear is influenced by many variables, some of which are difficult or impossible to measure. Thus, there is no general applicable equation to estimate the maximum volume of wear. On the basis of the adhesive mechanism, Archard (1980) developed the so-called adhesive wear or Archard model, in which the volume of wear W is determined as:

$$W = k\frac{Ld}{H} \qquad [1.4]$$

where L is the load, H is the hardness of the softer material and d is the sliding distance. The wear coefficient, k is a dimensionless constant that, as a first approximation, can be considered as the probability that a micro-

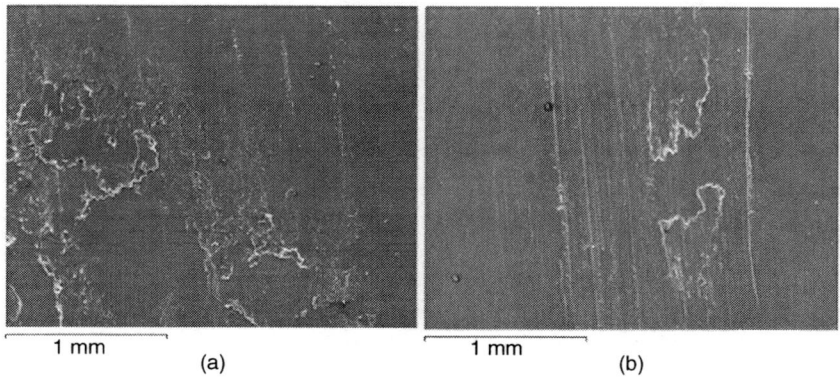

1.4 Examples of adhesive wear in hip implants: (a) SEM image of a metal femoral head; (b) SEM image of a ceramic femoral head.

junction is produced by a wear particle. The Archard assumptions have two limits. First, wear is not always inversely proportional to hardness but it depends on the way by which hardness is produced in the microstructure of the material. Second, the theoretical wear coefficient is always very far from actual results. Comparing the results of Rabinowicz (1965) and Archard (1980), the adhesive wear coefficient should be numerically equivalent to three times the abrasive wear coefficient.

The adhesion of a polyethylene surface to a metal counterface is an example of adhesive wear in orthopaedic implants. As a result of this adhesion, pits and voids appear on the polyethylene surface (Wang *et al.*, 1995). The articulating surface releases wear particles as a consequence of the accumulation of plastic strain over a limit and the existence of a plasticity-induced damage layer has been shown to be due to the reorientation of crystalline lamellae in the polyethylene structure (Kurtz *et al.*, 2000). Adhesive wear also affects both metal and ceramic components, as shown in Fig. 1.4.

1.2.3 Erosive wear

Erosive wear is typical of coupling in which one of the antagonists is in the fluid stage and is associated with the abrasion produced by particles contained in the fluid, often combined with a chemical action facilitating erosion of the metal matrix. Erosion can have different levels of severity and damage can occur as specular micro-cavities or unidirectional scratches. In a lubricated system, the erosion particles can be spheroids that impinge on a component surface or edge and remove material from that surface due to momentum effects (Archard, 1980; Peterson, 1980; Schmalzried and Callaghan, 1999). The phenomenon of erosive wear is shown in Fig. 1.5.

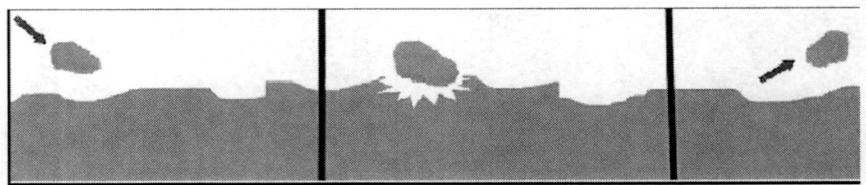

1.5 Schematic illustration of erosive wear mechanism.

When the angle of impingement is small, the wear produced is closely analogous to abrasion. When the angle of impingement is normal to the surface, material is displaced by plastic flow or is dislodged by brittle failure. This type of wear is especially noticed in components with high-velocity flows such as servo and proportional valves. Particles repeatedly striking the surface may also cause denting and eventual fatigue of the surface. It is a widely encountered mechanism in industry. A common example is the erosive wear associated with the movement of slurries through piping and pumping equipment.

Erosive wear closely depends on the material properties of the particles, such as hardness, impact velocity, shape and impingement angle. In particular, it was found that for ductile materials, the maximum wear rate is obtained when the impingement angle is approximately 30°. For non-ductile materials, the maximum wear rate occurs when the impingement angle is normal to the surface (Jones *et al.*, 1992; Lombardi *et al.*, 1989). Figure 1.6 shows two examples of erosive wear in retrieved ceramic femoral heads.

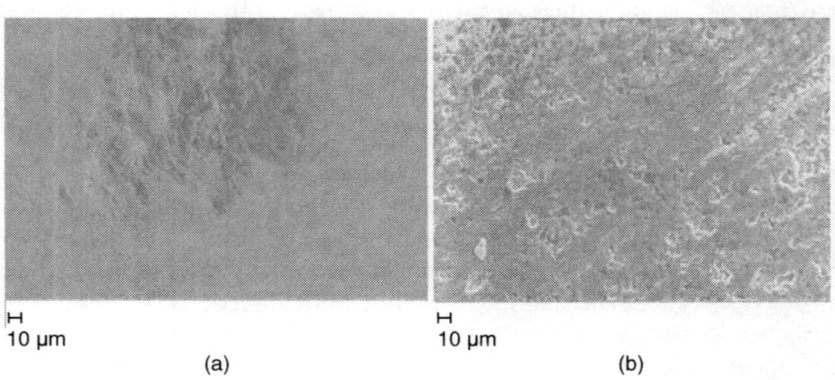

1.6 Examples of erosive wear in hip implant showing SEM images of a ceramic femoral head.

1.2.4 Corrosive wear

Corrosive wear is degradation of a material that involves both corrosion and wear mechanisms (ASTM, 1987). Corrosion is the deterioration that a material undergoes as a result of interaction with its environment and involves a chemical reaction on the wearing surface. The most common form of corrosion is oxidation and corrosion products, usually oxides, have shear strengths different to those of the metal wearing surfaces from which they derived. The oxides tend to flake away, resulting in the pitting of working surfaces, and act as an abrasive third body. Ball and roller bearings depend on extremely smooth surfaces to reduce frictional effects and corrosive pitting is especially detrimental to these types of bearings (Archard, 1980; ASM, 1998; ASTM, 1987; Peterson, 1980). Corrosive wear accelerates the mechanism of corrosion: owing to joint motion, corrosive products are removed from the surface together with the protective passive layer; in this way, protection against corrosion is reduced, thus promoting new material removal (Jacobs *et al.*, 1998).

The environment in contact with materials in the body comprises water, ions, organic compounds and dissolved oxygen; the temperature is around 37°C and pH is around 7.4. In these conditions, almost all metals (with the exception of a few particularly resistant alloys) will be significantly attacked after prolonged permanence in human tissue. Corrosion is a superficial phenomenon, so it is sufficient to use material with excellent surface properties even if it has intrinsically low resistance to corrosion. Mechanical stresses play a important role in accelerating or triggering specific corrosion mechanisms, while the biological environment interferes with the kinetics of the different types of corrosion (Thomann and Uggowitzer, 2000). Corrosive wear occurs in three forms.

> **Pitting** is a kind of localized corrosion manifested as small cavities more or less evenly distributed on the surface with a rate of penetration that increases exponentially with time (Flasker *et al.*, 2001). Pitting attack occurs in phases: (i) localization and triggering and (ii) propagation. Localization begins where the protective film is defective or less resistant because of a small imperfection of mechanical source. The attack is triggered when the electrochemical potential of the material reaches a critical value, called the pitting potential, which depends on the type of material, temperature and concentration of chlorides (Kwok *et al.*, 1998). Once triggered, pitting proceeds with a self-stimulating mechanism, producing a further increase in the number of chlorides and a decrease in pH.
>
> **Fretting** is a kind of corrosion that intervenes the mechanical component. When a metallic surface undergoes cyclic rubbing from another surface,

its protective film can be scratched, thus exposing the unprotected metal below (Hoeppner and Chandrasekaran, 1994). The attack is accelerated by abrasion of the mechanically removed oxides that are harder than the base metal and which have difficulty in moving away from the contact zone, owing to the limited amplitude of reciprocal movement between the surfaces and the cyclic behavior. Fretting corrosion is not very dangerous in terms of the resulting thickness loss, but can trigger a more insidious corrosion such as fatigue wear (Hurricks, 1970).

Stress corrosion takes place in some metals subjected to tensile stress and in the presence of a specific environment (Winzer *et al.*, 2005). It occurs as a crack that can penetrate the metal in an intergranular, transgranular or mixed way depending on the particular coupling between the metal and its environment. The stresses involved are lower than the yield stress and are due to the presence of internal stresses generated during production or assemblage. The corrosive environment can be very bland, with electrochemical conditions causing instability of the passive film. The trigger point is a mechanical defect or existing pit triggered by the environment. Indeed, the two corrosion mechanisms involved are, on the one hand, mechanical break accelerated by a corrosive environment and, on the other, localized corrosion accelerated by applied stress (Jones, 1992; Sieradzki and Newman, 1987).

Corrosion attack can occur in the head–neck taper connection of a modular hip implant. If the tolerance between the taper and the mating hole in the head is quite high, the mechanical stability of the connection will be low. Consequently, the interference fit of a modular connection can be removed by the loads applied during gait, producing disintegration of the metal surface and the triggering of corrosion (Jacobs *et al.*, 1998).

1.2.5 Fatigue wear

Fatigue wear is due to the application of cyclic loading on the material when the applied load is higher than the fatigue strength of the material (Stewart and Ahmed, 2002). Fatigue surface or subsurface cracks can grow and penetrate deeper, coalescing and producing separation of pieces of materials. Two forms of fatigue wear can be distinguished – macroscopic and microscopic. The former is connected with rolling contact fatigue, which results from the repeated mechanical stressing on the surface of a body rolling on another body. Repetitive stressing of the surface microstructure leads to accumulation of dislocations, nucleation of voids or micro-cracks where there are discontinuities, pores or inclusions. The damage can spread to areas close to the beginning of fatigue cracks from surface or subsurface defects, and can lead to catastrophic failure.

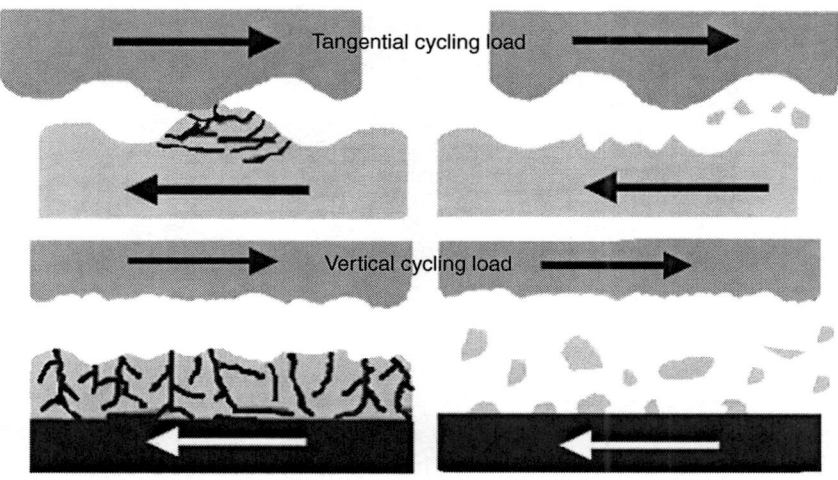

1.7 Schematization of fatigue wear.

Microscopic fatigue wear, on the other hand, is related to an individual asperity instead of a single large region (Miller *et al.*, 1985; Teoh, 2000). A schematization of the phenomenon is shown in Fig. 1.7.

It has been demonstrated that fatigue wear is responsible for orthopaedic implant failure. For metals used in hip and knee implants, such as stainless steel, cobalt chrome and titanium, it has been shown that fatigue strength is improved by post-processing treatment with respect to the cast component (Teoh, 2000). In orthopaedic prostheses, fatigue wear of polyethylene is predominant because it is the weaker material. The presence of defects and plastic flow parameters such as yield stress and ultimate stress can influence the wear behavior of polyethylene components, which also depends on patient activity, weight and duration of implantation. Furthermore, γ-radiation and oxidative ageing may affect the fatigue threshold and crack propagation resistance (Pruitt and Bailey, 1998). Figure 1.8 shows SEM images of fatigue wear of a retrieved ultra-high molecular weight polyethylene (UHMWPE) tibial insert.

1.2.6 Fretting wear

Fretting wear is a small-amplitude oscillatory motion, usually tangential, between two solid surfaces in contact (Peterson, 1980). When this kind of wear is associated with oxidation or corrosion, the phenomenon evolves in fretting corrosion. Fretting occurs when repeated loading and unloading

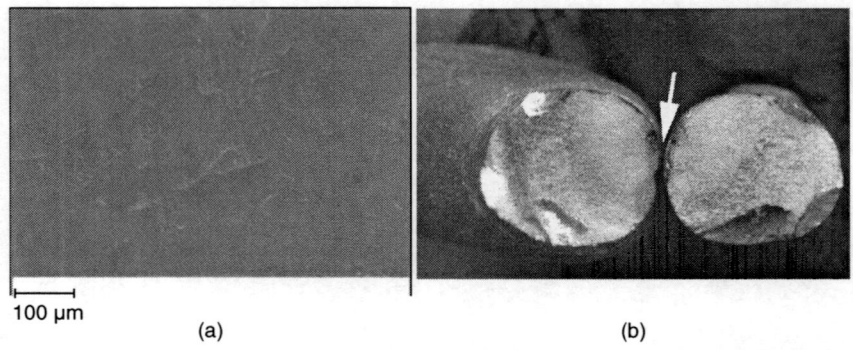

1.8 Fatigue wear in hip implants: SEM images of a retrieved polyethylene tibial insert of a knee implant.

causes cyclic stresses that induce a surface or subsurface break-up and loss of material (Archard, 1980; ASTM, 1987; Peterson, 1980). Vibration is a common cause of fretting wear. Couplings that are subject to fretting are a rotating system with little misalignment, bolted joints made to vibrate by different causes, etc. The fretting phenomenon is illustrated in Fig. 1.9.

The main wear mechanisms in fretting are adhesion, abrasion by oxidation products that are finely crushed due to rubbing, plastic

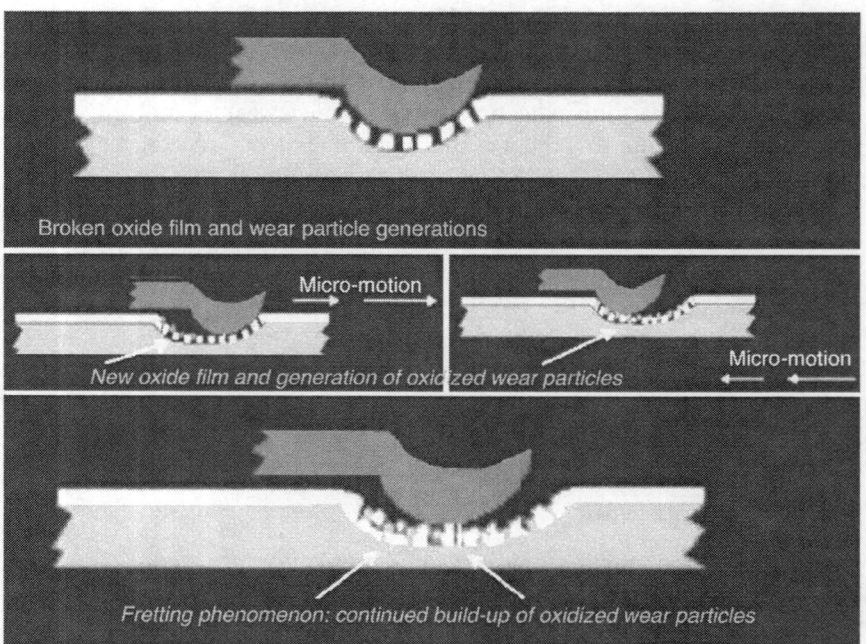

1.9 Schematic illustration of fretting.

Introduction to wear phenomena of orthopaedic implants 15

deformation and oxidation/corrosion of the environment, eventually triggered by contact temperature. Fretting damage is easily distinguishable from other types of damage. It is characterized by a zone of heavy plastic micro-deformation, leading to crumbling of the metal matrix concentrated around areas of adhesion between two surfaces, promoting micro-spalling and producing spherical particles with a matt surface, usually oxidized. When fretting evolves into fretting corrosion, the micro-spalling becomes full of broken corrosion products. Fretting evolving into fretting fatigue can lead to catastrophic failure of the bearing owing to the formation of cracks in the surfaces. Fretting has been noted in modular hip implants in which a cylindrical taper connects the head and the neck of the stem. This is due to the presence of side micro-movements at the stem fixation in the bone and at the head/neck contact that, together with corrosive action, can lead to the release of ions and particles, which is dangerous for bone tissue (Tritschler *et al.*, 1999). Figure 1.10 shows a SEM image of fretting wear in a hip stem.

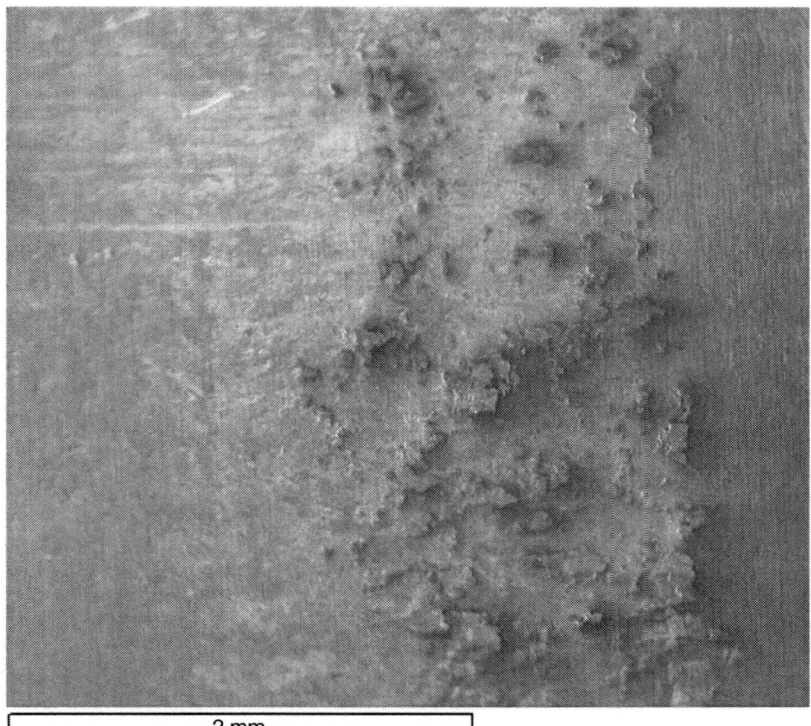

1.10 An example of fretting wear in a hip implant.

1.2.7 Delamination

In 1973, Suh developed the concept of delamination. He started from the observation that plastic deformations produced by adhesive micro-junctions and plowing on the surface are not confined to the surface but proceed in sub-superficial layers to certain depths depending on load, wear coefficient, local conditions and microstructural material properties (Suh, 1977). These deformations can be responsible for a flux of dislocations that accumulate on grain boundaries, micro-precipitates or existing defects, creating micro-voids. With continued plastic deformation, these micro-voids become oval, coalesce and nucleate in micro-cracks. If plastic deformation carries on, the crack tends to propagate in the direction of displacement until it reaches a length of instability, called the critical length. The crack then tends to resurface, causing the separation of a delaminated particle. Delamination is most evident in contact where superficial adhesion is not catastrophic. Indeed, delamination takes place under the surface and includes a stage of nucleation and one of evolution, in the same way as fatigue processes.

On the basis of this mechanism, reflecting the real behavior of materials to sliding wear, Suh developed a numeric model of delamination. The main assumption of this model is that delamination occurs by the removal of successive layers. The Suh model states that the wear volume W is determined as:

$$W = N_1 \frac{S}{S_{01}} A_1 h_1 + N_2 \frac{S}{S_{01}} A_2 h_2 \qquad [1.5]$$

where S is the total sliding distance, N is the number of delaminated particles, A is the particle surface and h the thickness of the particle layer. Subscripts 1 and 2 correspond to the elements of the coupling and the rate S/S_0 is the number of exported layers due to wear during the path S. From the theory of dislocations, h can be written as:

$$h = \frac{Gb}{4\pi(1-v)\sigma_F} \qquad [1.6]$$

where G is the shear modulus, b is Burger's vector of friction solicitation, v is Poisson's ratio and σ_F is the friction stress. The surface A of each delaminated particle is proportional to the real contact area A that in turn is proportional to the load L. In this way, the wear volume is:

$$W = \frac{K}{4\pi} \left(\frac{h_1 G_1}{\sigma_{f1} S_{01}(1-v_1)} + \frac{h_2 G_2}{\sigma_{f2} S_{02}(1-v_2)} \right) LS \qquad [1.7]$$

The Suh model does not consider the hardness of the material but refers to the microstructural properties of the materials in contact. This model allows

Introduction to wear phenomena of orthopaedic implants

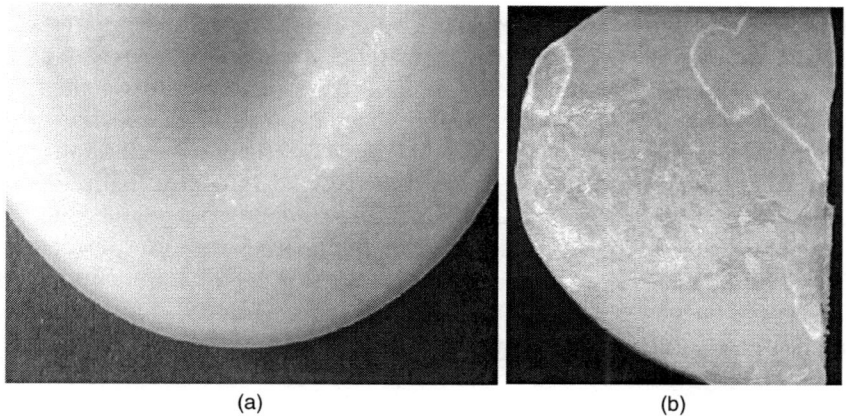

1.11 Examples of delamination in orthopaedic implants: (a) a retrieved polyethylene acetabular cup of a hip prosthesis; (b) a retrieved polyethylene tibial insert of a knee prosthesis.

interpretation of the tribological behavior of many couplings, but is rather complicated and of limited numerical reliability.

Delamination is frequent in polyethylene components, such as UHMWPE tibial inserts of knee prostheses, especially in bearings with lower conformity. High contact stresses and low mechanical properties due to oxidation can lead to the failure of polyethylene. The surface damage on total knee components has been found to be greater than that observed on total hip replacement components. This is because the contact area during flexion is smaller in the tibial component of a knee prosthesis than in the acetabular cup of a hip prosthesis, leading to more contact (Bartel *et al.*, 1986). Figure 1.11 shows the effect of delamination of retrieved UHMWPE components.

1.3 Importance of wear mechanisms and their evaluation

It has been agreed that wear cannot be totally prevented, but most wear mechanisms can be attenuated and, in some cases, avoided altogether. However, as long as load-bearing, interacting surfaces are in relative motion, some wear can be anticipated.

There is no specific standard for testing or measuring materials wear resistance. This can be attributed to the complex nature of wear and the difficulties associated with accurately simulating wear processes. A number of wear tests have been developed by committees in an attempt to standardise wear testing for specific applications. In the results of standard wear tests (such as those formulated by the respective subcommittees of ASTM Committee G-2), the loss of material during wear is expressed in terms of volume. The volume loss gives a truer picture than weight loss, particularly when comparing the wear resistance properties of materials with large differences in density. The working life of an engineering component is over when dimensional losses exceed the specified tolerance limits. Wear, along with other ageing processes such as fatigue, creep and fracture toughness, causes progressive degradation of materials with time, leading to failure of the material at an advanced age. Wear is one of a limited number of ways in which a material object loses its usefulness. The economic implications can be of enormous value to industry.

1.4 *In vivo* wear measurements

In vivo wear assessments have traditionally been based on radiography (Collier *et al.*, 2008). The degree of penetration of a femoral component into polyethylene on sequential radiography has been noted as linear wear. The most commonly used method of radiographic assessment is described by Livermore *et al.* (1990). In sequential radiography, the distance from the centre of the femoral head to a particular reference point on the acetabular cup is measured and corrected for magnification. The difference from the initial post-operative radiograph to the most recent radiograph represents linear wear as measured in millimetres. It has been calculated that clinical analysis of X-rays has an accuracy of 0.1–0.5 mm and gives a reliable measurement if penetration p is more than 0.5 mm, a condition verified only with polyethylene inserts (Barrack *et al.*, 2001). The linear wear rate is that measured over the period of implantation. Estimated values can be high because they include viscoelastic effects and smoothing. The difficulty with this technique for evaluating linear wear is that it cannot distinguish linear wear from creep or plastic deformation (Stilling *et al.*, 2009).

Volumetric wear is a measure of the volume of material removed from a bearing surface. With the assumption that wear is the only factor determining misalignment of the centres of a femoral head and acetabular cup, the worn volume V of the acetabular cup can be obtained as the difference between the volume of the cup sphere (with radius R_c) and the volume head sphere (with radius R_h), whose centres have a separation p. An analytically obtained expression does not exist but some simplified formulas are able to provide similar results (Charnley and Halley, 1975; Kabo *et al.*, 1993; Yamaguchi *et al.*, 1999). In this way, the worn volume could be represented by the formula (Raimondi *et al.*, 2000):

$$V = \pi \left[\frac{2}{3}(R_h^3 - R_c^3)^2 + \frac{(R_h^2 - R_c^2)^2}{4p} + p\left(\frac{R_c^2 + R_h^2}{2}\right) - \frac{p^3}{12} \right] \quad [1.8]$$

Linear and angular measurements can also be taken by means of software that is able to reconstruct a circumference on the digitized X-rays whose coordinates can be exported and analysed. Computer-assisted techniques with digitized radiography have been used with reasonable reliability; other techniques have included the shadowgraph technique and fluid displacement methods for retrieved specimens (Dowson, 1993; Dowson *et al.*, 1985; Kabo and Amstutz, 1993).

Radio-stereometric analysis (RSA) is a good way of measuring displacement and wear of articular prostheses, such as total hip arthroplasty, indicating how the body and the implant are interacting (Bottner *et al.*, 2005). RSA is based on the three-dimensional reconstruction of the position of segments within the human body from a two-dimensional X-ray film. Movement between segments is calculated by localizing each segment, marked with at least three tantalum beads, in a coordinate system. RSA is more accurate and precise than other methods (Onsten *et al.*, 2001). Some clinical studies have demonstrated an accuracy of approximately 0.2 mm, while *in vitro* studies have an accuracy of 0.047–0.121 mm (von Schewelov *et al.*, 2004).

Many variables affect *in vivo* wear; as a result, reports regarding wear rates have shown great variability (Nevelos *et al.*, 1999). Patient variables include age, sex, weight, general health and activity level. Variables related to the hip reconstruction include the choice of bearing material, the design and manufacturing of the prosthesis and characteristics of implantation (i.e. operative technique, biomechanical considerations, initial and long-term implant fixation) (Braunstein *et al.*, 2009; Clarke and Manley, 2008). Multiple assessments of wear over time are more valuable than a single measurement and comparing rates of linear penetration after different durations of implantation may be difficult (Affatato *et al.*, 2004; Manning *et al.*, 2005).

1.5 *In vitro* wear measurements

In vitro wear assessments have traditionally been based on the gravimetric method. This method is the standard measurement practice adopted by the orthopaedic industry for the development of new joints and materials in pre-clinical evaluations after testing according to ISO 14242-1: 2002 (ISO, 2002) for hip prostheses and ISO 14243-1: 2009 (ISO, 2009a) for knee prostheses. ISO 14242-2: 2000 (ISO, 2000) and ISO 14243-2: 2009 (ISO, 2009b) define a detailed gravimetric measurement procedure for hip and knee prostheses. The gravimetric method has some limitations, however. It does not provide information on change of form of the wear surface, it is not helpful in the case of clinically explanted prostheses and other damages not involving material loss (e.g. plastic deformations) are not measurable. In previous work, a gravimetric technique was used where the acetabular cups or tibial components were weighed on a micro-balance after a careful and rigorous preparation method; fluid absorption due to the hydrophilic nature of UHMWPE was also measured with unloaded and loaded soak controls and the mass gain due to fluid absorption was taken into account (Affatato et al., 2008, 2009).

Coordinate measuring machines (CMMs) have recently been used as an alternative to the gravimetric method (Spinelli, 2009). Use of a CMM is allowed by ISO 14242-2: 2000 (ISO, 2000). A CMM is a very precise Cartesian robot, equipped with a tactile probe and used as a three-dimensional digitizer. The probe, under computer control, touches a sequence of points on the surface of a physical object to be measured and the CMM produces a stream of x, y, z coordinates of the contact points. The coordinate stream is interpreted by algorithms that support applications (Carmignato et al., 2011). Although the major limitation to the use of this technique is that measurement uncertainty has not been evaluated (Smith and Unsworth, 1999), the analytical model produced has the advantage of giving an answer as a function of specific input for each patient, with high efficiency and reliable results. Some software programs simulate the biomechanics of joints by estimating the wear rate of prostheses using a finite-element modeling of dry sliding wear. In the literature, there are several mathematical models that simulate the wear behavior of the acetabular cup in hip prostheses, based on different assumptions. To introduce simplifying hypotheses and obtain more easily manageable models, it is important to fix *a priori* some characteristics and behavior because each complex phenomenon depends on a large variety of parameters. The mechanical behavior of the material constituting the coupling is one of the distinctive elements between the models. Contact can be considered rigid or deformable. In the latter case, elastic properties of materials play an important role.

The first models proposed were based on Hertz's theorem to calculate contact stress and on Archard's formula for the wear rate (Pietrabissa et al., 1996; Wang et al., 1998). The Hertz contact theorem applies under steady or static loading. When UHMWPE is coupled with metal or ceramic, the hypotheses of the Hertz model are not verified, owing to the high deformability of UHMWPE with respect to metal or ceramic. Indeed, the radii of the contact areas are of the same order of magnitude as the radii of the bodies, so another kind of formulation is necessary (Wu et al., 2003).

According to Archard's formula (Archard, 1980), the wear rate W can be calculated as:

$$W = KsP \qquad [1.9]$$

where K is the wear coefficient per unit load per sliding distance, s is the sliding distance and P is the applied load. In this way, the wear rate is not dependent on the apparent contact area and there is no consideration about surface topography in the variation of wear over time.

1.6 Socio-economic wear impact

Wear of an articular bearing surface is one of the main causes of failure after five years from the date of implant and, very often, wear is accepted as a natural consequence of use (Kurtz et al., 2007). Wear is not only just a failure mode, but can be a prime cause of secondary failures (Bozic et al., 2010). Worn parts lead to increased vibration and fatigue, shock loading and misalignment, all of which increase the probability of equipment failure. In addition, wear debris can cause seizure or spalling failures in other components. In these conditions, joint revision is necessary, incurring significant cost penalties (Oduwole et al., 2010). So, even if failure does not occur, wear causes deterioration in performance and this loss of 'efficient operation' may well be the major cost of wear (Burns et al., 2006).

Hip and knee revisions cost more than primary operations because of the complexity of the procedure and the possibility of complications, leading to longer operating times and hospital stays (Barrack, 1995; Bozic et al., 2005). In the USA, the median hospital charge for revision were estimated to be $38,000 and $35,000 for hips and knees respectively (Kim, 2008).

Innovations have significantly decreased the amount of wear particles created by friction on joint surfaces, thus delaying, and in some cases preventing, the need for revision surgery. In this way, the higher costs associated with the use of alternative bearings can be amortized by lower revision rates. The cost-effectiveness of alternative bearings is highly dependent on the age of the patient at the time of surgery and, additionally, the impact of unexpected events (e.g. instability, impingement, ceramic fracture, material failure of cross-linked polyethylene and potential biological responses to metal ions) on long-term revision rates and patient outcomes remains unknown (Bozic et al., 2006). It is thus very important for designers to know the amount of wear a component can sustain before it must be replaced. Since manufacturers must recommend replacement or overhaul times for equipment, they must be able to ascertain for each component not only the wear rate but also when sufficient wear has occurred so that the component is no longer usable.

1.7 Future trends

Hip and knee joint replacements have been two of the major successes of modern medicine. Their continued success depends on effective collaboration between clinicians and researchers across many different areas in science and medicine. Extensive study, development and new technologies have allowed developing and improving imaging and computer-assisted implant replacement with more precise reconstruction of the orthopaedic implants with less direct visualization. In addition, new implant designs and materials are being developed to facilitate minimally invasive surgery for hip and knee implants, prolonging the lifespan of replacements and improving the life of the patients.

1.8 References

Affatato, S., Bersaglia, G., Foltran, I., Emiliani, D., Traina, F. and Toni, A. (2004) The influence of implant position on the wear of alumina-on-alumina studied in a hip simulator. *Wear*, 256, 400–5.

Affatato, S., Cristofolini, L., Leardini, W., Erani, P., Zavalloni, M., Tigani, D. and Viceconti, M. (2008) A new method of in vitro wear assessment of the UHMWPE tibial insert in total knee replacement. *Artif Organs*, 32, 942–8.

Affatato, S., Traina, F., Mazzega-Fabbro, C., Sergo, V. and Viceconti, M. (2009) Is ceramic-on-ceramic squeaking phenomenon reproducible in vitro? A long-term simulator study under severe conditions. *J Biomed Mater Res B Appl Biomater*, 91, 264–71.

Archard, J. F. (1980) *Wear theory and mechanism*. In Peterson, M. B. and Winer, W. O. (Eds) *Wear Control Handbook*. New York, ASME.

ASM, H. (1998) *Friction, Lubrication and Wear Technology*. Materials Park, OH, ASM International.

ASTM (1987) Standard terminology relating to wear and erosion. *Annual Book of Standards*. West Conshohocken, PA, ASTM.

Barrack, R. L. (1995) Economics of revision total hip arthroplasty. *Clin Orthop Relat Res*, 209–14.

Barrack, R. L., Lavernia, C., Szuszczewicz, E. S. and Sawhney, J. (2001) Radiographic wear measurements in a cementless metal-backed modular cobalt-chromium acetabular component. *J Arthroplasty*, 16, 820–8.

Bartel, D. L., Bicknell, V. L. and Wright, T. M. (1986) The effect of conformity, thickness, and material on stresses in ultra-high molecular weight components for total joint replacement. *J Bone Joint Surg Am*, 68, 1041–51.

Bayer, R. G. (1994) *Mechanical Wear Prediction and Prevention*. New York, USA, Marcel Dekker.

Bhushan, B. (1999) Definition and history of tribology. *Principles and Applications of tribology*. New York, Wiley.

Bhushan, B. (2001) *Principles of Tribology*. Washington, DC, LLC.

Bottner, F., Su, E., Nestor, B., Azzis, B., Sculco, T. P. and Bostrom, M. (2005) Radiostereometric analysis: the hip. *HSS J*, 1, 94–9.

Bozic, K. J., Katz, P., Cisternas, M., Ono, L., Ries, M. D. and Showstack, J. (2005)

Hospital resource utilization for primary and revision total hip arthroplasty. *J Bone Joint Surg Am*, 87, 570–6.

Bozic, K. J., Kurtz, S. M., Lau, E., Ong, K., Chiu, V., Vail, T. P., Rubash, H. E. and Berry, D. J. (2010) The epidemiology of revision total knee arthroplasty in the United States. *Clin Orthop Relat Res*, 468, 45–51.

Bozic, K. J., Morshed, S., Silverstein, M. D., Rubash, H. E. and Kahn, J. G. (2006) Use of cost-effectiveness analysis to evaluate new technologies in orthopaedics. The case of alternative bearing surfaces in total hip arthroplasty. *J Bone Joint Surg Am*, 88, 706–14.

Braunstein, V., Sprecher, C. M., Wimmer, M. A., Milz, S. and Taeger, G. (2009) Influence of head size on the development of metallic wear and on the characteristics of carbon layers in metal-on-metal hip joints. *Acta Orthop*, 80, 283–90.

Brown, S. S. and Clarke, I. C. (2006) A review of lubricant conditions for wear simulation in artificial hip joint replacements. *Tribol Trans*, 49, 72–8.

Burns, A. W., Bourne, R. B., Chesworth, B. M., Macdonald, S. J. and Rorabeck, C. H. (2006) Cost effectiveness of revision total knee arthroplasty. *Clin Orthop Relat Res*, 446, 29–33.

Callaghan, J. J., Pedersen, D. R., Olejniczak, J. P., Goetz, D. D. and Johnston, R. C. (1995) Radiographic measurement of wear in 5 cohorts of patients observed for 5 to 22 years. *Clin Orthop Relat Res*, 317, 14–18.

Carmignato, S., Affatato, S. and Savio, E. (2011) Uncertainty evaluation of volumetric wear assessment from coordinate measurements of ceramic hip joint prostheses. *Wear*, doi:10.1016/j.wear.2011.01.012.

Charnley, J. and Halley, D. K. (1975) Rate of wear in total hip replacement. *Clin Orthop Relat Res*, 112, 170–9.

Clarke, I. C. and Manley, M. T. (2008) How do alternative bearing surfaces influence wear behavior? *J Am Acad Orthop Surg*, 16(Suppl 1), S86–93.

Collier, M. B., Engh, C. A., JR., Hatten, K. M., Ginn, S. D., Sheils, T. M. and Engh, G. A. (2008) Radiographic assessment of the thickness lost from polyethylene tibial inserts that had been sterilized differently. *J Bone Joint Surg Am*, 90, 1543–52.

Dowson, D. (1993) An evaluation of the penetration of ceramic femoral heads into polyethylene acetabular cups. *Wear*, 162–4, 880–9.

Dowson, D. (1998a) Tribology. In *History of Tribology*. London, Professional Engineering Publishing.

Dowson, D. (1998b) Towards tribology 1925–the present. In *History of Tribology*. London, Professional Engineering Publishing.

Dowson, D., Wallbridge, N. C., Atkinson, J. R., Wroblewski, B. M. and Isaac, J. H. (1985) Laboratory wear test and clinical observation of the penetration of femoral heads into acetabular cups in total hip replacement hip joints. *Wear*, 104, 203–44.

Flasker, J., Fajdiga, G., Glodez, S. and Hellen, T. K. (2001) Numerical simulation of surface pitting due to contact loading. *Int J Fatigue*, 23, 599–605.

Hoeppner, D. W. and Chandrasekaran, V. (1994) Fretting in orthopaedic implants: A review. *Wear*, 173, 189–97.

Holm, R. (1946) Electrical Contacts. In Bowden, F. P. and Tabor, D. (Eds) *The Friction and Lubrication of Solids, Part II*. New York, Springer-Verlag.

Hurricks, P. L. (1970) The mechanism of fretting – A review. *Wear*, 15, 389–409.
ISO (2000) ISO14242-2: 2000 Implants for surgery. Wear of total hip-joint prostheses. Part 2: Methods of measurement. Geneva, ISO.
ISO (2002) ISO14242-1: 2002 Implants for surgery. Wear of total hip-joint prostheses. Part 1: Loading and displacement parameters for wear-testing machines and corresponding environmental conditions for test. Geneva, ISO.
ISO (2009a) ISO14243-1: 2009 Implants for surgery. Wear of total hip-joint prostheses. Part 3: Loading and displacement parameters for orbital bearing type wear testing machines and corresponding environmental conditions for test. Geneva, ISO.
ISO (2009b) ISO14243-2: 2009 Implants for surgery. Wear of total knee-joint prostheses. Part 2: Methods of measurement. Geneva, ISO.
Jacobs, J. J., Gilbert, J. L. and Urban, R. M. (1998) Corrosion of metal orthopaedic implants. *J Bone Joint Surg Am*, 80, 268–82.
Jones, R. H. (1992) *Stress-Corrosion Cracking*. Materials Park, OH, ASM International.
Jones, S. M. G., Pinder, I. M., Moran, C. G. and Malcolm, A. J. (1992) Polyethylene wear in uncemented knee replacements. *J Bone Jt Surg Br*, 74B, 18–22.
Kabo, M. and Amstutz, H. C. (1993) *In vivo* wear of polyethylene acetabular components. *J Bone Joint Surg Br* 75, 254–58.
Kabo, J. M., Gebhard, J. S., Loren, G. and Amstutz, H. C. (1993) *In vivo* wear of polyethylene acetabular components. *J Bone Jt Surg Br*, 75, 254–258.
Kim, S. (2008) Changes in surgical loads and economic burden of hip and knee replacements in the US: 1997–2004. *Arthritis Rheum*, 59, 481–488.
Kurtz, S. M., Rimnac, C. M., Pruitt, L., Jewett, C. W., Goldberg, V. and Edidin, A. A. (2000) The relationship between the clinical performance and large deformation mechanical behavior of retrieved UHMWPE tibial inserts. *Biomaterials*, 21, 283–91.
Kurtz, S., Ong, K., Lau, E., Mowat, F. and Halpern, M. (2007) Projections of primary and revision hip and knee arthroplasty in the United States from 2005 to 2030. *J Bone Joint Surg Am*, 89, 780–5.
Kwok, C. T., Man, H. C. and Cheng, F. T. (1998) Cavitation erosion and pitting corrosion of laser surface melted stainless steels. *Surf Coat Technol*, 99, 295–304.
Lawn, B. R. (2002) Ceramic-based layer structures for biomechanical applications. *Curr Op Solid State Mater Sci*, 6, 229–35.
Livermore, J., Ilstrup, D. and Morrey, B. (1990) Effect of femoral head size on wear of the polyethylene acetabular component. *J Bone Jt Surg Am*, 72, 518–28.
Lombardi, A. V. J., Mallory, T. H., Vaughn, B. K. and Drouillard, P. (1989) Aseptic loosening in total hip arthroplasty secondary to osteolysis induced by wear debris from titanium-alloy modular femoral heads. *J Bone Jt Surg Am*, 71A, 1337–42.
Manning, D. W., Chiang, P. P., Martell, J. M., Galante, J. O. and Harris, W. H. (2005) *In vivo* comparative wear study of traditional and highly cross-linked polyethylene in total hip arthroplasty. *J Arthroplasty*, 20, 880–6.
Martorana, S., Fedele, A., Mazzocchi, M. and Bellosi, A. (2009) Surface coatings of bioactive glasses on high strength ceramic composites. *Appl Surf Sci*, 255, 6679–85.
McGee, M. A., Howie, D. W., Costi, K., Haynes, D. R., Wildenauer, C. I., Pearcy,

M. J. and McLean, J. D. (2000) Implant retrieval studies of the wear and loosening of prosthetic joints: a review. *Wear*, 241, 158–65.

McKellop, H. A., Campbell, P., Park, S.-H., Schmalzried, T. P., Grigoris, P., Amstutz, H. C. and Sarmiento, A. (1995) The origin of submicron polyethylene wear debris in total hip arthroplasty. *Clin Orthop Relat Res*, 311, 3–20.

Miller, G. R., Keer, L. M. and Cheng, H. S. (1985) On the mechanics of fatigue crack growth due to contact loading. *Proc Royal Soc London Ser A Math Phys Sci*, 397, 197–209.

Nevelos, J. E., Ingham, E., Doyle, C., Fisher, J. and Nevelos, A. B. (1999) Analysis of retrieved alumina ceramic components from Mittelmeier total hip prostheses. *Biomaterials*, 20, 1833–40.

Oduwole, K. O., Molony, D. C., Walls, R. J., Bashir, S. P. and Mulhall, K. J. (2010) Increasing financial burden of revision total knee arthroplasty. *Knee Surg Sports Traumatol Arthrosc*, 18, 945–8.

Onsten, I., Berzins, A., Shott, S. and Sumner, D. R. (2001) Accuracy and precision of radiostereometric analysis in the measurement of THR femoral component translations: human and canine in vitro models. *J Orthop Res*, 19, 1162–7.

Peterson, M. B. (1980) Classification of wear process. In Peterson, M. B. and Winer, W. O. (Eds) *Wear Control Handbook*. New York, NY, ASME.

Pietrabissa, R., Raimondi, M. and Di Martino, E. (1998) Wear of polyethylene cups in total hip arthroplasty: a parametric mathematical model. *Med Eng Phys*, 20, 199–210.

Pruitt, L. and Bailey, L. (1998) Factors affecting near-threshold fatigue crack propagation behavior of orthopedic grade ultra high molecular weight polyethylene. *Polymer*, 39, 1545–53.

Quinn, T. F. J., Rowson, D. M. and Sullivan, J. M. (1980) Application of the oxidational theory of mild wear to the sliding wear of low alloy steel. *Wear*, 65, 1–20.

Rabinowicz, E. (1965) *Friction and Wear of Materials*. New York, NY, Wiley.

Raimondi, M. T., Sassi, R. and Pietrabissa, R. (2000) A method for the evaluation of the change in volume of retrieved acetabular cups. *Proc Inst Mech Eng H*, 214, 577–87.

Santavirta, S. S., Lappalainen, R., Pekko, P., Anttila, A. and Konttinen, Y. T. (1999) The counterface, surface smoothness, tolerances, and coatings in total joint prostheses. *Clin Orthop Relat Res*, 369, 92–102.

Scherge, M., Shakhvorostov, D. and Pöhlmann, K. (2003) Fundamental wear mechanism of metals. *Wear*, 255, 395–400.

Schmalzried, T. P. and Callaghan, J. J. (1999) Current concepts review – wear in total hip and knee replacements. *J Bone Jt Surg Am*, 81, 115–36.

Sieradzki, K. and Newman, R. C. (1987) Stress-corrosion cracking. *J Phys Chem Solids*, 48, 1101–13.

Sin, H., Saka, N. and Suh, N. P. (1979) Abrasive wear mechanisms and the grit size effect. *Wear*, 55, 163–90.

Smith, S. L. and Unsworth, A. (1999) A comparison between gravimetric and volumetric techniques of wear measurement of UHMWPE acetabular cups against zirconia and cobalt–chromium–molybdenum femoral heads in a hip simulator. *Proc Inst Mech Eng H*, 213, 475–83.

Spinelli, M., Carmignato, S. Affatato, and Vicecontia, M. (2009) CMM-based procedure for polyethylene non-congruous unicompartmental knee prosthesis wear assessment. *Wear*, 267, 753–6.

Stewart, S. and Ahmed, R. (2002) Rolling contact fatigue of surface coatings–a review. *Wear*, 253, 1132–44.

Stilling, M., Soballe, K., Andersen, N. T., Larsen, K. and Rahbek, O. (2009) Analysis of polyethylene wear in plain radiographs. *Acta Orthop*, 80, 675–82.

Suh, N. P. (1973) The delamination theory of wear. *Wear* 25, 111–24.

Suh, N. P. (1977) An overview of the delamination theory of wear. *Wear*, 44, 1–16.

Teoh, S. H. (2000) Fatigue of biomaterials: a review. *Int J Fatigue*, 22, 825–37.

Thomann, U. I. and Uggowitzer, P. J. (2000) Wear-corrosion behavior of biocompatible austenitic stainless steels. *Wear*, 239, 48–58.

Tritschler, B., Forest, B. and Rieu, J. (1999) Fretting corrosion of materials for orthopaedic implants: a study of a metal/polymer contact in an artificial physiological medium. *Tribology Int*, 32, 587–96.

von Schewelov, T., Sanzen, L., Borlin, N., Markusson, P. and Onsten, I. (2004) Accuracy of radiographic and radiostereometric wear measurement of different hip prostheses: an experimental study. *Acta Orthop Scand*, 75, 691–700.

Wang, A., Stark, C. and Dumbleton, J. H. (1995) Role of cyclic plastic deformation in the wear of UHMWPE acetabular cups. *J Biomed Mater Res*, 29, 619–26.

Wang, A., Stark, C. and Dumbleton, J. H. (1996) Mechanistic and morphological origins of ultra-high molecular weight polyethylene wear debris in total joint replacement prostheses. *Proc Inst Mech Eng H*, 210, 141–55.

Winzer, N., Atrens, A., Song, G., Ghali, E., Dietzel, W., Kainer, K. U., Hort, N. and Blawert, C. (2005) A critical review of the stress corrosion cracking (SCC) of magnesium alloys. *Adv Eng Mater*, 7, 659–93.

Wu, J. S.-S., Hung, J.-P., Shu, C.-S. and Chen, J.-H. (2003) The computer simulation of wear behavior appearing in total hip prosthesis. *Comput Meth Prog Biomed*, 70, 81–91.

Yamaguchi, M., Hashimoto, Y., Akisue, T. and Bauer, T. W. (1999) Polyethylene wear vector in vivo: a three-dimensional analysis using retrieved acetabular components and radiographs. *J Orthop Res*, 17, 695–702.

2
Biology of implant wear

G. CIAPETTI, Istituto Ortopedico Rizzoli, Italy

Abstract: Periprosthetic osteolysis is a 'silent disease' that can progress without symptoms until catastrophic structural failure or mechanical loosening of the implant components occur. Arthroplasty is no doubt the most efficacious means to restore function of the degenerated joints, and it will continue to be the best treatment until tissue engineering strategies enter the clinics for joint replacement. Wear-mediated osteolysis is a clinical complication most frequently encountered in joint reconstruction, and the solution of this problem requires a joint effort of orthopaedic surgeons, bioengineers, and cell and molecular biologists. A deeper insight into the biology of wear has disclosed unexplored mechanisms to be modulated in order to escape particle-induced osteolytic disease. Therapeutic targets have already been identified following recognition of the molecular aspects of osteolysis initiation and progression, and several biological treatments are under trial. The combination of osteoclast-inhibiting factors and anabolic agents with new implant design and refined surgical techniques will lower, if not cancel, the incidence of wear-induced osteolysis.

Key words: wear particles, osteolysis, osteoclasts, inflammatory cytokines, arthroplasty, RANK/RANKL/OPG, macrophages.

2.1 Introduction

Wear-mediated osteolysis was first described by Sir John Charnley in 1975 as a 'cystic erosion of bone'; he found fragments of polymethylmethacrylate (PMMA) bone cement within the tissue surrounding fractured femoral stems and non-linear erosion of periprosthetic bone.[1] Later, in 1976, Harris et al. reported osteolysis at the proximal femur surrounding loose hip implants and characterized periprosthetic tissue histologically as 'sheets of macrophages, a few giant cells, and multiple small fragments of a birefringent material'.[2]

Periprosthetic osteolysis and aseptic loosening resulting from wear debris are still unresolved major complications of total joint arthroplasty. As defined by Marshall et al. in 2008, periprosthetic osteolysis is a 'silent disease' that can progress without symptoms until catastrophic structural failure or mechanical loosening of the implant components occur (Fig. 2.1).[3]

Although the success rate for total hip arthroplasty (THA) approaches 97% at 10–20 year follow-up, over 75% of THA implant failures are due to aseptic osteolysis, whereas infection accounts for 7%, recurrent dislocation for 6%, periprosthetic fracture for 5% and surgical error for 3%. As noted by Hallab and Jacobs, two types of debris are generated by implant wear – particles, ranging from nanometres to millimetres in size, and ions, which are soluble products usually bound to serum proteins.[4] Therefore, the tissue response to degradation products is different, depending on the nature and size of the debris, with a 'classical' granulomatous reaction to particles, whereas 'nanotoxicology' is more likely involved in the response to ions. It has to be remarked that multiple factors, including mechanical performance of the implant and host local conditions, are associated with the complex biological response to wear debris leading to periprosthetic osteolysis. However, the finding that osteolysis is correlated with a high wear rate and that a large number of wear particles is found to be associated with the periprosthetic interfacial membrane removed during revision surgery confirms that wear debris represents the most important underlying cause of periprosthetic osteolysis. Therefore, a better understanding of the biological scenario can aid in the search for an anti-osteolytic therapy.

2.2 Inflammatory reaction to particulate materials

2.2.1 Particle characteristics

The size of particles, as well as the amount, is a critical parameter in a discussion of tissue reaction to wear products. As a general rule, larger particles (micrometric) are generated by polyethylene (PE) bearings, ceramic particles are mainly of submicron size and metal particles range from nanometres to a few micrometres. Although a wide range of particles has been found, the majority of randomly shaped particles formed are less than 5 μm in diameter, with a mean size of of 0.5 μm for polymeric particles and 0.05 μm for metal or ceramic particles.[5]

There is consensus about the inflammatory activity of particles below 10 μm, that is, particles that can be phagocytosed by cells, but different results have been obtained concerning the dose that is likely to evoke an inflammatory response. Gallo et al. developed a computational algorithm to calculate the total number of PE particles for volumetric wear and

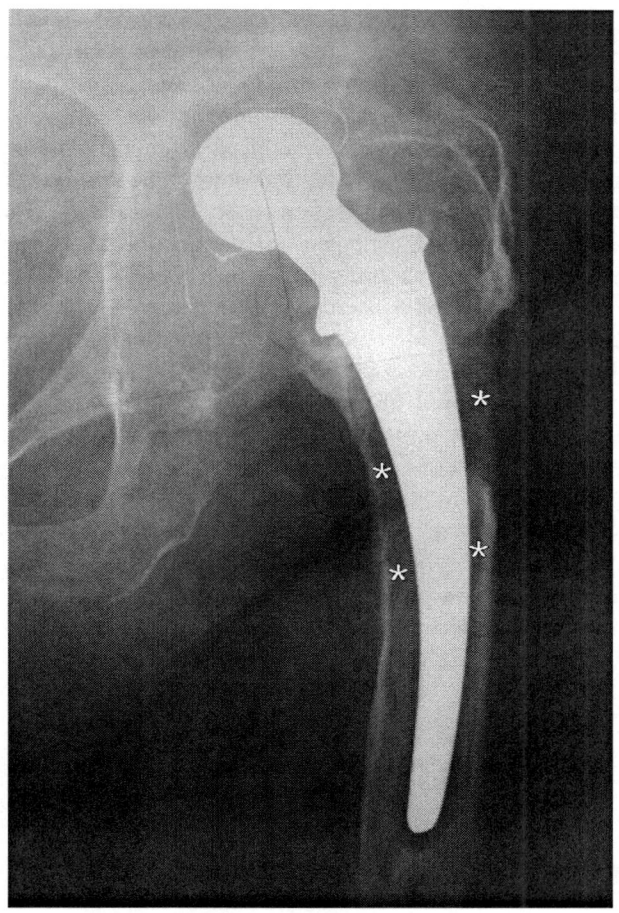

2.1 Radiolucent osteolytic areas (stars) along the stem of a Co–Cr hip prosthesis.

concluded that the risk for the development of osteolysis in THA cannot be simply estimated from volumetric wear.[6]

Biological activity is a measure of cytokine release after ingestion of the small wear debris particles by macrophages. The role of the size of the particles versus the chemistry in determining the type of cell response is still under discussion, and a clear prevalence of one factor has not been documented. Recently, it has been noted how the severity of the cell reaction can be related to the elemental composition of the particle surface, with surface cobalt more toxic to cells than titanium.[7] Even ceramic bearings may generate particles that cause an aspecific tissue reaction.[8]

New materials and couplings with a reduced volumetric wear rate are being developed, but if debris particles are small, the total surface area exposed may be large with high bioreactivity. Moreover, while large particles are entrapped in dense, collagen-rich connective tissue, submicron-sized particles are able to move and diffuse both locally and systemically. Following migration and local concentration of particles at an interface, a periprosthetic tissue reaction may be initiated; in systemic transportation, the likelihood of a tissue reaction is reduced, but lymph nodes, spleen and liver could become repositories of wear debris.[9]

In this respect, the danger represented by nanometre-sized wear particles, generated by different materials including ceramics, metals and polymers, is under investigation.[10] Nanometric PE particles were found in tissue samples retrieved from failed Charnley total hip replacements (THRs) and the biological response to this type of wear should be verified.[11] Maitra et al. described two different mechanisms – the direct binding of polymeric structures to the Toll-like receptor (TLR) signaling pathway and lysosomal damage by engulfed micrometric and nanometric particles with activation of the so-called 'inflammasome' (see Section 2.3.1).[12]

2.2.2 Tissue response

Several processes are recognized in the area of wear-induced osteolysis:

- local and systemic trafficking of inflammatory cells mediated by chemokines;
- inflammation, initiated and maintained by interleukin (IL)-1, IL-6, IL-8 and tumor necrosis factor alfa (TNF-α), as well as prostaglandins (PGE2);
- bone matrix destruction by metalloproteinases, including MT1-MMP, MMP-1, MMP-2, MMP-3 and MMP-9, with enlargement of the osteolytic areas;
- degradation of cell debris and molecules by lysosomal enzymes;
- increased osteoclastic activity.

As early as 1977, Willert observed the formation of a macrophage-based foreign body reaction to cobalt–chromium debris, while giant cells were prevalent in the foreign body reaction to PE particles.[13] The formation of granulation tissue is the 'usual' response to wear, as demonstrated by the finding of a granulomatous inflammation in stable implants as early as one year after implantation,[14] but the severity of such response has been found to be correlated with the extent of osteolysis and the amount of wear debris.[15] According to Gallo et al. particle disease may lead to increased and prolonged activity of 'bone multicellular units' (BMUs), resulting in periprosthetic osteolysis. Moreover, the expression and functional activity of the molecules involved in the pathways regulating BMU function, including RANKL/RANK/OPG/TRAF6, TNF-α/TNFR/TRAF1 and IL-6/CD126/JAK/STAT, can be affected by variations in their genes. These may explain the differences in severity of bone defects or prosthetic failure between patients with similar wear rates and the same prosthesis. There is an individual susceptibility to prosthetic failure: through a study of gene polymorphisms, it has been found that genetic variants of pro-inflammatory cytokines TNF-α and IL-6 confer susceptibility to severe osteolysis. Conversely, single-nucleotide polymorphisms in the IL-2 gene may protect carriers from the above THA complications.[16,17] Cells are recruited to the site of inflammation by chemotactic stimuli, which induce circulating cells to adhere to the vascular endothelium and, after rolling on the endothelial cells, to extravasate and reach the inflammatory site.[18]

The extent of the granulation tissue invasion depends on a variety of factors, including patient conditions or sensitivity, the type of particles, the rate of production/clearance of particles and the duration of the exposure, while the wear seems unrelated to the head diameter. Patient conditions include pre-operative diagnosis, body weight, lifestyle, etc., but implant-specific factors are no doubt main factors in wear onset. Interestingly, Gordon et al. compared individuals with a susceptibility to periprosthetic osteolysis after THA with individuals who remained osteolysis-free in the late period (~14 years) after primary THA, and suggested a quantitatively higher innate immune responses, in terms of cytokine gene expression, to pro-inflammatory stimuli in susceptible patients.[19] Under the microscope, the granulation tissue is composed of histiocytes (always observed when small wear debris was present) giant cells and sometimes necrosis, observed in the presence of small and large ultra-high molecular weight polyethylene (UHMWPE) wear debris.

The current view suggests that osteolysis occurs due to the chronic expression of inflammatory cytokines such as IL-1β and TNF-α in cells that are stimulated by either particle engulfment or particle surface contact. In patients revised for pain and suspected metal hypersensitivity with metal debris infiltrating the tissue, a unique picture of a perivascular infiltration of lymphocytes has been often observed. This tissue feature, termed 'aseptic lymphocytic vasculitis-associated lesion' (ALVAL) has been ranked using a score: patients with a high ALVAL may develop pseudotumor-like tissue.[20]

2.3 Cellular/molecular response to wear

Different cell types are implicated in progressive periprosthetic osteolysis in response to wear debris, with local bone resorption as a result of a complex network of cellular activities. Wear debris primarily targets macrophages residing in the reactive inflammatory membrane and osteoclast precursor cells, although mesenchymal stromal cells (MSC), osteoblasts, synovial fibroblasts and lymphocytes may also be involved. Cells have been shown to respond to size, chemistry, shape and charge of the particles.[21, 22]

However, the precise nature of the initial cellular interaction with wear debris and the subsequent pathways have been only partially disclosed, with a number of potential co-factors, including endotoxin contamination of particles,[23] protein-reactive response[24] and mechanical stress.[25] It has been shown that adherent endotoxin substantially enhances the effects of wear particles on pro-inflammatory cytokine production, osteoclast differentiation and osteolysis through stimulation of MAPK and NF-κB activation induced by wear particles.[26]

After release, wear particles may be coated by different molecules (e.g. lipids, carbohydrates, proteins) and this coating may then evoke a reaction of the innate or acquired immune system. The similarity between activation of macrophages through the macrophage complement-receptor proteins CD11b and CD18, and activation by particles in the absence of phagocytosis, confirms that particulate debris from orthopaedic biomaterials bind plasma proteins. The binding of five human plasma proteins (IgG, serum albumin, α(1)-acid glycoprotein, holo-transferrin and α(1)-antitrypsin) to UHMWPE wear particles (0.1–10 μm) isolated from hip periprosthetic tissues has been recently described: the unfolding of these proteins with exposure of active sites is bound to activate reactive cells as residing macrophages.[27]

Some groups have attempted to correlate wear-related osteolysis with serum and urine markers; that is, measuring the collagen fragments or bone proteins used for monitoring patients with Paget's disease or osteoporosis under treatment. Studies with larger control groups have identified high false-positive results, lowering the perception of test specificity, although Savarino et al. reported 33% sensitivity and 100% specificity of serum crosslinked N-terminal telopeptide of type I collagen (NTx) with respect to osteolysis.[28]

2.3.1 Monocytes/macrophages

It has been known since 1977 that monocytes (or tissue macrophages) are the cardinal cells activated by wear particles and are most likely responsible for the chronic inflammatory process.[13, 29–31] Monocytes move from blood to the site of wear by chemotaxis, with a chemokine-mediated mechanism that has been reviewed recently.[32] It has been shown recently that the infusion of clinically relevant PE particles in the femoral canal of mice stimulated the systemic recruitment and migration of remotely injected macrophages, as well as local bone resorption.[33] The interactions among particulate PMMA or titanium alloy, patient blood monocytes and periprosthetic tissues have recently been investigated using a SCID-hu model of aseptic loosening. Collectively, the results from this study showed that PMMA or titanium particles readily activate peripheral monocytes and promote cell trafficking to the debris-containing prosthetic tissues. The authors concluded that particle-provoked peripheral blood mononuclear cells participated in and promoted the local inflammatory process, osteoclastogenesis and bone resorption.[34]

The initiation of an inflammatory reaction is the first mechanism used by macrophages when challenged by wear particles. Macrophages, as well as the other responding cells, secrete a number of cytokines, metalloproteinases, prostaglandins, lysosomal enzymes and growth factors, whose collective activities lead to an inflammatory reaction against debris, which in turn stimulates focal bone resorption at the bone–implant interface. Although markers of bone turnover have thus far shown limited predictive value, several studies have quantified biochemical mediators associated with the inflammatory process.

Shanbhag et al. used a high-throughput protein chip to identify inflammatory markers in osteolytic tissues from around failed metal-on-polyethylene total joint arthroplasties. They identified several markers associated with osteolysis, including IL-8 and IL-6, which recruit osteoclast precursors and facilitate the maturation of osteoclasts. Additionally, various T cell chemotactic factors such as IP-10 (interferon γ-inducible protein of 10 kDa) and MIG (monokine induced by interferon γ) were significantly elevated in the osteolytic tissues.[35]

In fact, the finding of high levels of inflammatory cytokines is not a consistent finding in studies on wear-related osteolysis: only IL-6 was found to be elevated in patients with osteolysis by Hernigou et al.,[36] while Fiorito et al. found that serum levels of IL-1β, IL-6, TNF-α, MMP-1 and PGE2 in patients with osteolysis did not significantly differ from those of patients without osteolysis or normal subjects.[37] As reported by Purdue et al., the role of inflammatory cytokines has been largely assessed using in vitro models and animal experimentation, while direct evidence for similar involvement of pro-inflammatory cytokines in humans is far from conclusive. For example, although some reports of TNF-α elevation in synovial fluid and periprosthetic tissues with osteolysis have appeared, no increase in circulating TNF-α or in its expression has been demonstrated in patients suffering from osteolytic disease.[38] The presence of anti-inflammatory factors, i.e. IL-11 (a member of the IL-6 superfamily) and transforming growth factor beta (TGF-β), in the osteolytic areas has also been investigated. Interestingly, IL-11 was almost undetectable in the serum of patients with cementless hip prostheses in comparison with patients without osteolysis who had normal values: this unbalance between pro- and anti-inflammatory cytokines could be an additional factor in osteolysis persistence.[37]

Since osteoclasts are responsible for active bone resorption in wear-related osteolysis, several studies have investigated the RANK/RANKL/OPG (receptor activator of the nuclear transcription factor kappaB/receptor activator of the NFκB ligand/osteoprotegerin) system in osteoclast maturation (see later) and evaluated the clinical relevance of the circulating osteoprotegerin (OPG) and RANKL levels in a variety of human diseases including osteolysis.[39–41]

Granchi et al. measured serum OPG and receptor activator of the nuclear factor κB ligand (RANKL) in four groups of patients: healthy patients without implants; patients with osteoarthritis but no implants; patients with clinically stable hip arthroplasties; and patients with loose hip implants. The results showed significantly increased OPG in patients with osteoarthritis (but no arthroplasty) and in patients with loose implants, while RANKL was higher in patients without osteolysis compared to patients with loose implants. Even if serum levels of OPG and RANKL cannot be considered as specific markers of their activity in the bone because of the redundancy and pleiotropic effects of these molecules, the increase in OPG levels may reflect a protective mechanism of the skeleton to compensate for the osteolytic activity that occurs in severe osteoarthritis and in aseptic loosening.[42]

The molecular pathway of macrophage activation by wear particles up to inflammation-mediated osteolytic bone resorption has been described quite recently. Following surface interaction between macrophages and debris, or even phagocytosis, macrophages are activated through several receptors, including CD11b, CD14 and TLR family members. The signal is then transduced intracellularly via mitogen-activated protein kinases (MAPKs) to nuclear transcription factors, such as NFκB. This results in up-regulation of genes for pro-inflammatory cytokines and inhibition of the protective actions of anti-osteoclastogenic cytokines such as interferon gamma. These cytokines induce bone loss adjacent to the implant by promoting the differentiation of osteoclast precursors into mature osteoclasts, the cells responsible for the degradation of bone.[43, 44]

The molecular network activated in monocytes/macrophages facing wear particles is actually much more complicated. The large complex of proteins sensing the stress signals triggered by foreign agents in the cytoplasm of macrophages has been named 'inflammasome', and a variety of studies are currently exploring signaling pathways and molecules with the aim of identifying potential targets for anti-osteolytic therapy.[45] As an example, Hao *et al.* have recently found that Hsp60 is the specific heat shock protein produced by monocytes in response to UMHWPE particles. The stress caused by UMHWPE particle interaction with monocytes, through TLRs, is similar to that induced by heavy metal particle exposure, since this form of stress can activate immunoresponding cells to increase local and systemic cytokine concentrations.[46] TLRs, the key receptors that inform the immune system about the presence of a bacterial infection, have also been suggested to signal different molecules potentially noxious to the body, such as immunostimulatory molecules produced by both gram-negative and gram-positive bacteria. That the TLRs are the membrane structures involved in capturing the wear-associated signals to convey them to the cell nucleus through mitogen-activated protein kinase cascade and transcription factor activation, has been confirmed by many authors. In fact, TLR immunoreactivity has been recently shown in monocytes/macrophages infiltrating aseptic synovial membrane-like tissue, the major wear particle reactive cell population.[47] Among the thirteen types of TLRs identified, TLR4 has been recognized as the receptor involved in particle-mediated stimulation of monocytes/macrophages.

2.3.2 Lymphocytes

The finding of lymphocytes clustered around vessels or spread in periprosthetic tissue is mainly ascribed to the presence of metal ions or particles and to the potential hypersensivity of the patient against the metal.[48, 49] The perivascular infiltration of lymphocytes with plasma cells, also named aseptic lymphocytic vasculitis-associated lesion (ALVAL), has been ascertained even when wear is within normal reported range limit.[50] It has been reported that perivascular lymphocytic infiltration is more extensive in revisions of metal-on-metal (MoM) and in aseptic loosening, idiopathic pain or infection, but is also present in total knee arthroplasty (TKA), non-MoM and different reasons for revision. It correlates with other signs of metal hypersensitivity, but not with histologic measures of metal particulate load.[51] Interactions between macrophages and locally recruited lymphocytes, which may or may not give rise to an immunologically mediated process have been demonstrated, but it has not been definitely proven if this mechanism is present in individuals with aseptic loosening without clinical evidence of sensitization.[52] Cutaneous reactions to metal implants, orthopaedic or otherwise, are well documented in the literature; the first case of a dermatitis reaction over a stainless steel fracture plate was described in 1966. Nickel (Ni), cobalt (Co) and chromium (Cr) are the three most common metals that elicit both cutaneous and extracutaneous allergic reactions from chronic internal exposure, but other metal ions, as well as bone cement components, can cause such hypersensitivity reactions.[53] The role of lymphocytes in metal sensitivity mediated by metal particles is recurrently discussed, with contrasting results obtained from *in vitro* or *in vivo* testing. While some authors have observed a direct response of lymphocytes to metal particles, with a reduction in CD8+T cells in patients with MoM implants,[54] others have ruled out any potential inolvement of lymphocytes in particle-induced osteolysis.[55]

Measurement of the serum metal level may be used for diagnosing prosthetic loosening of metal appliances: in a study on patients with either stable ($n = 24$) or loosened ($n = 35$) total knee replacement, a significant increase in the mean level of Cr ions was seen in the group with failed implants ($p = 0.001$). Therefore, it was concluded that chromium ions, but not aluminum, titanium or cobalt, may be of value for diagnosing implant failure due to loosening.[56] There is some evidence that patients with MoM bearings and/or high serum metal levels elicit more response to metal antigen challenge measured as either patch test sensitivity or lymphocyte proliferation.[57, 58]

A study on the reliability of a skin test, i.e. patch test, in detecting the sensitization to the implant components in patients undergoing THR was undertaken. Sensitization to cobalt-based alloys (CoCrMo), Ti-based alloys (TiAlV) and bone cements was assessed in 66 candidates to THR, 53 with a stable implant and 104 with THR loosening (total number of patients, 223), to find that the frequency of positive patch testing in pre-implant patients did not differ from that observed after THR. With regard to the THR outcome, patch testing was not able to discriminate between stable and failed implants, but a medical history of hypersensitivity together with positivity to one metallic hapten negatively influenced the THR survival. In conclusion, the cause–effect relationship between sensitization and negative outcome cannot be established, but the shorter lifespan of THR in patients who have a positive patch testing supports the significant role of this event in contributing to implant failure.[59]

Unlike THR, high positivity to metallic haptens representative of cobalt-based alloys (CoCrMo), titanium-based alloys (TiAlV) and bone cements, was found using patch testing on 94 subjects including 20 patients without implant, 27 individuals with a well-functioning TKA and 47 patients with loosened TKA components. The frequency of positive skin reactions to metals increased significantly after TKA, either stable or loosened (no implant, 20%; stable TKA, 48.1%, $p = 0.05$; loosened TKA, 59.6%,

$p = 0.001$), and a higher frequency of positive response to vanadium was found in patients with a stable TKA. The authors concluded that the medical history for metal allergy is a risk factor, because TKA failure was fourfold more likely in patients who had symptoms of metal hypersensitivity before implantation.[59]

Hallab et al. found a debris-mediated upregulation of T cell co-stimulatory molecules and cytokines, and a T-helper type (Th1) response to metal debris. This suggests an adaptive (macrophage-recruiting) immune response rather than an innate (non-specific) immune response to metals.[60, 61] Roato et al., who noted a spontaneous transformation of peripheral blood mononuclear cells (PBMCs) from periprosthetic osteolysis patients in osteoclasts, and a close vicinity of lymphocytes and osteoclasts in periprosthetic tissue, suggest a temporal sequence where T cells initially proliferate and support osteoclastogenesis through RANK/RANKL pathway. Later, osteoclasts may provide a negative feedback on T cells, leading to activation of CD8 regulatory T cells and subsequent inhibition of effector CD4 T cells.[62]

Recent studies have shown that natural killer cells are a principal tissue-infiltrating lymphocyte subset in patients with osteoarthritis and patients with periprosthetic inflammation, and display a quiescent phenotype that is consistent with post-activation exhaustion.[63]

Some studies have reported local soft tissue pseudotumors in patients with MoM prostheses. In these cases, Co, Cr, Ni metal ion levels in serum/aspirate are often not increased,[64] and in vitro testing using a lymphocyte transformation test (LTT) in response to Co, Cr and Ni has shown no difference between patients with pseudotumors and those without. This suggests that a hypersensitivity type IV reaction is not the main reaction involved in pseudotumor formation following prolonged metal exposure.[65]

It has been ascertained that solid pseudotumors are nearly exclusively observed with resurfacing procedures, carrying a high annual revision rate in women under 40 years of age, occurring particularly in cases of acetabular malposition and with use of cast-molded Cr–Co alloys.[66]

It can be concluded that today there are no scientific or epidemiologic data supporting a risk of carcinogenesis or teratogenesis related to the use of a MoM bearings couple. However, according to some authors, patients bearing MoM may be more susceptible to periprosthetic infection.[67] Actually, bacterial molecules, such as lipoteichoic acid produced by gram-positive bacteria, subclinical biofilms tethered to prosthetic surfaces, lypopolysaccharide and endotoxin on wear particles are collectively known as 'pathogen-associated molecular patterns' (PAMPs); when adherent to wear particles, even at a low level, these molecules activate TLRs on macrophages in periprosthetic membranes of patients with aseptic loosening.[68, 69]

2.3.3 Fibroblasts

Fibroblasts are responsible for the production of connective tissue as a component of the interface and the particle-induced secretion of chemoattractive cytokines, including monocyte chemoattractant protein-1 (MCP-1), monocyte inflammatory protein-1α (MIP-1α) and IL-8. These chemokines recruit from circulation monocytes, which are the precursors of bone-resorbing mature osteoclasts.

When cultured *in vitro*, explanted fibroblasts from the interface release TNF-α, IL-1β, IL-6 and vascular endothelial growth factor; moreover, following stimulation with TNF-α, or IL-1β, they express receptor activator of the NFκB ligand (RANKL), which is the molecule required for osteoclast maturation from monocytic precursors.[70]

2.3.4 Endothelial cells

The main role of endothelial cells in the wear-induced tissue reaction is to recruit circulating cells, including monocytes and lymphocytes, to their surface: such cells then tether to and roll along the vessel surface so as to exit the bloodstream and reach the reactive site. This attractive mechanism is mediated by chemoattractive cytokines, or chemokines, such as MCP-1, MIP-1 and IL-8. These molecules are produced not only by endothelial cells but also by monocytes/macrophages, fibroblasts and osteoblasts. MCP-1 and MIP-1 regulate the migration and accumulation of monocyte/macrophages, dendritic cells, NK and memory T lymphocytes, as well as induce secretion of pro-inflammatory cytokines, while IL-8 is attracting mainly neutrophils.[32]

2.3.5 Osteoblasts/osteocytes

In the past decade, there have been major advances in the understanding of how osteoblasts regulate osteoclastogenesis.[71] The receptor activator of nuclear factor-kappa B (NFκB) ligand (RANKL) has been shown to play a fundamental role in regulating osteoclastogenesis (see Section 2.3.6). RANKL, which is also known as the osteoclast differentiation factor, binds two types of receptors. The first one is RANK, which is expressed in pre-osteoclasts. The binding of RANK with RANKL triggers a cascade of intracellular events that are essential to completing osteoclast differentiation and activation. The second type of RANKL receptor is osteoprotegerin (OPG), which is a decoy receptor that limits the biologic activity of RANKL. Activation of OPG suppresses the differentiation of osteoclasts, inhibits their activation and induces apoptosis. Therefore, the balance between OPG and RANKL is essential to regulate bone re-modeling, by controlling the activation state of RANK on osteoclasts. Interested readers are referred to the literature for a detailed description of the molecules and mechanisms of the RANK/RANKL/OPG system.[72–74]

Osteocytes, too, have been suggested to participate in wear-debris-induced osteolysis. Atkins et al.,[75] using a novel *in vitro* three-dimensional cell culture system, tested PE-particle-induced differentiation of normal human bone-derived cells (NHBC) into a mature osteocyte-like phenotype over a 21–28 day culture period. They found an increase in mRNA expression of the osteocyte markers E11, DMP-1 and SOST/sclerostin, an increase in mRNA expression of genes associated with osteoclast formation and activity (RANKL, IL-8 and M-CSF) and a decreased expression of the osteoclast antagonist, OPG. Overall, their data suggest that PE particles directly induce a change in the phenotype of mature osteoblasts and osteocytes, consistent with the net loss of bone near orthopaedic implants.[75] In another study, an inflammatory cytokine production and increased apoptosis has been recorded in the MLO-Y4 osteocytic cells after treatment with Co–Cr–Mo alloy particles.[76]

2.3.6 Osteoclasts

Osteoclasts are cells of haematopoietic origin and their precursors undergo proliferation and differentiation to become multi-nucleated bone-resorbing osteoclasts. It has been shown that osteoclast progenitors are recruited to the bone implant interface and maturation is regulated by two essential cytokines: receptor activator of NFκB ligand (RANKL) and macrophage colony-stimulating factor (M-CSF). Under physiologic conditions, osteoclasts are generated when their precursors are in direct contact with RANKL-generating supporting cells, e.g. osteoblasts and stromal cells and their precursors. These supporting cells secrete M-CSF and carry membrane-bound RANKL to initiate osteoclastogenesis by engaging the c-Fms and RANK receptors on osteoclast precursors, respectively. Osteoclasts carry on their membrane the RANK receptor, a type I transmembrane protein of the TNF receptor superfamily, able to bind RANKL molecule released by accessory cells. That the receptor activator of NFκB ligand (RANKL) is essential for osteoclastogenesis is demonstrated by the fact that mice deficient in the RANKL gene exhibit severe osteopetrosis, defects in tooth eruption and complete lack of osteoclasts because of impaired osteoclastogenesis. RANKL also induces expression of tartrate-resistant acid phosphatase and cathepsin K through NFATc1.

The molecule counteracting the formation of osteoclasts is OPG, which was first cloned as a potential inhibitor of osteoclastogenesis. OPG is a member of the TNF receptor superfamily, and is highly expressed in adult lung, heart, kidney, liver, spleen, thymus, prostate, ovary, small intestine, thyroid, lymph node, trachea, adrenal gland, testis and bone marrow. Molecular binding experiments showed that OPG associates with RANKL and functions as a decoy receptor. The RANK/RANKL/OPG system is central to periprosthetic osteolysis due to wear particles (Fig. 2.2).

Osteoclast differentiation into mature bone-resorbing osteoclasts may occur in response to several cytokines, including TNF-α, PGE2, IL-1, IL-6 and IL-11.[73] As responsible for bone resorption, osteoclasts play a pivotal role in the pathogenesis of osteolytic disorders, but other cells participate in the resorptive activity of osteoclasts. It has been reported that, in response to direct particulate exposure, bone marrow-derived cells may activate receptor activator of NFκB ligand (RANKL) production into the conditioned medium with increased formation of mature osteoclasts capable of active bone resorption.

It has also been reported that M-CSF and TNF-α induce human arthroplasty-derived macrophage differentiation *in vitro* into osteoclasts, expressing tartrate-resistant acid phosphatase and vitronectin receptor, and exhibiting a synergistic increase in lacunar bone resorption in response to TNF-α and IL-1.[77, 78] Lymphocytes, too, have been shown to differentiate into osteoclasts, as described in Section 2.3.2.[62]

2.4 Conclusion and therapeutic targets

Total joint replacement is one of the most successful and effective procedures developed for treatment of pain associated with end-stage arthritis. Unfortunately, after implant stabilization occurs, wear of the bearing surfaces is the major issue limiting longevity of the prosthesis.

Osteolytic response to implant wear is extremely variable among patients, suggesting a genetic contribution, in addition to clinical situation, implant design and surgical factors, which all contribute to the risk of osteolysis. As far as the patient is concerned, the innate immune response to pro-inflammatory stimuli, suggested by Gordon *et al.*,[19] which leads to a 'susceptibility' of individuals to periprosthetic osteolysis, could be an important factor in loosening promotion.

Moreover, sensitivity to implant materials is an unpredictable event, which may contribute to the process leading to the failure of the total hip replacement. In this context, the role of lymphocytes, which have been shown to be always present in the reactive tissue, has to be ascertained.

Concerning the implant/design, a number of important advances have been made in material manufacturing and processing, alternative bearing surfaces, low-wear implant design and revision techniques, and these improvements are expected to reduce the future burden of revision hip and knee arthroplasty. Synthesis and manufacturing of new materials and alloys with reduced wear is the first line of defence against osteolytic disease: recent

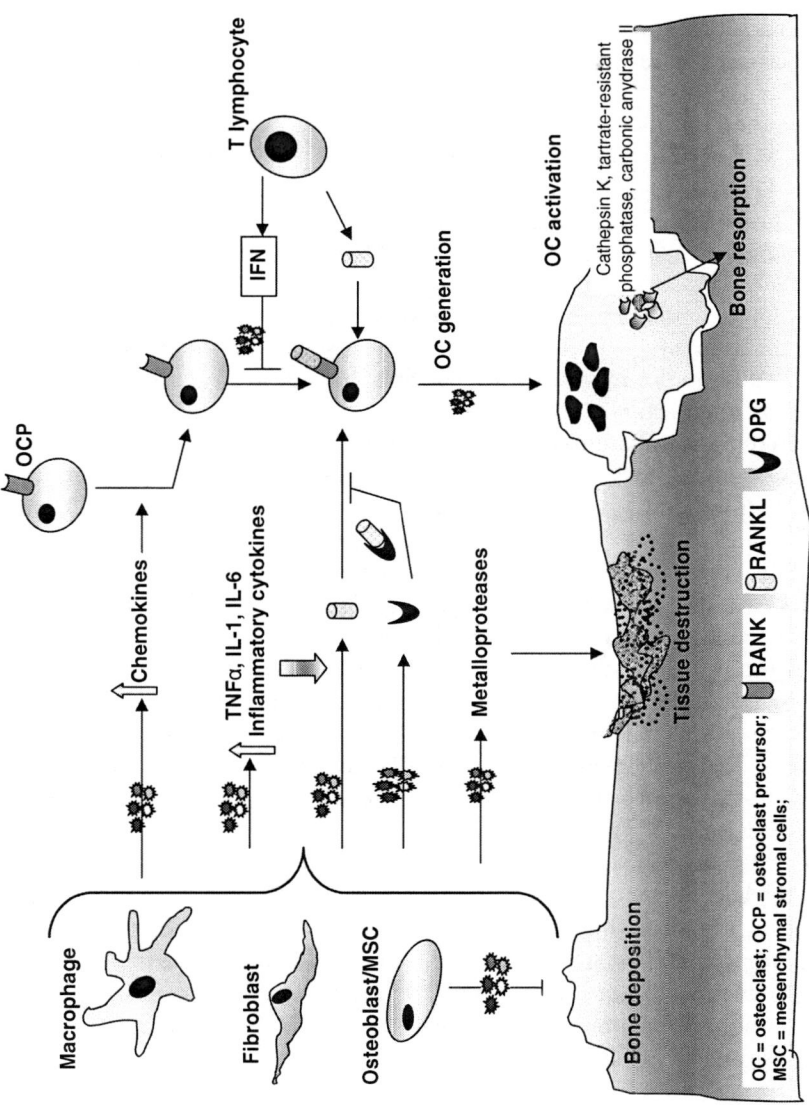

2.2 Role of the RANK/RANKL/OPG system in wear particle-induced osteolysis (adapted from Purdue PE et al., Human Soc Sci J, 2006, 2, 102–13).

studies focus on avoiding direct metal contact to reduce MoM wear,[79] the addition of free radical scavenger to reinforced UHMWPE[80] or the use of a plasma-sprayed surface to yield better implant integration.[81] Likewise, the continuous refining of implant design, taking into account anatomical differences among subjects, is another strategy to decrease the risk of wear and failure.[82]

However, it is not only the amount and size of particles (governed by device design) but several biological factors (which are poorly recognized) also influence the severity of wear-related osteolysis. Therefore, better understanding of the molecules and mechanisms involved in the tissue reaction to wear particles is essential to stop or at least reduce osteolytic disease. Discovery of the RANKL/RANK/OPG signaling system for skeletal homeostasis has been one of the most important advances in bone biology in the last decade and updated therapies are often centered on this system.

Potential biologic treatments for wear-related aseptic loosening block bone resorption or promote bone formation, so as to prevent osteolysis when administered intra- or short post-operatively or to stop progression of the disease when established. Traditional pharmacologic therapies employ non-steroidal anti-inflammatory drugs (NSAIDs) or selective cyclo-oxygenase (COX) inhibitors. Most recent strategies include bisphosphonates (BPs), anti-inflammatory agents and osteoclast-suppressing factors (Fig. 2.3).

To date, the most extensively investigated pharmacological strategy against wear-related osteolysis is the use of BPs, as it has long been known that BPs reduce periprosthetic bone loss at least in the short term after THR. A multitude of *in vitro* studies have tried to decipher the mechanism and pathways of BP activity on osteoclast differentiation and formation, but the results remain controversial. For example, BP effects on resorption have been attributed to differences in osteoclastic activity rather than their number, based on apparently normal osteoclast formation in isolated rat osteoclast cultures.

A pharmacological study has shown that BPs inhibit lipopolysaccharide- or parathyroid hormone-induced osteoclast differentiation, fusion, attachment, actin ring formation and activation. Moreover, it is apparent that one of the inhibitory effects of BPs on bone resorption might be the impairment of the production of osteopontin and its localization with integrin $a_v b_3$ at the cell periphery membrane. To resorb bone effectively, osteoclasts must attach themselves firmly to the bone surface using specialized actin-rich podosomes and integrins so as to form tight seals with the underlying bone matrix. Therefore, a lack of properly localized cell adhesive structures hampers the cytoskeletal rearrangement associated with cell attachment and resorption in osteoclasts.[83]

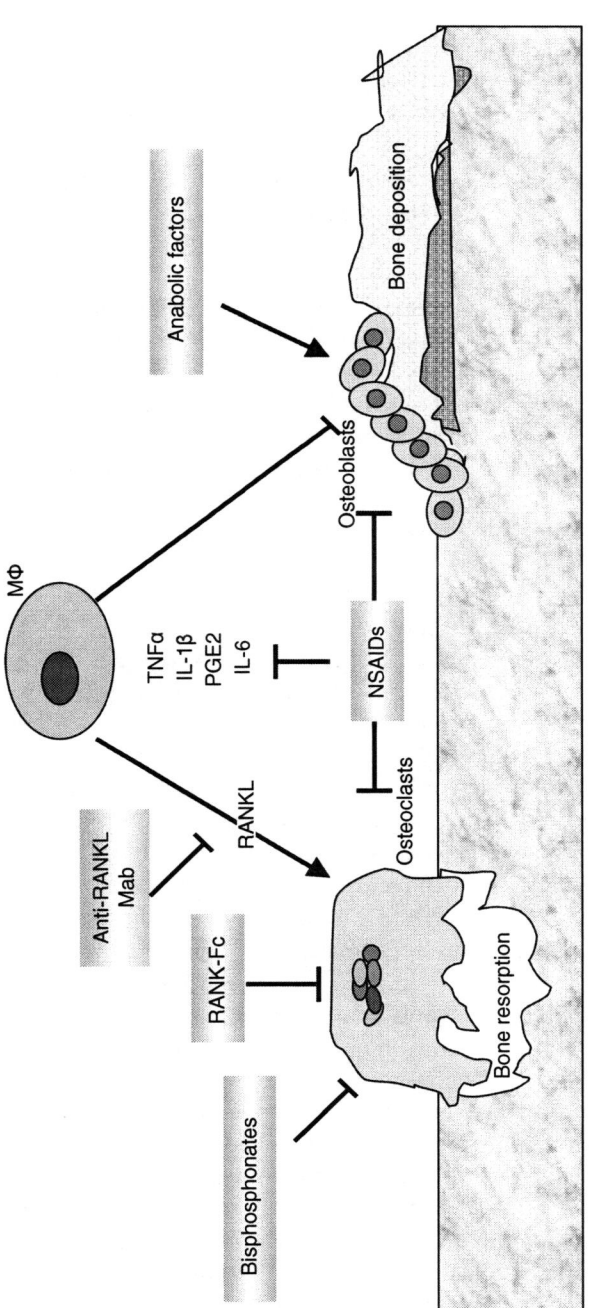

2.3 Potential biologic treatments for particle-induced osteolysis (adapted from Schwarz).[90]

The role of TNF-α as an anti-apoptotic signal, which renders osteoclasts insensitive to BP, has been advocated to justify the lack of efficacy of these drugs in inflammatory focal bone loss.[84] The resistance of osteoclasts to BP-induced apoptosis within the particle-mediated inflammatory site has been studied *in vitro*, and it was found that RANKL protects osteoclasts from the apoptosis-inducing and anti-resorptive effects of BPs.[85] The clinical outcome of a BP-based therapy to block or decrease particle-induced bone loss is highly debated.

The long-term effects of a single-dose therapy of pamidronate were analyzed in a study on 37 patients (out of 50 enrolled) at five years from drug administration, using a clinical/radiological score and bone mineral density assessment. The femoral and acetabular bone mineral density, as well as the Harris hip score, were similar in the pamidronate and placebo groups along the study duration and, at five years, two from each group (BP-treated and placebo) developed osteolysis. It was concluded that a single post-operative dose does not influence the clinical outcome or prevent osteolysis.[86]

A recent population-based association study analyzed retrospectively the use of BPs and the incidence of revision surgery after primary THA.[87] It was found that BP use was associated with an increased risk of revision for infection but a lower overall risk of revision for all causes with long-term use (240 days in the post-operative period). However, the robustness of these findings is unclear as the direction of the observed effects varied with post-surgery duration of BP therapy, and it is concluded that further research is warranted in order to clarify whether these associations are truly causal.

It can be concluded that although BPs are effective in preventing metabolic bone loss, they are less effective for inflammatory bone loss.

As noted earlier, at the core of the inflammatory reaction, host defense cells recognize particles and release large quantities of pro-inflammatory cytokines and factors such as TNF, IL-1α, IL-1β, IL-6, RANKL and PGE_2, among others. These factors recruit and stimulate bone loss by targeting osteoclasts and their monocytic precursors. As a consequence, local cytokine inhibition is a potential therapy that may reduce inflammation in the periprosthetic tissue, and several biological mediators have been identified as useful for clinical application. TNF-α and IL-1β are the key cytokines that play a critical role in the development of inflammatory bone resorption, as the NFκB pathway is activated after stimulation of these cytokines. Pharmacological therapies targeted at such cytokines have scored some success in studies *in vitro* and animal models, but anti-TNF therapies to treat osteolysis have largely been unsuccessful in human clinical trials.[32] This may be due to the fact that inflammatory pathways are very redundant, as well as issues related to timing and dosing of specific pharmacological agents, which would probably have to be continued indefinitely.[88]

The IL-1 receptor antagonist protein and the anti-inflammatory cytokine IL-10 appear to possess the capacity to reduce cell-mediated inflammatory reactions, but the delivery of appropriate doses of pro-inflammatory cytokine inhibitors to the periprosthetic tissue remains a challenge. An alternative may be gene therapy with Etanecerpt, a TNF-α receptor fusion protein (sTNF:Fc) acting as soluble inhibitor of TNF, which has been shown to prevent wear-induced osteolysis in mice. But the efficacy of such TNF inhibitors, though verified in rats or mice, failed to show an obvious effect in patients with osteolysis.[89, 90] Furthermore, many of the inflammatory mediators are important to general immune surveillance and tissue homeostasis, making their blockage controversial for a non-life-threatening condition such as periprosthetic osteolysis.

Statins (inhibitors of the mevalonate pathway) have been indicated because of their role against inflammatory cytokines. An *in vitro* model of the human monocyte/macrophage inflammatory response to PMMA particles has been studied: the production of inflammatory cytokines TNF-α and MCP-1 by human monocytes in response to PMMA particle activation was abrogated by pre-treatment with cerivastatin.[91]

As already remarked, periprosthetic membrane particles activate macrophages and osteoclasts, leading to a significant bone loss, with RANK/RANKL as the principal axis that regulates the osteoclastogenic event, and the transcription factor NFκB, involved in both inflammatory and osteolytic responses, at the center of this process. Moreover, the NFκB signaling pathway regulates the synthesis and action of inflammatory cytokines including IL-1β and TNF-α, with a paracrine feedback mechanism that amplifies the reaction.[92] Direct inhibition of osteoclast differentiation may therefore be achieved by application of RANKL decoy molecules such as OPG.[93]

In vivo micro-CT and traditional histology have been used in a murine calvaria model to test OPG efficacy versus zoledronic acid (BP) in preventing wear titanium (Ti) and PE-debris-induced osteolysis. Traditional histomorphometry of the sagittal suture area of calvaria from Ti- and PE-treated mice confirmed the remarkable suppression of resorption by OPG versus the lack of effect by physiological BPs. The result was confirmed by the significant difference in osteoclast numbers observed between OPG versus BPs in both Ti- and PE-treated calvaria.[94]

An alternative is Denosumab, a fully human monoclonal antibody obtained by injecting mice with human RANKL, which binds to and inactivates RANKL, similar to the action of OPG. Compared with OPG:Fc (OPG construct), Denosumab has a long circulating half-life and a prolonged effect to reduce serum levels of markers of bone resorption and formation.[95] The relative efficacy, cost-effectiveness and side-effects of targeted RANKL inhibition compared with conventional anti-resorptive drugs (i.e. BPs) should be resolved by clinical trials in coming years.[96]

Another RANKL decoy molecule is the soluble fusion protein RANK-Fc. It has been developed to treat severe bone losses, such as cancer lesion or osteosarcoma metastasis in bone, and suggested as a potential osteoclastic blocking agent in wear-mediated osteolysis.[97, 98]

IFN-γ is a cytokine secreted primarily by activated T cells and NK cells, and was originally characterized as a powerful macrophage activator that upregulated nitric oxide production and MHC class II expression in macrophages. Then it was reported to be a strong suppressor of osteoclastogenesis *in vitro* through inhibition of RANKL signaling. However, its effects on osteoclast formation are controversial. It is likely that the effects of IFN-γ on osteoclast formation are complex and will depend on specific conditions in the bone micro-environment and relative concentrations of other cytokines that can affect the differentiation of the osteoclast precursors.[72]

As discussed earlier, altered NFκB signaling in osteoclasts has been associated with excessive osteoclastic activity and frequently observed in periprosthetic osteolysis. Therefore, modification of NFκB signaling may represent a new approach to retard wear-debris-induced prosthetic loosening.[73]

Doxycycline (DOX), a semi-synthetic tetracycline, was shown to effectively inhibit *in vitro* osteoclastogenesis (from blood monocytes), affect the fate of mature osteoclasts and inhibit bone resorption by mature osteoclasts. *In vivo* data indicated that DOX strongly inhibited PMMA- or UHMWPE-induced osteolysis and osteoclastogenesis.[99]

A promising therapy includes the use of erythromycin (EM), an inhibitor of the transcription factor NFκB.[100, 101] EM, an antibiotic used for the treatment of infectious disease for over 50 years, has attracted a great deal of attention because of its anti-inflammatory effects at sub-anti-microbial doses. EM shows a unique 'phagocyte targeted delivery' property, with a tropism for monocytes and macrophages in bone marrow and inflammatory tissues. The study analyzed 32 patients with a total hip prosthesis, thought to be loose without a suspicion of infection. Exclusion criteria included rheumatoid arthritis and other auto-immune diseases and the diagnosis of aseptic loosening in all patients was confirmed at revision surgery and by subsequent histological analysis.

Oral EM has been shown to reduce the inflammation of periprosthetic tissues, as the numbers of infiltrating cells, CD68+ macrophages, RANKL + cells, and TRAP+ cells, as well as TNF-α, IL-1β and RANKL gene transcripts, and serum levels of TNF-α and IL-1β, are decreased. Therefore, EM represents a biological cure or prevention for those patients who might need repeated revision surgeries and/or show the early signs of progressive osteolysis after TJR.

Gene therapy is a technique that draws on the introduction of new genes into cells for the purpose of treating disease by restoring or adding gene expression. By delivering the relevant genes to the site to be treated, the therapeutic substances thereby can be persistently produced directly by local cells at the site of diseases. Recent advances in gene therapy techniques suggest that anti-inflammatory cytokine or anti-resorptive factor genes may be delivered to the periprosthetic tissues by viral vectors, to control the local reaction and extend the life of the prosthesis.

Gene transfer of OPG using an adeno-associated virus vector was shown to be protective against orthopaedic wear-debris-induced bone loss. In osteoclastogenesis and in bone wafer resorption assays, the bioactivity of the transgene OPG was proven by depletion of osteoclastogenesis and reduced bone resorption. Using an *in vivo* model of debris-induced bone resorption, complete inhibition of osteolysis in animals receiving AAV–OPG gene therapy was demonstrated.[102]

The feasibility and efficacy of a cell-based OPG gene delivery approach has been recently investigated using a murine model of prosthesis failure.[103] To mimic a weight-bearing knee arthroplasty, a titanium pin was implanted into mouse proximal tibia, followed by titanium particles challenge to induce periprosthetic osteolysis. Following *in vitro* transduction of mouse fibroblast-like synoviocytes with OPG, these cells were transfused in the osteolytic joint three weeks post-surgery. By histological observation, inflammatory pseudomembranes at the bone–implant interface were constantly seen in control groups, whereas only sporadically in OPG gene-modified groups. Moreover, TRAP-positive osteoclasts and TNF-α, IL-1β, CD68+ expressing cells were significantly reduced in periprosthetic tissues of OPG gene-modified mice. This suggests that cell-based *ex vivo* OPG gene therapy was as efficient as *in vivo* local gene transfer technique to deliver functional therapeutic OPG activities, halting the debris-induced osteolysis.

Translation of the gene therapies inhibiting osteolysis from experimental trials to the clinics is subjected to conclusive proofs of safety and efficiency in transfection procedures. Future therapeutic treatments include stimulation of osteogenic activity to improve bone quality.

An *in vitro* study has shown that OP-1 stimulates osteogenesis in MC3T3-E1 osteoprogenitor cells that have been inhibited by PMMA particles. Therefore, local administration of OP-1 to the site of osteolysis may be a potential adjunctive therapy to reverse the bone destruction due to wear particles.[104]

Recent studies have demonstrated that endogenous parathyroid hormone (PTH), the active form of vitamin D, 1,25-dihydroxyvitamin D [1,25(OH)

2D] and PTH-related peptide (PTHrP), known for their osteolytic activity, also exert bone anabolic activity. Such molecules may be suggested to counteract bone erosion due to wear.[105]

In conclusion, periprosthetic wear-induced osteolysis is the product of enhanced osteoclast formation and activation prompted by inflammatory cytokines. Effective therapies for reducing osteolytic areas are bound to hit the mechanisms of periprosthetic inflammation, osteoclastic recruitment, the RANKL/RANK/OPG axis of osteoclast activation and bone resorption. Control of these aspects will ultimately lead to a decreased bone loss with major stability of the prosthetic device.

2.5 References

1. Charnley J. Fracture of femoral prostheses in total hip replacement: A clinical study. *Clin Orthop Rel Res*, 1975, 111, 105–20.
2. Harris WH, Schiller AL, Scholler JM, Freiberg RA, Scott R. Extensive localized bone resorption in the femur following total hip replacement. *J Bone Joint Surg Am*, 1976, 58, 612–8.
3. Marshall A, Ries MD, Paprosky W. How prevalent are implant wear and osteolysis, and how has the scope of osteolysis changed since 2000? *J Am Acad Orthop Surg*, 2008, 16, S1–S6.
4. Hallab NJ, Jacobs JJ. Biologic effects of implant debris. *Bull NYU Hosp Joint Dis*, 2009, 67, 182–8.
5. Jacobs JJ, Shanbhag A, Glant TT, Black J, Galante JO. Wear debris in total joint replacements. *J Am Acad Orthop Surg*, 1994, 2, 212–20.
6. Gallo J, Slouf M, Goodman SB. The relationship of polyethylene wear to particle size, distribution, and number: A possible factor explaining the risk of osteolysis after hip arthroplasty. *J Biomed Mater Res B Appl Biomater*, 2010, 94, 171–7.
7. Mostardi RA, Kovacik MW, Ramsier RD, Bender ET, Finefrock JM, Bear TF, Askew MJ. A comparison of the effects of prosthetic and commercially pure metals on retrieved human fibroblasts: the role of surface elemental composition. *Acta Biomater*, 2010, 6, 702–7.
8. Savarino L, Baldini N, Ciapetti G, Pellacani A, Giunti A. Is wear debris responsible for failure in alumina-on-alumina implants? *Acta Orthop*, 2009, 80, 162–7.
9. Baxter RM, Ianuzzi A, Freeman TA, Kurtz SM, Steinbeck MJ. Distinct immunohistomorphologic changes in periprosthetic hip tissues from historical and highly crosslinked UHMWPE implant retrievals. *J Biomed Mater Res Part A*, 2010, 95A, 68–78.
10. Billi F, Campbell P. Nanotoxicology of metal wear particles in total joint arthroplasty: a review of current concepts. *J Appl Biomater Biomech*, 2010, 8, 1–6.
11. Richards L, Brown C, Stone MH, Fisher J, Ingham E, Tipper JL. Identification of nanometre-sized ultra-high molecular weight polyethylene wear particles in samples retrieved *in vivo*. *J Bone Joint Surg Br*, 2008, 90, 1106–13.
12. Maitra R, Clement CC, Scharf B, Crisi GM, Chitta S, Paget D, Purdue PE,

Cobelli N, Santambrogio L. Endosomal damage and TLR2 mediated inflammasome activation by alkane particles in the generation of aseptic osteolysis. *Mol Immunol*, 2009, 47, 175–84.
13. Willert HG, Semlitsch M. Reactions of the articular capsule to wear products of artificial joint prostheses. *J Biomed Mater Res*, 1977, 11, 157–64.
14. Nygaard M, Bastholm L, Elling F, Soballe K, Borgwardt A. Can ultrastructural particle location predict aseptic loosening? A biopsy study of nonloose hip implants one year postoperative using three bearing material combinations. *J Long Term Eff Med Implants*, 2007, 17, 321–34.
15. Jasty M, Bragdon C, Jiranek W, Chandler H, Maloney W, Harris WH. Etiology of osteolysis around porous-coated cementless total hip arthroplasties. *Clin Orthop Relat Res*, 1994, 308, 111–26.
16. Gallo J, Raška M, Mràzek F, Petřek M. Bone remodeling, particle disease and individual susceptibility to periprosthetic osteolysis. *Physiol Res*, 2009, 57, 339–49.
17. Gallo J, Mràzek F, Petřek M. Variation in cytokine genes can contribute to severity of acetabular osteolysis and risk for revision in patients with ABG 1 total hip arthroplasty: a genetic association study. *BMC Med Genet* 2009, 10, 109, DOI 10.1186/1471-2350-10-109.
18. Huang Z, Ma T, Ren PG, Smith RL, Goodman SB. Effects of orthopedic polymer particles on chemotaxis of macrophages and mesenchymal stem cells. *J Biomed Mater Res A*, 2010, 94, 1264–9.
19. Gordon A, Greenfield EM, Eastell R, Kiss-Toth E, Wilkinson JM. Individual susceptibility to periprosthetic osteolysis is associated with altered patterns of innate immune gene expression in response to pro-inflammatory stimuli. *J Orthop Res*, 2010, 28, 1127–35.
20. Campbell P, Ebramzadeh E, Nelson S, Takamura K, De Smet K, Amstutz HC. Histological features of pseudotumor-like tissues from metal-on-metal hips. *Clin Orthop Relat Res*, 2010, 468, 2321–7.
21. Gonzalez O, Smith RL, Goodman SB. Effect of size, concentration, surface area, and volume of polymethylmethacrylate particles on human macrophages in vitro. *J Biomed Mater Res*, 1996, 30, 463–73.
22. Sabokbar A, Pandey R, Athanasou NA. The effect of particle size and electrical charge on macrophage-osteoclast differentiation and bone resorption. *J Mater Sci Mater Med*, 2003, 14, 731–8.
23. Greenfield EM, Bi Y, Ragab AA, Goldberg VM, Nalepka JL, Seabold JM. Does endotoxin contribute to aseptic loosening of orthopedic implants? *J Biomed Mater Res B Appl Biomater*, 2005, 72, 179–85.
24. Sun DH, Trindade MC, Nakashima Y, Maloney WJ, Goodman SB, Schurman DJ, Smith RL. Human serum opsonization of orthopedic biomaterial particles: protein-binding and monocyte/macrophage activation in vitro. *J Biomed Mater Res A*, 2003, 65, 290–8.
25. De Jong PT, Tigchelaar W, Van Noorden CJ, Van der Vis HM. Polyethylene wear particles do not induce inflammation or gelatinase (MMP2 and MMP9) activity in fibrous tissue interfaces of loosening total hip arthroplasties. *Acta Histochem*, 2011, 113, 556–63.
26. Beidelschies MA, Huang H, McMullen MR, Smith MV, Islam AS, Goldberg VM, Chen X, Nagy LE, Greenfield EM. Stimulation of macrophage TNFα

production by orthopaedic wear particles requires activation of the ERK1/2/ Egr-1 and NF-κB pathways but is independent of p38 and JNK. *Cell Physiol*, 2008, 217, 652–66.
27. Zolotarevová E, Hudeček J, Spundová M, Entlicher G. Binding of proteins to ultra high molecular weight polyethylene wear particles as a possible mechanism of macrophage and lymphocyte activation. *J Biomed Mater Res A*, 2010, 95, 950–5.
28. Savarino L, Granchi D, Cenni E, Baldini N, Greco M, Giunti A. Systemic cross-linked N-terminal telopeptide and procollagen I C-terminal extension peptide as markers of bone turnover after total hip arthroplasty. *J Bone Joint Surg Br*, 2005, 87, 571–6.
29. Shanbhag AS, Jacobs JJ, Black J, Galante JO, Glant TT. Human monocyte response to particulate biomaterials generated *in vivo* and *in vitro*. *J Orthop Res*, 1995, 13, 792–801.
30. Daniels AU, Barnes FH, Charlebois SJ, Smith RA. Macrophage cytokine response to particles and lipopolysaccharide *in vitro*. *J Biomed Mater Res*, 2000, 49, 469–78.
31. Haynes DR, Boyle SJ, Rogers SD, Howie DW, Vernon-Roberts B. Variation in cytokines induced by particles from different prosthetic materials. *Clin Orthop Relat Res*, 1998, 352, 223–30.
32. Goodman SB, Ma T. Cellular chemotaxis induced by wear particles from joint replacements. *Biomaterials*, 2010, 31, 5045–50.
33. Ren PG, Irani A, Huang Z, Ma T, Biswal S, Goodman SB. Continuous infusion of UHMWPE particles induces increased bone macrophages and osteolysis. *Clin Orthop Rel Res*, 2011, 469, 113–22.
34. Yang SY, Zhang K, Bai L, Song Z, Yu H, McQueen DA, Wooley PH. Polymethylmethacrylate and titanium alloy particles activate peripheral monocytes during periprosthetic inflammation and osteolysis. *J Orthop Res*, 2011, 29, 781–6.
35. Shanbhag AS, Kaufmann AM, Hayata K, Rubash HE. Assessing osteolysis with use of high-throughput protein chips. *J Bone Joint Surg Am*, 2007, 89, 1081–9.
36. Hernigou P, Intrator L, Bahrami T, Bensussan A, Farcet JP. Interleukin-6 in the blood of patients with total hip arthroplasty without loosening. *Clin Orthop Relat Res*, 1999, 366, 147–54.
37. Fiorito S, Magrini L, Goalard C. Pro-inflammatory and antiinflammatory circulating cytokines and periprosthetic osteolysis. *J Bone Joint Surg Br*, 2003, 85, 1202–6.
38. Purdue PE, Koulouvaris P, Potter HG, Nestor BJ, Sculco T. The cellular and molecular biology of periprosthetic osteolysis. *Clin Orthop Rel Res*, 2007, 454, 251–61.
39. Haynes DR, Crotti TN, Potter AE, Loric M, Atkins GJ, Howie DW, Findlay DM. The osteoclastogenic molecules RANKL and RANK are associated with periprosthetic osteolysis. *J Bone Joint Surg Br*, 2001, 83, 902–11.
40. Grimaud E, Soubigou L, Couillaud S, Coipeau P, Moreau A, Passuti N, Gouin F, Redini F, Heymann D. Receptor activator of nuclear factor kappaB ligand (RANKL)/osteoprotegerin (OPG) ratio is increased in severe osteolysis. *Am J Pathol*, 2003, 163, 2021–31.

41. Granchi D, Amato I, Battistelli L, Ciapetti G, Pagani S, Avnet S, Baldini N, Giunti A. Molecular basis of osteoclastogenesis induced by osteoblasts exposed to wear particles. *Biomaterials*, 2005, 26, 2371–9.
42. Granchi D, Pellacani A, Spina M, Cenni E, Savarino L, Baldini N, Giunti A. Serum levels of osteoprotegerin and receptor activator of nuclear factorkappa B ligand as markers of periprosthetic osteolysis. *J Bone Joint Surg Am*, 2006, 88, 1501–9.
43. Schwarz EM, Lu AP, Goater JJ, Benz EB, Kollias G, Rosier RN, Puzas JE, O'Keefe RJ. Tumor necrosis factor-alpha/nuclear transcription factor-kappaB signaling in periprosthetic osteolysis. *J Orthop Res*, 2000, 18, 472–80.
44. Greenfield EM, Bi Y, Ragab AA, Goldberg VM, VanDeMotter RR. The role of osteoclast differentiation in aseptic loosening. *J Orthop Res*, 2002, 20, 1–8.
45. Caicedo MS, Desai R, McAllister K, Reddy A, Jacobs JJ, Hallab NJ. Soluble and particulate Co–Cr–Mo alloy implant metals activate the inflammasome danger signaling pathway in human macrophages: a novel mechanism for implant debris reactivity. *J Orthop Res*, 2009, 27, 847–54.
46. Hao HN, Zheng B, Nasser S, Ren W, Latteier M, Wooley Pl, Morawa L. The roles of monocytic heat shock protein 60 and Toll-like receptors in the regional inflammation response to wear debris particles. *J Biomed Mater Res*, 2010, 92A, 1373–81.
47. Pajarinen J, Cenni E, Savarino L, Gomez-Barrena E, Tamaki Y, Takagi M, Salo J, Konttinen YT. Profile of toll-like receptor-positive cells in septic and aseptic loosening of total hip arthroplasty implants. *J Biomed Mater Res A*, 2010, 94, 84–92.
48. Hallab NJ, Anderson S, Stafford T, Glant T, Jacobs JJ. Lymphocyte responses in patients with total hip arthroplasty. *J Orthop Res*, 2005, 23, 384–91.
49. Goodman SB, Goldberg V, O'Keefe R. Biology summary. *J Am Acad Orthop Surg*, 2008, 16(suppl.1), S76–S78.
50. Nich C, Hamadouche M. Cup loosening after cemented Metasul® total hip replacement: a retrieval analysis. *Int Orthop*, 2011, 35, 965–70.
51. Ng VY, Lombardi AV Jr, Berend KR, Skeels MD, Adams JB. Perivascular lymphocytic infiltration is not limited to metal-on-metal bearings. *Clin Orthop Relat Res*, 2011, 469, 523–9.
52. Revell PA. The combined role of wear particles, macrophages and lymphocytes in the loosening of total joint prostheses. *J R Soc Interface*, 2008, 5, 1263–78.
53. Basko-Plluska JL, Thyssen JP, Schalock PC. Cutaneous and systemic hypersensitivity reactions to metallic implants. *Dermatitis*, 2011, 22, 65–79.
54. Ogunwale B, Schmidt-Ott A, Meek RM, Brewer JM. Investigating the immunologic effects of CoCr nanoparticles. *Clin Orthop Relat Res*, 2009, 467, 3010–16.
55. Taki N, Tatro JM, Nalepka JL, Togawa D, Goldberg VM, Rimnac CM, Greenfield EM. Polyethylene and titanium particles induce osteolysis by similar, lymphocyte-independent, mechanisms. *J Orthop Res*, 2005, 23, 376–83.
56. Savarino L, Tigani D, Greco M, Baldini N, Giunti A. The potential role of metal ion release as a marker of loosening in patients with total knee replacement: a cohort study. *J Bone Joint Surg Br*, 2010, 92, 634–8.
57. Hallab NJ, Anderson S, Caicedo M, Skipor A, Campbell P, Jacobs JJ. Immune

responses correlate with serum-metal in metal-on-metal hip arthroplasty. *J Arthroplasty*, 2004, 19, 88–93.
58. Granchi D, Cenni E, Trisolino G, Giunti A, Baldini N. Sensitivity to implant materials in patients undergoing total hip replacement. *J Biomed Mater Res B Appl Biomater*, 2006, 77, 257–64.
59. Granchi D, Cenni E, Tigani D, Trisolino G, Baldini N, Giunti A. Sensitivity to implant materials in patients with total knee arthroplasties. *Biomaterials*, 2008, 29, 1494–500.
60. Caicedo MS, Pennekamp PH, McAllister K, Jacobs JJ, Hallab NJ. Soluble ions more than particulate cobalt-alloy implant debris induce monocyte costimulatory molecule expression and release of proinflammatory cytokines critical to metal-induced lymphocyte reactivity. *J Biomed Mater Res A*, 2010, 93, 1312–21.
61. Hallab NJ, Caicedo M, Finnegan A, Jacobs JJ. Th1 type lymphocyte reactivity to metals in patients with total hip arthroplasty. *J Orthop Surg Res*, 2008, 3, 6, DOI 10.1186/1749-799X-3-6.
62. Roato I, Caldo D, D'Amico L, D'Amelio P, Godio L, Patanè S, Astore F, Grappiolo G, Boggio M, Scagnelli R, Molfetta L, Ferracini R. Osteoclastogenesis in peripheral blood mononuclear cell cultures of periprosthetic osteolysis patients and the phenotype of T cells localized in periprosthetic tissues. *Biomaterials*, 2010, 31, 7519–25.
63. Huss RS, Huddleston JI, Goodman SB, Butcher EC, Zabel BA. Synovial tissue–infiltrating natural killer cells in osteoarthritis and periprosthetic inflammation. *Arthritis Rheum*, 2010, 62, 3799–805.
64. Kwon YM, Ostlere SJ, McLardy-Smith P, Athanasou NA, Gill HS, Murray DW. "Asymptomatic" pseudotumors after metal-on-metal hip resurfacing arthroplasty prevalence and metal ion study. *J Arthroplasty*, 2011, 26, 511–8.
65. Kwon YM, Thomas P, Summer B, Pandit H, Taylor A, Beard D, Murray DW, Gill HS. Lymphocyte proliferation responses in patients with pseudotumors following metal-on-metal hip resurfacing arthroplasty. *J Orthop Res*, 2010, 28, 444–50.
66. Delaunay C, Petit I, Learmonth ID, Oger P, Vendittoli PA. Metal-on-metal bearings total hip arthroplasty: The cobalt and chromium ions release concern. *Orthop Traumatol Surg Res*, 2010, 96, 894–904.
67. Hosman AH, van der Mei HC, Bulstra SK, Busscher HJ, Neut D. Effects of metal-on-metal wear on the host immune system and infection in hip arthroplasty. *Acta Orthop*, 2010, 81, 526–34.
68. Greenfield EM, Beidelschies MA, Tatro JM, Goldberg VM, Hise AG. Bacterial pathogen-associated molecular patterns stimulate biological activity of orthopaedic wear particles by activating cognate toll-like receptors. *J Biol Chem*, 2010, 285, 32378–84.
69. Lhdeeoja T, Pajarinen J, Kouri VP, Sillat T, Salo J, Konttinen YT. Toll-like receptors and aseptic loosening of hip endoprosthesis – a potential to respond against danger signals? *J Orthop Res*, 2010, 28, 184–90.
70. Koreny T, Tunyogi-Csapó M, Gál I, Vermes C, Jacobs JJ, Glant TT. The role of fibroblasts and fibroblast-derived factors in periprosthetic osteolysis. *Arthritis Rheum*, 2006, 54, 3221–32.

71. Filvaroff E, Derynck R. Bone remodelling: a signalling system for osteoclast regulation. *Curr Biol*, 1998, 8, R679–82.
72. Boyce BF, Xing L. Review-functions of RANKL/RANK/OPG in bone modeling and remodeling. *Archiv Biochem Biophys*, 2008, 473, 139–46.
73. Xu J, Wu HF, Ang ESM, Yip K, Woloszyn M, Zheng MH, Tan RX. Survey. NF-kB modulators in osteolytic bone diseases. *Cytokine & Growth Factor Reviews*, 2009, 20, 7–17.
74. Granchi D, Pellacani A, Spina M, Cenni E, Savarino L, Baldini N, Giunti A. Serum levels of osteoprotegerin and receptor activator of nuclear factor-{kappa}B ligand as markers of periprosthetic osteolysis. *J Bone Joint Surg Am*, 2006, 88, 1501–9.
75. Atkins GJ, Welldon KJ, Holding CA, Haynes DR, Howie DW, Findlay DM. The induction of a catabolic phenotype in human primary osteoblasts and osteocytes by polyethylene particles. *Biomaterials*, 2009, 30, 3672–81.
76. Kanaji A, Caicedo MS, Virdi AS, Sumner DR, Hallab NJ, Sena K. Co–Cr–Mo alloy particles induce tumor necrosis factor alpha production in MLO-Y4 osteocytes: a role for osteocytes in particle-induced inflammation. *Bone*, 2009, 45, 528–33.
77. Sabokbar A, Kudo O, Athanasou NA. Two distinct cellular mechanisms of osteoclast formation and bone resorption in periprosthetic osteolysis. *J Orthop Res*, 2003, 21, 73–80.
78. Wang ML, Sharkey PF, Tuan RS. Particle bioreactivity and wear-mediated osteolysis. *J Arthropl*, 2004, 19, 1028–38.
79. Wimmer MA, Fischer A, Büscher R, Pourzal R, Sprecher C, Hauert R, Jacobs JJ. Wear mechanisms in metal-on-metal bearings: the importance of tribochemical reaction layers. *J Orthop Res*, 2010, 28, 436–43.
80. Gómez-Barrena E, Medel F, Puértolas JA. Polyethylene oxidation in total hip arthroplasty: evolution and new advances. *Open Orthop J*, 2009, 3, 115–20
81. Lombardi AV Jr, Berend KR, Mallory TH, Skeels MD, Adams JB. Survivorship of 2000 tapered titanium porous plasma-sprayed femoral components. *Clin Orthop Relat Res*, 2009, 467, 146–54.
82. Manley MT, Sutton K. Bearings of the future for total hip arthroplasty. *J Arthropl*, 2008, 23, 47–50.
83. Suzuki K, Takeyama S, Sakai Y, Yamada S, Shinoda H. Current topics in pharmacological research on bone metabolism: inhibitory effects of bisphosphonates on the differentiation and activity of osteoclasts. *J Pharmacol Sci*, 2006, 100, 189–94.
84. Zhang Q, Badell IR, Schwarz EM, Boulukos KE, Yao Z, Boyce BF, Xing L. Tumor necrosis factor prevents alendronate-induced osteoclast apoptosis *in vivo* by stimulating Bcl-xL expression through Ets-2. *Arthritis Rheum*, 2005, 52, 2708–18.
85. Sutherland KA, Rogers HL, Tosh D, Rogers MJ. RANKL increases the level of Mcl-1 in osteoclasts and reduces bisphosphonate-induced osteoclast apoptosis *in vitro*. *Arthritis Res Ther*, 2009, 11, R58.
86. Shetty N, Hamer AJ, Stockley I, Eastell R, Willkinson JM. Clinical and radiological outcome of total hip replacement five years after pamidrate therapy. A trial extension. *J Bone Joint Surg Br*, 2006, 88, 1309–15.
87. Thillemann TM, Pedersen AB, Mehnert F, Johnsen SP, Soballe K.

Postoperative use of bisphosphonates and risk of revision after primary total hip arthroplasty: A nationwide population-based study. *Bone*, 2010, 46, 946–51.
88. Schwarz EM, Looney RJ, O'Keefe RJ. Anti-TNF-alpha therapy as a clinical intervention for periprosthetic osteolysis. *Arthritis Res*, 2000, 2, 165–8.
89. Tuan RS. What are the local and systemic biologic reactions and mediators to wear debris, and what host factors determine or modulate the biologic response to wear particles? *J Am Acad Orthop Surg*, 2008, 16 (suppl.1), S42–S48.
90. Schwarz EM. What potential biologic treatments are available for osteolysis? *J Am Acad Orthop Surg*, 2008, 16(suppl 1), S72–S75.
91. Laing AJ, Dillon JP, Mulhall KJ, Wang JH, McGuinness AJ, Redmond PH. Statins attenuate polymethylmethacrylate-mediated monocyte activation. *Acta Orthop*, 2008, 79, 134–40.
92. Abu-Amer Y, Darwech I, Clohisy JC. Aseptic loosening of total joint replacements: mechanisms underlying osteolysis and potential therapies. *Arthritis Res Ther*, 2007, 9 (Suppl 1), S6.
93. Ulrich-Vinther M, Carmody EE, Goater JJ, Sballe K, O'Keefe RJ, Schwarz EM. Recombinant adeno-associated virus-mediated osteoprotegerin gene therapy inhibits wear debris-induced osteolysis. *J Bone Joint Surg Am*, 2002, 84-A, 1405–12.
94. Tsutsumi R, Hock C, Bechtold CD, Proulx ST, Bukata SV, Ito H, Awad HA, Nakamura T, O'Keefe RJ, Schwarz EM. Differential effects of biologic versus bisphosphonate inhibition of wear debris-induced osteolysis assessed by longitudinal micro-CT. *J Orthop Res*, 2008, 26, 1340–6.
95. Pageau SC. Denosumab. *Mabs*, 2009, 1, 210–5.
96. Romas E. Clinical applications of RANK-ligand inhibition. *Int Med J*, 2009, 39, 110–6.
97. Akiyama T, Choong PF, Dass CR. RANK-Fc inhibits malignancy *via* inhibiting ERK activation and evoking caspase-3-mediated anoikis in human osteosarcoma cells. *Clin Exp Metastasis*, 2010, 27, 207–15.
98. Childs L, Paschalis E, Xing L, Dougall W, Anderson D, Bosky A, Puzas J, Rosier R, O'Keefe R, Boyce B. *In vivo* RANK signaling blockade using the receptor activator of NF-κB:Fc effectively prevents and ameliorates wear debris-induced osteolysis via osteoclast depletion without inhibiting osteogenesis. *J Bone Miner Res*, 2002, 17, 192–9.
99. Zhang C, Tang TT, Ren WP, Zhang XL, Dai KR. Inhibiting wear particles-induced osteolysis with doxycycline. *Acta Pharmacol Sin*, 2007, 28, 1603–10.
100. Ren W, Blasier R, Peng X, Shi T, Wooley PH, Markel D. Effect of oral erythromycin therapy in patients with aseptic loosening of joint prostheses. *Bone*, 2009, 44, 671–7.
101. Ren W, Markel DC. Emerging ideas: can erythromycin reduce the risk of aseptic loosening? *Clin Orthop Relat Res*, 2011, 469, 2399–403.
102. Ulrich-Vinther M. Gene therapy methods in bone and joint disorders. Evaluation of the adeno-associated virus vector in experimental models of articular cartilage disorders, periprosthetic osteolysis and bone healing. *Acta Orthop Suppl*, 2007, 78, 1–64.
103. Zhang L, Jia TH, Chong AC, Bai L, Yu H, Gong W, Wooley PH, Yang SY. Cell-based osteoprotegerin therapy for debris-induced aseptic prosthetic loosening on a murine model. *Gene Ther*, 2010, 17, 1262–9.

104. Kann S, Chiu R, Ma T, Goodman SB. OP-1 (BMP-7) stimulates osteoprogenitor cell differentiation in the presence of polymethylmethacrylate particles. *J Biomed Mater Res A*, 2010, 94, 485–8.
105. Goltzman D. Emerging roles for calcium-regulating hormones beyond osteolysis. *Trends Endocrinol Metab*, 2010, 21, 512–8.

3
Biomechanics of the hip and knee: implant wear

F. E. KENNEDY, Dartmouth College, USA

Abstract: The hip and knee joints are the most heavily loaded movable joints in the human body and they allow relatively complex motions that enable human motion to take place unimpeded. When the natural joints are replaced by artificial joint prostheses, those implants are expected to encounter the same loads and motions that the natural joint had seen. This chapter focuses on the motions, loads and tribological conditions that are encountered by the joint surfaces *in vivo*. The implications of the tribological contact conditions for wear of the contacting implant materials are also discussed.

Key words: hip and knee joints, joint kinematics, joint forces, joint lubrication, contact conditions.

3.1 Introduction

Replacements of hip and knee joints make up the vast majority of total joint arthroplasty in the world today. For example, in the USA in 2004, hip and knee replacement procedures accounted for 95% of all arthroplasty procedures, with shoulder replacements (4%) and all other joint replacement procedures (1%) being much less common (Jacobs, 2008). Success or failure of total hip or knee joint replacement, particularly in the long term, is dependent on how well the contacting surfaces of the implanted prosthesis are able to resist wear in the demanding conditions encountered *in vivo*. The focus of this chapter will be on the tribological conditions that are faced by the implant surfaces.

The chapter will begin with a look at the motions seen by typical hip and knee joints during walking and other everyday activities. Modern hip and knee prostheses aim to give the patients' joints the same degrees of freedom they had naturally, so most of the motions seen in joint prostheses are similar to those found in natural joints. Following the kinematics discussion, there will be a review of the forces seen by human hip and knee joints. The primary force of interest is the resultant contact force between the two contacting components of the joint, but those contact forces depend on ground reaction forces and the forces applied to the joints by muscles and tendons. All of these forces are transient in nature and depend on the activity being performed. There will then be a discussion of the influence of contact forces and motions on the tribological conditions encountered at the contact surfaces of prosthetic hip and knee joints during normal activities. Since the joint surfaces are deformable and are lubricated by synovial fluid, determination of the contact conditions requires an elastohydrodynamic lubrication (EHL) analysis. Results of EHL analyses will be presented for both hip and knee joints, and the consequences of the lubricated contact conditions, including contact pressure and lubricant film thickness, for potential wear of the joint materials will be considered. There will be coverage of the more conventional prosthesis materials, polymer (ultra-high molecular weight polyethylene (UHMWPE)) in contact with metal (cobalt–chromium–molybdenum), as well as for other material combinations, such as metal-on-metal, ceramic-on-polyethylene and ceramic-on-ceramic.

3.2   Kinematics of hip and knee joints

The hip and knee joints are diarthrodial joints that allow relative movement of the connected bones. These movements are usually defined in three mutually perpendicular anatomic planes (Stedman, 2006): the coronal or frontal plane, in which the individual is facing the observer; the sagittal plane, in which the observer is facing the side of the individual; and the transverse or horizontal plane, in which the observer looks down at the individual from directly above. Rotations of the leg in the coronal plane are abduction, in which the leg is raised outward away from the center of the body, and adduction, in which the leg rotates back toward the center of the body. Rotations in the sagittal plane are flexion, which is a folding movement in which for the knee the rear surfaces of the femur and tibia are becoming closer together or for the hip the femur rotates forward, and extension, in which the bones rotate back toward their straightened position. Rotations in the transverse plane are internal rotation, in which the bone rotates about its own longitudinal axis toward the center of the body, and external rotation, in which the bone rotates outward. The hip joint is a ball-in-socket joint that allows all three of these rotations, so it has three degrees of freedom. The knee joint also allows all three rotations but, in addition, the joint allows relative translation in up to three directions between the contacting surfaces of the femur and tibia; therefore the knee joint can have six degrees of freedom. Current hip and knee prostheses are designed to maintain all of the degrees of freedom of the natural joints as much as possible.

Measurements of joint motions during walking and other activities may be made by several methods. Triaxial electrogoniometers have been developed to measure the three rotations at knee and hip joints and they have been used successfully in gait analysis (Chao et al., 1980). Strain gages or accelerometers are used to determine the angle changes. The instruments have been found to give precise angle measurements, both statically and dynamically, but they cannot measure translation. Many studies of hip and/ or knee kinematics have used optoelectronic photogrammetric systems (e.g. Andriacchi et al., 1998; Antonsson and Mann, 1989), in which the motion of markers placed on the skin near the joints is tracked using one or more video cameras. The markers may be either light emitting diodes (LEDs), infrared (IR) emitters or pieces of reflective tape. The imaging system keeps track of the coordinate locations of each marker and computer software processes this information to determine the kinematics of the body segments of interest. With advances in processing software, these optoelectronic systems offer good precision, but errors may be introduced by the relative motion that occurs between the skin on which the markers are placed and the underlying bone (Ramakrishnan and Kadaba, 1991). The errors due to skin movement can be minimized by placing a cluster of points on the thigh and using computer software to analyze the complete six degree of freedom joint kinematics (Andriacchi et al., 1998).

X-ray fluoroscopy has been used to measure three-dimensional kinematics of knee and hip joints, including all six degrees of freedom of knee joints (Banks and Hodge, 1996). The technique involves computer analysis of the images from a single-plane (two-dimensional, sagittal plane) X-ray fluoroscope to develop information about all six degrees of freedom, although translations perpendicular to the sagittal plane are less accurate (Banks and Hodge, 1996). The fluoroscopy method exposes the individual to radiation, particularly during prolonged gait analysis. Other methods have also been used successfully to determine the complete kinematics of hip and knee joints, including dynamic magnetic resonance imaging (Woltring et al., 1990), along with invasive methods such as implanting intra-cortical traction pins in the bones and following them using radiography and high-speed cameras (Lafortune et al., 1992).

Whatever technique is used to gather kinematic data for the human leg, the motions must be determined with respect to a well-defined coordinate system that is physically meaningful to biomechanics researchers and clinicians alike. Most analyses of knee kinematics now use a three-dimensional joint coordinate system, originally proposed by Grood and Suntay (1983), in which unit base vectors are defined relative to commonly employed anatomic reference points. All six degrees of freedom of the knee

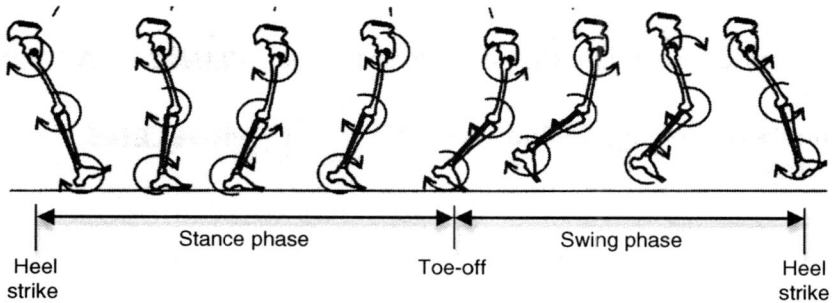

3.1 Typical human walking cycle.

joint, three rotations and three translations, can then be defined precisely relative to the joint coordinates, and those motions can be described in terms familiar to clinicians. Guidance has been given in the selection of the anatomic reference points (Andriacchi *et al.*, 1998; Grood and Suntay, 1983). The International Society of Biomechanics has developed a similar definition of a joint coordinate system for the hip (Wu *et al.*, 2002). That recommendation defines anatomical landmarks that should be used as a standard for the location of the hip joint coordinate system.

Most studies of hip and knee joint kinematics focus primarily on the normal walking cycle or gait. For the vast majority of individuals, normal gait is very reproducible and follows the pattern shown in Fig. 3.1. The gait cycle consists of two phases, the stance and swing phases. The stance phase begins when the heel strikes the ground and continues until the foot leaves the ground at the toe-off point. For a short period during the initial and final segments of the stance phase, i.e. near heel strike and toe-off, both feet are on the ground and both legs bear a portion of the individual's weight. During the remainder of the stance phase, only one foot is on the ground while the contralateral leg is in the swing phase. In the swing phase the foot is off the ground. For most individuals, the stance and swing phases occupy about 60–65% and 35–40% respectively of the normal gait cycle.

When an individual is running, toe-off occurs before 50% of the gait cycle is completed, so there are no periods when both feet are on the ground. It has been found that during moderate running the stance phase may only occupy 35–40% of the gait cycle, and the stance phase becomes shorter as the individual runs faster or sprints (Novacheck, 1998).

3.2.1 Kinematics of the hip joint

The hip joint is subjected to rotation about three axes during normal activities. The three rotations, flexion–extension, abduction–adduction and internal–external rotation, have been measured for a variety of individuals during normal gait as well as during other activities, including running and stair climbing.

Typical hip joint rotation data for a normal walking gait are shown in Fig. 3.2, based on gait data from Ramamurti *et al.* (1996), who used electrogoniometric measurements by Johnston and Smidt (1969). It can be seen that the hip joint extends continuously in the sagittal plane by nearly 40° during the stance phase and flexes back during the swing phase. Abduction–adduction and internal–external rotation angles both cover a span of about 10° during a gait cycle, with the hip abducting and rotating internally during the first half of the stance phase and returning during the last half of stance.

Table 3.1 summarizes the results from several investigators for the span of rotations in each plane during the complete gait cycle, as well as spans for each rotation during only the stance phase during a normal walking cycle. Data are also included for typical ranges of the rotations during the stance phase while running, ascending stairs and descending stairs. It should be noted that these motions might differ between individuals. For example, female runners tend to have greater adduction and internal rotations than

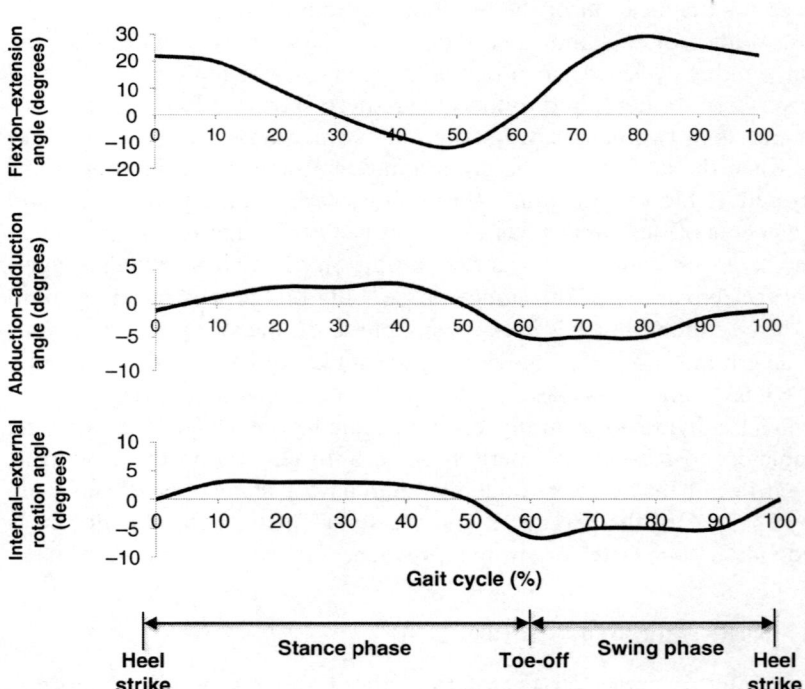

3.2 Typical hip rotations during normal gait. Data from Johnston and Smidt (1969) and Ramamurti *et al.* (1996).

Table 3.1 Typical ranges of flexion–extension angle, internal–external rotation angle and abduction–adduction angle for the hip joint during normal walking, running and stair climbing

	Normal walking		Running stance phase	Stairs stance phase	
	Complete cycle	Stance phase		Up	Down
Flexion–extension	50–55°	35–40°	35–45°	34°	13°
Internal–external rotation	13°	5–10°	7–11°		
Abduction–adduction	12°	6–8°	5–9°		

Note: data from Johnston and Smidt (1969); Andriacchi *et al.* (1980); Novacheck (1998) and Ferber *et al.* (2003).

male runners (Ferber *et al.*, 2003), and an increase in running speed generally leads to increased extension and adduction during the stance phase (Novacheck, 1998).

Since the hip joint is a conformal ball-in-socket configuration, any of the rotations of the femoral head relative to the acetabular socket generate sliding at the contact interface. From Fig. 3.2 and Table 3.1 it can be concluded that substantial relative sliding of the femoral head within the acetabular socket in the hip joint occurs during daily activities, with the flexion–extension motion being particularly important. Because of the combination of rotations in the hip, the center of contact between the femoral head and acetabular cup of a hip joint prosthesis will move around on the acetabular cup surface. This motion was plotted by Ramamurthi *et al.* (1996) using kinematic data from Johnston and Smidt (1969); a typical result is shown in Fig. 3.3. It is seen that two adjacent points on the femoral head trace out similar quasi-rectangular paths on the acetabular surface and, at the point where those paths cross, material on the acetabular cup surface will be subjected to multi-directional shear forces. As will be seen later, this multi-directional motion can affect the wear of the polyethylene used in many acetabular cups.

3.2.2 Kinematics of the knee joint

Many researchers have studied the relatively complex motions of the knee, both during normal gait and in other activities (e.g. Andriacchi *et al.*, 2005; Banks and Hodge, 1996; Chao *et al.*, 1983). Typical flexion–extension, internal–external rotation and anterior–posterior translation data for normal walking are shown in Fig. 3.4, which is based on data from ISO 14243-3 (ISO, 2004). This standard is derived from average patient data and is used for programming the motion of knee simulators for wear testing

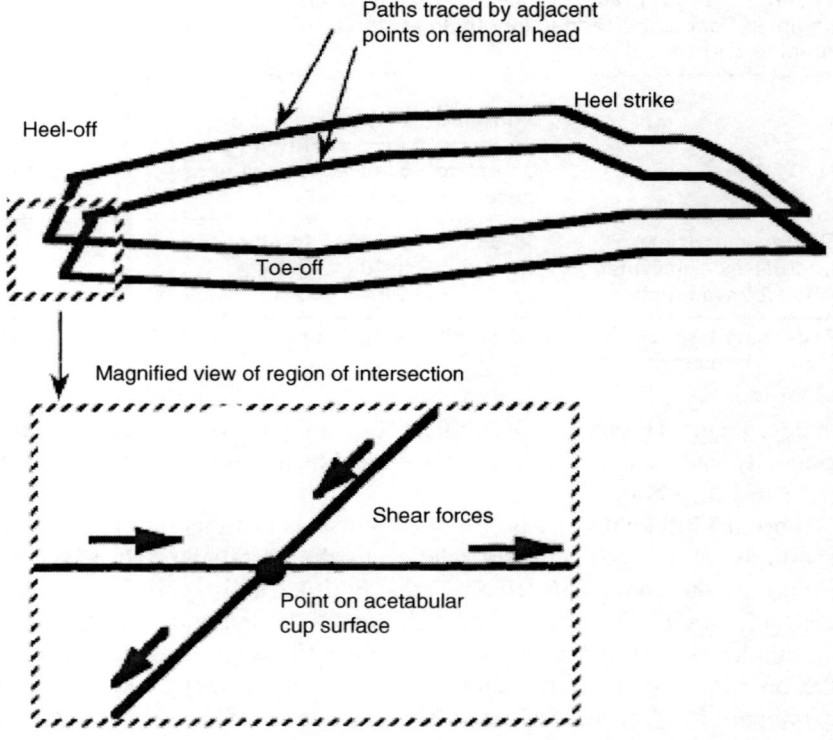

3.3 Paths traced out on acetabular cup by two adjacent points on femoral head during a single normal walking cycle. Path is traced counter-clockwise. Adjacent paths intersect during stance phase, creating multi-directional shear forces on surface of actetabular cup. From Ramamurti *et al.* (1996), with permission.

of knee prostheses. There is some debate about whether the ISO standard accurately mimics the kinematics seen in typical patients with well-functioning total knee replacements (DesJardins *et al.*, 2007), but it is widely used as a test protocol.

For the gait cycle shown in Fig. 3.4, at heel strike the knee joint is nearly fully extended (approximately zero degrees of flexion–extension) and the tibia is rotated slightly relative to the femur. During the first half of the stance phase, the knee flexes up to about 20° while the tibia rotates internally and displaces forward (anteriorly) relative to the femur. During the last half of the stance phase, the knee returns to almost full extension while the tibia rotates externally and displaces posteriorly relative to the femur. During the swing phase, there is a large flexion (of nearly 60°) before it returns to full extension in time for the next strike of the heel. It should be noted that individuals may have different gait cycles from the one shown here, but the total spans of motion are rather consistent. Those spans are shown in Table 3.2. During normal gait, the stance phase is the only part of the cycle in which the leg is in contact with the ground, so it is during that

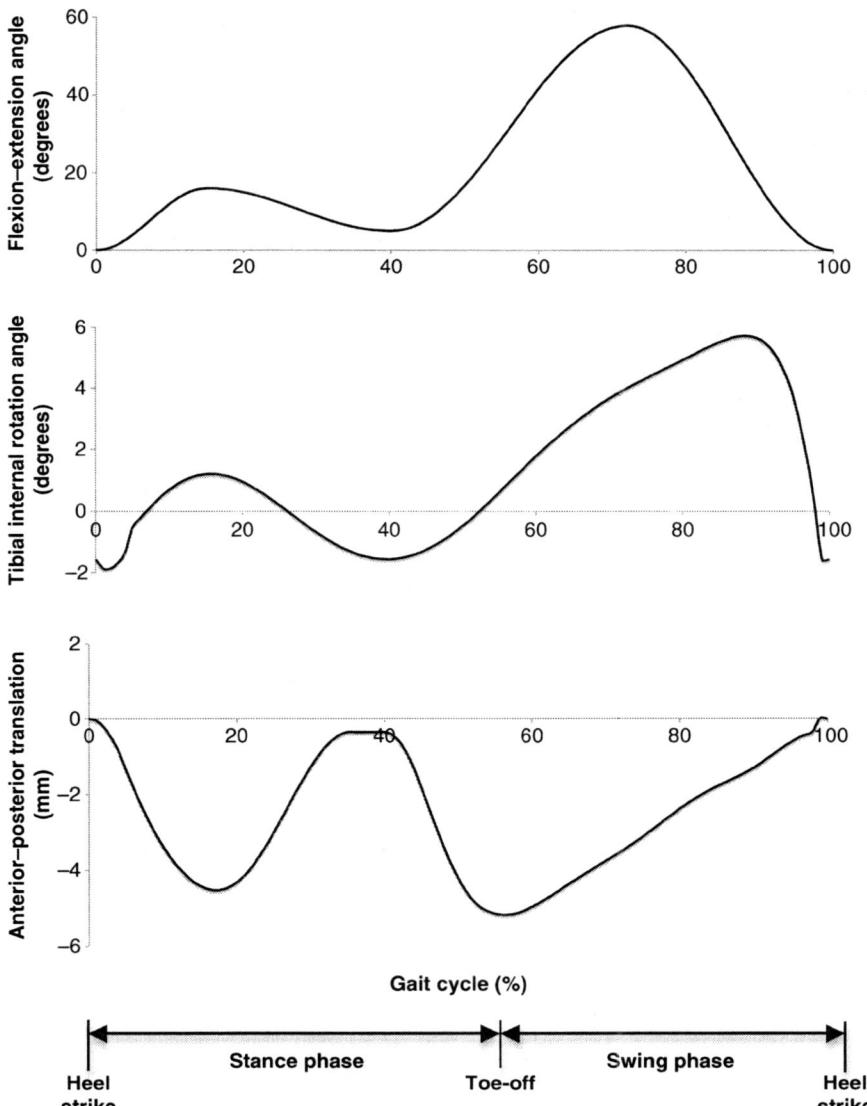

3.4 Typical rotations (flexion–extension and internal–external rotation) and anterior–posterior translation for knee joint during walking cycle. Data from ISO 14243-3 (ISO, 2004).

Table 3.2 Typical spans of flexion–extension angle, internal–external rotation angle, abduction–adduction angle and anterior–posterior (AP) translation distance for the knee joint during normal walking, running and stair climbing activities

	Normal walking		Running (stance phase)	Stair climbing (stance phase)
	Complete cycle	Stance phase		
Flexion–extension	65–70°	15–30°	44–47°	65–70°
Internal–external rotation	9–11°	9–10°	1–3°	8–12°
Abduction–adduction	10–12°	7–8°	4–7°	
AP translation	5.5–7.0 mm	3–5 mm		6–9 mm

Note: data from Chao *et al.* (1983); Ferber *et al.* (2003); Fregly *et al.* (2005); Andriacchi *et al.* (2005); DesJardins *et al.* (2007) and Moro-oka *et al.* (2008).

period that the largest loads and contact stresses occur in the knee joint. Data are also included in Table 3.2 for knee motions for the stance phase of running and stair climbing activities.

Owing to the combination of rotations and translation, the knee joint sees a combination of rolling and sliding motion and, as a result, the location of contact between femoral and tibial components of a knee prosthesis will move during a typical gait cycle. The exact motion will depend on the design of the two components. One example of the motion pattern that can occur is shown in Fig. 3.5 (DesJardins *et al.*, 2007). As can be seen, the contact pathway usually follows a narrow 'figure 8' shape, with there often being a difference between the pathways on the medial and lateral condyles. As will be seen later, load, pressure and lubrication conditions within this moving patch of contact are responsible for wear of the components of prostheses.

3.3 Kinetics and joint forces

The loads acting on hip and knee joints during normal activities have contributions from the ground reaction force during the stance period, when the foot is in contact with the ground, as well as from the muscles that apply forces and moments to the joints. From the point of view of tribology or failure of the implant surfaces, the most important force is the resultant contact force acting at the interface between the contacting components of the prosthesis. Researchers have determined the forces acting on knee and hip joints using both experimental and analytical methods. It is relatively easy to measure the ground reaction force using an instrumented force plate, but *in vivo* contact forces are much more difficult to measure, particularly for the knee joint.

Experimental methods that utilize instrumented implants with telemetric transmission of load, strain or pressure data have been successful in the hip

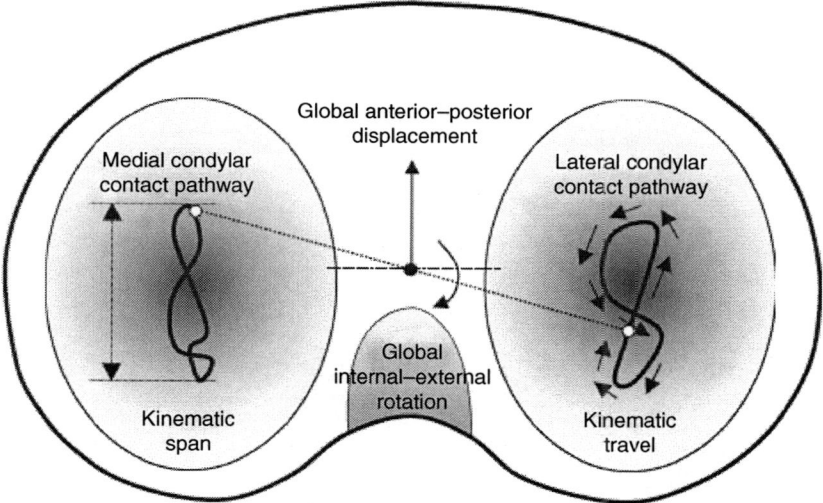

3.5 Typical motions of contact paths on medial and lateral condyles of total knee replacement from kinematic measurements during normal gait cycle. From DesJardins *et al.* (2007), with permission.

joint (e.g. Bergmann *et al.*, 2001; Rydell, 1966). In most of these experimental studies, strain gages are placed on the neck of the femoral component of a total hip replacement and the strain gage output is transmitted wirelessly to a receiver where analysis of the data can provide all three components of force acting on the femoral head, along with the resultant hip joint contact force. Results of some of these studies will be discussed below.

For the knee, though, experimental methods have been less successful; among the few studies that have been somewhat fruitful are one that tested instrumented replacements of the distal portion of the femur, with telemetric transmission of the strain measurements (Taylor and Walker, 2001), and another that used a specially instrumented tibial knee prosthesis (D'Lima *et al.*, 2008). Owing to the problems with experimental measurement of knee forces, most investigators have relied on analytical methods in their studies of knee joint forces. Analytical methods can also be used effectively for determining hip joint forces.

Analytical studies of joint forces require analysis of the freebody diagrams of the lower leg as the leg moves through the gait cycle. This is a difficult task because the human leg contains over 45 muscles and each joint is acted upon by three resultant force components and three resultant moment components. The primary muscles and their insertion points have been characterized by Duda *et al.* (1996) and Viceconti *et al.* (2003) and they are shown in Fig 3.6 (Heller *et al.*, 2001). The system of forces acting on a model

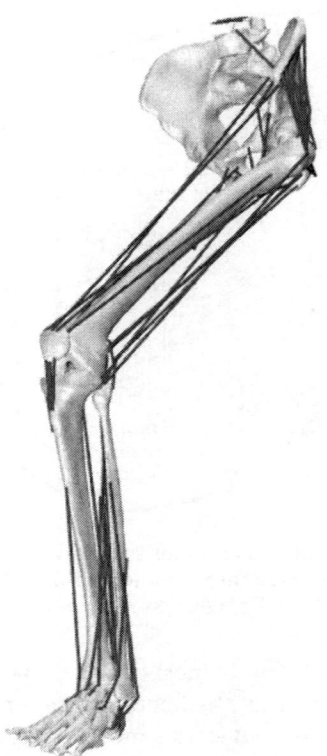

3.6 Model for musculoskeletal analysis of lower limb loads, showing major muscles acting on femur and tibia and their attachments. From Heller *et al.* (2001), with permission.

of the human leg, such as that shown in Fig 3.6, is statically indeterminate, and solutions must be determined for many orientations of the leg during a gait cycle or any other activity. Two main techniques have been implemented to solve this complex system of equations for the unknown joint force components.

1. *Optimization* criteria (e.g. satisfying a condition such as maximizing efficiency) have been used to solve for the unknown forces and moments in the indeterminate system. (Brand *et al.*, 1982; Seireg and Arvikar, 1973).
2. *Reduction* methods, in which muscles are grouped into functional sets, can be used to minimize the number of muscle forces so that the number of unknowns equals the number of available equations of motion. This enables the system of equations to be solved for the unknown joint forces (Komistek *et al.*, 1998; Morrison, 1970; Paul, 1976).

Use of either of these methods in a musculoskeletal analysis to determine forces in knee or hip joints first requires the determination of joint kinematics, as outlined in Section 3.2, followed by solution for the unknown forces at each orientation of the limbs. Successful analytical techniques are reviewed and described by Komistek *et al.* (2005), Prendergast *et al.* (2005) and Andriacchi *et al.* (2005).

3.3.1 Forces acting on hip joints

A number of investigators have studied the contact forces that occur in hip joints during a walking cycle. Perhaps the most complete study was that of Bergmann *et al.* (2001), who used instrumented hip prostheses to measure hip joint forces in a series of individuals during walking and other activities. An example of their results is shown in Fig. 3.7. It can be seen that all three components of the hip joint force, along with the resultant hip contact force, vary considerably during a typical gait cycle. The orientation of the resultant force may also change slightly during the walk cycle as the femur goes through flexion–extension, abduction–adduction and internal–external

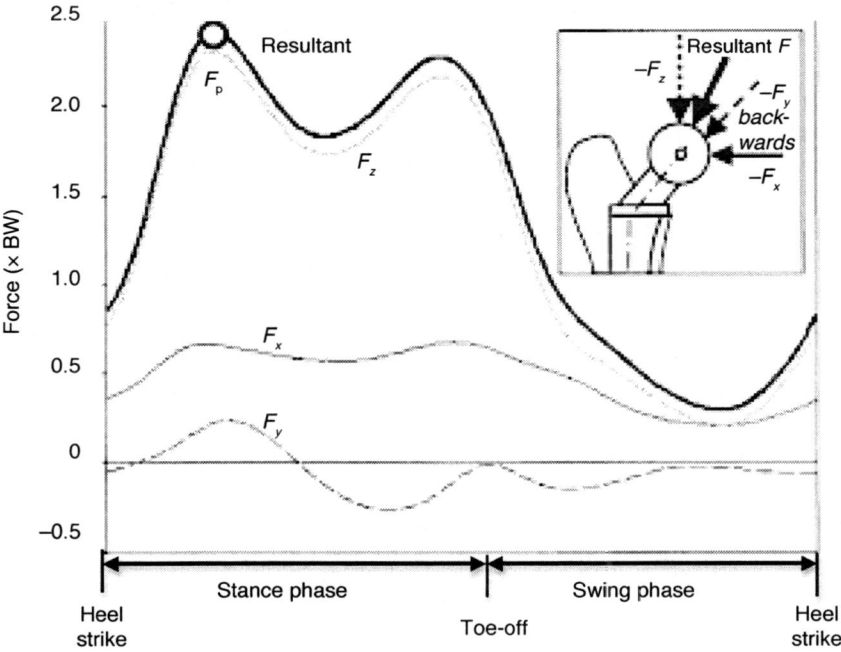

3.7 Hip joint contact force components and resultant, as a multiple of body weight (BW), for average individual during normal walking cycle.

Table 3.3 Peak hip joint forces reported by various authors as a multiple of body weight for a variety of daily activities

Activity	Reference	Maximum hip joint force (multiple of body weight)
Level walking (slow)	Paul (1976)	4.9
Level walking (slow)	Bergmann et al. (2001)	2.4
Level walking (normal)	Bergmann et al. (2001)	2.4
Level walking (normal)	Prendergast et al. (2005)	3.0–3.3
Level walking (fast)	Paul (1976)	7.6
Level walking (fast)	Bergmann et al. (2001)	2.5
Downhill walking	Paul (1976)	5.1
Uphill walking	Paul (1976)	5.9
Descending stairs	Paul (1976)	7.2
Descending stairs	Bergmann et al. (2001)	2.6
Ascending stairs	Paul (1976)	7.1
Ascending stairs	Bergmann et al. (2001)	2.5
Ascending stairs	Prendergast et al. (2005)	2.8–3.3

rotation motions, but the dominant force component is the vertical component (F_z), so the resultant contact force is generally oriented close to vertically down. For the typical patient whose forces are shown in Fig. 3.7, the peak resultant hip joint contact force (F_p) occurs just after heel strike and its magnitude is about 2.5 times body weight (BW).

Table 3.3 summarizes many of the values of peak hip joint force reported by various authors for walking and other common daily activities. The peak forces are given as a multiple of body weight. The data reported by Bergmann et al. (2001) were measured experimentally, while the other data were from musculoskeletal analyses coupled with kinematic measurements. One reason for the variability of the data is the methodology, while other differences may stem from whether or not the individual had been subjected to surgery that may have disturbed muscle function. Despite the variability, it is apparent that the peak hip joint forces are much higher than body weight. Since the contribution from the ground reaction force is approximately equal to body weight during the stance phase, the largest contributors to the peak hip joint contact force are the muscle forces acting on the hip joint. From Table 3.3 it can be seen that the peak hip joint force increases somewhat as the pace of walking quickens, and that stair climbing and downhill/uphill walking can result in high hip joint contact forces.

3.3.2 Forces acting on knee joints

Determination of knee joint forces during walking or other daily activities has generally relied on kinematic measurements in combination with one of the musculoskeletal analysis techniques, either optimization or reduction, mentioned earlier. Many of the studies have also used force plates to determine ground reaction force during an activity. The results of these studies have shown that both ground reaction and the sum of muscle forces acting on the bones surrounding the joint contribute to the resultant knee joint contact force. Usually, the contribution of the ground reaction to the knee contact force during walking amounts to approximately the individual's body weight for most of the stance phase (Chao et al., 1983; Komistek et al., 2005). There is a short period at the beginning and end of the stance phase (during heel strike and toe-off) when the ground reaction force contribution ramps up from zero to about 1.1 times body weight (BW) or down from $1.1 \times BW$ to zero, while at mid-stance the ground reaction force may diminish to about $0.8 \times BW$ (Chao et al., 1983). Studies have shown elevated ground reaction force and consequent increased contribution to knee forces during some other activities. For example, Kuster et al. (1997) measured a peak ground force contribution of about $1.6 \times BW$ during downhill walking and Novacheck (1998) found peak ground reaction forces of about $3 \times BW$ during running.

When the muscle force contributions are considered as well as the ground force contribution, one can obtain the resultant knee joint contact force for a typical gait cycle. An example of this is shown in Fig. 3.8, which is based on data from ISO 14243-3 (ISO, 2004) for an individual weighing 750 N.

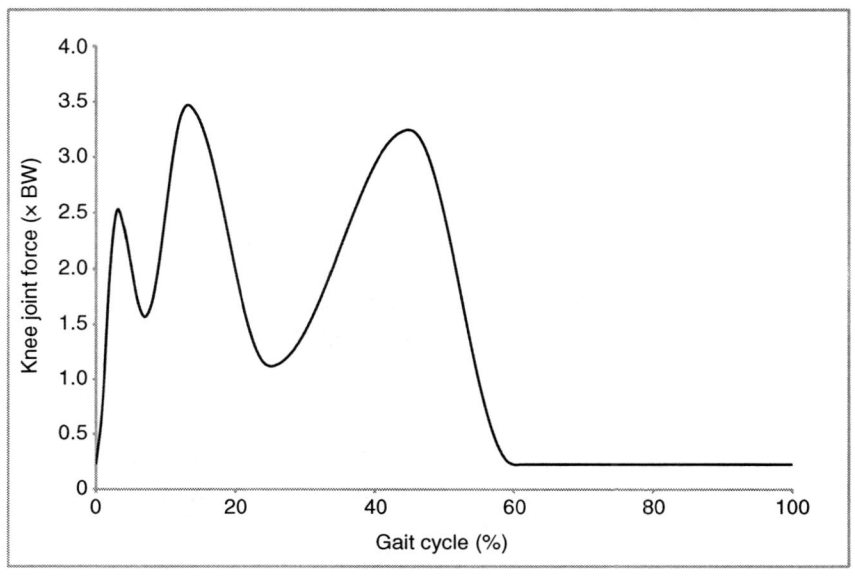

3.8 Typical knee joint contact force, as a multiple of body weight (BW), during a gait cycle. Data from ISO 14243-3 (ISO, 2004) for individual weighing 750 N.

Table 3.4 Peak knee joint forces reported by various authors as a multiple of body weight for a variety of daily activities

Activity	Authors	Maximum knee joint force (multiple of body weight)
Level walking	Morrison (1970)	2.1–4.0
Level walking	Paul (1976)	2.7–4.3
Level walking	Wimmer and Andriacchi (1997)	3.3
Level walking	Kuster et al. (1997)	3.4–3.9
Level walking	Taylor and Walker (2001)	2.6–2.8
Level walking	Komistek et al. (2005)	2.1–3.4
Downhill walking	Paul (1976)	4.4
Downhill walking	Kuster et al. (1997)	7.0–8.0
Uphill walking	Paul (1976)	3.7
Descending stairs	Paul (1976)	4.9
Descending stairs	Taylor and Walker (2001)	2.9–3.1
Ascending stairs	Paul (1976)	4.4
Ascending stairs	Taylor and Walker (2001)	2.4–2.5
Jogging	Taylor and Walker (2001)	3.1–3.6
Jogging	D'Lima et al. (2008)	4.1–4.5

The loads given in ISO 14243-3 are frequently used in programming force-controlled knee joint simulators for wear testing of knee prostheses.

From Fig. 3.8 it can be seen that the knee joint force reaches several peaks during the stance phase. Researchers have found that a primary contributor to the first peak (just after heel strike) is the hamstring muscles, while the second peak (at mid-stance) is influenced primarily by the quadriceps and the third (near toe-off) is principally from the gastrocnemius muscle (Andriacchi et al., 2005). In the curve in Fig. 3.8, the largest of the peaks was the second one, reaching nearly $3.5 \times BW$. It should be noted that variants of the knee joint force curve during a gait cycle have been found by different researchers, with some of them having the highest peak being the one just after heel strike and others having the highest peak near toe-off.

Table 3.4 presents a summary of the peak knee joint forces, as a multiple of body weight, which have been determined by various investigators for normal walking and other activities. It is apparent that there is some disagreement among researchers about the exact magnitude of the peak knee joint contact force; the differences stem partly from the different methods used to determine the force and partly by differences in the physiology of the individuals. For example, the data from Taylor and Walker (2001) were measured experimentally just above the knee using an instrumented distal femoral replacement, whereas most of the other data were determined at the tibial/femoral contact using a musculoskeletal analysis of measured kinematic data. In addition, in some of the studies, the patients had been subjected to surgery, such as total knee replacement, that may have disturbed some of the muscles and ligaments that normally apply forces to the knee joint. Komistek *et al.* (2005) reported that loads on the knee are increased if the kinematics of the patella are modified during surgery and Andriacchi *et al.* (2005) discuss how knee kinematics and forces are modified if the posterior cruciate ligament is removed during knee replacement surgery.

From the data in Table 3.4, it is apparent that activities that are more strenuous cause greater knee joint forces. Paul's studies (1976), for example, found that knee joint force increased from $2.7 \times BW$ for slow walking to $4.3 \times BW$ for rapid walking and Novacheck (1998) describes how muscle forces, and the resultant knee joint force, increase with speed during running. In addition, studies have shown that knee joint forces are higher when descending a slope or stairs than when ascending.

3.4 Lubrication and contact conditions in hip and knee implants

During implantation of an artificial hip or knee joint, the synovial membrane that surrounds the natural joint is disrupted and the synovial fluid that serves to lubricate natural diarthrodial joints is drained. After implantation of the joint prosthesis, the synovial membrane is re-attached and, within a month or so, the membrane is once again producing a type of synovial fluid called periprosthetic synovial fluid, a viscous fluid that lubricates artificial joint replacements (Delecrin *et al.*, 1994). As with other synovial fluids, periprosthetic fluid contains hyaluronic acid in a concentration of protein (mucin) (Dumbleton, 1981). Because of the long-chain protein molecules, the fluid's viscous behavior is non-Newtonian; it is a thixotropic fluid – that is, its viscosity decreases and the fluid thins when subjected to increased shear rate (Schurz and Ribitsch, 1987). In addition to hyaluronic acid, synovial fluids contain other components, including lubricin, albumin and phospholipid bilayers, that play important roles in the lubrication of artificial joints (Fam *et al.*, 2007; Schurz and Ribitsch, 1987). Although periprosthetic synovial fluid lubricant is a non-Newtonian fluid, it may often be approximated with reasonable accuracy as Newtonian for the purposes of artificial joint analysis because its viscosity does not change substantially at the shear rates and pressures encountered in prosthetic joints (Jin *et al.*, 1997). The viscosity of periprosthetic synovial fluid is a strong function of patient age and health, as well as of the velocity of joint motion. A viscosity of between 0.0025 and 0.01 Pa s is usually selected for analysis of artificial joint lubrication (Fam *et al.*, 2007; Yao *et al.*, 2003).

In order to get a good understanding of the contact conditions that exist

Table 3.5 Mechanical properties of orthopaedic prosthesis materials

Material	ASTM designation	Modulus of elasticity (GPa)	Ultimate tensile strength (MPa)	Tensile yield strength (MPa)	Hardness (GPa)
Polymers					
Unirradiated UHMWPE	ASTM F648	0.85	46–58	22	—
Irradiated UHMWPE	—	0.94	43–55	24	—
Highly cross-linked UHMWPE	ASTM F2565	0.74	43–51	19–21	—
Ceramics					
Al_2O_3	ASTM F603	366	500	—	20–30
ZrO_2	—	201	800	—	15
Al_2O_3/ZrO_2 composite	—	350	1390	—	17.2
Metals					
Stainless steel	ASTM F138	190	930	241–820	1.3–1.8
CoCrMo	ASTM F75	210–250	655–1275	207–950	5.5
Ti–6Al–4V	ASTM 136	116	965–1100	897–1034	3
Zr–2.5Nb (oxidized surface)	—	98	—	—	Bulk: 3 Surface: 12.1

Note: data from Long *et al.* (1998), Collier *et al.* (2003); Ratner *et al.* (2004); Currier *et al.* (2007); Kurtz (2009) and Kuntz *et al.* (2009).

in implanted hip and knee joints, it is necessary to analyze the contact pressure between load-bearing components of the implant and the thickness of the film of synovial fluid lubricant that is meant to separate those two surfaces. Such an analysis requires information about the loads acting at the joint, the relative velocities of the contacting surfaces, the geometry of those surfaces, the properties of the contacting solids and the properties of the synovial fluid lubricant. The load variation in hip and knee joints during typical activities was discussed in Section 3.3. The relative sliding velocities can be determined by knowing the displacements during the walking or other activity cycles (Section 3.2) and by knowing the speed at which the activities are performed.

Because both hip and knee implants have relatively high contact pressures, resulting in some deformation of the contacting solids, it is necessary to include deformation in analyzing the pressure and film thickness distributions in the film of synovial fluid that may separate the solid surfaces. This is best done by an EHL analysis in which the prediction of lubricant film thickness and pressure distribution requires simultaneous analysis of the elasticity equations for solid deformation analysis and the Reynolds equation for analyzing the fluid film lubricant behavior

(Hamrock, 1994). In such an analysis, the properties of the contacting solids must be used along with the properties of the synovial fluid lubricant. The properties of typical artificial hip and knee joint materials are given in Table 3.5.

The pressure distribution within an EHL film, and therefore the contact pressure distribution acting on the circular (hip) or elliptical (knee) contact area between the solid knee implant components, is well approximated by a Hertzian contact analysis. The peak contact pressure for an elliptical contact is given by (Greenwood, 1997):

$$p_{max} = \frac{1}{\pi}\left(\frac{6WE^{*2}}{R_e^2}\right)^{1/3} \quad [3.1]$$

where W is the applied force, R_e is the effective radius, which is a function of the radii of curvature of the contacting solids, E^* is the effective elastic modulus given by:

$$\frac{1}{E^*} = \frac{1-v_1^2}{E_1} + \frac{1-v_2^2}{E_2} \quad [3.2]$$

and v_1 and E_i are Poisson's ratio and the modulus of elasticity, respectively, of the two contacting solids. Although the geometry (i.e. radii of curvature) of implants changes when wear occurs, nearly all EHL analyses have relied on original unworn implant dimensions and most have assumed that the contacting surfaces of the implant are smooth.

3.4.1 Hip prostheses

Many artificial hip joints are so-called metal-on-polyethylene (MoP) joints, consisting of a polished metallic femoral head in contact with an acetabular cup or socket made of UHMWPE. Most metallic femoral heads in use today are made of a hardened cobalt–chromium–molybdenum alloy (CoCrMo), although some implant manufacturers offer femoral heads made of a stainless steel alloy (e.g. ASTM F138) or a zirconium alloy with an oxidized surface (OXINIUM™). In recent years, in an attempt to avoid the problems related to wear of the polyethylene acetabular components, three other material combinations have become popular for total hip replacements: metal-on-metal (MoM), ceramic-on-ceramic (CoC) and ceramic-on-metal (CoM).

In MoM designs, both acetabular socket and femoral head are made of a metal such as CoCrMo. For CoC designs, both femoral head and acetabular cup are made of either a monolithic ceramic such as alumina (Al_2O_3) or zirconia (ZrO_2), or possibly a ceramic composite such as an alumina/zirconia composite (e.g. BIOLOX™delta). The femoral head fits on a metallic (CoCrMo or Ti-6Al4V) femoral stem. CoM designs have a monolithic ceramic (Al_2O_3 or ZrO_2) or ceramic composite (e.g. Al_2O_3/ZrO_2) femoral head in contact with an acetabular socket made of a metal such as CoCrMo. These implant materials are discussed in more detail in Chapter 6 of this volume. No matter what the prosthesis material, the hip implant is lubricated *in vivo* by periprosthetic synovial fluid. EHL analysis is the most appropriate way to study the contact and lubrication conditions.

MoP hip implants have been the subject of EHL analysis by a number of investigators in recent years, particularly by Jin and colleagues (Jalali-Vahid and Jin, 2002; Jalali-Vahid *et al.*, 2001; Wang and Jin, 2005). Transient analyses of physiologically relevant hip joint rotations and time-varying loads have shown that the minimum thickness of the synovial fluid lubricant ranges from 0.15 to 0.4 µm, with the predicted cyclic film thickness remaining relatively constant owing to the combined effects of fluid entrainment and squeeze-film (Jalali-Vahid and Jin, 2002). The calculated minimum film thickness is often smaller than the surface roughness of the UHMWPE surface, which is usually in the order of 1 µm (Jin *et al.*, 1997), so the hip joint contact region is likely to be in the mixed lubrication regime during much of the walking cycle. As a result, some solid–solid contact would be anticipated and wear of the polyethylene would result, as will be discussed in Section 3.5.1.

Transient EHL studies of typical MoP hip implants have shown that the average transient minimum film thickness predicted throughout a walking cycle was very close to that determined under quasi-static conditions based on average velocity and load (Jalali-Vahid and Jin, 2002). For this reason, simpler steady-state EHL analysis can be carried out to determine the effect of geometric and operational variables on minimum film thickness. Sensitivity analyses of steady-state conditions (constant velocity and constant load) showed that the lubricant film thickness increases with a decrease in radial clearance or an increase in femoral head radius (Jalali-Vahid *et al.*, 2001), but inclination angle of the acetabular cup has a negligible effect on film thickness or contact pressure (Wang and Jin, 2005). The dominant kinematic influence on the lubricant film was found to be flexion–extension, with only a small contribution from internal–external rotation (Wang and Jin, 2005).

Since about the year 2000, many hard-on-hard hip prostheses, particularly MoM or CoC, have been implanted in an attempt to avoid problems related to wear of UHMWPE acetabular cups. MoM hip joints have been especially popular, but their failure for wear-related reasons has recently become a concern, as will be discussed in later chapters of this volume. For this reason, many researchers have recently carried out EHL analyses of MoM hip implants, and those studies have been reviewed in a comprehensive report by Mattei *et al.* (2011). Some of the transient EHL studies of

MoM hip joints have used kinematic and load data prescribed by ISO 14242-1 (ISO, 2002), while others have simplified the loading conditions by assuming that only the vertical load and flexion–extension rotations were of importance. Perhaps the most complete analysis of a MoM hip to date is that by Gao *et al.* (2009), who determined the transient film thickness for physiological motions and loads such as those shown in Figs 3.2 and 3.7. Their resulting variation of central, average and minimum film thickness during a walking cycle is shown in Fig. 3.9. It can be seen that the thinnest film occurs in the stance phase (between 0 and 0.6 s), with the minimum film thickness becoming as low as 10–15 nm. Even in the swing phase the minimum film thickness is less than 0.05 μm. Since these film thicknesses are of the same order as the surface roughness of the metallic components, it is likely that the fluid film will be insufficiently thick to prevent metal–metal contact and wear during a typical walking cycle. Although the vertical component of hip joint force is by far the largest contributor to the resultant contact force (see Fig. 3.7), it was found necessary to include all three force components in order to correctly predict the film thickness throughout the

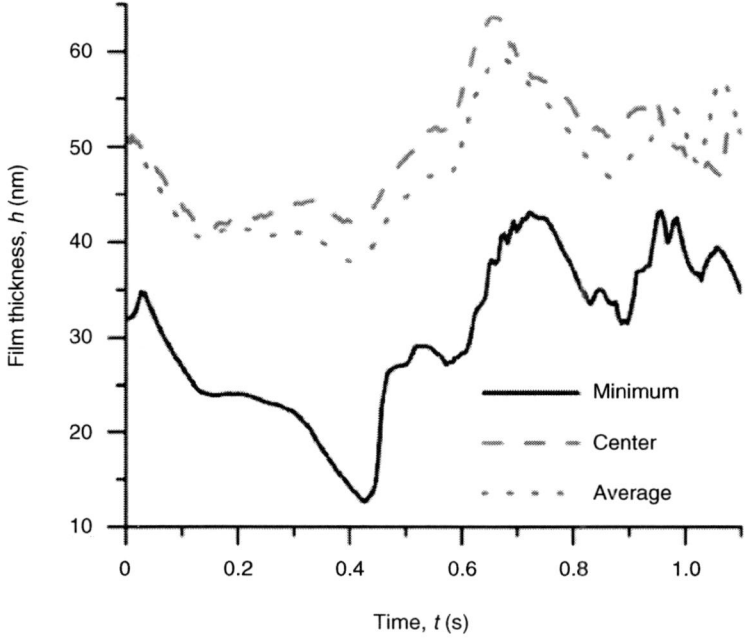

3.9 Minimum, center and average thickness of lubricant film in MoM hip implant during a walking cycle under transient three-dimensional loading and motion. From Gao *et al.* (2009), with permission.

walking cycle (Gao *et al.*, 2009). For example, the lowest point in the minimum film thickness plot in Fig. 3.9 occurs just after the point when the anterior–posterior load component (F_y in Fig. 3.7) changes direction. It might be noted that the film thickness never decreases to zero, even at the lowest point in the cycle, because there is a squeeze-film effect that helps maintain a very thin film of periprosthetic synovial fluid between the surfaces.

Another transient EHL study of MoM hip joints looked at the influence of start-up conditions and gait initiation on lubricant film thickness (Jalali-Vahid *et al.*, 2006). It was found that the variations in film thickness at start-up gradually disappear after two or three gait cycles, so they probably have only a small effect on the life of the implant.

Other studies have used simplifying assumptions or quasi-static analyses to study the effect of various geometric parameters on lubricant effectiveness. Mattei *et al.* (2011) showed that an equivalent ball-on-plane configuration can be used in lubrication modeling of hard-on-hard implants, including MoM, as long as the equivalent radius R_e of the ball-on-plane is equal to that of the hip joint's ball-in-socket. Using a ball-on-plane model, it was found that hip joint designs with a larger equivalent radius, attained by either larger femoral head radius or smaller radial clearance between femoral head and acetabular cup, will produce a thicker lubricant film and a lower contact pressure (Mattei *et al.*, 2011). Wang *et al.* (2009) studied the effect of a non-spherical bearing surface geometry on EHL in hip implants and found that the effect was dependent on the orientation, the magnitude and the deviation direction of the non-sphericity; a well-controlled non-sphericity was seen to be beneficial for improving the lubrication.

Other hard-on-hard hip implants, including CoC, have been studied in the ball-on-plane configuration by Mattei *et al.* (2009). It was found that the CoC bearing had similar lubrication characteristics to the MoM, with both having a much thinner lubricant film than MoP bearings for the same load and velocities. This is primarily because the equivalent modulus of elasticity of the hard-on-hard couples is so much higher than that of MoP, according to Table 3.5 and equation 3.2. The film thickness with a CoC couple is generally even smaller than that determined for a MoM, because of the higher modulus of elasticity for the ceramic materials (Table 3.5). However, ceramics can often be polished to a smaller surface roughness than the metals used in hip joints and they generally retain their low roughness longer than metals, so the resulting lubrication condition may more likely remain in the hydrodynamic regime longer for the CoC couple, while the MoM and MoP couples are more likely to spend a lot of time in the mixed lubrication regime (Mattei *et al.*, 2009, 2011). This means that there may be less likelihood of solid–solid contact in CoC hip implants.

3.4.2 Knee prostheses

Most artificial knee joints today are MoP joints, consisting of a polished metallic femoral component, generally made of a hard metal alloy such as CoCrMo or oxidized zirconium, in contact with a tibial bearing made of UHMWPE. The implant is lubricated *in vivo* by periprosthetic synovial fluid. Deformation of low-modulus UHMWPE can have a significant influence on the thickness of the lubricant film, so EHL analysis is necessary to study the contact and lubrication conditions.

EHL analyses of the oscillatory lubricated conjunctions between the polymer bearing and a polished metallic femoral component of total knee prostheses have been carried out by Murakami and Ohtsuki (1987), Jin *et al.* (1998) and Mongkolwongrojn *et al.* (2010). These studies reported transient analyses of the fluid film thickness and film pressure in lubricated conjunctions in knee prostheses for a walking cycle, using kinematic data similar to those discussed in Section 3.2.2 and load data similar to those described in Section 3.3.2. Results of the EHL analyses have been found to

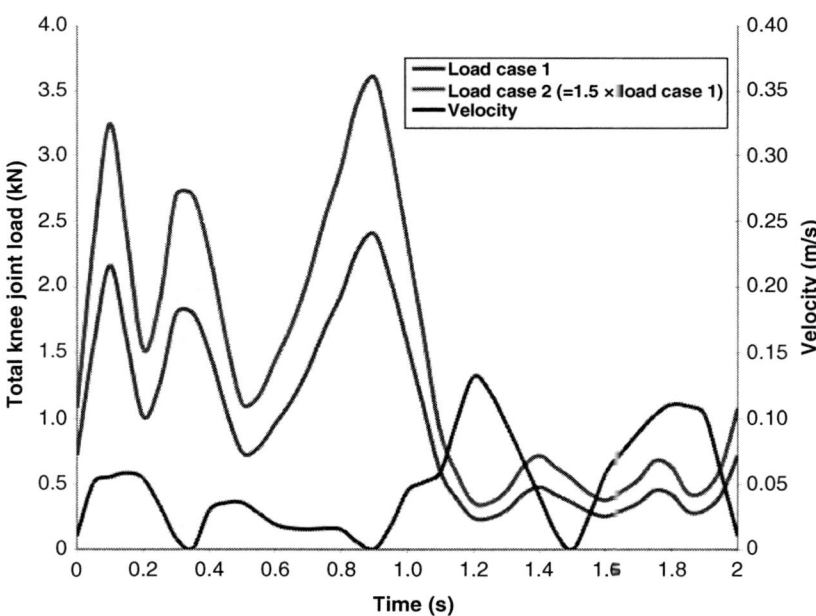

3.10 Loads and velocity used in elastohydrodynamic analysis of MoP knee prosthesis during typical gait cycle. Two load cases were analyzed, one with 50% higher load than the typical load. During the analysis, the total load was divided by two to give the load on each condyle. Data provided by K. Wongseedakaew.

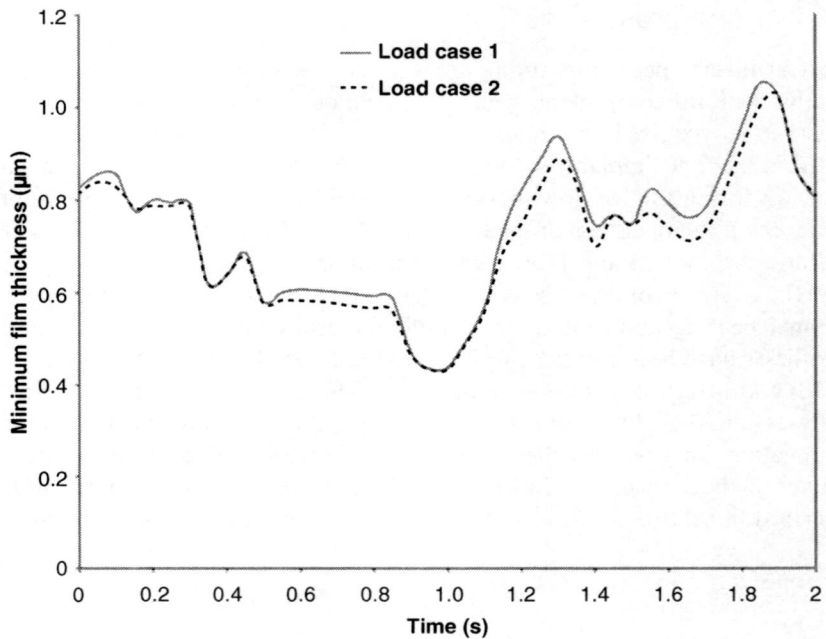

3.11 Transient plots of minimum thickness of synovial lubricant film in MoP knee implant during typical gait cycle. Two loading cases were analyzed, as in Fig. 3.10. Results provided by K. Wongseedakaew.

agree well with fluid film thickness measurements made using an electrical resistance technique in a knee simulator (Jin *et al.*, 1998).

Typical input to an EHL analysis of a knee implant is shown in Fig. 3.10 and results of the analysis are shown in Fig. 3.11. Two different load cases were used (Fig. 3.10). In load case 1, the peak knee joint force was 2.4 kN, or 3.2 × BW for an individual weighing 750 N. It was assumed that the joint force was equally distributed between the medial and lateral condyles. A second load case with a 50% increase in joint force (load case 2) was also carried out to determine contact conditions in more strenuous activities. Load case 2 also serves to analyze the lubrication and contact conditions if one condyle sees a higher load than the other. It has been found that the medial condyle often carries more than half of the joint force (Morrison, 1970), especially at high loads. The solution methodology used in the analysis was that developed by Mongkolwongrojn *et al.* (2010). It should be noted that the knee component dimensions used in the analysis were typical unworn dimensions similar to those given by Bartel *et al.* (1986). As will be seen in Section 3.5.2, those dimensions change after wear occurs.

It is apparent in Fig. 3.11 that the film thickness in the conjunction follows the changes in load and velocity during a walking cycle; the lowest value of film thickness occurs at the point in the walking cycle (at toe-off) when the highest load and lowest velocity occur. It can also be seen that there is a squeeze-film effect at the zero-velocity portion of the motion, which can prevent the film thickness from ever decreasing to zero during a cycle. It is interesting to note that the lubricant film is not much thinner for the higher load case (load case 2) than for the lower load case, especially during the high-load portions of the gait cycle; this is partly due to the squeeze-film effect. Despite the added benefit of a squeeze-film, the lubricant film, especially near the change of motion direction, is quite thin ($<0.5\,\mu m$), so it is unlikely that the lubricant film thickness is sufficient to prevent solid–solid contact; the conjunction probably spends much of its time in the mixed lubrication regime and enters the boundary lubrication regime during the low-velocity/high-load periods.

The maximum contact pressure within the elliptical contact area between the metallic and polyethylene components for load case 1 is 12.5 MPa, acting at the center of the contact area. For load case 2, the maximum pressure was 14.3 MPa. These two values agree very well with calculations using equation 3.1, which says that a 50% increase in joint force will lead to a 14.5% increase in contact pressure.

An alternative material combination in use today is ceramic-on-polyethylene (CoP), in which a femoral component made from alumina, zirconia or alumina/zirconia composite is in contact with a tibial tray made from UHMWPE (Benazzo et al., 2007). An analysis was performed for the same knee implant design analyzed above but using an alumina/zirconia composite femoral component instead of a CoCrMo material. The CoP analysis used the same velocity and load (load case 1) shown in Fig. 3.10, and the same polyethylene tibial component. It was found that the results were almost identical to those for the MoP combination described above: there was less than 1% difference between minimum film thickness for the two material combinations and maximum contact pressure also differed by less than 1%. This is to be expected because the deformation of the polyethylene component is dominant and the effective elastic modulus E^* for MoP and CoP differs by much less than 1%, according to equation 3.2 (using material properties from Table 3.5).

It may be of interest to see what would happen if a CoC knee joint were to be implanted (none have yet been reported). Using equation 3.2, one can see that the effective elastic modulus E^* for a CoC pair would be more than 167 times the E^* value for MoP. Using equation 3.1, one finds that the maximum contact pressure for a CoC pair would be more than 30 times the maximum contact pressure for an otherwise identical CoP knee implant. The resulting contact pressure in the CoC joint would be over 375 MPa for load case 1, and this would almost certainly cause some potential fracture concerns for the ceramic components.

3.5 Implications for implant wear

One of the primary reasons for failure of both hip and knee prostheses is wear of the contacting materials (Bozic et al., 2009; Sharkey et al., 2002). These failures will be discussed in some detail in later chapters of this volume. As was apparent from Section 3.4, although hip and knee implants are lubricated by synovial fluid, the lubricant film is often insufficiently thick to separate the solid surfaces completely, so solid–solid contact occurs during a substantial portion of the implant's life *in vivo*. This will result in gradual wear of one or both of the contacting surfaces; such wear can result in failure of the device, as will be discussed in later chapters of this book.

3.5.1 Hip prostheses

Metal-on-polyethylene hip prostheses often fail because of wear of the polyethylene acetabular liner, which results in the production of millions of small wear particles (Ries *et al.*, 2001). These small wear particles can be responsible for osteolysis, which can ultimately result in loosening of the prosthesis, a major cause of hip implant failure (Ulrich *et al.*, 2008). As was seen in Section 3.4.1, the thickness of the periprosthetic synovial fluid lubricant film in a MoP hip prosthesis may be smaller than the average surface roughness of the polyethylene acetabular cup. As a result, solid–solid contact would occur during a good portion of the implant's *in vivo* life and the solid–solid contact would cause gradual wear of the polyethylene.

It was seen in Fig. 3.3 that sliding motion within the contact area between the femoral head and acetabular liner in a hip joint is multi-directional in nature. Studies have shown that wear of the UHMWPE component is significantly affected by multi-directional motion, with wear rates being higher than in unidirectional reciprocating motion (Bragdon *et al.*, 1996; Wang, 2001). For this reason, the wear behavior of potential materials for MoP hip implants is usually evaluated using multi-directional pin-on-disk test devices (Burroughs and Blanchet, 2001; Saikko and Ahlroos, 1999). A more accurate indication of UHMWPE's *in vivo* wear rate for typical hip joint applications can be determined by the use of multi-directional hip simulators that employ load and motion variation of the types discussed in Sections 3.3.1 and 3.2.1 respectively (Affatato *et al.*, 2008). The tests must be done in a lubricated environment, since the *in vivo* tribological performance of the prosthetic bearings is determined by the material's lubricated wear resistance and not by dry sliding behavior. While periprosthetic synovial fluid is the biological joint lubricant, it is not available in sufficient quantities to be used in wear testing or simulation. Studies of a number of possible lubricant alternatives have shown that bovine serum produces wear rates and wear debris that are similar to those that occur *in vivo* (Brown and Clarke, 2006; Saikko and Ahlroos, 1999). As a result, nearly all testing of hip joint materials is carried out in bovine serum.

Numerous investigators around the world have used hip joint simulators to get an *in vitro* measure of the amount of wear that might occur *in vivo* with a given hip implant design or with a given combination of hip implant materials (Affatato *et al.*, 2008). However, such tests are often complex and expensive. As a complement to wear testing, or as an alternative, it is often useful to model the wear process so the amount of wear may be predicted analytically and the effect of different materials or operating variables can be determined. The methodologies that have been used in modeling wear of hip prostheses have been discussed in the review paper by Mattei *et al.* (2011), along with some of the wear predictions that have been developed by various wear models. A typical contact-coupled wear model methodology for MoP hip implants is described by Kang *et al.* (2006). In that model, as in many other contact-coupled wear models in use today, the joint motions and the transient load on the joint are assumed to follow the patterns described in Sections 3.3.1 and 3.3.2 respectively. The contact pressure is determined at each time interval, usually using a numerical method such as a finite-element method as described by Mattei *et al.* (2011), and the sliding distance in an interval is then calculated (Kang *et al.*, 2006). Then, the wear volume and linear wear depth during the interval are determined at nodal locations around the implant surface. The wear at a point is generally determined using a wear equation originally developed by Archard (1953), which states that the linear wear (or wear depth) at a point is given by

$$U_1 = kps \qquad [3.3]$$

where U_1 is the linear wear depth at the point, k is the wear coefficient for the material combination, p is the contact pressure calculated at the point and s is the sliding distance at the point during the interval.

The wear coefficient k can be found from data gathered in either hip simulator tests or multi-directional pin-on-disk wear tests of the same materials in bovine serum. After the calculation of wear at each nodal point on the surface, the geometry of the worn material (the UHMWPE acetabular cup in MoP hip implants) is updated and the calculation process moves to the next interval in the simulated cycle.

The result of a typical MoP wear simulation for a walking cycle is shown in Fig. 3.12 (from Kang *et al.*, 2006). It can be seen that the maximum contact pressure in the MoP hip implant during a gait cycle generally follows the transient hip joint contact force (Fig. 3.7), but the magnitude of

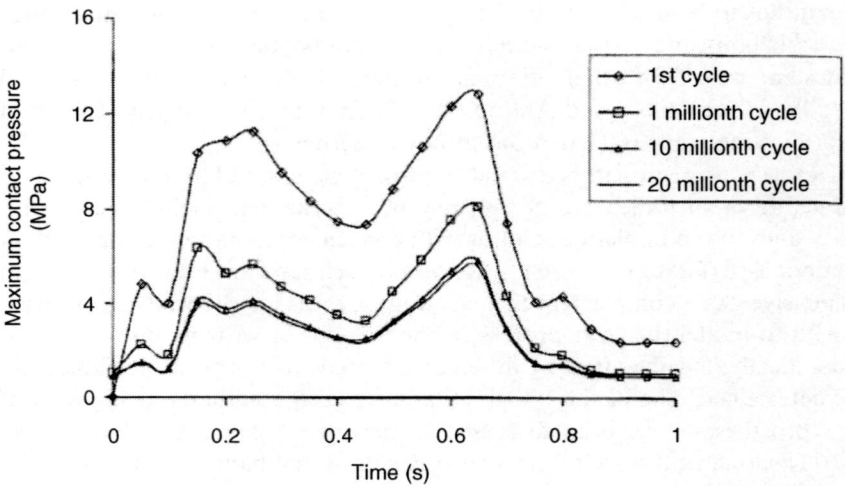

3.12 Predicted variation of maximum contact pressure in MoP hip implant during walking cycles over the 20 million cycle life of the implant. From Kang *et al.* (2006), with permission.

the contact pressure decreases as wear of the polyethylene acetabular cup occurs and the worn surface of the acetabular cup becomes more conformal with the surface of the metallic femoral head. Wear (both linear and volumetric) predicted by the model has been found to be in good agreement with experimental data for UHMWPE acetabular cups, and the relationship between wear and geometric variables such as femoral head diameter and diametral clearance was found to agree well with experimental results (Kang *et al.*, 2006). Therefore, wear modeling can provide useful information for hip implant designers about the effect of various design or material changes on anticipated wear performance.

MoM hip prostheses have been implanted in large numbers in the past decade in an attempt to avoid the wear problems encountered with MoP hip implants. However, the *in vivo* performance of MoM hip implants has been disappointing for many patients (MacDonald and Hanssen, 2004; Mikhael *et al.*, 2009). As was seen in Section 3.4.1, the thickness of the lubricant film in an MoM prosthesis is very small (less than 50 nm) and, since the surface roughness of the metallic components is generally of the order of 15–70 nm (Mattei *et al.*, 2011), it is expected that mixed lubrication will prevail in the contact and some solid–solid contact will occur. This will inevitably result in small amounts of metallic wear debris being liberated within the contact region. Although the wear rates for MoM hip designs may be much lower than for MoP, it has been found that even small amounts of wear in metallic sliding components of MoM hip implants cause the release of metal ions, particularly Co and Cr, at levels that can result in implant failure (Dumbleton and Manley, 2005; Mikhael et al., 2009).

In an attempt to gather more information about the wear of MoM hip implants, many retrieved MoM implants that failed in service have been analyzed (e.g. Sieber et al., 1999) and numerous in vitro experimental tests, generally using hip simulators, have been run (e.g. Fisher et al., 2006). As is the case with MoP hip simulations, the hip simulators usually use bovine serum as the lubricant and use load and kinematic cycles such as ISO standard 14242-1 to simulate a typical walking cycle (Affatato et al., 2008). Results of the simulations have shown that the wear rates of MoM prostheses are generally quite low, and much lower than for MoP hip implants (Fisher et al., 2006). However, wear rate information by itself does not give an indication of how well the implant materials will perform in the body. In particular, the biological reaction of an individual patient to metallic wear debris cannot be determined by any in vitro wear test.

Wear models have been developed for MoM hip implants and they can be useful in predicting the amount of wear (volumetric or linear) that will occur in typical walking cycles (Mattei et al., 2011). For example, a model developed by Harun et al. (2009), which used procedures very similar to those described above for MoP hip implants, was successful in predicting wear volumes similar to those found in hip simulator wear tests. Contact pressures in the MoM hip implant were found to decrease substantially over 50 million simulated walk cycles (Harun et al., 2009). Such numerical wear models can be useful in predicting the effect of various design changes on wear and contact pressure changes.

CoC hip prostheses have been found to have even lower wear rates in hip simulation tests than MoM implants, and much lower than MoP designs (Williams et al., 2007). This is partly because of the high hardness of the ceramic materials (Table 3.5) and partly because those materials can be polished to a very low surface roughness, enabling them to maintain a hydrodynamic lubricant film better than rougher MoM or MoP bearings. This prevents solid–solid contact from occurring as frequently in CoC designs. This is despite the fact that the minimum film thickness may be smaller and the maximum contact pressures may be higher in the ceramic designs than for MoM hip implants. Long-term resistance of ceramic hip components to fracture has yet to be determined, but it may be a concern if the hip encounters excessive impact loads.

An additional clinical complication that has been receiving increased attention and documentation over the past few years is the phenomenon of friction-induced squeaking in CoC hips. The squeaking can be persistent and audible, representing an unacceptable outcome for some patients. Recent studies have shown that the squeaking is a result of friction-induced vibration that is driven by the rotation of the hip during walking and is related to the small diametral clearance between femoral head and acetabular cup (Currier *et al.*, 2010).

3.5.2 Knee prostheses

A primary cause of failure of MoP knee implants is wear of the polyethylene tibial tray (Currier *et al.*, 2005). Much of the wear occurs at the articular surface where the metallic femoral component contacts the UHMWPE tibial tray. As was seen in Section 3.4.2, the lubricant film in the contact is insufficiently thick to prevent solid/solid contact during typical activities such as walking. The liberated wear particles can cause osteolysis, which often results in loosening of the knee prosthesis. The articular surface of the polyethylene tibial bearing is subjected to oscillatory rolling/sliding motion during joint motion at a rate of one to several hertz. Much tribotesting of total knee prostheses is done in knee simulators that attempt to duplicate the kinematics of the knee and the load cycle that is applied to it during walking (e.g. Young *et al.*, 2000). Such knee simulator tests are done with bovine serum as the joint lubricant. Contact in a typical knee joint is relatively concentrated, with a high contact pressure, and the contact location moves on the surface of the tibial bearing during a typical walking cycle, as was shown in Fig. 3.5. It has been found that most of the sliding motion in the locations of highest contact stress in knee prostheses is very close to unidirectional reciprocation, with little cross-motion (Hamilton *et al.*, 2005). To further reduce the contact stress on the articular surface of knee prostheses, mobile bearing knee implant designs have been created that allow the UHMWPE bearing to rotate against the metallic tibial backplate (Hamelynck and Stiehl, 2002). One outcome of the mobile bearing design is that wear can then occur on the back (non-articulating) surface as well as on the articulating surface (Conditt *et al.*, 2004). The back surface of the mobile tibial bearing sees only oscillatory rotation, with no crossing motion of the type that occurs in hip joints. As a result, preliminary wear testing of materials for knee prosthesis applications can be done in either an oscillatory rolling/sliding tester for articular surfaces (Van Citters *et al.*, 2007) or in an oscillatory pin-on-disk tester for back surfaces (e.g. Atwood *et al.*, 2006).

Fixed bearing designs are supposed to have no relative sliding motion between the back surface of the modular polyethylene tibial bearings and the metallic tibial plates into which they are snapped into 'fixed' position; therefore it was expected that there would be no wear of the back surface of the polyethylene. Analysis of retrieved bearings, however, showed that there was unexpected relative motion of up to ± 0.5 mm at the backside interface, leading to fretting-type wear (Engh *et al.*, 2001). The particles produced by backside wear could be sufficient in number to be responsible for some of the osteolysis and implant loosening that occurs *in vivo*.

Simulations of wear of MoP knee prostheses have been developed to predict the wear of UHMWPE bearings during typical walking cycles and other daily activities (Fregly *et al.*, 2005; Miura *et al.*, 2002). The model of Fregly *et al.* (2005) couples dynamic contact analysis with computational wear prediction; it uses patient-specific transient kinematic data for walking and stair climbing, along with typical knee joint forces for those activities. The methodology is somewhat similar to that described earlier for hip joint wear models, including the use of the Archard-type equation (equation 3.3) to determine wear at nodal points on the articular surface of the polyethylene tibial bearing. In the knee joint, there can be a difference between load carried by the medial and lateral condyles, so a load split can be built into the model. The output of the model is a prediction of transient linear wear distribution on both condyles of the articular surface of the knee prosthesis for both walking and stair climbing cycles. It has been found that the model could predict wear damage distribution and wear depths that were consistent with damage on a tibial insert retrieved from a patient whose kinematic data were used in the model (Fregly *et al.*, 2005).

CoP knee prostheses have been used in Japan since the 1980s, where it has been found that, although UHMWPE showed considerably less wear against alumina femoral components than against CoCrMo components in knee simulator testing, retrieval analysis has shown that there has been little difference in the *in vivo* wear performance of MoP and CoP knee implants (Oonishi *et al.*, 2009). More recently, advances in ceramic processing and properties and the use of more ceramic composite femoral components have led to successful implementation of CoP knee implants in a number of European countries (Benazzo *et al.*, 2007).

As was discussed in Section 3.4.2, it is predicted that the lubricant film thickness in a CoP knee implant would be similar to that in a MoP knee prosthesis. Because of the relatively large roughness of the UHMWPE tibial bearing, the lubricated CoP conjunction could very well be in the mixed lubrication regime for much of its time *in vivo*, as is the case for MoP prostheses. However, the low surface roughness of the ceramic component could lead to a bit less wear by abrasion of the polyethylene in the CoP design than in a MoP knee prosthesis. It should be noted that one of the metallic materials used in MoP knee implants, oxidized zirconium, has a thin (about 5 μm thick) layer of zirconium oxide on the articulating surface of the femoral component. As a result, the contact in such an implant is actually ceramic (ZrO_2) against UHMWPE. It has been found in knee simulator testing that polyethylene wear can be considerably lower against the oxidized zirconium component than against a similar CoCrMo component, presumably because the hard oxide surface retains its smooth surface finish better than does CoCrMo, resulting in less abrasion of the polyethylene (Spector *et al.*, 2001). It remains to be seen, however, whether the oxide layer will resist spalling during long-term *in vivo* use.

3.6 Future trends in biomechanics of hip and knee joints

In recent years, many advances in experimental and analytical methods have been made that have improved our understanding of the kinematics, kinetics, contact mechanics and lubrication of artificial knee and hip joints. Those new techniques have enabled implant designers and clinicians to provide better, longer lasting prostheses for many thousands of individuals. Further advances continue to be made and they will influence research, implant design and failure analysis in future years. Among the areas in which further advances are anticipated are the following.

- Improved methodology for *in vivo* kinematic measurements will enable more patient-specific joint kinematics to be used in the design and selection of implants and in the modeling of wear for realistic conditions.
- As kinetic models of joint forces become more sophisticated, there should be improved analysis of contact forces in hip and knee joints, particularly for activities other than normal walking. This will enable researchers to eliminate some of the wide variability in predicted knee and hip joint contact loads that is evident in Tables 3.3 and 3.4.
- Improved measurements of the viscous and boundary lubricant properties of periprosthetic synovial fluid will allow better EHL analysis of hip and knee implants. Micro-EHL models that incorporate mixed lubrication, with some solid–solid contact, will be developed and these will allow even better understanding of the behavior of the lubricated conjunctions in hip and knee implants.
- Contact-coupled models of wear will continue to be improved, probably with more accurate patient-specific models of relative motions and sliding velocities within the contact for different activities. These will enable better prediction of wear rates for a specific patient's implant.
- With the continuing development of new implant materials, it is anticipated that future hip and knee implants will show better resistance to wear and other modes of failure than has been the case up until now. However, as prostheses begin to be implanted in younger and more active patients, in whom they will likely be subjected to more severe contact loads, reductions in wear and increases in durability may not always occur.

3.7 Sources of further information

Books

Mow VC and Huiskes R (eds) (2005) *Basic Orthopædic Biomechanics and Mechano-Biology*, 3rd edition. Philadelphia, PA, Lippincott, Williams & Wilkins.

This book covers a range of topics in orthopaedic biomechanics, from basic concepts and the properties of living tissues to the normal functions and pathologies of the musculoskeletal system to biomechanical factors influencing implant design. The following chapters could be of particular interest.

- Chapter 2, Analysis of muscle and joint loads, by PJ Prendergast, FCT van der Helm and GN Duda. This chapter contains a good review of musculoskeletal analysis techniques, with application to the hip.
- Chapter 3, Musculoskeletal dynamics, locomotion, and clinical applications, by TP Andriacchi, TS Johnson, DE Hurwitz and RN Natarajan. This chapter contains a good discussion of the kinetics of the lower limb, particularly for the knee.
- Chapter 15, Biomechanics of total knee replacement designs, by PS Walker provides a discussion of the various types of knee implants and how they can be tested.

Review papers

Komistek RD, Kane TR, Mahfouz M, Ochoa JA and Dennis DA (2005) Knee mechanics: a review of past and present techniques to determine in vivo loads. *J Biomech*, 38, 215–28.

A review of the various techniques that have been used to determine *in vivo* loads in the human knee joint.

Mattei L, Di Puccio F, Piccigallo B and Ciulli E (2011) Lubrication and wear modelling of artificial hip joints: A review. *Tribol Int*, 44, 532–49.

A review of lubrication and wear models for hip implants, including both MoP and MoM. Operating conditions (load and motion) in the hip are also reviewed.

3.8 References

Affatato S, Spinelli M, Zavalloni M, Mazzega-Fabbro C and Viceconti M (2008) Tribology and total hip joint replacement: Current concepts in mechanical simulation. *Med Eng Phys*, 30, 1305–17.

Andriacchi TP, Anderson BJ, Fermier BW, Stern D and Galante JO (1980) A study of lower-limb mechanics during stair-climbing. *Bone Joint Surg*, 62A, 749–57.

Andriacchi TP, Alexander EK and Toney MK (1998) A point cluster method for *in vivo* motion analysis. *ASME J Biomech Eng*, 120, 743–49.

Andriacchi TP, Johnson TS, Hurwitz DE and Natarajan RN (2005) Musculoskeletal dynamics, locomotion, and clinical applications. In Mow VC and Huiskes R (eds) *Basic Orthopaedic Biomechanics and Mechano-Biology*, 3rd edn. Philadelphia PA, Lippincott Williams & Wilkins. pp. 90–121.

Antonsson EK and Mann RW (1989) Automatic 6-DOF kinematic trajectory acquisition and analysis. *ASME J Dyn Sys Meas Control*, 111, 31–9.

Archard JF (1953) Contact and rubbing of flat surfaces. *J Appl Phys*, 24, 981–8.

Atwood, SA, Kennedy FE, Currier JH, Van Citters DW and Collier JP (2006) In-vitro study of backside wear mechanism on mobile knee bearing components. *ASME J Tribology*, 12, 275–81.

Banks SA and Hodge WA (1996) Accurate measurement of three-dimensional knee replacement kinematics using single-plane fluoroscopy. *IEEE Trans Biomed Eng*, 43, 638–49.

Bartel DL, VL Bicknell VL and Wright TM (1986) The effect of conformity, thickness, and material on stresses in ultra-high molecular weight components for total joint replacement. *J Bone Joint Surg Am*, 68, 1041–51.

Benazzo F, Macchi F, Rossi S and Dalla Pria P (2007) Ceramic total knee arthroplasty – an update. *Eur Musculoskeletal Rev*, 2, 59–62.

Bergmann G, Deuretzbacher G, Heller M, Graichen F, Rohlmann A, Strauss J and Duda GN (2001) Hip contact forces and gait patterns from routine activities. *J Biomech*, 34, 859–71.

Bozic KJ, Kurtz SM, Lau E, Ong K, Vail TP and Berry DJ (2009) The epidemiology of revision total hip arthroplasty in the United States. *J Bone Joint Surg Am*, 91, 128–33.

Bragdon CR, O'Connor DO, Lowenstein JD, Jasty M and Syniuta WD (1996) The importance of multidirectional motion on the wear of polyethylene. *IMechE J Eng Med*, 210, 157–66.

Brand RA, Crowninshield RD, Wittstock CE, Pederson DR Clark CR and van Krieken FM (1982) A model of lower extremity muscular anatomy. *ASME J Biomech Eng*, 104, 305–10.

Brown SS and Clarke IC (2006) A review of lubrication conditions for wear simulation in artificial hip replacements. *Tribology Trans*, 49, 72–8.

Burroughs BR and Blanchet TA (2001) Factors affecting the wear of irradiated UHMWPE. *Tribology Trans*, 45, 215–23.

Chao EY, Laughman RK and Stauffer RN (1980) Biomechanical gait evaluation of pre and postoperative total knee replacement patients. *Arch Orthop Traumat Surg*, 97, 309–17.

Chao EY, Laughman RK, Schneider E and Stauffer RN (1983) Normative data of knee joint motion and ground reaction forces in adult level walking. *J Biomechanics*, 16, 219–33.

Collier JP, Currier BH, Kennedy FE, Currier JH, Timmins G, Jackson SK and Brewer RL (2003) Comparison of cross-linked polyethylene materials for orthopedic applications. *Clin Orthop Relat Res*, 414, 289–304.

Conditt MA, Ismaily SK and Alexander JW (2004) Backside wear of modular ultra-high molecular weight polyethylene tibial inserts. *J Bone Joint Surg Am*, 86-A, 1031–7.

Currier JH, Bill MA and Mayor MB (2005) Analysis of wear asymmetry in a series of 94 retrieved polyethylene tibial bearings. *J Biomechanics*, 38, 367–75.
Currier BH, Currier JH, Mayor MB, Lyford KA, Van Citters DW and Collier JP (2007) In vivo oxidation of γ-barrier–sterilized ultra–high-molecular-weight polyethylene bearings. *J Arthroplasty*, 22, 721–31.
Currier JH, Anderson DE and Van Citters DW (2010) A proposed mechanism for squeaking of ceramic-on-ceramic hips. *Wear*, 269, 782–9.
Delecrin J, Oka M, Takahashi S, Yamamuro T and Nakamura T (1994) Changes in joint fluid after total arthroplasty: a quantitative study on the rabbit knee joint. *Clin Ortho Rel Res*, 307, 240–9.
DesJardins JD, Banks SA, Benson LC, Pace T and LaBerge M (2007) A direct comparison of patient and force-controlled simulator total knee replacement kinematics. *J Biomechanics*, 40, 3458–66.
D'Lima DD, Steklov N, Patil S and Colwell CW (2008) Knee forces during recreation and exercise after knee arthroplasty. *Clin Orthop Relat Res*, 466, 2605–11.
Duda GN, Brand D, Freitag S, Lierse W and Schneider E (1996) Variability of femoral muscle attachments. *J Biomechanics*, 29, 1185–90.
Dumbleton JH (1981) *Tribology of Natural and Artificial Joints*. London, Elsevier.
Dumbleton JH and Manley MT (2005) Metal-on-metal total hip replacement: what does the literature say? *J Arthroplasty*, 20, 174–8.
Engh GA, Lounici S, Rao AR and Collier MB (2001) In vivo deterioration of tibial baseplate locking mechanisms in contemporary modular total knee components. *J Bone Joint Surg Am*, 83, 1660–5.
Fam H, Bryant JT and Kontopoulou M (2007) Rheological properties of synovial fluids. *Biorheology*, 44, 59–74.
Ferber R, Davis IM and Williams DS (2003) Gender differences in lower extremity mechanics during running. *Clin Biomech*, 18, 350–7.
Fisher J, Jin ZM, Tipper J, Stone M and Ingham E (2006) Tribology of alternative bearings. *Clin Orthop Relat Res*, 453, 25–34.
Fregly BJ, Sawyer WG, Harman MK and Banks SA (2005) Computational wear prediction of a total knee replacement from in vivo kinematics. *J Biomechanics*, 38, 305–14.
Gao L, Wang F, Yang P and Jin Z (2009) Effect of 3D physiological loading and motion on elastohydrodynamic lubrication of metal-on-metal total hip replacements. *Med Eng Phys*, 31, 720–9.
Greenwood JA (1997) Analysis of elliptical Hertzian contacts. *Tribology Int*, 30, 235–7.
Grood ES and Suntay WJ (1983) A joint coordinate system for the clinical description of three-dimensional motions: application to the knee. *ASME J Biomech Eng*, 105, 136–44.
Hamelynck KJ and Stiehl JB (2002) *LCS Mobile Bearing Knee Arthroplasty*. Berlin, Springer.
Hamilton MA, Sucec MC, Fregly BJ, Banks SA and Sawyer WG (2005) Quantifying multidirectional sliding motions in total knee replacements. *ASME J Tribology*, 127, 280–6.
Hamrock BJ (1994) *Fundamentals of Fluid Film Lubrication*. New York, NY, McGraw-Hill.

Harun MN, Wang FC, Jin ZM and Fisher J (2009) Long-term contact-coupled wear prediction for metal-on-metal total hip joint replacement. *IMechE J Eng Trib*, 223J, 993–1001.

Heller MO, Bergmann G, Deuretzbacher G, Durselen L, Pohl M, Claes L Haas NP and Duda GN (2001) Musculo-skeletal loading conditions at the hip during walking and stair climbing. *J Biomechanics*, 34, 884–93.

ISO (2002) ISO 14242-1: *Implants for surgery. Wear of total hip-joint prostheses – Part 1*. Geneva, International Organization for Standardization.

ISO (2004) ISO 14243-3: *Implants for surgery. Wear of total knee-joint prostheses – Part 3*. Geneva, International Organization for Standardization.

Jacobs JJ (ed) (2008) *The Burden of Musculoskeletal Diseases in the United States*. Rosemont, IL, American Academy of Orthopaedic Surgeons.

Jalali-Vahid D and Jin ZM (2002) Transient elastohydrodynamic lubrication analysis of ultra-high molecular weight polyethylene hip joint replacements. *IMechE J Mech Eng Sci*, 216, 409–20.

Jalali-Vahid D, Jagatia M, Jin ZM and Dowson D (2001) Prediction of lubricating film thickness in UHMWPE hip joint replacement. *J Biomechanics*, 34, 261–6.

Jalali-Vahid D, Jin ZM and Dowson D (2006) Effect of start-up conditions on elastohydrodynamic lubrication of metal-on-metal hip implants. *IMechE J Eng Tribology*, 220, 143–50.

Jin ZM, Dowson D and Fisher J (1997) Analysis of fluid film lubrication in artificial hip joint replacements with surfaces of high elastic modulus. *IMechE J Eng Med*, 211H, 247–56.

Jin ZM, Dowson D, Fisher J, Ohtsuki N, Murakami T, Higaki H and Moriyama S (1998) Prediction of transient lubricating film thickness in knee prostheses with compliant layers. *IMechE J Eng Med*, 212, 157–64.

Johnston RC and Smidt GL (1969) Measurement of hip-joint motion during walking. *J Bone Joint Surg Am*, 51, 1083–94.

Kang I, Galvin AL, Jin ZM and Fisher F (2006) A simple fully integrated contact-coupled wear prediction for ultra-high molecular weight polyethylene hip implants. *IMechE J Eng Med*, 220H, 33–46.

Komistek RD, Stiehl JB and Dennis DA (1998) Mathematical model of the lower extremity joint reaction forces using Kane's method of dynamics. *J Biomechanics*, 31, 185–9.

Komistek RD, Kane TR, Mahfouz M, Ochoa JA and Dennis DA (2005) Knee mechanics: a review of past and present techniques to determine in vivo loads. *J Biomechanics*, 38, 215–28.

Kuntz M, Masson B and Pandorf T (2009) Current state of the art of the ceramic composite material BIOLOX™ delta. In Mendes G and Lago B (eds) *Strength of Materials*. Hauppauge, NY, Nova Science Publishers, pp. 133–55.

Kurtz SM (2009) *UHMWPE Biomaterials Handbook*, 2nd Edn. London, Elsevier.

Kuster MS, Wood GA, Stachowiak GW and Gachter A (1997) Joint load considerations in total knee replacement. *J Bone Joint Surg*, 79-B, 109–13.

Lafortune MA, Cavanagh PR, Sommer HJ and Kalenak A (1992) Three dimensional kinematics of the human knee during walking. *J Biomechanics*, 25, 347–57.

Long M, Riester L and Hunter G (1998) Nano-hardness measurements of oxidized Zr-2.5Nb and various orthopaedic materials. *Trans Soc Biomater*, 21, 528.

MacDonald SJ and Hanssen AD (2004) Metal-on-metal total hip arthroplasty: the concerns. *Clin Orthop Relat Res*, 429, 86–93.

Mattei L, Piccigallo B, Stadler K, Ciulli E and Di Puccio F (2009) EHL modeling of hip implants based on a ball-on-plane configuration. *Proceedings XIX Congresso AIMETA, Ancona, Italy*, pp.161–73.

Mattei L, Di Puccio F, Piccigallo B and Ciulli E (2011) Lubrication and wear modelling of artificial hip joints: a review. *Tribology Int*, 44, 532–49.

Mikhael MM, Hanssen SD and Sierra RJ (2009) Failure of metal-on-metal total hip arthroplasty mimicking hip infection: a report of two cases. *J Bone Joint Surg Am*, 91, 443–46.

Miura H, Higaki H, Nakanishi Y, Mawatari T, Moro-oka T, Murakami T and Iwamoto Y (2002) Prediction of total knee arthroplasty polyethylene wear using the wear index. *J Arthroplasty*, 17, 760–66.

Mongkolwongrojn MK, Wongseedakaew K and Kennedy FE (2010) Transient elastohydrodynamic lubrication in artificial knee joint with non-Newtonian fluids. *Tribology Int*, 43, 1017–26.

Moro-oka T, Hamai S, Miura H, Shimoto T, Higaki H, Fregly BJ, Iwamoto Y and Banks SA (2008) Dynamic activity dependence of in vivo normal knee kinematics. *J Orth Res*, 26, 428–34.

Morrison JB (1970) The mechanics of the knee joint in relation to normal walking. *J Biomechanics*, 3, 51–61.

Murakami T and Ohtsuki N (1987) The evaluation of lubricating film formation in knee prostheses under walking conditions. In Berthe D and Dowson D (eds). *Fluid Film Lubrication–Osborne Reynolds Centenary*. London, Elsevier, pp. 387–94.

Novacheck TF (1998) The biomechanics of running. *Gait Post*, 7, 77–95.

Oonishi H, Ueno M, Kim SC, Oonishi Hiroyuki, Iwamoto M and Kyomoto M (2009) Ceramic versus cobalt-chrome femoral components; Wear of polyethylene insert in total knee prosthesis. *J Arthroplasty*, 24, 374–82.

Paul JP (1976) Approaches to design – force actions transmitted by joints in human body. *Proc Royal Soc London B*, 192, 163–72.

Prendergast PJ, van der Helm FCT and Duda GN (2005) Analysis of muscle and joint loads. In Mow VC and Huiskes R (eds) *Basic Orthopaedic Biomechanics and Mechano-Biology*, 3rd edn. Philadelphia, PA, Lippincott Williams & Wilkins, pp. 29–89.

Ramakrishnan HK and Kadaba MP (1991) On the estimation of joint kinematics during gait. *J Biomechanics*, 10, 969–71.

Ramamurti BS, Bragdon CR, O'Connor DO, Lowenstein JD, Jasty M, Estok DM and Harris WH (1996) Loci of movement of selected points on the femoral head during normal gait. *J Arthroplasty*, 11, 845–52.

Ratner, BD, Hoffman AS, Schoen FJ and Lemons JE (2004) *Biomaterials Science*, 2nd edn. London, Elsevier, pp. 535–6.

Ries, MD, Scott NK and Jani S (2001) Relationship between gravimetric wear and particle generation in hip simulators: conventional compared with cross-linked polyethylene. *J Bone Joint Surg*, 83A, 116–22.

Rydell NW (1966) *Forces acting on the femoral head-prosthesis: a study on strain gauge supplied prostheses in living persons*. Doctoral thesis, University of Gothenburg, Sweden.

Saikko V and Ahlroos T (1999) Type of motion and lubricant in wear simulation of pylyethylene acetabular cup. *Proc Inst Mech Eng H*, 123, 301–10.

Schurz J and Ribitsch V (1987) Rheology of synovial fluid. *Biorheology*, 24, 385–99.

Seireg A and Arvikar RJ (1973) A mathematical model for evaluation of forces in lower extremeties of the musculo-skeletal system. *J Biomechanics*, 6, 313–26.

Sharkey PF, Hozack WJ, et al. (2002) Why are total knee arthroplasties failing today? *Clin Orthop Relat. Res* 404, 7–13.

Sieber, H-P, Rieker CB and Kottig P (1999) Analysis of 118 second-generation metal-on-metal retrieved hip implants. *J Bone Joint Surg Br*, 81, 46–50.

Spector M, Ries MD, Bourne RB, Sauer WS, Long M and Hunter G (2001) Wear performance of ultra-high molecular weight polyethylene on oxidized zirconium total knee femoral components. *J Bone Joint Surg*, 83A, 80–6.

Stedman TL (2006) *Stedman's Medical Dictionary*, 28th edn. Baltimore, MD, Lippincott, Williams & Wilkins.

Taylor SJG and Walker PS (2001) Forces and moments telemetered from two distal femoral replacements during various activities. *J Biomechanics*, 34, 839–48.

Ulrich SD, Seyler TM, et al. (2008) Total hip arthroplasties: what are the reasons for revision? *Int Orth (SICOT)*, 32, 597–604.

Van Citters DW, Kennedy FE and Collier JP (2007) Rolling sliding wear of UHMWPE for knee bearing applications. *Wear*, 263, 1087–94.

Viceconti M, Ansaloni, M, Beleani M and Toni A (2003) The muscle standardized femur: a step forward in the replication of numerical studies in biomechanics. *IMechE J Eng Med*, 217H, 105–10.

Wang A (2001) A unified theory of wear for ultra-high molecular weight polyethylene in multi-directional sliding. *Wear*, 248, 38–47.

Wang FC and Jin ZM (2005) Elastohydrodynamic lubrication modelling of artificial hip joints under steady-state conditions. *ASME J Tribology*, 127, 729–39.

Wang FC, Zhao SX, Quinonez AF, Xu H, Mei XS and Jin ZM (2009) Nonsphericity of bearing geometry and lubrication in hip joint implants. *ASME J Tribology*, 131, 031201-1–11.

Williams S, Schepers A, Isaac G, Hardaker C, Ingham E, van der Jagt D, Breckon A and Fisher J (2007) Ceramic-on-metal hip arthroplasties: a comparative in vitro and in vivo study. *Clin Orthop Relat Res*, 465, 23–32.

Wimmer MA and Andriacchi TP (1997) Tractive forces during rolling motion in total knee replacement. *J Biomechanics*, 30, 131–8.

Woltring HJ, Roy PV, Hebbelinck M Osteaux M and Verbruggen L (1990) 3-D knee joint kinematics by magnetic resonance imaging. *J Biomechanics*, 23, 384.

Wu G, Siegler S, et al. (2002) ISB recommendation on definitions of joint coordinate system of various joints for the reporting of human joint motion – part I: ankle, hip, and spine. *J Biomechanics*, 35, 543–8.

Yao JQ, Laurent MP, Johnson TS, Blanchard CR and Crowinshield RD (2003) The influence of lubricant and material on polymer/CoCr sliding friction. *Wear*, 255, 780–4.

Young SK, Keller TS, et al. (2000) Wear testing of UHMWPE tibial components: influence of oxidation. *ASME J Tribology*, 122, 323–31.

4
Anatomy of the hip and suitable prostheses

F. TRAINA, M. DE FINE and S. AFFATATO
Istituto Ortopedico Rizzoli, Italy

Abstract: The hip joint is the articulation between the coxal bone and the femur. The hip is a ball-and-socket joint realized by the acetabulum (the socket) and the head of the femur (the ball). As any ball-and-socket type joint, the hip has a wide range of motion, including flexion, extension, abduction, adduction, internal rotation and external rotation. The function of the hip is to withstand body weight during standing and walking; during single-leg stance the hip joint must carry a load three times greater the body weight. Total joint replacements have been developed in an effort to eliminate pain and improve function of damaged joints. Total hip replacement is indicated for patients 60 to 75 years of age, with severe and debilitating hip pain that does not recede with non-surgical treatment and significant functional impairment. Contraindications for total hip replacement are the presence of an acute infection in any region of the body and any medical pathology able to unacceptably increase the operative risks. Total hip arthroplasty includes a femoral component (the stem) and an acetabular component (the socket or the cup). The method of fixation of cup and stem to the bone distinguishes between cemented and cementless total hip arthroplasty. Different options are available for the bearing surfaces. A polyethylene liner coupled with a metallic (cobalt–chromium) head represents the most widely used system.

Key words: hip anatomy, femur, acetabulum, body weight, prostheses.

4.1 Anatomy of the hip

The hip joint is the articulation between the coxal bone, also called the hip bone or innominate bone, and the femur (the thigh bone). The coxal bone (Fig. 4.1) is a flat bone that forms the pelvis, along with the contralateral coxal bone and the sacrum (Fig. 4.2). The ilium, ischium and pubis are three

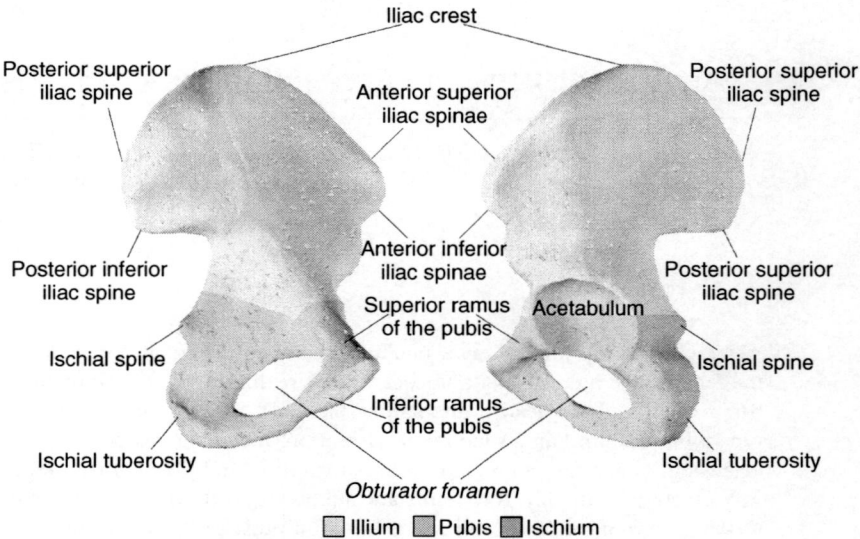

4.1 The coxal bone.

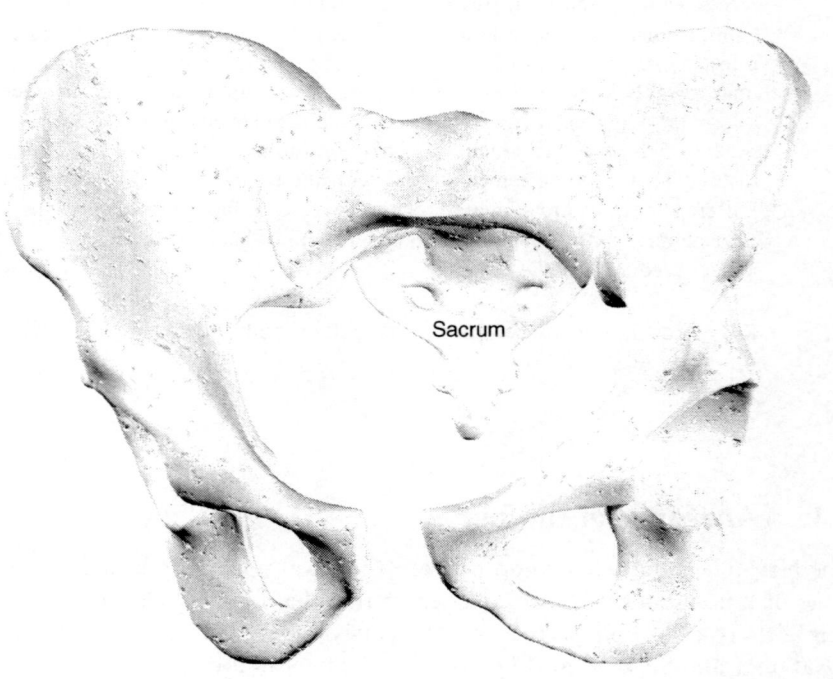

4.2 The pelvis.

different bones that contribute to the formation of the coxal bone during skeletal growth, fusing to each other at skeletal maturity.

The ilium is formed by two main parts: the ala superiorly and the body inferiorly. The ala is irregularly shaped and its internal surface is smooth and covered by the iliopsoas muscle whereas the external surface gives attachment to the gluteal muscles. A longitudinal crest with an internal and an external lip runs along its superior margin. The anterior margin presents two eminences separated by a notch, the anterior superior iliac spine and the anterior inferior iliac spine. The posterior superior iliac spine and the posterior inferior iliac spine are the most proximal prominences of the posterior margin of the ala. Below the latter structures, the greater sciatic notch divides the ilium from the ischium. The body of the ilium forms the upper part of the acetabulum.

The ischium provides the lower and posterior part of the coxal bone. Along the posterior aspect of the ischium, the first visible structure is the ischial spine. Below the ischial spine, the lesser sciatic notch precedes the ischial tuberosity, which is a large and strong apophysis where the posterior muscles of the thigh originate. The inferior ramus starts from the ischial tuberosity and goes upward and medially, connecting the ischium to the pubis.

The pubis forms the medial and anterior part of the coxal bone and it articulates with the contralateral pubis, closing the anterior part of the pelvis. It is connected to the ischium by means of the inferior and superior ramus. The hole described by these rami is called the *obturator foramen*.

The acetabulum is a hemispherical cavity located at the center of the outer surface of the coxal bone. It is directed downward, lateralward and forward. A cartilage layer covers the inner surface of the acetabulum with the exception of its central part, which is the site of origin of the *ligamentum teres*. The inferior part of the outer rim of the cavity is interrupted by the acetabular notch. The glenoidal labrum is a fibrocartilagineous structure attached to the outer rim of the acetabulum, which improves the acetabular depth. The transverse acetabular ligament is the part of the glenoidal labrum contributing to close the acetabular notch.

The femur is a long bone formed by a body (diaphysis) and two expanded extremities (epiphyses) (Fig. 4.3). The body is cylindrical in shape and a longitudinal crest, the *linea aspera*, goes through its posterior aspect. The proximal epyphisis includes the head of the femur, the neck of the femur and two eminences, the greater and the lesser trochanter. The head of the femur is hemispherical and it is almost fully covered by cartilage, with the exception of its central part, the *fovea capitis*, which represents the insertion of the *ligamentum teres*. The neck of the femur connects the head to the diaphysis. The greater and the lesser trochanter are two prominences, acting as points of insertion of different muscular groups that move the hip joint.

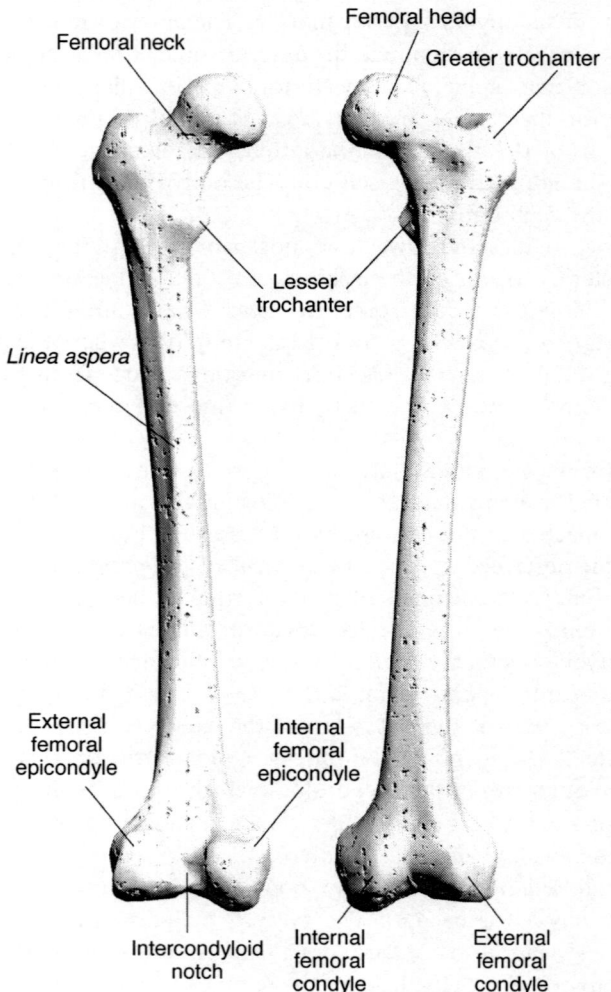

4.3 The femur: posterior view on the left, anterior view on the right.

The distal epyphisis consists of two large eminences, the femoral condyles, divided by a notch called the intercondyloid fossa. Above each femoral condyle there are further two little eminences, the medial and lateral epicondyles.

The hip joint is a subtype of diarthrodial joint (ball-and-socket joint) (Fig. 4.4). The joint is realized by the acetabulum (the socket) and the head of the femur (the ball). The articular capsule is a fibrous structure going from the origin of the glenoidal labrum to the base of the femoral neck. It is stronger in its anterior and superior aspect rather than in the inferior and posterior part. Three strong ligaments, the iliofemoral, the ischiofemoral and the pubofemoral ligaments reinforce the articular capsule.

The *ligamentum teres* warrants an additional link between the head of the femur and the acetabulum. The capsule, the ligaments and the muscles

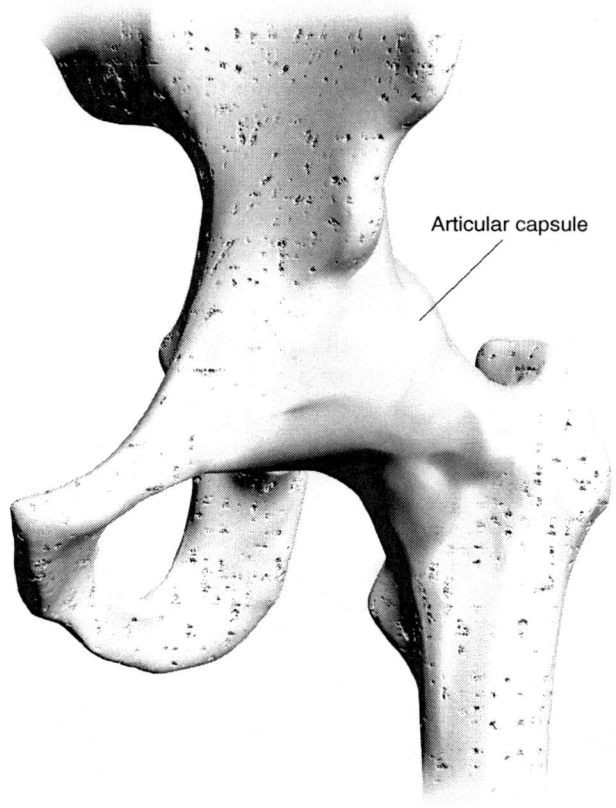

4.4 The hip joint.

around the hip keep joint stability, holding the bones in place and avoiding dislocation. The smooth cartilage layer over the head of the femur and the acetabulum cushions the compressive forces acting on the hip joint during weight bearing. The inner surface of the articular capsule is coated by the synovial membrane, which produces synovial fluid. The synovial fluid lubricates the joint, allowing hip motion with very low friction and without pain, even under great pressure (Gray, 1918; Thompson, 2002).

4.2 Kinematics of the hip

As with any ball-and-socket type joint, the hip has a wide range of motion, including flexion, extension, abduction, adduction, internal rotation and external rotation.

- Flexion is the movement that allows bringing the thigh towards the abdomen (Fig. 4.5). The extent of hip flexion is 0–130°. The main hip flexors are the iliopsoas muscle and the *quadriceps femoris*. The iliopsoas starts from the anterolaral aspect of the lumbar vertebrae and the inner part of the ala of the ilium, passes through the pelvic cavity and finally inserts on the lesser trochanter. The *quadriceps* lies on the anterior aspect of the thigh and is divided into four different muscles (*rectus femoris*, *vastus lateralis*, *vastus medialis* and *vastus intermedius*). It originates from the anterior superior iliac spine and from the femoral diaphysis and it inserts through the patellar tendon on the proximal part of the tibia.
- Hip extension is the opposite of hip flexion (Fig. 4.6). The arch of hip extension is 0–30°. The main hip extensor is the *gluteus maximus*, which originates from the outer surface of the ala and inserts on the proximal part of the *linea aspera* in the femoral diaphysis.
- Hip abduction is the movement to take the leg away from the body (Fig.

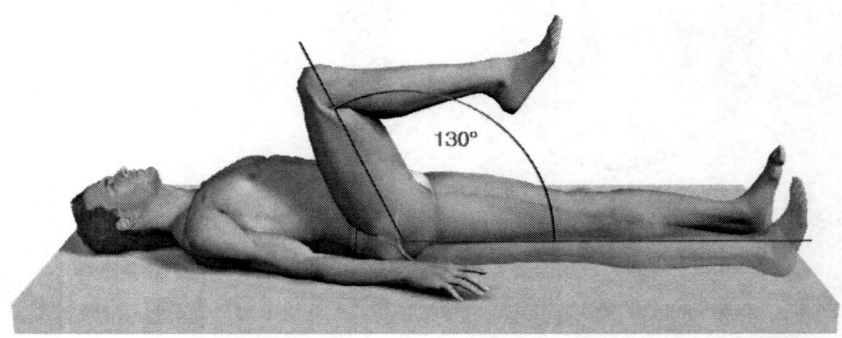

4.5 Hip flexion.

Anatomy of the hip and suitable prostheses 99

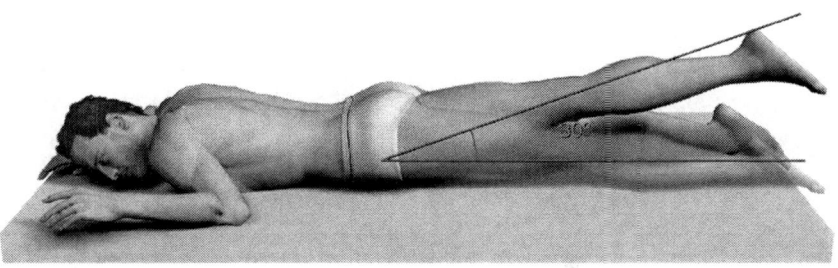

4.6 Hip extension.

4.7). Hip abduction is allowed from 0 to 45°. The most important abductors are the gluteal muscles. The *gluteus medius* and the *gluteus minimus* originate from the outer surface of the ala, below and behind the *gluteus maximus*, inserting on the greater trochanter. The gluteal muscles play a key role in the biomechanics of the hip. Further abduction is warranted by the tensor muscle of the *fascia lata*, which starts from the anterior superior iliac spine and inserts on the proximal and lateral part of the tibia.

- Hip adduction is the movement to bring the leg back toward the body (Fig. 4.8). The extent of this movement is 0–30°. The most important adductors are the *adductor longus, adductor brevis* and *adductor magnus*. The origin of the *adductor longus* and *adductor brevis* is the inferior ramus of the pubis, whereas the *adductor magnus* stars from the ischial tuberosity. The large area of insertion of these muscles is the *linea aspera* and the internal part of the femur.
- Hip internal and external rotation are the movements that make the foot turn in and out respectively (Fig. 4.9 and 4.10). As a secondary function,

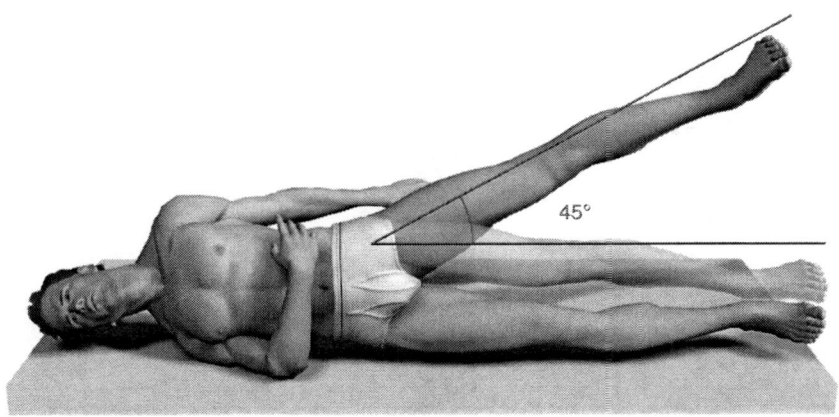

4.7 Hip abduction.

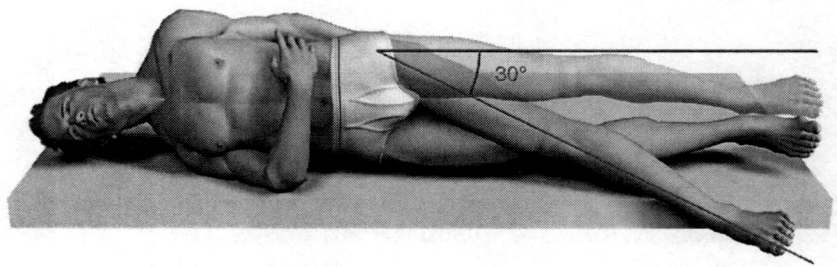

4.8 Hip adduction.

the *gluteus medius* and *minimus* act as internal rotators. External rotators are a group of muscles located in the buttock; in a proximal to distal direction, these muscles are the *piriformis*, the *superior gemellus*, the *obturator externus*, the *obturator internus*, the *inferior gemellus* and the *quadratus femoris*. These muscles originate from the anterior surface

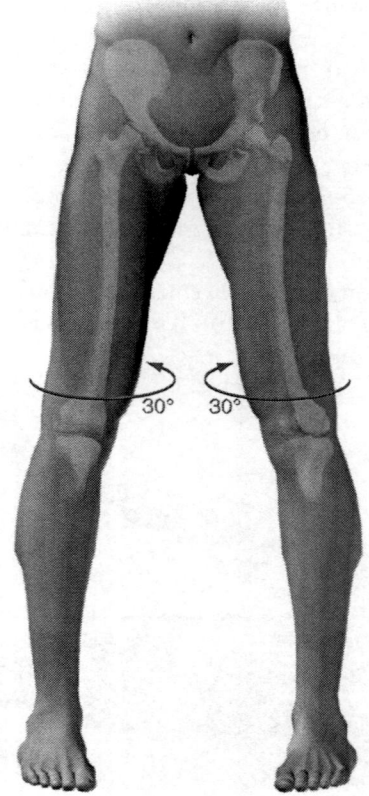

4.9 Hip internal rotation.

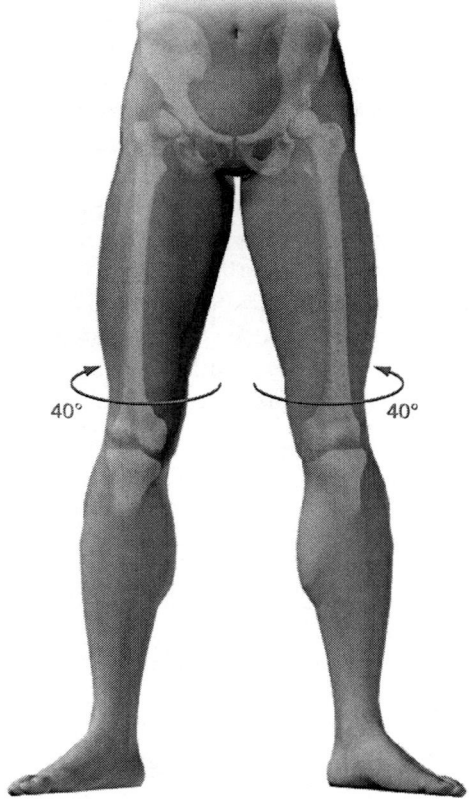

4.10 Hip external rotation.

of the sacrum, from the ischial tuberosity and from the obturator foramen and inserts on the posterior aspect of the greater trochanter and on the *linea aspera* (Kapandji, 1998).

4.3 Biomechanics of the hip

The function of the hip is to withstand body weight during standing and walking. The body weight is a load applied to the body's center of gravity. In a model subject, the center of gravity is located in the region just anterior to the top of the second sacral vertebra; the center of gravity is the point around which a body will rotate assuming no external forces are currently being applied. During single-leg stance, the body's center of gravity moves distally and away from the supporting leg, allowing the body weight to act on a lever arm going from the center of gravity to the hip center of rotation

(Canale and Beaty, 2007; Delp *et al.*, 1994). To avoid pelvic tilt during gait, the supporting leg has to counterbalance the body weight by means of the abductor muscles. Since the abductor muscles lever arm, which is the distance between the lateral aspect of the greater trochanter and the center of rotation of the hip, is about one third of the body weight lever arm, the abductor musculature needs to exert a force three times greater than the body weight (Traina *et al.*, 2008; Vasavada *et al.*, 1994) (Fig. 4.11).

The sum of all these forces produces a force directed towards the fulcrum of this balance, which is the hip center of rotation. Therefore, during single-leg stance, the hip joint must carry a load three times greater than the body weight, and this load can be significantly greater during jumping or running (Canale and Beaty, 2007). The abductor muscle lever arm depends on the femoral offset, which is the perpendicular distance between the hip center of

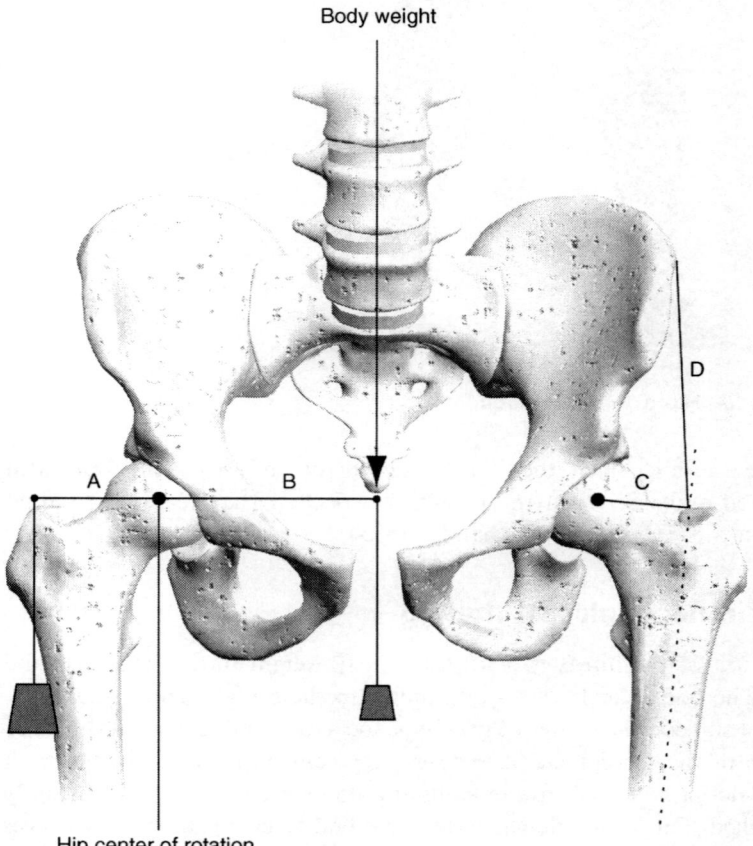

4.11 Biomechanics of the hip. A, abductor muscles lever arm; B, body weight lever arm; C, femoral offset; D, abductor vector.

Anatomy of the hip and suitable prostheses

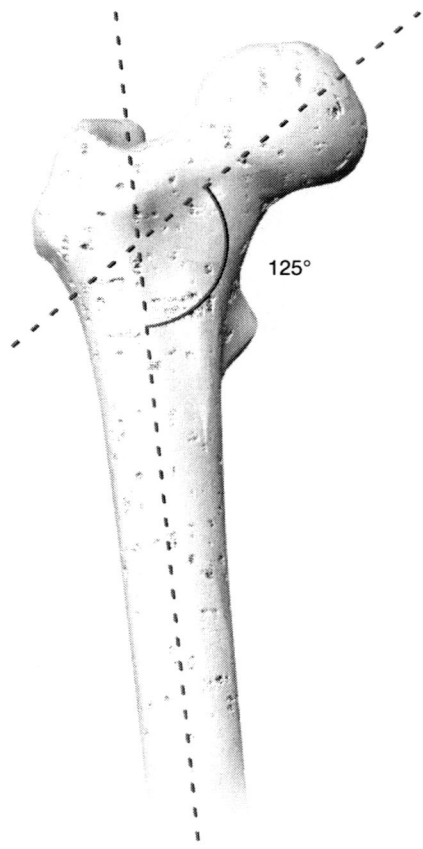

4.12 Inclination angle.

rotation and a line drawn down the femoral shaft (Charles *et al.*, 2005). The length and orientation of the femoral neck can modify the femoral offset. The angle between the femoral neck and the femoral shaft, called the neck–shaft angle or inclination angle, is normally about 125° (Fig. 4.12).

A valgus angle is an inclination angle greater than 125° and a varus angle is less than 125°. If the length of the femoral neck is the same, increasing the inclination angle reduces the femoral off-set and vice versa. The anteversion angle is the angle between the long axis of the neck of the femur and a line tangent to the posterior femoral condyles (Argenson *et al.*, 2007) (Fig. 4.13). The normal value of this angle is about 15° (Kapandji, 1998) and any increase in this value reduces femoral offset, subsequently reducing the abductor muscle lever arm (Argenson *et al.*, 2007). Many pathologic conditions affects the inclination and anteversion angle, reducing femoral offset and increasing the abductors' work (Argenson *et al.*, 2007; Noble

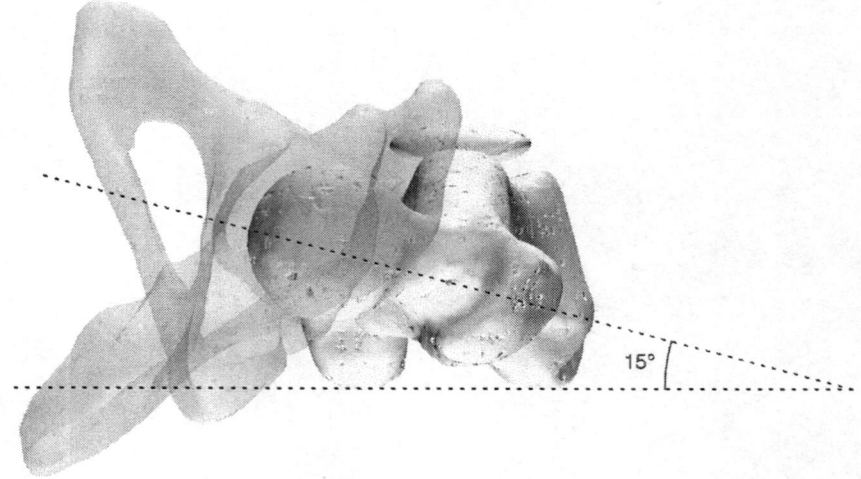

4.13 Anteversion angle.

et al., 2003). If pelvic tilt cannot be avoided during single-leg stance, limping occurs during walking (Kapandji, 1998).

4.4 History and indications for total hip replacement

Total joint replacements have been developed in an effort to eliminate pain and improve the function of damaged joints. The history of total hip arthroplasty began in 1923, when Smith-Pethersen implanted the first femoral cup made of glass. However, the modern concept of total hip arthroplasty is due to the work of Sir John Charnley in the 1960s and the 1970s. Charnley introduced cement to fix prosthetic components to bone and he used Teflon, the ancestress of modern polyethylene, as the bearing surface. Furthermore, he popularized concepts about hip biomechanics applied to total hip replacement, the design of prosthetic components, surgical technique, wear, implant loosening, the operating environment and many more. Until recently, a metal-on-polyethylene coupling was considered the gold standard for total hip replacement, but over the last three decades, many innovations have been developed. Surgical technique has been progressively modified toward less invasive and tissue-sparing approaches in order to reduce rehabilitation time. Furthermore, cementless fixation has been promoted to facilitate revision surgery and the use of hard-on-hard bearing surfaces such as metal-on-metal or ceramic-on-ceramic has been proposed with the aim of overcoming the problem of implant loosening due to polyethylene wear. The discovery of resurfacing hip replacements and the development of modular necks represent the latest evolutions in this field (Canale and Beaty, 2007; Chapman, 2001).

Total hip replacement is indicated to relieve pain and improve hip function. The ideal candidate was originally considered to be a patient of 60 to 75 years of age, with severe and debilitating hip pain that did not recede with non-surgical treatment and significant functional impairment (Charnley, 1961). However, in recent years, new materials and techniques have improved implant longevity and reduced possible complications, with total hip replacement being proposed to younger patients (Kearns *et al.*, 2006; Thillemann *et al.*, 2008). Furthermore, ageing of the population has seen this operation being performed in patients aged 80 years old or older.

The most common pathologic condition leading to total hip replacement is primary osteoarthritis, which is a degenerative process affecting different joints due to cartilage degeneration with age. Any condition that changes hip anatomy, producing an altered load distribution over the joint, can cause secondary osteoarthritis (Canale and Beaty, 2007; Chapman, 2001). This can be due to congenital pathologies (developmental dysplasia of the hip (Bernasek *et al.*, 2007, Biant *et al.*, 2009; Erdemli *et al.*, 2005), Legg–Calvè–Perthes disease (Traina *et al.*, 2011), slipped capital femoral epiphysis (Gent and Clarke, 2004), achondroplasia, hemophilia) or post-traumatic disorders (femoral neck fractures, acetabular fractures) (Ranawat *et al.*, 2009). Another possible indication for total hip replacement is osteonecrosis of the femoral head (Brinker *et al.*, 1994; Hartley *et al.*, 2000). This disease can develop without any provoking event (idiopathic), but can also be related to many different conditions and diseases (femoral neck fracture, traumatic hip dislocation, sickle cell disease, caisson disease, alcoholism, cortisone therapy, gaucher disease, lupus, etc.). Further indications for total hip replacement are rheumatologic diseases (rheumatoid arthritis (Lachiewicz *et al.*, 1986), ankylosing spondylitis), sequelae of septic hip arthritis (pyogenic arthritis, tubercolosis) and bone tumors involving the proximal femur. Contraindications for total hip replacement are the presence of an acute infection in any region of the body and any medical pathology (cardiac diseases, pulmonary diseases, liver disease, etc.) that unacceptably increases the operative risks (Canale and Beaty, 2007; Chapman, 2001).

4.5 Prosthetic designs and bearing surfaces

Total hip arthroplasty includes a femoral component (the stem) and an acetabular component (the socket or cup). The articular coupling of total hip arthroplasty is realized by means of the femoral head, which is taper locked to the neck of the stem, and the inner part of the acetabular cup, which in modular cups is a liner seated into the inner surface of the cup metal back (Fig. 4.14). Femoral stems can be made of cobalt–chromium or titanium alloys, whereas acetabular components can be made of either titanium or polyethylene.

The method of fixation of cup and stem to the bone distinguishes between cemented and cementless total hip arthroplasty. If a different method of fixation is chosen for each component (i.e. a cementless cup and a cemented stem) the result is called a hybrid total hip arthroplasty (Canale and Beaty, 2007; Chapman, 2001).

Bone cement is a polymer (polymethylmethacrylate, PMMA), which was

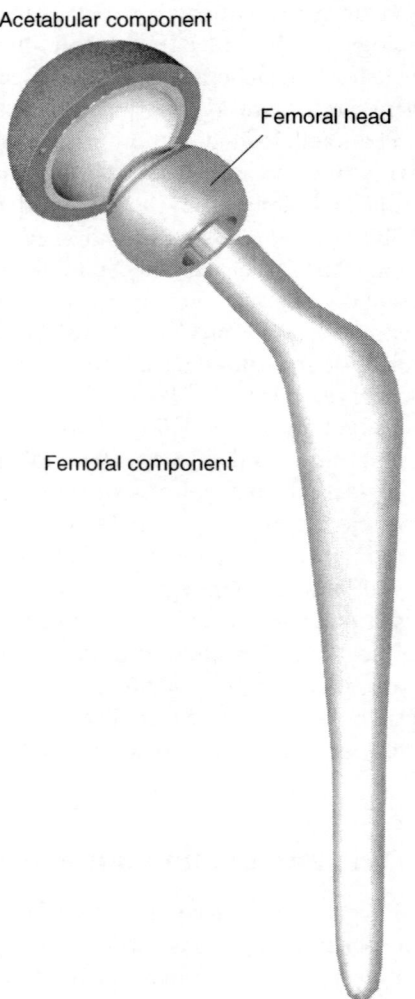

4.14 Components of a standard total hip arthroplasty.

first used to fix prosthetic components to bone. Due to a lack of adhesive properties, the bonding of cement to bone is realized by means of the interdigitation of the cement mantle within the cancellous bone (Jaeblon, 2010). Considering a cemented femoral stem, both the bone–cement interface and the stem–cement interface must to be taken into account. Different approaches exist with regard to the best stem design with which to achieve durable fixation at the stem–cement interface. Femoral components with textured or roughened surfaces have been produced to improve bonding between cement and implant (Berger et al., 1996; Clohisy and Harris, 1999; Crowninshield et al., 1998), similarly to what happens at the bone–cement interface. Since surface roughness enhances debris formation due to friction at the stem–cement interface, polished tapered stems have been proposed. This system means that the stem subsides slightly into the cement mantle, taking advantage of the viscoelastic properties of cement (Berry et al., 1998; Collis and Mohler, 1998). Even if a bond between the cement and the stem is not achieved, stem subsidence generates hoop stresses that increase stability at the bone–cement interface. Although there is no definitive consensus about the better stem design, the use of polished tapered stems has gained increasing popularity over recent years.

Problems related to the mechanical loosening of cemented implants have led to the development of a biological fixation. The aim of the cementless fixation is to improve implant longevity and facilitate revision surgery for stem loosening. Bone ingrowth at the bone–implant interface is obtained using stems with porous metal surfaces (Engh et al., 1987, 1997) or using biologically active materials such as grit-blasted titanium or hydroxyapatite coatings (Callaghan, 1993; Jaffe and Scott, 1996). The long time required for complete biological osteointegration of the implant makes the immediate mechanical stability of the stem during implantation an irremissible requisite. The press-fitting insertion of the stem into the femoral canal allows this goal to be attained. In terms of shape, a cementless femoral component can be anatomical or straight. Anatomical stems try to reproduce the femoral anatomy so that, after insertion, the loads applied to the implant can be uniformly transferred to the host bone, thus encouraging osteointegration. Anatomical stems are necessarily different for the right-hand and left-hand sides. Straight stems have a symmetrical cross-section and can be used for both sides, thus reducing inventory and costs; furthermore, straight stems make contact with the inner femur just at specific points. The long-term outcomes of total hip replacement with cementless stems do not show any relevant differences between anatomical and straight stems, but the use of straight stems is most popular among surgeons.

Acetabular components can be either cemented or cementless. All-polyethylene cups are used for cemented fixation. They present some longitudinal grooves on the outer surface to improve cement filling. Cementless cups consist of a generally hemispherical metal shell (titanium) with a porous surface to promote bone ingrowth. Additional flares or pegs can be used to improve mechanical stability on rotation and, in some models, two or more holes are available for the insertion of screws (Canale and Beaty, 2007; Chapman, 2001).

As a general rule, cementless fixation is preferable in young and active patients, whereas cemented fixation is generally used in older or less active patients or when poor bone quality contraindicate press-fit insertion of the implants.

Different options are available for the bearing surfaces. A polyethylene liner coupled with a metallic (cobalt–chromium) head represents the most widely used system. The problem of metal-on-polyethylene articulations is the creation of polyethylene wear debris that can lead to osteolysis and implant loosening (Heisel *et al.*, 2004). Hard-on-hard bearing surfaces (metal or ceramic) have been introduced to avoid debris formation but, despite the good long-term outcomes using these new bearing couplings (Amstutz and Grigoris, 1996; Baek and Kim, 2008; Hannouche *et al.*, 2005; Murphy *et al.*, 2006; Schmalzried *et al.*, 1996), further questions have arisen. For example an increase of the serum levels of cobalt and chromium has been reported after metal-on-metal total hip arthroplasty (Brodner *et al.*, 2003). The significance of this phenomenon is still unclear, but chromosomal aberrations have been recorded in patients with metal articulations (Dunstan *et al.*, 2008) and the risk of carcinogenesis has been postulated (Tharani *et al.*, 2001). Although this risk has not been demonstrated (Visuri *et al.*, 1996), hypersensitivity to metals has been proposed as a mechanism of implant loosening in sporadic cases (Thyssen *et al.*, 2009). The possible effects of metal ions warm against the use of metal couplings in fertile women or patients with kidney diseases (Canale and Beaty, 2007; Chapman, 2001).

Ceramic-on-ceramic articulation has excellent tribological properties (Bal *et al.*, 2007; Bierbaum *et al.*, 2002), but there is a risk of sudden failure due to the brittleness of the material (Diwanji *et al.*, 2007; Hannouche *et al.*, 2003; Min *et al.*, 2007). When cyclic loads are applied to a ceramic component, microscopic flaws that may be created during material manufacturing or during implantation can act as stress risers, leading to the propagation of cracks throughout the material and finally to catastrophic failure (Bal *et al.*, 2007; D'Antonio and Sutton, 2009; Diwanji *et al.*, 2007). Despite the very low incidence of ceramic fractures, the risk of sudden failure has not been avoided even with the use of newer ceramic materials (Hamilton *et al.*, 2010). Highly cross-linked polyethylene is a new type of polyethylene characterized by higher wear resistance. However, despite good results obtained *in vitro* (Glyn-Jones *et al.*, 2008) and satisfactory mid-term *in vivo* outcomes (Bascarevic *et al.*, 2010), long-term results are lacking. Further more, the chemical processes required to produce this material can affect its strength and fatigue resistance (Baker *et al.*, 2003) and some cases of sudden failure have been reported (Moore *et al.*, 2008).

4.6 Future trends

Newer prosthetic designs have been introduced to further improve the effectiveness of total hip replacement. The main innovations are in modular stem prostheses and resurfacing hip replacements.

Modular stem prostheses provide different modular solutions for the proximal part of the stem. After stem insertion into the femoral canal, a modular neck is taper-locked to the stem, allowing the surgeon to intraoperatively correct femoral anteversion, femoral offset and leg length independently by the type and size of the stem used (Traina *et al.*, 2004, 2009). The ability of this modularity in restoring hip biomechanics is particularly useful in the case of altered hip anatomy and good long-term results have been reported using modular necks in patients affected with developmental dysplasia of the hip (Traina *et al.*, 2011). A different type of modularity involves a modular proximal sleeve mated with a previously inserted femoral stem (Buly, 2005), and good results have been achieved in dysplastic patients (Biant *et al.*, 2009).

Resurfacing hip replacement is a procedure realized through coupling a traditional acetabular socket with a metallic femoral component, which is applied to the femoral head (Fig. 4.15).

This procedure was first used in the late 1970s (Trentani and Vaccarino, 1978), but poor surgical technique and fixation methods led to inadequate results. Renewed interest in re-surfacing hip replacement techniques over recent years is due to the good results achieved with newer materials and cemented fixation of the femoral component. The bone-preserving nature of the procedure makes resurfacing a reasonable option for young and active patients, because the femoral neck is preserved and revision surgery, if necessary, is straightforward (McGrory *et al.*, 2010). Nowadays, resurfacing necessarily requires metal-on-metal coupling, thus producing concerns about metal ions.

The ceramic-on-metal bearing option is an innovative solution involving the use of a metallic liner and a ceramic head. The objective of this new bearing coupling is to reduce wear and the risk of liner fractures compared with metal-on-metal and ceramic-on-ceramic articulations respectively. Since clinical data are lacking and *in vitro* studies have produced contrasting results (Barnes *et al.*, 2008; Cristofolini *et al.*, 2009), further investigations are needed to confirm the feasibility of this approach.

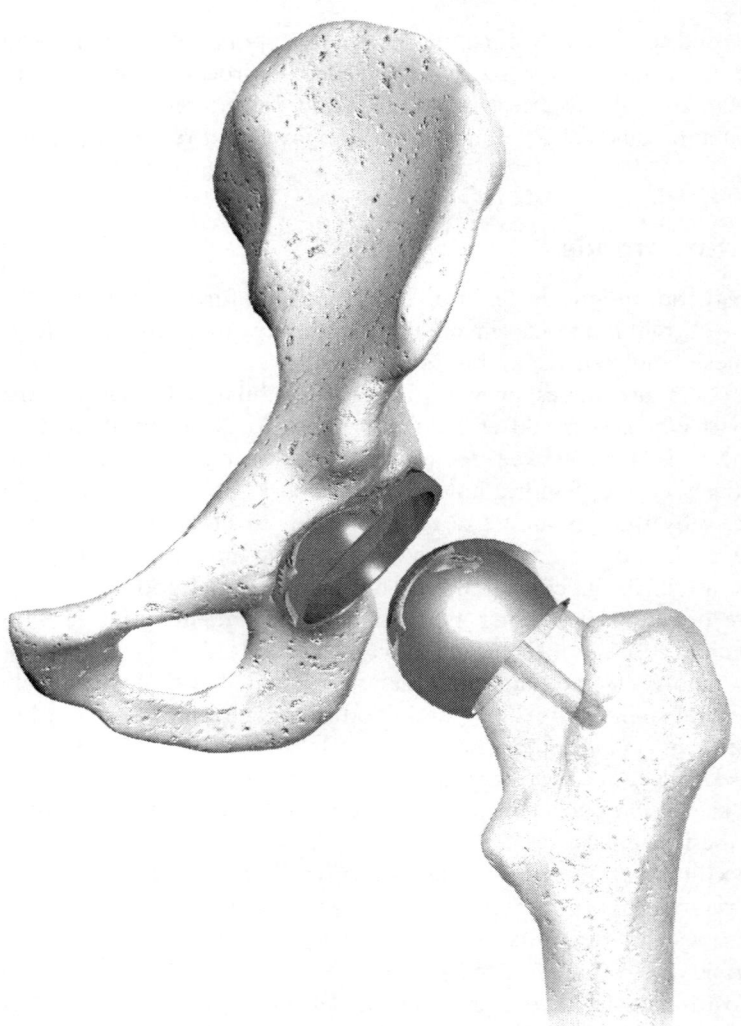

4.15 Resurfacing prosthesis.

4.7 Acknowledgments

We would like to thank Luigi Lena (Rizzoli Orthopaedic Institute) for his valuable help with the creation and processing of all the images in this chapter.

4.8 References

Amstutz, H. C. and Grigoris, P. (1996) Metal on metal bearings in hip arthroplasty. *Clin Orthop Relat Res*, 329, S11–34.

Argenson, J. N., Flecher, X., Parratte, S. and Aubaniac, J. M. (2007) Anatomy of the dysplastic hip and consequences for total hip arthroplasty *Clin Orthop Relat Res*, 465, 40–5.

Baek, S. H. and Kim, S. Y. (2008) Cementless total hip arthroplasty with alumina bearings in patients younger than fifty with femoral head osteonecrosis. *J Bone Joint Surg Am*, 90, 1314–20.

Baker, D. A., Bellare, A. and Pruitt, L. (2003) The effects of degree of crosslinking on the fatigue crack initiation and propagation resistance of orthopedic-grade polyethylene. *J Biomed Mater Res A*, 66, 146–54.

Bal, B. S., Garino, J., Ries, M. and Rahaman, M. N. (2007) A review of ceramic bearing materials in total joint arthroplasty. *Hip Int*, 17, 21–30.

Barnes, C. L., Deboer, D., Corpe, R. S., Nambu, S., Carroll, M. and Timmerman, I. (2008) Wear performance of large-diameter differential-hardness hip bearings. *J Arthroplasty*, 23, 56–60.

Bascarevic, Z., Vukasinovic, Z., Slavkovic, N., Dulic, B., Trajkovic, G., Bascarevic, V. and Timotijevic, S. (2010) Alumina-on-alumina ceramic versus metal-on-highly cross-linked polyethylene bearings in total hip arthroplasty: a comparative study. *Int Orthop*, 34, 1129–35.

Berger, R. A., Kull, L. R., Rosenberg, A. G. and Galante, J. O. (1996) Hybrid total hip arthroplasty: 7- to 10-year results. *Clin Orthop Relat Res*, 333, 134–46.

Bernasek, T. L., Haidukewych, G. J., Gustke, K. A., Hill, O. and Levering, M. (2007) Total hip arthroplasty requiring subtrochanteric osteotomy for developmental hip dysplasia: 5- to 14-year results. *J Arthroplasty*, 22, 145–50.

Berry, D. J., Harmsen, W. S. and Ilstrup, D. M. (1998) The natural history of debonding of the femoral component from the cement and its effect on long-term survival of Charnley total hip replacements. *J Bone Joint Surg Am*, 80, 715–21.

Biant, L. C., Bruce, W. J., Assini, J. B., Walker, P. M. and Walsh, W. R. (2009) Primary total hip arthroplasty in severe developmental dysplasia of the hip. Ten-year results using a cementless modular stem. *J Arthroplasty*, 24, 27–32.

Bierbaum, B. E., Nairus, J., Kuesis, D., Morrison, J. C. and Ward, D. (2002) Ceramic-on-ceramic bearings in total hip arthroplasty. *Clin Orthop Relat Res*, 405, 158–63.

Brinker, M. R., Rosenberg, A. G., Kull, L. and Galante, J. O. (1994) Primary total hip arthroplasty using noncemented porous-coated femoral components in patients with osteonecrosis of the femoral head. *J Arthroplasty*, 9, 457–68.

Brodner, W., Bitzan, P., Meisinger, V., Kaider, A., Gottsauner-Wolf, F. and Kotz, R. (2003) Serum cobalt levels after metal-on-metal total hip arthroplasty. *J Bone Joint Surg Am*, 85-A, 2168–73.

Buly, R. (2005) The S-ROM stem: versatility of stem/sleeve combinations and head options. *Orthopedics*, 28, S1025–32.

Callaghan, J. J. (1993) The clinical results and basic science of total hip arthroplasty with porous-coated prostheses. *J Bone Joint Surg Am*, 75, 299–310.

Canale. S.T. and Beaty, J. H. (2007) *Campbell's Operative Orthopaedics*, 11th edn. Philadelphia, PA, Mosby Elsevier.

Chapman, M. W. (2001) *Chapman's Orthopaedic Surgery*, 3rd edn. Philadelphia, PA, Lippincott Williams & Wilkins.

Charles, M. N., Bourne, R. B., Davey, J. R., Greenwald, A. S., Morrey, B. F. and Rorabeck, C. H. (2005) Soft-tissue balancing of the hip: the role of femoral offset restoration. *Instr Course Lect*, 54, 131–41.

Charnley, J. (1961) Arthroplasty of the hip. A new operation. *Lancet*, 1, 1129–32.

Clohisy, J. C. and Harris, W. H. (1999) Primary hybrid total hip replacement, performed with insertion of the acetabular component without cement and a precoat femoral component with cement. An average ten-year follow-up study. *J Bone Joint Surg Am*, 81, 247–55.

Collis, D. K. and Mohler, C. G. (1998) Loosening rates and bone lysis with rough finished and polished stems. *Clin Orthop Relat Res*, 355, 113–22.

Cristofolini, L., Affatato, S., Erani, P., Tigani, D. and Viceconti, M. (2009) Implant fixation in knee replacement: preliminary in vitro comparison of ceramic and metal cemented femoral components. *Knee*, 16, 101–8.

Crowninshield, R. D., Jennings, J. D., Laurent, M. L. and Maloney, W. J. (1998) Cemented femoral component surface finish mechanics. *Clin Orthop Relat Res*, 355, 90–102.

D'Antonio, J. A. and Sutton, K. (2009) Ceramic materials as bearing surfaces for total hip arthroplasty. *J Am Acad Orthop Surg*, 17, 63–8.

Delp, S. L., Komattu, A. V. and Wixson, R. L. (1994) Superior displacement of the hip in total joint replacement: effects of prosthetic neck length, neck-stem angle, and anteversion angle on the moment-generating capacity of the muscles. *J Orthop Res*, 12, 860–70.

Diwanji, S. R., Seon, J. K., Song, E. K. and Yoon, T. R. (2007) Fracture of the ABC ceramic liner: a report of three cases. *Clin Orthop Relat Res*, 464, 242–6.

Dunstan, E., Ladon, D., Whittingham-Jones, P., Carrington, R. and Briggs, T. W. (2008) Chromosomal aberrations in the peripheral blood of patients with metal-on-metal hip bearings. *J Bone Joint Surg Am*, 90, 517–22.

Engh, C. A., Bobyn, J. D. and Glassman, A. H. (1987) Porous-coated hip replacement. The factors governing bone ingrowth, stress shielding, and clinical results. *J Bone Joint Surg Br*, 69, 45–55.

Engh, C. A., Jr., Culpepper, W. J., 2nd and Engh, C. A. (1997) Long-term results of use of the anatomic medullary locking prosthesis in total hip arthroplasty. *J Bone Joint Surg Am*, 79, 177–84.

Erdemli, B., Yilmaz, C., Atalar, H., Guzel, B. and Cetin, I. (2005) Total hip arthroplasty in developmental high dislocation of the hip. *J Arthroplasty*, 20, 1021–8.

Gent, E. and Clarke, N. M. (2004) Joint replacement for sequelae of childhood hip disorders. *J Pediatr Orthop*, 24, 235–40.

Glyn-Jones, S., Isaac, S., Hauptfleisch, J., Mclardy-Smith, P., Murray, D. W. and Gill, H. S. (2008) Does highly cross-linked polyethylene wear less than conventional polyethylene in total hip arthroplasty? A double-blind, randomized, and controlled trial using roentgen stereophotogrammetric analysis. *J Arthroplasty*, 23, 337–43.

Gray, H. (1918) *Anatomy of the Human Body*. Philadelphia, PA, Lea and Febiger.

Hamilton, W. G., Mcauley, J. P., Dennis, D. A., Murphy, J. A., Blumenfeld, T. J. and Politi, J. (2010) THA with Delta ceramic on ceramic: results of a multicenter investigational device exemption trial. *Clin Orthop Relat Res*, 468, 358–66.

Hannouche, D., Nich, C., Bizot, P., Meunier, A., Nizard, R. and Sedel, L. (2003) Fractures of ceramic bearings: history and present status. *Clin Orthop Relat Res*, 417, 19–26.

Hannouche, D., Hamadouche, M., Nizard, R., Bizot, P., Meunier, A. and Sedel, L. (2005) Ceramics in total hip replacement. *Clin Orthop Relat Res*, 430, 62–71.

Hartley, W. T., Mcauley, J. P., Culpepper, W. J., Engh, C. A., Jr. and Engh, C. A., Sr. (2000) Osteonecrosis of the femoral head treated with cementless total hip arthroplasty. *J Bone Joint Surg Am*, 82-A, 1408–13.

Heisel, C., Silva, M. and Schmalzried, T. P. (2004) Bearing surface options for total hip replacement in young patients. *Instr Course Lect*, 53, 49–65.

Jaeblon, T. (2010) Polymethylmethacrylate: properties and contemporary uses in orthopaedics. *J Am Acad Orthop Surg*, 18, 297–305.

Jaffe, W. L. and Scott, D. F. (1996) Total hip arthroplasty with hydroxyapatite-coated prostheses. *J Bone Joint Surg Am*, 78, 1918–34.

Kapandji, I. A. (1998) *The Physiology of Joints, Volume Two: Lower Limb*, 5th edn. New York, NY, Churchill Livingstone.

Kearns, S. R., Jamal, B., Rorabeck, C. H. and Bourne, R. B. (2006) Factors affecting survival of uncemented total hip arthroplasty in patients 50 years or younger. *Clin Orthop Relat Res*, 453, 103–9.

Lachiewicz, P. F., McCaskill, B., Inglis, A., Ranawat, C. S. and Rosenstein, B. D. (1986) Total hip arthroplasty in juvenile rheumatoid arthritis. Two to eleven-year results. *J Bone Joint Surg Am*, 68, 502–8.

McGrory, B., Barrack, R., Lachiewicz, P. F., Schmalzried, T. P., Yates, A. J., Jr., Watters, W. C., 3rd, Turkelson, C. M., Wies, J. L. and St Andre, J. (2010) Modern metal-on-metal hip resurfacing. *J Am Acad Orthop Surg*, 18, 306–14.

Min, B. W., Song, K. S., Kang, C. H., Bae, K. C., Won, Y. Y. and Lee, K. Y. (2007) Delayed fracture of a ceramic insert with modern ceramic total hip replacement. *J Arthroplasty*, 22, 136–9.

Moore, K. D., Beck, P. R., Petersen, D. W., Cuckler, J. M., Lemons, J. E. and Eberhardt, A. W. (2008) Early failure of a cross-linked polyethylene acetabular liner. A case report. *J Bone Joint Surg Am*, 90, 2499–504.

Murphy, S. B., Ecker, T. M. and Tannast, M. (2006) Two- to 9-year clinical results of alumina ceramic-on-ceramic THA. *Clin Orthop Relat Res*, 453, 97–102.

Noble, P. C., Kamaric, E., Sugano, N., Matsubara, M., Harada, Y., Ohzono, K. and Paravic, V. (2003) Three-dimensional shape of the dysplastic femur: implications for THR. *Clin Orthop Relat Res*, 417, 27–40.

Ranawat, A., Zelken, J., Helfet, D. and Buly, R. (2009) Total hip arthroplasty for posttraumatic arthritis after acetabular fracture. *J Arthroplasty*, 24, 759–67.

Schmalzried, T. P., Peters, P. C., Maurer, B. T., Bragdon, C. R. and Harris, W. H. (1996) Long-duration metal-on-metal total hip arthroplasties with low wear of the articulating surfaces. *J Arthroplasty*, 11, 322–31.

Tharani, R., Dorey, F. J. and Schmalzried, T. P. (2001) The risk of cancer following total hip or knee arthroplasty. *J Bone Joint Surg Am*, 83-A, 774–80.

Thillemann, T. M., Pedersen, A. B., Johnsen, S. P. and Soballe, K. (2008) Implant survival after primary total hip arthroplasty due to childhood hip disorders: results from the Danish Hip Arthroplasty Registry. *Acta Orthop*, 79, 769–76.

Thompson, J. C. (2002) *Netter's Concise Atlas of Orthopaedic Anatomy*, 1st edn. Philadelphia, PA, Saunders Elsevier.

Thyssen, J. P., Jakobsen, S. S., Engkilde, K., Johansen, J. D., Soballe, K. and Menne, T. (2009) The association between metal allergy, total hip arthroplasty, and revision. *Acta Orthop*, 80, 646–52.

Traina, F., Baleani, M., Viceconti, M. and Toni, A. (2004) Modular neck primary prosthesis: experimental and clinical outcomes. *Scientific Exhibit at the 71st AAOS Annual Meeting*, San Francisco.

Traina, F., De Fine, M., Biondi, F., Tassinari, E., Galvani, A. and Toni, A. (2008) The influence of the centre of rotation on implant survival using a modular stem hip prosthesis. *Int Orthop*, 33, 1513–8.

Traina, F., De clerico, M., Biondi, F., Pilla, F., Tassinari, E. and Toni, A. (2009) Sex differences in hip morphology: is stem modularity effective for total hip replacement? *J Bone Joint Surg Am*, 91 (Suppl 6), 121–8.

Traina, F., De Fine, M., Tassinari, E., Sudanese, A., Calderoni, P. P. and Toni, A. (2011) Modular neck prostheses in DDH patients: 11-year results. *J Orthop Sci*, 16, 14–20.

Traina, F., De. Fine, M., Sudanese, A., Calderoni, P. P., Tassinari, E. and Toni, A. (2011) Long-term result of total hip replacement in Legg–Calvè–Perthes disease. *J Bone Joint Surg Am*, 93, e25.

Trentani, C. and Vaccarino, F. (1978) The Paltrinieri–Trentani hip joint resurface arthroplasty. *Clin Orthop Relat Res*, 134, 36–40.

Vasavada, A. N., Delp, S. L., Maloney, W. J., Schurman, D. J. and Zajac, F. E. (1994) Compensating for changes in muscle length in total hip arthroplasty. Effects on the moment generating capacity of the muscles. *Clin Orthop Relat Res*, 302, 121–33.

Visuri, T., Pukkala, E., Paavolainen, P., Pulkkinen, P. and Riska, E. B. (1996) Cancer risk after metal on metal and polyethylene on metal total hip arthroplasty. *Clin Orthop Relat Res*, 329, S280–9.

5
Anatomy of the knee and suitable prostheses

F. TRAINA, M. DE FINE and S. AFFATATO,
Istituto Ortopedico Rizzoli, Italy

Abstract: The knee joint can be divided into two different joints, the patello-femoral joint and the tibio-femoral joint. The most important ligaments of the knee are the anterior and posterior cruciate ligaments, the internal and external collateral ligaments and the patellar tendon. The external and internal menisci are two fibrocartilagineous disks that improve the articular congruity between the femur and the tibia. The main movement of the knee is flexion and extension, although a little degree of rotation is allowed. The goal of total knee replacement is pain relief and restoration of knee function. Modern total knee arthroplasty consists of a femoral component, a tibial component, a tibial platform/ insert and a patellar component. Both femoral and tibial components are generally made of cobalt–chromium alloys, whereas the tibial insert and the patellar component are made of polyethylene. Component fixation to bone is usually achieved using bone cement (polymethylmethacrylate). Recent trends toward minimally invasive surgery and tissue-sparing procedures have led to the idea of replacing only one damaged compartment, in so-called unicompartimental knee replacement. The introduction of computer-aided systems such as surgical navigation and the use of oxidized zirconium or ceramic femoral components are the more recent developments.

Key words: knee anatomy, femur, tibia, meniscus, knee prostheses.

5.1 Bones and ligaments

The knee is a joint formed by four different bones: the femur (thigh bone), the tibia (shin bone), the patella (knee cap) and the proximal part of the fibula. The femur is a long bone that contributes to the formation of this joint through its distal extremity (Fig. 5.1). The main structures of the distal femoral epiphysis are the femoral condyles, which are two oblong prominences separated anteriorly by a groove, the patellar surface, and

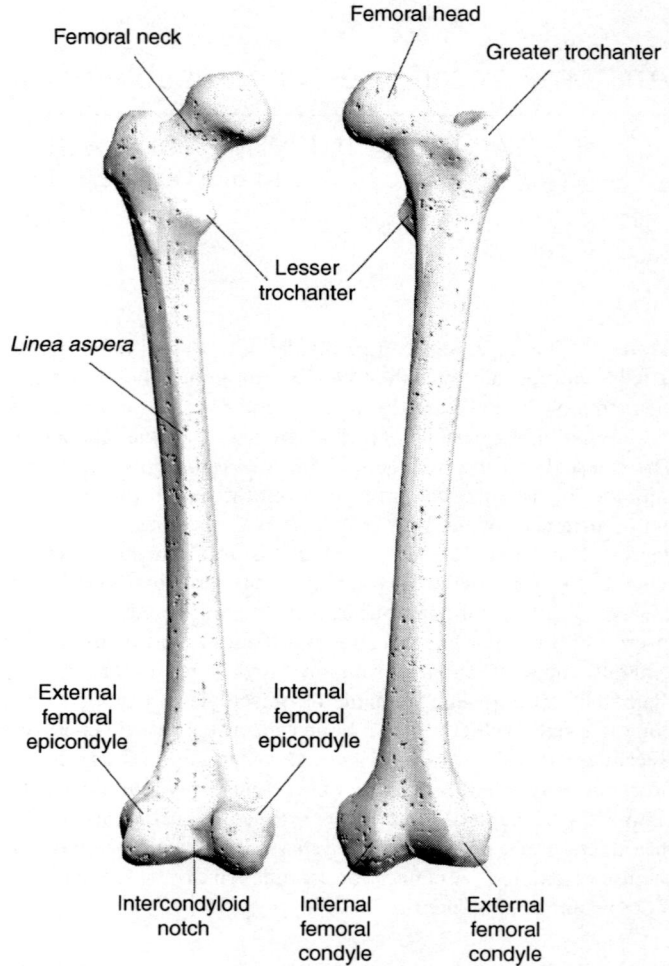

5.1 The left femur: posterior view on the left-hand side; anterior view on the right.

inferiorly and posteriorly by a deep notch, the intercondyloid fossa. The femoral condyles are convex and covered with smooth cartilage. The anterior aspect of the lateral condyle is most prominent with respect to that of the medial condyle. Above and laterally each femoral condyle are two small bony eminences, the medial and the lateral femoral epicondyles.

The tibia is also a long bone, which comprises a shaft and two enlarged epiphyses (Fig. 5.2). The proximal epiphysis makes contact with the distal femur by means of two tibial condyles. The superior part of the condyles consists of two articular facets for the femoral condyles; the medial facet is larger and has a slight concavity, whereas the lateral is concave in the coronal plane but slightly convex in the sagittal plane. In the mid-line of the superior articular surface of the proximal tibia, between the articular facets of the two condyles, is the intercondyloid eminence, which is a bony prominence surmounted by two tubercles, the spines of tibia. Along the anterior aspect of the proximal epiphysis, the tibial condyles are separated by an apophysis, the tibial tuberosity, whereas the intercondyloid fossa is a notch providing separation along the posterior surface of the proximal epiphysis. The lateral surface of the lateral condyle presents an articular facet for the head of the fibula.

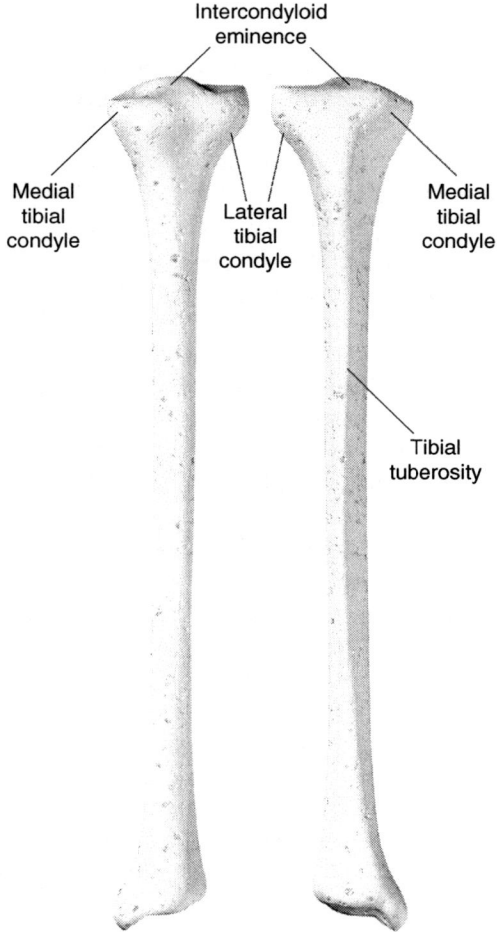

5.2 The right tibia: posterior view on the left-hand side; anterior view on the right.

The patella is a flat bone localized in front of the knee joint. Because it is a bone developed in the context of the *quadriceps femoris* tendon, the patella is considered a sesamoid bone. It has a triangular shape and a convex anterior surface. The posterior surface represents the articular surface of the patella, with the exception of its lower non-articular 25%. The articular area is further divided into two different facets by a longitudinal crest. The patella is embedded in the context of the quadriceps tendon, which inserts into its superior pole. The patella is connected to the tibia by the distal part of this tendon, the so-called patellar tendon, which inserts into the tibial tuberosity.

The fibula (calf bone) is a long bone extending laterally and parallel to the tibia. It has a body and two epiphyses. The proximal epiphysis, the head of the fibula, articulates with the tibia through an articular facet in its lateral aspect, forming the proximal tibio-fibular joint. The degree of movement of this joint is so slight that it can be regarded as motionless.

The knee is thus a very complex joint that has not been exhaustively classified. It is frequently considered as a ginglymus (hinge joint), but a different approach divides the knee into two different joints, the patello-femoral joint and the tibio-femoral joint (Fig. 5.3). The patello-femoral joint is an arthrodial joint (a gliding joint) that allows the articular surface of the patella to glide over the patellar groove of the distal femur. The tibio-femoral joint can be further divided into two condyloid joints between each femoral and tibial condyle. Therefore, the knee can be finally identified as a single joint composed of three different compartments – the patello-femoral compartment and the internal and exernal tibio-femoral compartments.

The articular capsule is a fibrous membrane that wraps around the knee, joining the bones to each other. Posteriorly, the capsule arises from the posterior aspect of the femoral condyles and inserts along the borders of the intercondyloid fossa of the tibia, and ligaments that restrain overextension of the knee reinforce it. The synovial membrane lies on the internal surface of the articular capsule, coating the articular cavity and particularly in the great recess beneath the quadriceps tendon. This membrane produces synovial fluid, which is a joint lubricant and provides nutrients for articular cartilage. Ligaments and tendons provide additional stability to the joint. The most important ligaments of the knee are the anterior and posterior cruciate ligaments and the internal and external collateral ligaments, the patellar tendon.

The internal collateral ligament, also called the medial or tibial collateral ligament, is a strong cord connecting the femur to the tibia; its origin is the medial femoral epicondyle and the medial aspect of the proximal tibia represents its insertion. The external collateral ligament, also called the lateral or fibular collateral the ligament, starts from the lateral femoral epicondyle and inserts into the head of the fibula. The cruciate ligaments are localized in the center of the knee joint. The anterior cruciate ligament arises

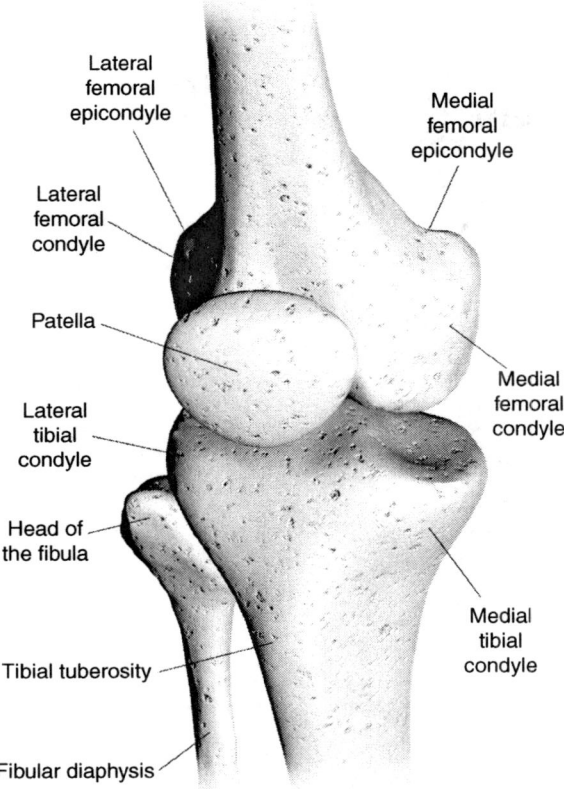

5.3 The knee joint.

just anteriorly with repsect to the intercondyloid eminence of the tibia and then it goes upward, inserting into the internal aspect of the lateral femoral condyle. The posterior cruciate ligament takes origin from the posterior part of the tibia, the intercondyloid fossa, and it inserts into the internal part of the medial femoral condyle. These ligaments owe their name to the fact that they form an 'X', crossing each other. The collateral ligaments resist lateral displacement of the tibia with respect to the femur, whereas the cruciate ligaments provide restrain to anteroposterior displacement. This complex system of ligaments also adds rotational stability to the knee.

To improve the articular congruity between the femur and the tibia, two fibrocartilagineous disks, the external and internal meniscus, are localized above each tibial condyle, increasing the depth of the tibial articular facets. These structures cover the outer part of the tibial facets and resemble a wedge that is thicker toward the periphery of the tibial condyles. The

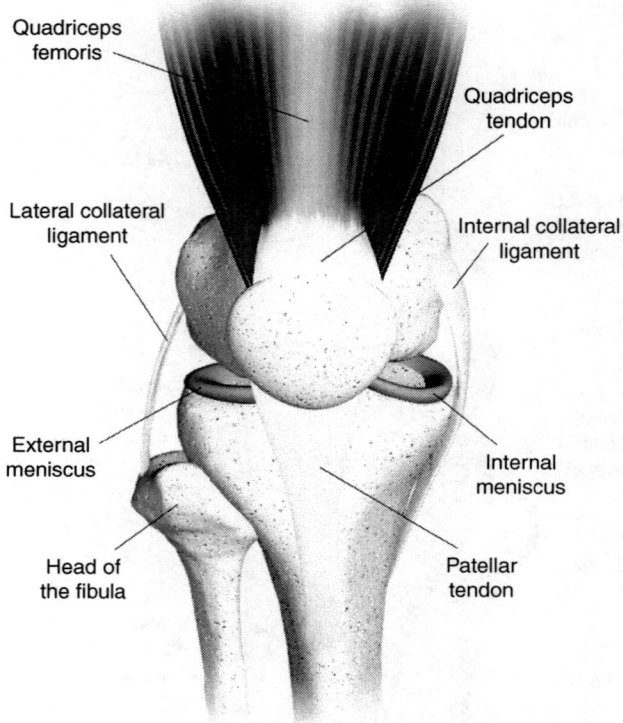

5.4 Ligaments and tendons around the knee.

internal meniscus has a semi-circular shape, whereas the external meniscus is nearly circular. The menisci are connected to the tibia along its periphery by means of the coronary ligaments, which are part of the articular capsule, and they are connected to each other anteriorly by the transverse ligament. The menisci act to cushion compressive forces and increase the stability of the joint (this is expecially true for the internal meniscus, which is firmly anchored to the bone) (Gray, 1918; Kapandji, 1998) (Fig. 5.4).

5.2 Kinematics

Although the main movement of the knee is around the transverse axis of the joint (flexion and extension), a little degree of rotation is allowed. Flexion is the movement by which the calf touches the posterior thigh (the extent of active flexion is 140°). Extension is the movement by which the leg returns to a straight position (at 0°) (Fig. 5.5), nevertheless a small degree (5–10°) of hyperextension could be possible. If more than 10° of hyperextension is allowed, the knee is defined as *genu recurvatum*, and it

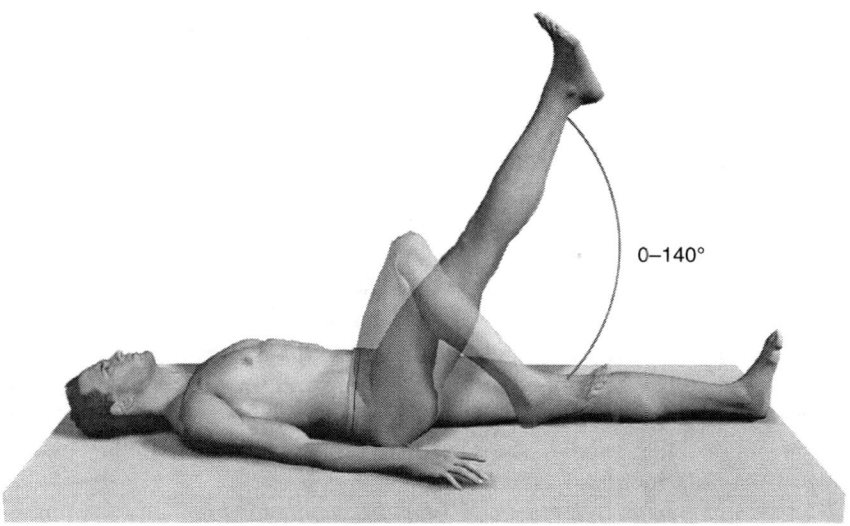

5.5 The range of knee extension and flexion.

is generally due to ligamentous laxity. The mechanism of knee flexion implies a combined movement of rolling and sliding of the distal femur over the proximal tibia. In fact, if it were just a simple rolling of the femoral condyles over the tibia, the knee would dislocate posteriorly before complete flexion; the forward sliding associated with the posterior rolling allows the maximum extent of flexion to be achieved without affecting knee stability.

Internal rotation is the movement to take the foot inward and external rotation moves the foot outward. The amount of rotation depends on the degree of flexion and therefore full knee extension is associated with a slight external rotation of the foot whereas a small degree of internal rotation is visible during full flexion (Fig. 5.6). These movements are considered automatic rotation because they are due to the anatomic conformation of the knee. The medial tibio-femoral compartment has a greater stability because of the closer articular congruity between the femoral and the tibial articular surfaces and the presence of the internal meniscus, which is more stable with respect to the lateral.

During extension, the medial compartment acts as a pivot while the lateral compartment slides forward, causing internal rotation of the femur over the tibia which consequently rotates outward. The opposite sequence is produced by knee flexion. Full extension locks the intercondyloid eminence of the tibia into the intercondyloid fossa of the femur, the collateral ligaments become taut and the posterior capsule and, to a lesser extent, the cruciate ligaments stretch, thus generating a position of greater knee stability. During flexion, there is a greater amount of joint laxity; external rotation of the tibia to 45° and internal rotation to 30° are allowed. Twisting around each other, the cruciate ligaments provide restraint to the internal rotation, whereas the internal collateral ligament checks the external rotation becoming tense. Flexion is associated with downward gliding of the patella over the patellar groove, whereas extension leads the patella to glide upward. In the straight leg position, the patella lies in front of the distal part of the femur, being completely disengaged from the patellar groove.

Knee extension is due to the action of the quadriceps femoris, which lies on the anterior aspect of the thigh, and is divided into four different muscles (rectus femoris, vastus lateralis, vastus medialis, vastus intermedius). It originates from the anterior superior iliac spine and the proximal part of the femur, inserting through the quadriceps tendon into the proximal pole of the patella. Below the patella, the tendon continues as the patellar tendon toward the anterior tibial tuberosity.

The *biceps femoris, sartorious, gracilis, semitendinosus* and *semimembranosus* are the main knee flexors. The *biceps femoris* originates with two

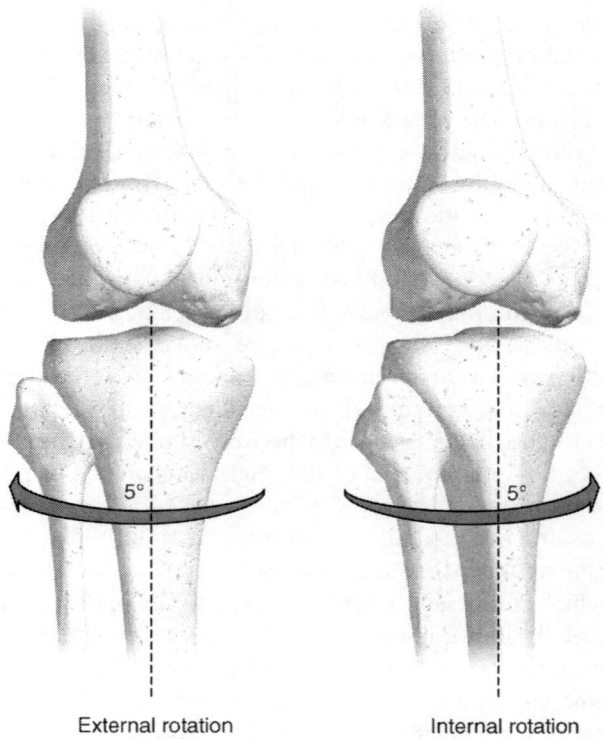

5.6 The amount of knee rotation.

heads from the ischial tuberositiy and from the posterior part of the femoral diaphysis, inserting into the head of the fibula. This muscle flexes and rotates outward the knee. The *sartorious* originates from the anterior superior iliac spine, the *gracilis* from the pubis, whereas the *semitendinosus* takes origin from the ischial tuberosity: these three muscles insert into the anterior and internal aspect of the proximal tibia through a common tendon, the *pes anserinus*. The *semimembranosus* connects the ischial tuberosisty with the posterior and internal part of the tibia and with the internal meniscus. These muscles provide flexion and inward rotation of the knee.

5.3 Biomechanics

The anatomical alignment of the lower limb results from the angle formed by the long axis of the femur and the long axis of the tibia. When the value is lower than 180° the knee is valgus, when it is higher than 180° it is varus. The extent of valgus angulation is controlled by the tension of the internal collateral ligament, while the external collateral ligament provides a restraint to varus angulation (Gray, 1918; Kapandji, 1998). Since the value of this angle averages 6°, the physiologic anatomical alignment of the lower limb is considered to be valgus.

The mechanical axis of the lower limb is the line by which body weight is transmitted to the joints of the lower limb. This line connects the center of the hip to the center of the ankle (Canale and Beaty, 2007; Chapman, 2001). If this line passes through the center of the knee, the resulting mechanical axis can be considered neutral (Fig. 5.7). If the line lies internally with respect to the center of the knee, there is a varus alignment of the lower limb; vice versa, a line passing externally with respect to the center of the knee produces a valgus alignment. The amount of varus or valgus deviation with respect to the neutral mechanical axis can be assessed by evaluating the angle formed by a line connecting the center of the hip to the intercondylar notch of the femur and a line connecting the center of the ankle to the intercondyloid eminence of the tibia. Unlike the anatomical valgus alignment, the average value of this angle in the normal population is 1° of varus angulation, thus resulting in a mechanical varus alignment. Due to different weight distribution, osteoarthritis affects the internal tibio-femoral compartment much more frequently. Since osteoarthritis causes damage to the cartilage layer and to the subcondral bone, the height of the internal tibio-femoral compartment decreases, increasing the extent of varus deformation and creating a vicious circle that progressively worsens knee function.

The patella transmits the quadriceps's strength to the tibia, acting as a pulley. Furthermore, moving this muscle away from the femur, the patella increases the quadriceps lever arm, improving the efficiency of the extensor

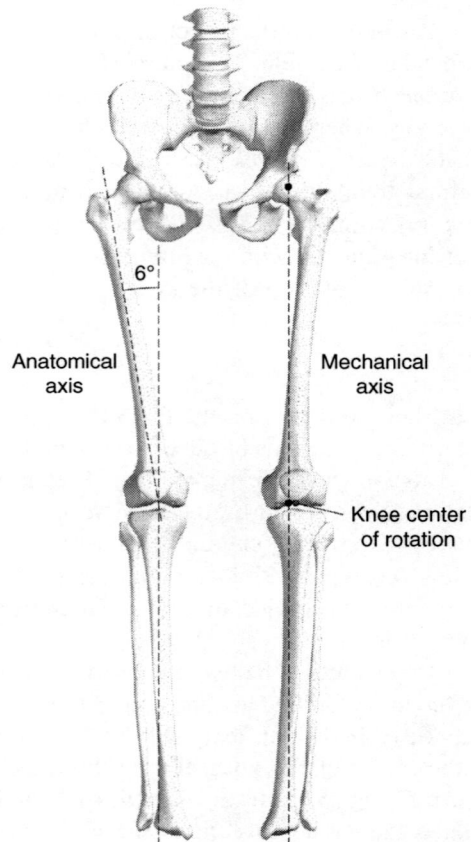

5.7 The anatomical and the mechanical axis. The mechanical axis lies just internally with respect to the knee center of rotation, thus producing a mechanical varus alignment.

mechanism (Fig. 5.8). Finally, the patella provides protection for the knee (Insall and Scott, 2006).

5.4 History and indications for total knee replacement

The first attempt at total knee replacement was carried out at the end of the nineteenth century by a German surgeon, Theophilus Gluck, who fixed ivory prosthetic components to the bone by means of plaster. Since this pioneer trial, no significant evolutions were made until 1973, when John Insall and colleagues popularized a knee prosthesis named 'total condylar knee'. This prosthesis is considered the prototype of modern knee prostheses and consisted of a metallic femoral component, a plastic tibial and patellar components, all fixed to the bone with cement. Cruciate ligaments were both sacrificed and joint stability was ensured by the geometry of the prosthetic components. After a few years, further evolutions led to the development of a total knee prosthesis with a metal back for the tibial component, and posterior cruciate ligament retention. In an effort to realize bone-sparing techniques, surgical procedures involving the substitution of only one tibio-femoral compartment – unicompartmental knee arthroplasty – was subsequently proposed.

In recent years, computer-aided systems to help surgeons achieve proper prosthetic component positioning have gained increasing popularity and cementless fixation and newer bearing options have been introduced (Ranawat, 2002). Due to excellent long-term clinical results, total knee replacement is now a successful operation and the rate of such prostheses is expected to grow in the future (Culliford et al., 2010).

The goal of total knee replacement is pain relief and restoration of knee function. Because the survival of knee prostheses is adversely influenced by the patient's activity level, the operation is usually proposed to patients in the sixth or seventh decade of life (Canale and Beaty, 2007; Chapman,

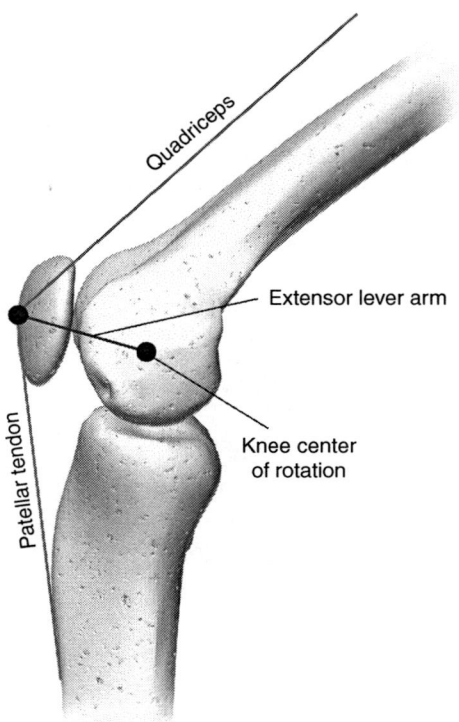

5.8 The patella acts to improve the extensor lever arm.

2001), although, good clinical outcomes have been reported in younger patients (Duffy *et al.*, 1998).

The main reason for total knee replacement is primary osteoarthritis, which is a degenerative process due to ageing and leads to joint impairment. Secondary osteoarthritis occurs as a result of an altered load distribution around the knee and is generally due to post-traumatic disorders (fractures of the distal femur or proximal tibia) or congenital anomalies that produce varus or valgus alignments. Further indications for total knee replacement include osteonecrosis of the femoral condyles (Radke *et al.*, 2005), rheumatoid arthritis (Meding *et al.*, 2004) and hemophilic arthropathy (Goddard *et al.*, 2010).

5.5 Prosthetic designs and bearing surfaces

Modern total knee arthroplasty consists of a femoral component, a tibial component, a tibial platform/insert and a patellar component (Fig. 5.9). Both femoral and tibial components are generally made of cobalt–chromium alloy, whereas the tibial insert and the patellar component are made of polyethylene. The femoral component reproduces the anatomy of the distal femur; it has an asymmetrical anterior flange similar to the patellar grove, which is useful to avoid lateral dislocation of the patella. The tibial component looks like the tibial platform and is further stabilized by means of a short stem that fits into the tibial medullary canal. The tibial insert is secured to the tibial component and its superior surface is congruent with the outer surface of the femoral component. The patellar component is an all-polyethylene dome.

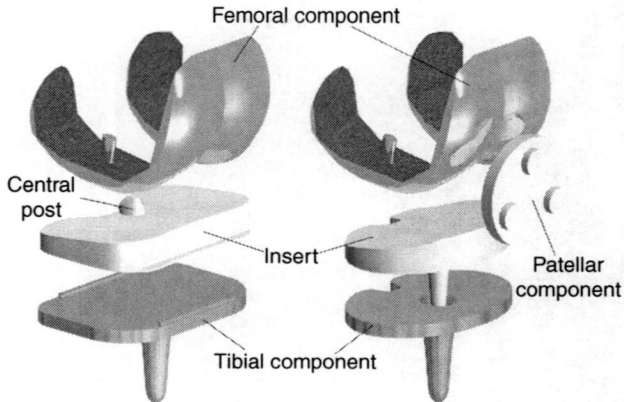

5.9 Components of a standard total knee arthroplasty. The left-hand side shows a posterior-stabilized prosthesis while the right image is of a cruciate-retaining model.

Component fixation to bone is usually achieved using bone cement (polymethylmethacrylate). Unlike total hip arthroplasty, cemented fixation is considered the gold standard (Font-Rodriguez *et al.*, 1997; Malkani *et al.*, 1995; Scuderi *et al.*, 1989) as most reports on cementless prostheses indicate poorer outcomes (Meneghini and Hanssen, 2008) in comparison with the excellent results of cemented prostheses (Callaghan and Liu, 2010).

Two different designs of standard total knee arthroplasty are currently available: posterior-stabilized prostheses and cruciate-retaining prostheses (Fig. 5.9). Posterior-stabilized designs require both cruciate ligaments to be sacrificed and introduce a cam mechanism to reproduce the combined movement of rolling and sliding of the distal femur over the proximal tibia. At about 70° of flexion, the cam, which is a box localized in the center of the femoral component, engages a central post in the tibial insert, thus preventing the femur from dislocating posteriorly during flexion.

Cruciate-retaining designs leave the posterior cruciate ligmanet *in situ*. The main theoretical advantage of this design is a greater amount of knee flexion. Numerous studies have compared the degree of flexion of posterior-stabilized and cruciate-retaining prostheses, but no conclusive statements confirming the supposed superior performance of cruciate-retaining designs have been reported (Seon *et al.*, 2011). Further questions have arisen about patellar resurfacing. Some researchers advise performing tricompartmental knee arthroplasties, implanting the patellar component any time during the primary operation, whereas others advise patellar resurfacing only in selected cases. Since patellar pain is the most common complication after total knee replacement, patellar resurfacing can be also regarded as a salvage procedure. This matter remains under debate (Canale and Beaty, 2007; Chapman, 2001; Fu *et al.*, 2011; He *et al.*, 2011; Li *et al.*, 2011).

Both cruciate-retaining and posterior-stabilized knees can be associated with mobile tibial inserts. Because of the possibility of the tibial insert slightly rotating over the tibial component during flexion and extension, mobile bearing prostheses are characterized by the high congruence between the tibial platform and femoral component, allowing the load to be distributed over the largest area and contact stresses to be reduced. This mechanical behavior should theoretically decrease the polyethylene wear rate, but even in this case there is no agreement in the literature (Kelly *et al.*, 2011; Smith *et al.*, 2011).

Specific types of knee prostheses are useful in cases of difficult knee surgery. The constrained condylar knee was developed by Insall and colleagues as an evolution of the traditional total condylar knee (Donaldson *et al.*, 1988). This model was realized by increasing the depth of the femoral cam and enlarging the tibial post. Furthermore, a femoral stem and a longer tibial stem were added to restrain varus or valgus stresses, further improving stability. These features allow the constrained condylar knee to be used in

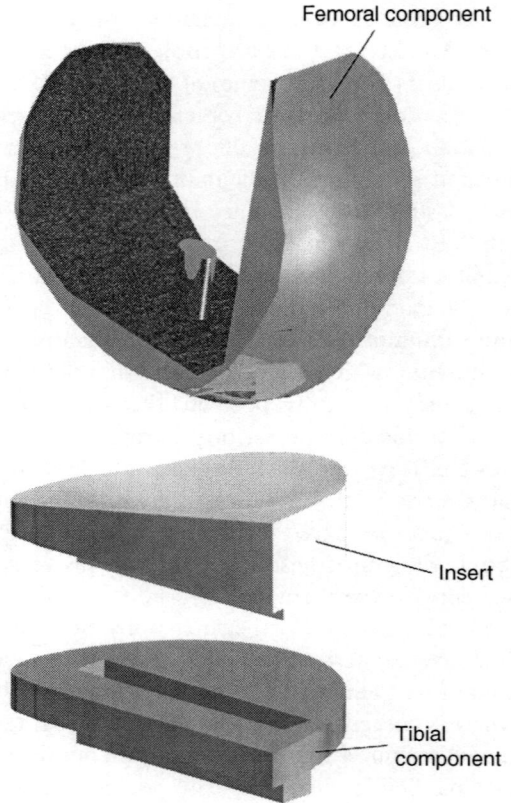

5.10 Unicompartmental knee arthroplasty.

cases of severe valgus deformity (Sculco, 1989; Stern *et al.*, 1991) or revision knee surgery (Rand, 1991). Hinged prostheses represent alternative models that are especially useful in cases of revision surgery. These designs incorporate the longest femoral and tibial stems and a central hinge, allowing flexion and rotatory movements by means of a rotating platform (Barrack *et al.*, 2000; Jones, 2006). Unlike constrained prostheses, which tolerate a little degree of varus or valgus tilting, hinged implants completely eliminate these movements.

Recent trends toward minimally invasive surgery and tissue-sparing procedures led to the idea of replacing only one damaged compartment, the so-called unicompartmental knee replacement (Fig. 5.10). Reduced blood loss, less hospitalization time and quicker rehabilitation are some of the purported advantages of this surgical approach. Due to the bone-preserving nature of unicompartmental knee replacement, straightforward revision to a standard total knee arthroplasty was advocated as another favorable feature. The unicompartmental model can be proposed to older patients, giving them less surgical trauma in comparison with a standard total knee replacement, or to young people with unicompartmental knee disease (e.g. osteonecrosis of one femoral condyle) considering the high probability of a second operation during their lifetime (Jamali *et al.*, 2009; McAllister, 2008; Repicci and Hartman, 2004; Vince and Cyran, 2004). However, since there is no consensus with regard to the advantages of unicompartmental knee arthroplasty, the choice of knee implant design is left to the personal surgeon's perspective. In this model, the metallic femoral component articulates with the tibial polyethylene insert; thus metal-on-polyethylene coupling is generally accepted as the most widely used bearing option.

5.6 Future trends

The introduction of computer-aided systems such as surgical navigation and the use of oxidized zircomium or ceramic femoral components are some of the more recent inventions.

Surgical navigation was introduced in an effort to improve the accuracy of implant positioning and component alignment during a total knee replacement procedure. Various systems for surgical navigations are available and this tool was thought to be of paramount importance, especially for young, less experienced surgeons. Although navigation seems to help surgeons achieve better component positioning, long-term studies that demonstrate the superior outcomes of navigated total knee replacements are lacking (Deirmengian and Lonner, 2009; Haaker *et al.*, 2005; Lutzner *et al.*, 2008, 2010).

Considering the outstanding results achieved with ceramic bearing surfaces in total hip arthroplasty, the use of ceramics has been proposed recently to reduce the problem of polyethylene wear and implant loosening in total knee replacements. All-ceramic femoral components have been used with encouraging results, but concerns about ceramic brittleness led to a newer approach involving the use of oxidized zirconium. This is a zirconium – niobium alloy thermally treated in the presence of oxygen, thus resulting in a oxidized layer with surface characteristics similar to those of ceramics but without the brittleness (Cristofolini *et al.*, 2009; Heyse *et al.*, 2011; Innocenti *et al.*, 2010; Majima *et al.*, 2008).

Further developments in these areas and their role in knee replacement surgery remain interesting for the future.

5.7 Acknowledgment

We would like to thank Luigi Lena (Rizzoli Orthopaedic Institute) for his valuable assistance with all the images presented in this chapter.

5.8 References

Barrack, R. L., Lyons, T. R., Ingraham, R. Q. and Johnson, J. C. (2000) The use of a modular rotating hinge component in salvage revision total knee arthroplasty. *J Arthroplasty*, 15, 858–66.

Callaghan, J. J. and Liu, S. S. (2010) Cementless tibial fixation in TKA: not a second coming. *Orthopedics*, 33, 655.

Canale S.T. and Beaty, J. H. (2007) *Campbell's Operative Orthopaedics*, 11th edn. Philadelphia, PA, Mosby Elsevier.

Chapman, M. W. (2001) *Chapman's Orthopaedic Surgery*, 3rd edn. Philadelphia, PA, Lippincott Williams & Wilkins.

Cristofolini, L., Affatato, S., Erani, P., Tigani, D. and Viceconti, M. (2009) Implant fixation in knee replacement: preliminary in vitro comparison of ceramic and metal cemented femoral components. *Knee*, 16, 101–8.

Culliford, D. J., Maskell, J., Beard, D. J., Murray, D. W., Price, A. J. and Arden, N. K. (2010) Temporal trends in hip and knee replacement in the United Kingdom: 1991 to 2006. *J Bone Joint Surg Br*, 92, 130–5.

Deirmengian, C. A. and Lonner, J. H. (2009) What's new in adult reconstructive knee surgery? *J Bone Joint Surg Am*, 91, 3008–18.

Donaldson, W. F., 3rd, Sculco, T. P., Insall, J. N. and Ranawat, C. S. (1988) Total condylar III knee prosthesis. Long-term follow-up study. *Clin Orthop Relat Res*, 226, 21–8.

Duffy, G. P., Trousdale, R. T. and Stuart, M. J. (1998) Total knee arthroplasty in patients 55 years old or younger. 10- to 17-year results. *Clin Orthop Relat Res*, 356, 22–7.

Font-Rodriguez, D. E., Scuderi, G. R. and Insall, J. N. (1997) Survivorship of cemented total knee arthroplasty. *Clin Orthop Relat Res*, 345, 79–86.

Fu, Y., Wang, G. and Fu, Q. (2011) Patellar resurfacing in total knee arthroplasty for osteoarthritis: a meta-analysis. *Knee Surg Sports Traumatol Arthrosc*, 19, 1460–6.

Goddard, N. J., Mann, H. A. and Lee, C. A. (2010) Total knee replacement in patients with end-stage haemophilic arthropathy: 25-year results. *J Bone Joint Surg Br*, 92, 1085–9.

Gray, H. (1918) *Anatomy of the Human Body*. Philadelphia, PA, Lea and Febiger.

Haaker, R. G., Stockheim, M., Kamp, M., Proff, G., Breitenfelder, J. and Ottersbach, A. (2005) Computer-assisted navigation increases precision of component placement in total knee arthroplasty. *Clin Orthop Relat Res*, 345, 152–9.

He, J. Y., Jiang, L. S. and Dai, L. Y. (2011) Is patellar resurfacing superior than nonresurfacing in total knee arthroplasty? A meta-analysis of randomized trials. *Knee*, 18, 137–44.

Heyse, T. J., Chen, D. X., Kelly, N., Boettner, F., Wright, T. M. and Haas, S. B. (2011) Matched-pair total knee arthroplasty retrieval analysis: Oxidized zirconium vs. CoCrMo. *Knee*, 18, 448–52.

Innocenti, M., Civinini, R., Carulli, C., Matassi, F. and Villano, M. (2010) The 5-year results of an oxidized zirconium femoral component for TKA. *Clin Orthop Relat Res*, 468, 1258–63.

Insall J. N. and Scott N. (2006) *Surgery of the Knee*, 4th edn. Philadelphia, PA, Churchill Livingstone.
Jamali, A. A., Scott, R. D., Rubash, H. E. and Freiberg, A. A. (2009) Unicompartmental knee arthroplasty: past, present, and future. *Am J Orthop (Belle Mead NJ)*, 38, 17–23.
Jones, R. E. (2006) Total knee arthroplasty with modular rotating-platform hinge. *Orthopedics*, 29, S80–2.
Kapandji, I. A. (1998) *The Physiology of Joints. Volume Two: Lower Limb*, 5th edn. New York, NY, Churchill Livingstone.
Kelly, N. H., Fu, R. H., Wright, T. M. and Padgett, D. E. (2011) Wear damage in mobile-bearing TKA is as severe as that in fixed-bearing TKA. *Clin Orthop Relat Res*, 469, 123–30.
Li, S., Chen, Y., Su, W., Zhao, J., He, S. and Luo, X. (2011) Systematic review of patellar resurfacing in total knee arthroplasty. *Int Orthop*, 35, 305–16.
Lutzner, J., Gunther, K. P. and Kirschner, S. (2010) Functional outcome after computer-assisted versus conventional total knee arthroplasty: a randomized controlled study. *Knee Surg Sports Traumatol Arthrosc*, 18, 1339–44.
Lutzner, J., Krummenauer, F., Wolf, C., Gunther, K. P. and Kirschner, S. (2008) Computer-assisted and conventional total knee replacement: a comparative, prospective, randomised study with radiological and CT evaluation. *J Bone Joint Surg Br*, 90, 1039–44.
Majima, T., Yasuda, K., Tago, H., Aoki, Y. and Minami, A. (2008) Clinical results of posterior cruciate ligament retaining TKA with alumina ceramic condylar prosthesis: comparison to Co-Cr alloy prosthesis. *Knee Surg Sports Traumatol Arthrosc*, 16, 152–6.
Malkani, A. L., Rand, J. A., Bryan, R. S. and Wallrichs, S. L. (1995) Total knee arthroplasty with the kinematic condylar prosthesis. A ten-year follow-up study. *J Bone Joint Surg Am*, 77, 423–31.
McAllister, C. M. (2008) The role of unicompartmental knee arthroplasty versus total knee arthroplasty in providing maximal performance and satisfaction. *J Knee Surg*, 21, 286–92.
Meding, J. B., Keating, E. M., Ritter, M. A., Faris, P. M. and Berend, M. E. (2004) Long-term followup of posterior-cruciate-retaining TKR in patients with rheumatoid arthritis. *Clin Orthop Relat Res*, 428, 146–52.
Meneghini, R. M. and Hanssen, A. D. (2008) Cementless fixation in total knee arthroplasty: past, present, and future. *J Knee Surg*, 21, 307–14.
Radke, S., Wollmerstedt, N., Bischoff, A. and Eulert, J. (2005) Knee arthroplasty for spontaneous osteonecrosis of the knee: unicompartimental vs bicompartimental knee arthroplasty. *Knee Surg Sports Traumatol Arthrosc*, 13, 158–62.
Ranawat, C. (2002) History of total knee replacement. *J South Orthop Assoc*, 11, 218–26.
Rand, J. A. (1991) Revision total knee arthroplasty using the total condylar III prosthesis. *J Arthroplasty*, 6, 279–84.
Repicci, J. A. and Hartman, J. F. (2004) Minimally invasive unicondylar knee arthroplasty for the treatment of unicompartmental osteoarthritis: an outpatient arthritic bypass procedure. *Orthop Clin North Am*, 35, 201–16.
Scuderi, G. R., Insall, J. N., Windsor, R. E. and Moran, M. C. (1989) Survivorship of cemented knee replacements. *J Bone Joint Surg Br*, 71, 798–803.

Sculco, T. P. (1989) Total condylar III prosthesis in ligament instability. *Orthop Clin North Am*, 20, 221–6.

Seon, J. K., Park, J. K., Shin, Y. J., Seo, H. Y., Lee, K. B. and Song, E. K. (2011) Comparisons of kinematics and range of motion in high-flexion total knee arthroplasty: cruciate retaining vs. substituting designs. *Knee Surg Sports Traumatol Arthrosc*, 19, 2016–22.

Smith, H., Jan, M., Mahomed, N. N., Davey, J. R. and Gandhi, R. (2011) Meta-analysis and systematic review of clinical outcomes comparing mobile bearing and fixed bearing total knee arthroplasty. *J Arthroplasty*, 26, 1205–13.

Stern, S. H., Moeckel, B. H. and Insall, J. N. (1991) Total knee arthroplasty in valgus knees. *Clin Orthop Relat Res*, 273 5–8.

Vince, K. G. and Cyran, L. T. (2004) Unicompartmental knee arthroplasty: new indications, more complications? *J Arthroplasty*, 19, 9–16.

6
Orthopaedic implant materials and design

D. TIGANI, Santa Maria alle Scotte Hospital, Italy,
M. FOSCO, R. BEN AYAD and R. FANTASIA,
Istituto Ortopedico Rizzoli, Italy

Abstract: Knee and hip arthroplasties are designed to replace biological materials that have been damaged, to relieve pain and improve joint function and quality of life. This chapter discusses modern designs of prosthetic components for hip and knee replacement and considers the evolution of prosthetic models in the past. The chapter reviews all biomaterials used in contemporary total joint designs: metals, polymers, ceramics and composites.

Key words: knee arthroplasty, hip arthroplasty, ceramic, trabecular metal, ultra-high molecular weight polyethylene (UHMWPE).

6.1 Introduction

Joint implants are designed to replace biological materials that have been damaged, to relieve pain and to improve joint function and patient quality of life. In most cases, injured cartilage and bone are removed from the articulating surfaces of the joint and synthetic materials are used in their place. The major design objectives in artificial joint replacement are: (1) the geometry and material design of the articulating surfaces; (2) the design of the surface contact between the artificial component and the host bone. Modern design of prosthetic components for joint replacement involves functional and structural considerations about the evolution of prosthetic models in the past.

Materials used in prosthetic joints must be able to transmit normal loads and provided laxity and range of motion, while structurally they must be durable for a long time (Bahraminasa and Jahan, 2011; Bureau, 2005). Black (1992) defined biomaterials as materials of natural or manmade origin that are used to direct, supplement or replace the functions of living tissues. Trial tests and errors that have occurred in the past, in both laboratory and clinical settings, have restricted the possible biomaterials used in contemporary total joint designs to four categories: (1) metals; (2) polymers (acrylic, nylon, silicone, polyurethane, ultra-high molecular weight polyethylene (UHMWPE) and polypropylene; (3) ceramics; (4) composites.

6.2 Materials in knee and hip arthroplasty

Materials used in orthopaedic implants should represent three main criteria of load transfer capacity, good fixation and biocompatibility. Another important non-mechanical requirement of an orthopaedic biomaterial is 'inertness' (www.fda.org). However, in reality, such a state is unachievable and a relative degree of implant degradation is therefore considered acceptable.

6.2.1 Metals and alloys

Metals and alloys require particular treatments to achieve biocompatibility. The alloys currently used as orthopaedic biomaterials are protected from accelerated corrosion by a passive oxide layer that acts like an electrical resistor to retard the anodic dissolution of metal.

Cobalt–chromium

There are basically two types of cobalt (Co) chromium (Cr) alloys: CoCrMo (Mo, molybdenum) alloy and CoNiCrMo (Ni, nickel) alloy. Cast CoCrMo alloys have been used for many decades in dentistry and, recently, as biomaterials for prosthetic components of artificial joints. Nickel–chromium alloys have a chromium content of at least 20% in order for these alloys to be corrosion-resistant and thus biocompatible. Chromium protects the underlying metal through the formation of mechanically and chemically stable oxide layers. Alloys with less than 0.1% nickel can be designated nickel-free. The claim that a cobalt–chromium alloy is absolutely nickel-free would be objectively false.

An important property of a cobalt-based alloy is its high resistance to corrosion; moreover, such alloys are quite resistant to fatigue and cracking caused by corrosion and they are not brittle, having a minimum elongation of 8%. However, cobalt-based alloys can fail because of fatigue fracture (but this occurs less often than for stainless steel stems).

The wrought CoNiCrMo alloy is a relative newcomer, now used to produce prosthesis stems for heavily loaded joints such as the knee and hip. It is similar to the CoCrMo alloy in abrasive wear properties, although it is not recommended for the bearing surfaces of artificial joints because of its poor frictional properties with other materials (Alvarado *et al.*, 2003).

Stainless steel

Stainless steel is the generic name for a number of different steels all sharing a minimum percentage of chromium, added to improve corrosion resistance. Other elements, particularly nickel and molybdenum, could be added. The principal properties of stainless steel are corrosion resistance, fire and heat resistance, hygiene (the easy cleaning ability of stainless steel makes it the first choice for strict hygiene conditions), strength-to-weight advantage (allowing reduced material thickness compared with conventional grades, thus yielding cost savings), ease of fabrication, impact resistance and long-term durability (http://www.avestapolarit.com/template).

All grades of stainless steel can be divided into five classes; each is identified by the alloying elements that affect their microstructure and for which each is named. Stainless steel 316L is the type mainly used for joint replacements.

Titanium and titanium alloys

Titanium (Ti) has been used for more than 30 years for implants and surgical devices. It is the most biocompatible of all metals because of its resistance and tolerance to body fluids. The high strength, low weight and outstanding corrosion resistance possessed by Ti and Ti alloys has led to a diverse range of successful applications. Pure Ti metal has a relatively low density, a high melting point (1668°C) and an elastic modulus of 107 GPa (15.5×10^6 psi).

The mechanical and physical properties of Ti alloys combine to provide implants that are highly damage-tolerant. The lower modulus of elasticity of Ti alloys compared with steel is a positive factor in reducing bone resorption (Table 6.1). Two further parameters define the usefulness of an implantable alloy – notch sensitivity (the ratio of tensile strength versus un-notched condition) and resistance to crack propagation (or fracture toughness) (Burstein *et al.*, 2000). There are three structural types of titanium alloys.

1 Alpha (α) alloys are non-heat-treatable and are generally very weldable. They possess excellent mechanical properties at cryogenic temperatures.
2. Alpha–beta (α–β) alloys are heat-treatable and most are weldable. Their strength levels are medium to high. Their hot-forming qualities are good, but their high-temperature creep strength is not as good as most alpha alloys.
3. Beta (β) alloys, or near-beta alloys, are readily heat-treatable, are generally weldable and have high strengths and good creep resistance at intermediate temperatures.

Ti alloys are excellent biomaterials, especially when direct contact with

Table 6.1 Names and properties of prosthetic biomaterials

Material/alloy	Corrosion resistance	Osteointegration	Wear resistance	Modulus of elasticity (GPa)	Elongation (%)
Stainless steel L316 (annealed)	High	Above average	Above average	200	40
Stainless steel L316 (cold-worked)	High	Above average	Very high	200	12
Co-Cr alloys (wrought Co–Ni–Cr–Mo)	Very high	High	Extremely high	240	10–30
Co-Cr alloys (cast Co–Cr–Mo)	Very high	High	Extremely high	240	10–30
Ti alloys (pure Ti)	Exceptionally high	Very high	Above average	100	54
Ti alloys (Ti-6Al-4V)	Exceptionally high	Very high	High	112	12
Ti-6Al-7Nb (IMI-367 wrought)	Exceptionally high	Very high	High	105–120	≥10
Ti-6Al-7Nb (Protasul-100 hot-forged)	Exceptionally high	Average	High	110	10–15
NiTi shape memory alloy	Extremely high	Exceptionally high	Exceptionally high	≥48	12
Porous NiTi shape memory alloy	Very high		Exceptionally high	15	12

tissue or bone is required. The poor shear strength of Ti alloys makes them unsuitable for bone screws or plates. They also have poor surface wear properties and tend to seize when in sliding contact with another Ti alloy or other metal. Surface treatments such as nitriding and oxidizing can improve the surface wear properties.

6.2.2 Ceramics

Ceramics are brittle, polycrystalline solids, used in orthopaedics by fusing or sintering microscopic grains of alumina (Al_2O_3) and/or zirconia (ZrO_2) ceramic powder into a consolidated product. The powder composition (i.e. purity and size of granular powder particles) determines the strength of the ceramic component. Ceramics have several outstanding tribological properties including hardness, which contributes to wear and scratch resistance. Ceramic surfaces are also more hydrophilic than CoCr surfaces; the improved wettability of ceramics leads to lower friction than CoCr when articulated against UHMWPE under physiologic loading and lubrication conditions (Morlock *et al.*, 2002).

There are four types of ceramics that are clinically used in prosthetic joint replacements. These are alumina, zirconia and zirconia-toughened alumina (ZTA) composites, oxidized zirconium and silicon nitride.

1. Alumina is the ceramic composite with the oldest history of use in orthopaedic implants. Currently, CeramTec AG (Plochingen, Germany) is the world's largest supplier of medical-grade alumina.
2. Zirconia was initially chosen for commercialization largely due to its higher strength relative to alumina. Zirconia particles, which are finely distributed in a stable aluminia matrix, will change phase from tetragonal to monoclinic once there is a crack. This phase change increases the particle volume up to approximately 5%, which helps reduce energy consumption and can stop crack propagation by closing the crack space (Dalla Pria, 2007). For articulations with UHMWPE, or for use in ceramic-on-ceramic (CoC) alternate bearings, a newer and more complex alumina composite incorporating zirconia has emerged as the current state-of-the-art biomaterial. Zirconia-toughened alumina (ZTA) matrix composite (BIOLOX Delta, CeramTec AG, Plochingen, Germany) consists of an alumina matrix (82% by volume) reinforced with zirconia (17%), strontium aluminate (0.5%) and chromium oxide (0.5%). The additives are incorporated into the alumina matrix to provide crack tip blunting and toughening mechanisms, as well as to increase the hardness of the composite (Fig. 6.1).
3. Oxidized zirconium is a ceramic implant material marketed under the

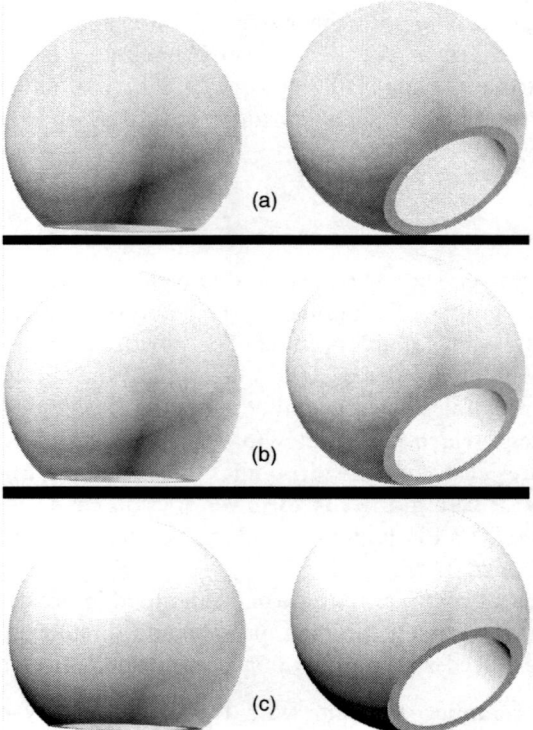

6.1 Alumina (a), zirconia (b) and zirconia-toughened alumina (ZTA) (c) femoral head components.

trade name Oxinium (Smith & Nephew Orthopedics, Memphis, Tennessee, USA) (Sheth *et al.*, 2008). Clinically introduced for the knee in December 1997 and for the hip in October 2002, oxidized zirconium is intended only for hard-on-soft bearings in both total hip arthroplasty (THA) and total knee arthroplasty (TKA) (Fig. 6.2). The ceramic surface of Oxinium provides increased scratch resistance and is more wettable and provides lower UHMWPE wear in a hip simulator than that provided by a CoCr alloy femoral head, without the negative risks associated with ceramic fracture because of the ductile zirconium alloy substrate (Bourne *et al.*, 2005; Li *et al.*, 2006).

4. Silicon nitride is a ceramic composite recently introduced in hip arthroplasty. With an elastic modulus of 300 GPa and a fracture toughness of 10 MPa m$^{1/2}$, this material provides a higher strength than alumina. Wear testing of ceramic-on-metal (CoM) and CoC bearings in a hip simulator demonstrated ultra-low wear rates, comparable to or

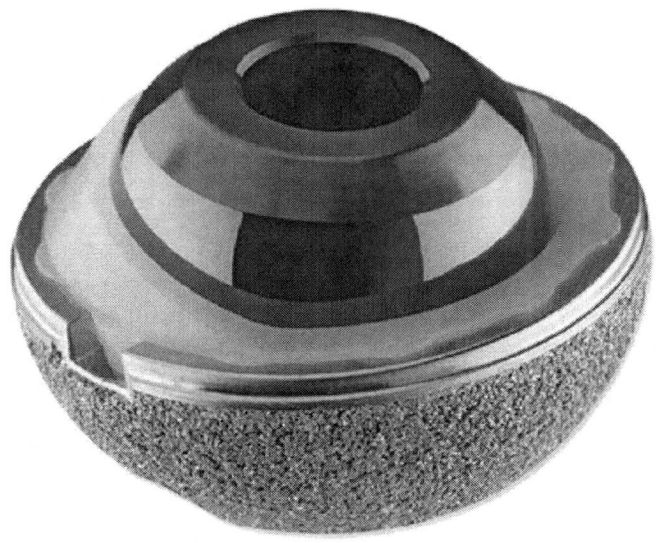

6.2 Oxidized zirconium femoral head component coupled with polyethylene insert (courtesy of Smith & Nephew).

lower than alumina–alumina (Bal *et al.*, 2009). Nevertheless, clinical results of implanted components of this material are not yet available.

Ceramics in hip arthroplasty

The application of ceramic materials in hip arthroplasty has its origins in Europe and Japan. Pierre Boutin, in collaboration with Ceraver Inc., France, first reported clinical results of CoC hip arthroplasty in the early 1970s (Boutin, 1971, 1972). In 1977 Shikata, in Japan, introduced the concept of using alumina femoral heads with UHMWPE acetabular components.

The first generation of CoC components consisted of a monolithic acetabular component, fabricated entirely from alumina (Al_2O_3), articulating against an alumina femoral head, fitted using a tapered interlock to the metallic femoral stem. The potential for extremely low clinical wear rates exhibited by those early components (Bizot *et al.*, 2000; Jazrawi *et al.*, 1999; Nevelos *et al.*, 1993) inspired increased interest in the development of new CoC designs during the 1990s (second-generation ceramic bearings) (Boehler *et al.*, 2000).

Laboratory tests have demonstrated that the harder surfaces of ceramic biomaterials should theoretically be more scratch-resistant than CoCr femoral heads for articulation against UHMWPE (Cuckler *et al.*, 1995; Lancaster *et al.*, 1997). However, the real clinical benefit of ceramic femoral heads in hip arthroplasty has not been fully established. For reasons associated with *in vivo* phase transformation and surface roughening of zirconia, clinical wear studies published in the past 5 years with zirconia heads have reported mixed results in the literature, ranging from no significant difference to inferior performance relative to CoCr heads.

Ceramics in knee arthroplasty

Ceramic implant designs for TKA have been developed mainly to address the potential problem of allergic reactions in patients due to the release of wear particles from modern titanium or cobalt–chromium alloy components (Bader *et al.*, 2008; Dalla Pria, 2007; Kircher *et al.*, 2007; Rack and Pfaff, 2001).

The first biocompatible ceramic product was implanted as a unicondylar tibial surface replacement by G. Langer in 1972 and resulted in limited wear between the ceramic and cartilage (Langer, 2002). The first alumina total knee prosthesis was realized by the Kyocera Corp. (Kyoto, Japan) and implanted by Oonishi in the early 1980s (Oonishi *et al.*, 1992). First-generation TKA from 1981 to 1985 consisted of alumina femoral and tibial components and an UHMWPE insert (Fig. 6.3).

Second-generation TKA, from 1990 to 1996, consisted of an alumina femoral component, a titanium alloy tibial component and an UHMWPE insert (Fig.6.4). The alumina tibial component used in first-generation TKA was changed to a titanium alloy component to be fixed with bone cement because alumina tibial components were thick and brittle, and a relatively

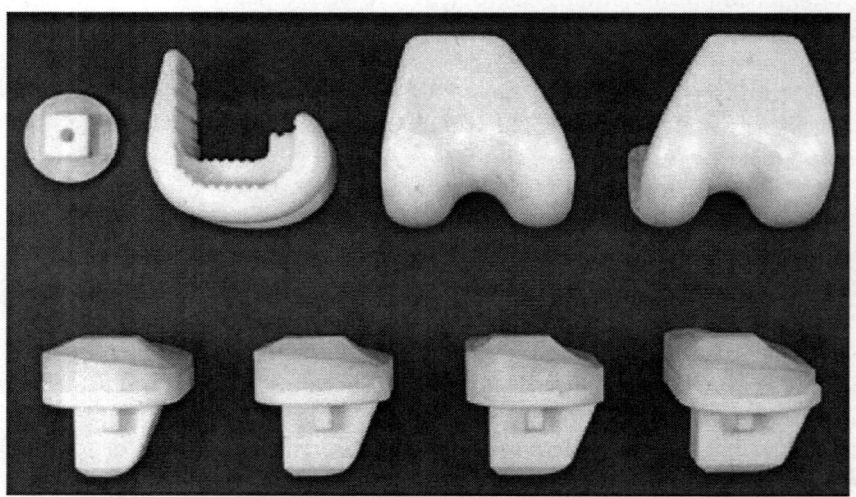

6.3 First-generation ceramic components for knee arthroplasty (1981–1985) (modified from Oonishi *et al.*, 2006).

Orthopaedic implant materials and design 141

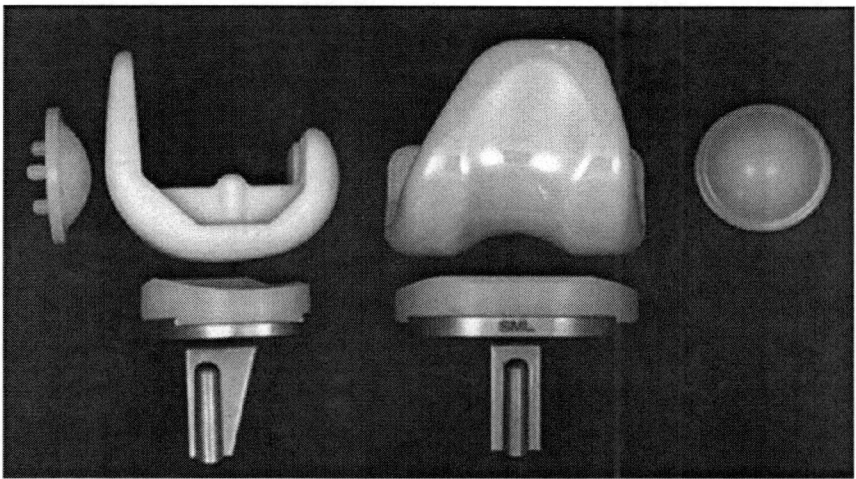

6.4 Second-generation femoral ceramic components for knee arthroplasty (1990–1996) (modified from Oonishi *et al.*, 2006).

high incidence of sinking and occurrence of radiolucent lines were observed when cementless fixation was used.

In third-generation TKA, used from 1993 to 1998, a porous coating of ceramic beads was applied to the surface of the femoral component to improve fixation between the bone cement and the ceramic (Fig. 6.5).

Long-term results (follow-up ranging from 5 to 10 years) of 105 cemented alumina ceramic knee prostheses (Kryocera Corp., Kyoto, Japan) showed a tibial plate fracture in one case; however the fracture of metal implants has also been reported (Abernethy *et al.*, 1996; Majima *et al.*, 2008; Yasuda, 2004). While the use of ceramics in THA was worldwide, there was extreme resistance to the use of ceramic knee arthroplasty outside Japan, mainly due to some unfavourable mechanical properties of ceramics – high brittleness, the absence of plastic deformation in comparison with ductile materials and low tensile strength.

In THA, articulating components are used with optimum contact contributions, resulting in low stresses, even if joint loads are very high. On the contrary, total knee replacements require components (especially the femoral component) with shapes and contact conditions that necessarily result in high stresses near the corners of femoral resections (tension stress) and at the points of contact with the polyethylene (shear stress). New alternative strategies include the use of a ZTA composite with which it is possible to develop a femoral component with a tensile strength that meets the demands for application in total knee replacement (Fig. 6.6).

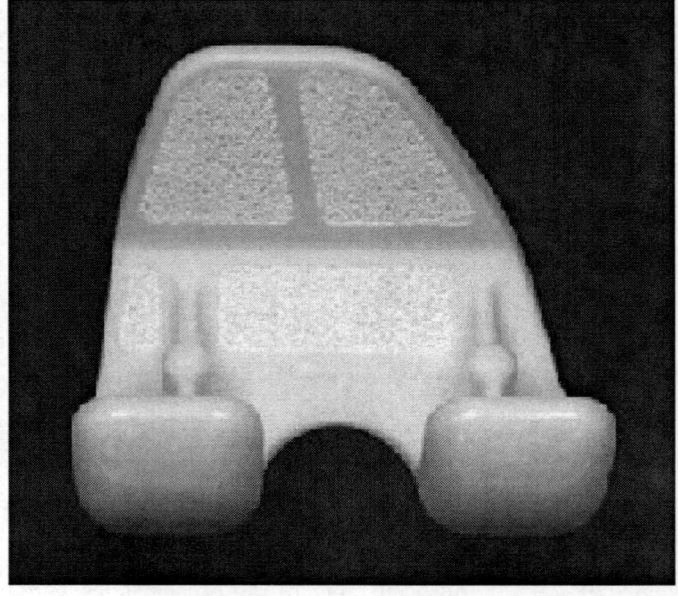

6.5 Third-generation femoral ceramic component for knee arthroplasty (1993–1998) (modified from Oonishi *et al.*, 2006).

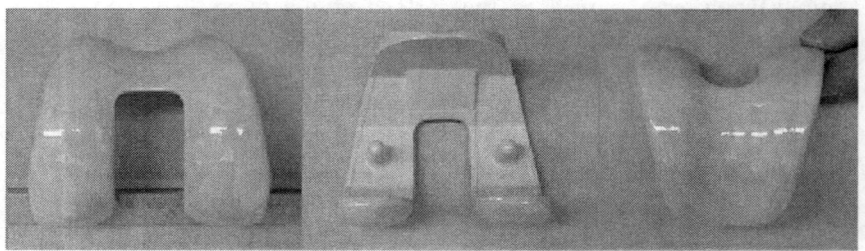

6.6 Multigen Plus TKR (Lima, San Daniele, Italy) symmetric femoral component made with Biolox® Delta ceramic (CeramTec AG, Polchingen, Germany).

6.2.3 Polyethylene

Each year, about two million joint replacement procedures are performed around the world and the majority of these incorporate UHMWPE (Li and Burstein, 1994). UHMWPE, a member of the polyethylene family, is made from the polymerization of ethylene, with a deceptively simple chemical composition, consisting of only hydrogen and carbon. The different types of polyethylene can be classified into: (i) low density; (ii) linear low density; (iii) high density; (iv) ultra-high molecular weight (Stephen, 1999).

The manufacturing processes of components differ with respect to the type of radiation used (gamma radiation or electron beam), the radiation dose, the method of thermal stabilization (remelting or annealing), machining and final sterilization (McKellop et al., 1999; Muratoglu et al., 2001). Most notable properties of UHMWPE are its chemical inertness, lubricity, higher impact strength and toughness, and abrasion resistance. Wear and damage of UHMWPE components have historically been factors that limit implant longevity (Hood et al., 1983). Damage to UHMWPE is different in total knee and total hip replacements. In a total hip prosthesis, the main types of damage are burnishing and abrasion of the acetabular insert and pitting, delamination, deformation and fracture of the tibial insert. This difference has been attributed to differences in kinematics, loading and geometry of joint components (Wright et al., 1988).

As a consequence of polyethylene evolution, and in the first 30 years of its use as a bearing surface, UHMWPE was primarily sterilized by gamma irradiation treatment in the presence of oxygen. Over the last 10 years, however, it has been realized that this irradiation renders the material unstable, causes chain scission and the formation of free radicals that induce oxidative degradation; this leads to delamination and fatigue failure, particularly in non-conforming highly stressed designs (Bell et al., 1998; Goodfellow, 1992; Reeves et al., 2000).

Stabilized polyethylene was thus introduced to reduce the incidence of oxidative degradation. Methods of stabilization include irradiation in an inert atmosphere or sterilization by other methods such as in ethylene oxide or gas plasma. In laboratory tests and clinical applications, these stabilized materials have shown resistance to delamination and fatigue failure (Bell et al., 1998; Reeves et al., 2000). Cross-linking has been used to improve the wear resistance of polyethylene; approximately 10- Mrad electron beam or gamma radiation is used to produced highly cross-linked polyethylene. Wear simulator studies have indicated that cross-linking can reduce polyethylene wear up to 80–90% (McKellop et al., 1999; Muratoglu et al., 2001, 2003). The advantages of highly cross-linked polyethylene are improved wear resistance, improved oxidative resistance and potentially lower susceptibility of third-body wear (Rajadhyaksha et al., 2009).

6.2.4 Trabecular Metal Technology (TMT)/non–TMT augments

Conventional orthopaedic implants have typically been fashioned from stainless steel or cobalt–chromium and titanium alloys. Because conventional metals used for fabrication of orthopaedic devices are typically unable to directly bond to living bone, numerous surface coatings and porous designs have been developed to enhance the biological fixation of implants to bone (Levine et al., 2006). Hydroxyapatite and other ceramics have been shown to spontaneously bond to bone, but these materials are brittle and cannot be used as bone substitutes for high-load bearing joints. These bioactive materials have also been shown to degrade over time and have the potential to debond from the underlying metallic surface (Bleobaum et al., 1994; Miyazaki et al., 2000). Moreover, as an increasingly younger patient population undergoes TKA, the orthopaedic surgery community must consider techniques and implants that may preserve bone for a potential revision TKA.

Tantalum, a transition metal, has shown favorable biological and mechanical characteristics in this regard (Levine et al., 2006). In vitro, tantalum shows a modulus of elasticity similar to that of subchondral bone and lower than that of conventional implant materials (i.e. titanium and cobalt–chromium); its fatigue properties and endurance limits are greater than those of cancellous bone, freeze-dried bone fragments, ceramic granules or composite calcium salt pastes (Shimko et al., 2005; Zardiackas et al., 2001). The biological advantages include its negative charge and interconnective pores, which form a scaffolding and surface for osteoblast-mediated bone ingrowth (Bobyn et al., 1999; Levine et al., 2007). With biomaterial properties similar to those of host bone, stress shielding is minimized and load transfer across the implant should be more uniform, thus resulting in an increase in the loading of the bone in contact with the whole implant.

These inherent properties and proven *in vivo* biocompatibility make porous tantalum a useful metal for the design and manufacture of press-fit or cementless components for total joint arthroplasty (Levine et al., 2006). The mechanical properties of the components allow this material to be used in orthopaedic applications requiring immediate weight bearing (given its high frictional characteristics) and bone ingrowth, while its corrosion resistance could be associated with less peri-implant stress shielding (Levine et al., 2006; Zhang et al., 1999). Porous tantalum components and augments are currently available for use in both primary and revision THA (Fig. 6.7) and TKA.

In knee arthroplasty, the use of metal augments for bone deficiencies has become quite popular since the mid-1980s after work by Brooks et al. (1984) indicated that, biomechanically, the modular augments are equivalent to a custom implant. Nevertheless, the first reported use of modular metal augments to augment bone stock deficiencies in TKA was by Brand et al. in 1989 (Brand et al., 1989).

A new class of prosthetic porous metal augments has been recently introduced, trabecular metal (TM) (Zimmer, Warsaw, IN, USA). TM is available in many shapes and forms (porous or solid, rectangular or wedge shaped, metaphyseal cones or patella buttons) and can be attached with the use of cement or screws (Fig. 6.8).

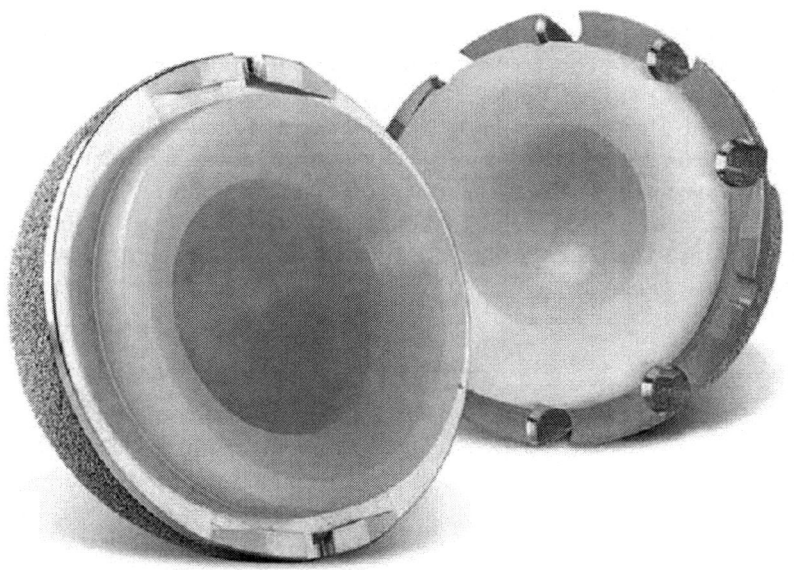

6.7 Acetabular polyethylene component with metal back, coated by tantalum surface (courtesy of Zimmer, Warsaw, IN, USA).

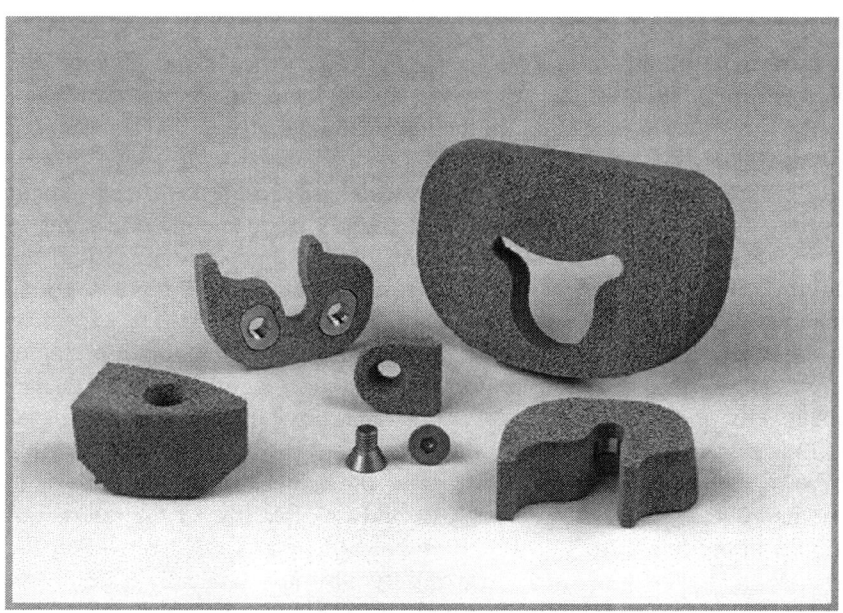

6.8 TM modular augments (courtesy of Zimmer, Warsaw, IN, USA).

TM has gained popularity because it can be applied quickly, allows intraoperative custom fabrication, supplies excellent biomechanical properties and requires minimal bone resection as the augments attach on the residual bone. However, a lack of long-term follow-up studies in comparison with alternative reconstructive techniques has limited its widespread acceptance. In the future, the perspective of the fibrous ingrowth potential of this metal makes it an option for coating specific regions of a prosthesis requiring soft tissue fixation (i.e. tendinous and muscular attachments).

6.2.5 Cement

Total joint replacements generally involve implantation of components held in place in a press-fit manner or by a cement mantle. Polymethylmethacrylate (PMMA) was developed by Charnley and firstly used for cementation in THA in 1969 (Charnley, 1970). PMMA is a derivative of acrylic acid that is formed by the combination of a monomer liquid mixed with polymer powder, thus leading to an exothermic reaction with a change into a solid state. Barium sulfate is often added to produce radiopacity for roentgenographic evaluation of the bone cement and metal–cement interfaces; although the addition of barium changes the properties slightly, the ability to visualize interfaces is of great importance.

The polymerization process takes several minutes, with a change from the liquid state (early state) through a doughy period (intermediate state) to a solid material (final state). Various physical factors can influence the polymerization process; for example, lower temperature and humidity lengthen the elapsed time between the liquid and doughy states (Hansen and Jensen, 1990).

All cements are not identical. In particular, the viscosity of the cement and the particle size of the powder vary slightly from one manufacturer to another. Surgical technique can also contribute to correct cementation: the ideal thickness of the cement mantle around a prosthesis is a major concern, recommended to be between 2 and 5 mm (Boss et al., 1993). The cement is not an adhesive agent and performs best under conditions of compression; moreover, slight compression after implantation contributes to deeper cement penetration in the bone, which can theoretically lead to firmer fixation and less chance of prosthetic loosening over time. It has been argued that the exothermic reaction occurring as the cement sets within the bone may theoretically lead to bone necrosis and possible loss of the interstitial complex in the bone (Boss et al., 1993). Nevertheless, it now seems that the thermal effects of cemented arthroplasty are not clinically significant. Antibiotics could be added to the cement mixture, usually in the setting of a revision procedure or after a previous infection. Although cement properties change with this addition, the fatigue properties are not changed at all.

Due to the limited mechanical properties of PMMA, the incorporation of hydroxyapatite in PMMA has been investigated. It has been shown that this not only improves the mechanical properties of PMMA but the osteoblast response of PMMA is also enhanced (Moursi et al., 2002; Vallo et al., 1999).

The elastic modulus of PMMA is higher than that of cancellous bone and slightly higher than that of polyethylene, so that loosening of the components often occurs at the interface between cement and bone. Although deeper penetration of cement into the interstices of cancellous bone should improve the mechanical interlock, subsequent bone resorption often results due to the modulus mismatch between cancellous bone and cement.

6.3 Evolution of total knee arthroplasty

Many current knee prostheses are derived from models designed in the 1960s and 1970s. The first models (Polycentric, Geomedic, Duocondylar) were considered unsatisfactory because of a high percentage of component mobilizations, component breakages and infection. However, the experience acquired with these systems allowed resurfacing prostheses planning to occur in successive design phases in two different ways: the anatomical approach and the functional approach (Robinson, 2005).

6.3.1 Anatomical approach

Advocators of the anatomical approach studied prostheses that preserve one or both cruciate ligaments and allow the femur to roll back on the tibia. At the Hospital for Special Surgery (HSS) in New York, during the early 1970s, the Duocondylar knee was completely redesigned in an anatomical and symmetrical design, resulting in the Duopatella. An anterior femoral flange, a patellar button and a more dished tibial surface were added. The tibial component had a fixation peg and, for the first time, a posterior rectangular cutout specifically designed for the preserved posterior cruciate ligament.

Although the results of the Duopatella were extremely good at the HSS, the posterior cruciate-preserving approach was developed in Boston at the Robert Breck Brigham Hospital (RBBH) (Scott, 1982; Sledge and Ewald, 1979). The posterior cruciate-retaining version developed at RBBH would later evolve into the PFC knee (Cintor Division of Codman; later, DePuy, Johnson & Johnson, Warsaw, IN, USA). At the same time, Peter Walker, Clement Sledge and Fred Ewald continued the Duopatella concept in the posterior cruciate-retaining version of the Kinematic knee (Howmedica, New York, NY, USA), which was implanted by Ewald in June 1978. This would evolve into the posterior cruciate-sparing versions of the Kinematic II, Kinemax and Kinemax Plus systems (Howmedica).

The 1980s saw significant advances in knee arthroplasty, particularly in the areas of surgical technique and instrumentation. Kenna, Hungerford and Krackow participated in the design of instruments that were later called Universal Instruments. Their tools were based on the anatomical concept of the measured resection technique. The principal aspect of this new conception was that the bone and cartilage removed were to equal the thickness of the prosthetic material replacing them.

In January 1980, the first porous-coated anatomical (PCA) knee was implanted by Hungerford at Johns Hopkins Hospital in Baltimore (Hungerford et al., 1982). The implant was anatomical with asymmetric medial and lateral femoral condyles and, for the first time, it introduced porous coating in a total condylar knee for a cementless fixation. Each of the three components was backed with metal and a 1.5 mm thick sintered porous coating of cobalt–chromium beads.

The Miller–Galante total knee, one of the first knee replacements designed for use with both cement and cementless fixation, was first implanted in 1986. The principal innovation of this implant was the choice of a titanium fiber composite for the bony ingrowth surface, because of its well-recognized biocompatibility, and the use of a titanium–aluminum–vanadium alloy (Ti_6Al_4V). The implant is fixed to the tibia with titanium screws and pegs.

'Cruciate-retaining' prostheses developed from the anatomical concept were different (Fig. 6.9): some consisted of a relatively flat surface on the sagittal and transversal plane (Kinemax and PCA Howmedica, Warsaw, IN, USA) while others maintained a more congruent surface on the sagittal plane. Genesis II (Smith & Nephew, Warsaw, IN, USA), Duracon (Howmedica), Nexgen CR (Zimmer), PFC CR (DePuy) represent some actual examples of this conception.

6.3.2 Functional design

Designers of the functional approach tried to simplify the knee biomechanics by removing both cruciate ligaments. The first system derived from the functional concept is represented by the total condylar (TC) prosthesis developed in 1973 at the HSS (Insall et al., 1976). The TC prosthesis consisted of two symmetric condylar surfaces with a posterior decreasing radius of curvature and an articular surface made of polyethylene, perfectly congruent in extension and partially congruent in flexion. The TC knee would prove to be highly successful and widely used, and would later demonstrate long survival (Vince et al., 1989). However, two concerns, were noted in the early phases of its clinical use. The first was that the femoral

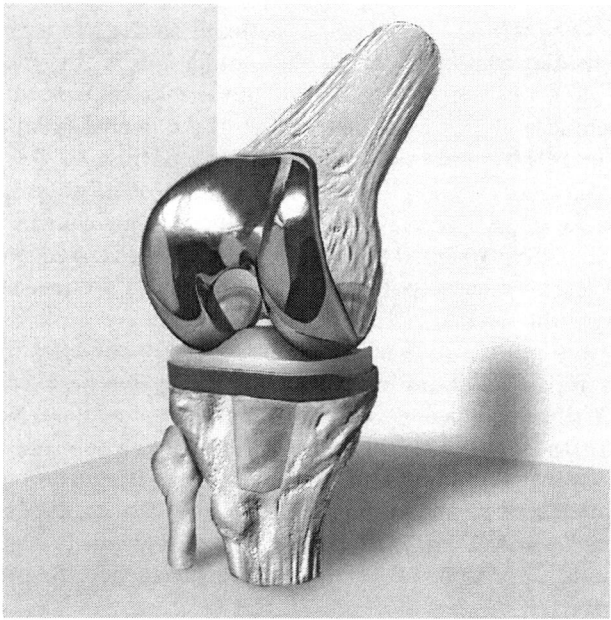

6.9 Model resembling a modern cruciate-retaining knee prosthesis (courtesy of Fabio Catani, MD).

component would shift forward, particularly in flexion. The second concern was the limited flexion achieved; average knee flexion with the TC knee was, in fact, 90° (Robinson, 2005).

In 1978, the Insall–Burstein prosthesis (IBPS) was designed to correct these problems by replacing the posterior cruciate ligament with a mechanical lock to reduce posterior translation of the femoral component by using a mechanism of a cam articulated with a post on the tibial component. The cam of the femoral component connected with the tibial central spine at about 70° of flexion and then the femur could roll back so to increase flexion (average flexion would be 115°) (Abdeen *et al.*, 2010). The HSS posterior-stabilized knee design would evolve into the Insall–Burstein Modular (IBPS II) knee (Zimmer) in 1988, the Optetrak Posterior-Stabilized knee (Exactech) in 1994 and the Advance Posterior-Stabilized knee (Wright Medical, Peschiera Borromeo, Italy) in 1994.

In the 1980s and 1990s, many variations of these functional designs were introduced by different manufacturers. All of them had the characteristic of producing motion through a so-called 'guided motion', which means that some characteristics of the motion, such as roll-back, are produced by mechanical interaction between the femoral and tibial components. An example of the guided motion knee was the Medial Pivot knee (Wright Mfg

Co, Memphis, TN, USA), in which a ball-and-socket configuration is present in the medial compartment. In that configuration, the medial side remains in the same position during flexion, but the lateral femoral condyle can displace behind with flexion. The purpose of the medial pivot design is to reproduce more physiological kinematics. In contrast to this type of solution, the 3D Knee was introduced. This provides anteroposterior stability similar to anterior cruciate ligament-deficient valgus knees through a concave lateral compartment. The aim of the, 3D Knee is to accommodate and control cruciate-deficient patterns of motion without constraints in a way to reproduce the normal kinematics of the knee.

One of the most innovative functional approaches to condylar total knee design evolved from a collaboration between Frederic Buechel (orthopaedic surgeon) and Michael Pappas (professor of mechanical engineering) at the New Jersey Medical School. Their project to achieve a low polyethylene contact stress while maintaining knee flexion and avoiding overload of the implant bone interfaces started in 1977 (Buechel and Pappas, 1986) with the introduction of the Low Contact Stress (LCS) knee system. It was the first complete systems approach to total knee replacement using meniscal bearing surfaces.

6.3.3 Mobile bearing (MB) knees

The principal characteristic of the femoral component was based on the same spherical surface on the mediolateral plane while a decreasing radius of curvature from extension to flexion was present on the lateral side. This shape maintained full area contact on the upper meniscal bearing from the 0 to 45° at which walking loads are encountered, maintaining a least spherical line at deeper flexion angles. In its origin, the LCS was proposed as a system inclusive of both the cruciate-sparing meniscal bearing and posterior cruciate ligament-sacrificing rotating platform variant, with the latter gaining the majority of popular usage over time. After the introduction of the LCS system, several types of MB knees were produced. They are categorized according to their conformity, either partially or fully conforming, and a third group represented by the posterior-stabilized MB.

Partially conforming MB

The LCS, other than being the ancestor of all MB prostheses is also, with its second version featuring a single plastic bearing that freely rotates about its post seated within a hole in the tibial tray, the prototype of the partially conforming MB. Partially conforming knees include the Self Aligning MB (Sulzer Orthopedics, Austin, TX, USA) designed by Bourne and Rorabeck in 1987, the MB knee called TACK produced in 1990 (Waldemar Link,

Hamburg, Germany) and the Interax Integrated Secure Asymmetric prosthesis (Howmedica). In Italy, Professor Ghisellini designed the Total Rotating Knee (TRK) (Cremascoli Ortho, Verona, Italy), characterized by a central tibia post projecting from the center of the tibial tray.

Fully conforming MB

The progenitor of fully conforming MB knees is certainly the Rotaglide Total Knee System (Corin, Cirencester, UK) designed in 1986 by Polyzoides and Tsakonas. The rotaglide femoral component has a constant flexion radius of curvature in the femoro-meniscal articulation, each condyle being part of a sphere of 24 mm radius. This design ensures that congruency is retained throughout the range of flexion. The tibial plateau has an anterior bollard that prevents anterior dislocation while restricting the rotation of the platform and another bollard in the middle of the tray that resists posterior dislocation.

The Medially Based Kinematics (MBK) knee was developed by Insall, Aglietti and Walker in 1992. The design concept of this prosthesis is complete conformity between the femoral component and the polyethylene insert at any degree of flexion and during rotation and anteroposterior translation of the tibial insert on the tibial tray. The prosthesis design allows medially based kinematics guided by the natural knee's stronger medial structures and greater lateral mobility.

Posterior-stabilized MB

These design are based on the 'cam and post' mechanism on a rotating polyethylene platform. The common feature is the presence of a cam situated between the posterior femoral condyles that engages a post projecting from the mobile polyethylene platform. The cam and post mechanism acts as a third weight-bearing condyle to help improve load transfer and minimize polyethylene stress. Belonging to this category are the Two Radii Area Contact (TRAC, Biomet, Warsaw, IN, USA), introduced in 1997, and the more recent designs P.F.C. Sigma RPF (DePuy) and the LPS mobile Flex (Zimmer).

6.4 History of total hip arthroplasty

Total replacement arthroplasty of the hip can be considered one of the great biomedical successes of the twentieth century. The design and manufacture of the components, surgeon skill level, patient disease and use of the implant after surgery (everyday activity) are the most important aspects for the longevity of implants.

The first attempt at hip replacement was carried out in Germany by Gluck in 1890, who used ivory to replace a femoral head. Before him, other surgeons dealt with arthritis of the hip using different methodologies. Excision arthroplasty is probably the earliest recorded procedure: resection of the proximal femur by White in 1822 restored some mobility at the expense of marked shortening.

Interposition arthroplasty was the next development in surgery for hip arthritis. This consisted of separation of the arthritic joint surfaces by a layer of material to prevent further degeneration and ankylosis. In this operation, the surgeons attempted to produce an extrarticular pseudoarthrosis. Many organic and inorganic materials were tried, including skin, fascia lata, silver, gold foil, rubber, celluloid and tanned pig bladder. In 1927, Hey-Groves, who had already used intramedullary ivory rods to fix femoral shaft fractures, described an uncemented short-stemmed ivory prosthesis with a hemispherical head (Hey-Groves, 1927). In 1943, the Judet brothers developed a similar prosthesis in acrylic, later modified to include metal reinforcement in the stem (Judet and Judet, 1950) (Fig. 6.10); very soon these prostheses were developed in acrylic, steel and vitallium. All had a similar design – a short stem inserted in the axis of femoral neck so that weight bearing tended to shear the head off the stem. The high failure rate of the short stem design led surgeons to experiment with long-stemmed prostheses that could transmit weight physiologically down the femoral shaft, virtually introducing the so-called endoprostheses.

Frederick Thompson developed a vitallium prosthesis in 1950 that had a flared collar below the head and a vertical cemented intramedullary stem

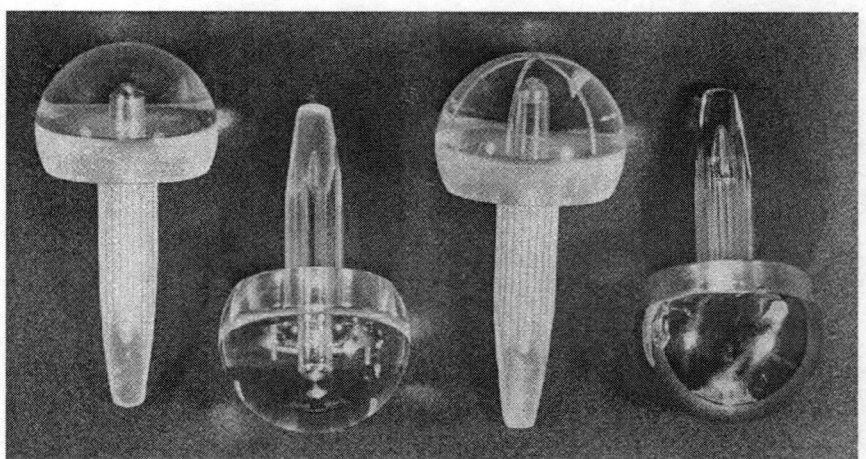

6.10 Resection–reconstruction of hip joint with a synthetic plastic material designed by Judet and Judet in 1943 (modified from Nissen, 1952).

(Thompson, 1952) while Austin Moore described a 'self-locking' prosthesis in 1952 that featured a fenestrated stem to allow bone ingrowth (Moore, 1952). Total hip replacement dates from 1958 when Wiles implanted a prosthesis consisting of precisely fitting stainless steel femoral and acetabular components, reporting good short-term results (Wiles, 1958). Other designs, followed by McKee and Watson-Farrar in 1951 (McKee and Watson-Farrar, 1966), Ring in 1964 (Ring, 1968) and Muller in 1966 (Muller, 1970). Unfortunately, all suffered from failure rates as high as 50% due to loss of fixation.

The modern artificial joint replacement procedure is largely based on the work of Sir John Charnley in the 1970s. Charnley's design consisted of three parts: (1) a metal (originally stainless steel) femoral component and (2) an UHMWPE acetabular component, both of which were fixed to the bone using (3) special bone cement. The replacement joint, which was known as 'low-friction arthroplasty', was lubricated with synovial fluid; the small femoral head resulted in a low friction rate but was suitable only for sedentary patients. For over two decades, the Charnley low-friction arthroplasty design was the most used system in the world, far surpassing the other available options (http://www.articlebase.com/advertising-articles/a-brief-history-of-hip-replacement-surgery-38958.html).

Total hip femoral and acetabular components of various materials and a multitude of designs are currently available. Properly selected and correctly implanted, total hip components of almost any design can be expected to yield satisfactory results in a high percentage of patients. No implant design is appropriate for every patient and therefore general knowledge of the characteristics of the available implants is essential for each surgeon. Selection is mainly based on patient needs, life expectancy and activity level, as well as bone quality and dimensions.

6.4.1 Acetabular components

In the past, acetabular and femoral components were commonly marketed together as total hip systems. With extension of the modularity of both femoral and socket implants, it is now possible to use different types of implants. In particular, acetabular components can be categorized as cemented and cementless.

Cemented acetabular components

The original socket for cemented use is a bulky polyethylene cup with vertical and horizontal groves located on the external surface to increase the stability within the cement mantle (Fig. 6.11). Generally, wire markers are

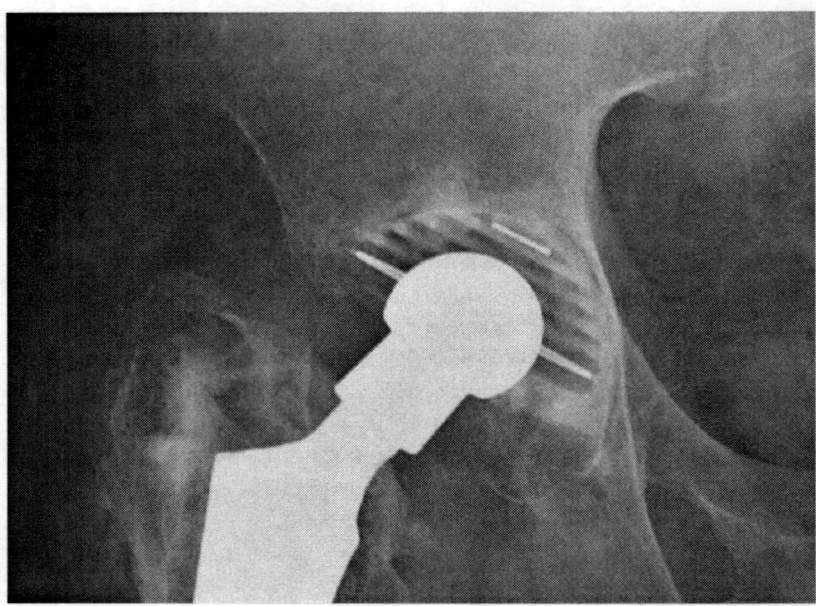

6.11 Total hip arthroplasty with cemented 'all-polyethylene' acetabular cup.

embedded in the polyethylene to allow better assessment of position on X-rays.

More recent designs are characterized by the presence of a PMMA spacer to ensure a uniform cement mantle. Another important characteristic of recent designs is the presence of a flange at the rim, ensuring better pressurization of the cement as the cup is pressed into position. Cemented metal-backed acetabular components have features similar to polyethylene components, from which they differ because of the possibility of being able to substitute the liner component without having to revise the entire acetabulum. The addition of a metal back support to the polyethylene was developed as an attempt to improve the longevity of socket fixation. Some studies have demonstrated that creating a more rigid implant construct could more evenly distribute stresses to the surrounding acetabular bone (Carter, 1983; Dalstra *et al.*, 1995).

Cementless acetabular components

From a general point of view, cementless acetabular components are divided into devices designed to achieve mechanical fixation to the pelvis, generally via the geometric shape of the implant, large pegs or treated rings (Fig. 6.12 (a)), and designs able to achieve biologic fixation due its porous surface (Fig.

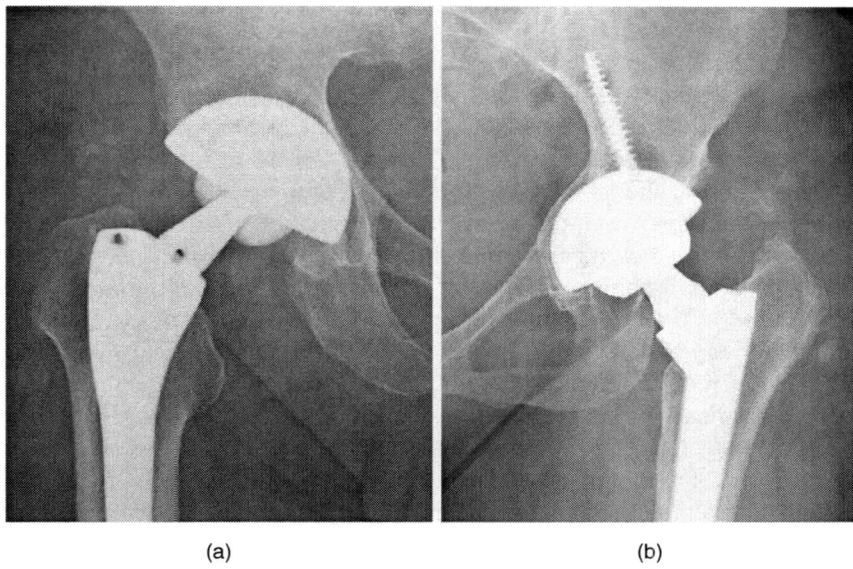

(a) (b)

6.12 (a) Mechanical fixation in which initial stability lies on cup positioning and two-screw fixation. (b) Biologic fixation in which initial fixation is obtained by press-fitting a slightly oversized cup; late stability requires bone integration by a porous-coated surface. Note the areas of osteolysis around the screws.

6.12(b)). Other devices designed for revisions in cases of severe bone loss are stemmed cups characterized by the conical shape of the socket, which is connected with a shaft designed for cementless press-fit into the dorsocranial ilium. Finally, there are the so-called reinforcement rings and cages (Fig. 6.13).

As biological fixation requires initial implant stability such that bone growth and remodeling will occur, threaded titanium cups were seen in a positive light because of the mechanical interlock that is created between the implant and the bone. The threaded-ring designs (so-called first-generation threaded rings) are no longer in use (Morscher, 1992); they included either truncated cones or hemispherical designs with smooth, polished threads. Several studies have demonstrated that these implants have initial satisfactory results but longer-term follow-up studies showed they exhibited an unacceptably high migration rate of up to 56% and early revision rates for aseptic loosening from 4% to 31% at mean follow-ups of 3.5–7 years (Bruijn *et al.*, 1995; Engh *et al.*, 1990; Fox *et al.*, 1994; Lord and Bancel, 1983; Malchau *et al.*, 1997; Peters and Miller, 2007; Pupparo and Engh, 1991). Second-generation threaded cups, characterized by the addition of a porous coating or blasting to provide for bone ingrowth or ongrowth, has improved the performance of threaded acetabular components. These surface-prepared threaded cups rely on the threads for initial mechanical stability and on biological fixation for long-term stability. Components with this design include the Zweymuller threaded cup (grit-blasted titanium) (Delaunay and Kapandji, 1998) and the S-ROM super cup (titanium beads) (Pupparo and Engh, 1991).

Many resurfacing methods for acetabular components are now available, including the most common surface treatments (fibermesh, sintered beads and plasma spray coatings) or more recent components with porous metal surfaces (titanium mesh or beads and porous tantalum) (Jafari *et al.*, 2010; Klika *et al.*, 2007). Virtually all porous-coated acetabular components available today have a hemispherical or modified hemispherical shape and are made of pure titanium, a titanium alloy or tantalum.

Hemispherical porous-coated alloys have been in use for THA for more than 20 years. Cook *et al.* (1988) and Bobyn *et al.* (1980) reported bone ingrowth into these implants through retrieval analysis. Options for initial fixation of acetabular cups include macrothreads, pegs, spikes, pins and screws.

Implant stability at the time of surgery and intimate contact between the implant surface and viable host bone are critical to gain success. Better fixation in torsion and less micromotion has been demonstrated with the use of two central screws than with press-fit cups or cups with pegs or spikes, in

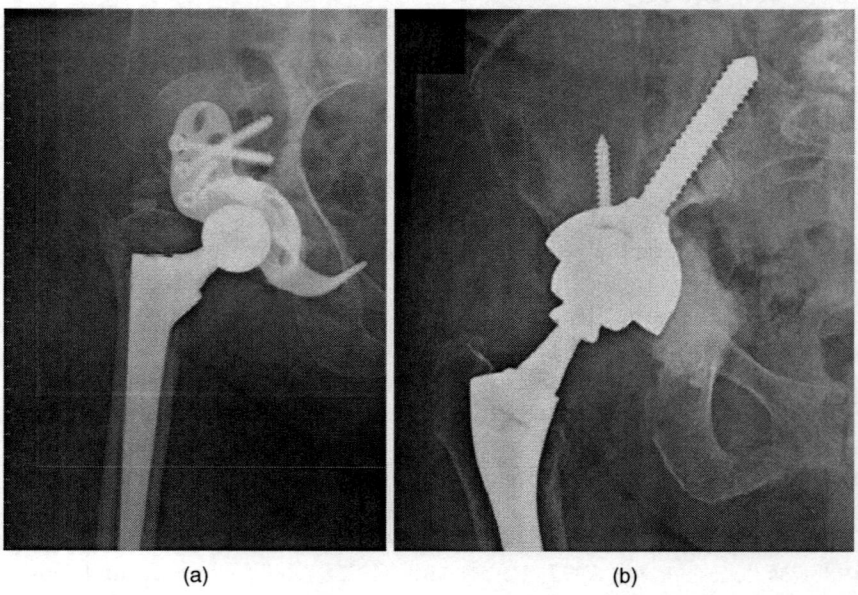

(a) (b)

6.13 (a) Revision stemmed cup with polar stem that provides accessory stability. (b) Severe bone loss requires additional fixation provided by a reinforced ring with various screws.

both laboratory (Lachiewicz *et al.*, 1989) and clinical studies (Stiehl *et al.*, 1991). Screws, however, may increase the effective joint space, decrease the acetabular surface area for bony ingrowth and potentially increase the extent of osteolysis. In addition, screw backout onto the backside of the polyethylene insert has been demonstrated to cause backside wear. Press-fit systems where the bone is reamed to 1–2 mm smaller than the actual component depend on hoop stresses to achieve primary stability and do not require supplemental fixation. However, care must be taken with regard to the risk of fracture.

Biological fixation is based on osteointegration between bone and prosthetic implant, defined as the attachment of lamellar bone to implants without intervening fibrous tissue (Albrektsson *et al.*, 1981). The surface characteristics of an implant are important to determine how bone attaches to the prosthesis: ingrowth occurs when bone grows inside a porous surface (ingrowth surfaces include sintered beads, fibermesh and porous metals), while ongrowth occurs when bone grows onto a roughened surface. Ongrowth surfaces are created by grit blasting or plasma spraying. Grit blasting creates a textured surface by bombarding the implant with small abrasive particles such as aluminum oxide (Corundum). Plasma spraying involves mixing metal powders with an inert gas that is pressurized and ionized, forming a high-energy flame (Klika *et al.*, 2007; Rodriguez, 2006).

The titanium fibermesh fixation surface has the longest published follow-up of all of these fixation surfaces, and numerous studies from throughout the world have come to a mechanical failure rate of 1% at 10–15 years (Della Valle *et al.*, 2004; Gonzalez *et al.*, 2004). The titanium-sintered bead fixation surface has demonstrated long-term fixation. Engh *et al.* (2004) reported only three sockets revised for loosening in a series of 427 acetabular components with a sintered bead surface and peripheral screws at an average 9.5-year follow-up. The titanium plasma spray surface is a so-called bony ongrowth fixation surface. There is less long-term published data with this surface, but the results are similar to the other fixation surfaces. Reina *et al.* (2005) studied a series of 145 hips in an active population with an average age of 63 years. At an average 8-year follow-up, there were no shell revisions, although there were two cases of polyethylene liner revisions for severe osteolysis.

6.4.2 Femoral components

In hip prostheses, cementless femoral fixation is the most commonly used technique. Cemented fixation is usually reserved for older patients or in cases with poor-quality host bone.

Femoral components used with cement

Cemented THA was first carried out by Sir John Charnley in 1961 (Charnley, 1961). Since then, reports on primary cemented femoral components have varied considerably, more because of the characteristics of the cementing technique rather than the design. Before considering the design of contemporary cemented implants it is thus important to summarize the evolution of cementing techniques. The first generation of cementing involved inserting doughy cement, using a finger, into an unplugged femoral canal. The second generation of the technique introduced the plug, the pulsatile lavage in order to clean the femoral canal and the retrograde introduction of cement using a cement gun. Third and fourth generations added pressurization of the cement and stem centralization proximally and distally.

From a general point of view, the most important characteristic of a cemented stem should be to transmit torsional as well axial load to the cement and to the bone without excessive micromotion or damaging. In other words, the stem should remain stable in the long term. Two methods have been adopted to achieve this goal – load-taper or force-closed fixation and composite-beam or shaped-closed fixation.

In the first model, a stem with a tapered shape in two or three planes is seated as a wedge in a mantle cement. Low peak stresses are present in the proximal and distal part of the cement and the stem is allowed to subside at the beginning until radial compressive forces are created in the cement and transferred to the bone. An air-filled distal centralizer is used to facilitate subsidence (Scheerlinck and Casteleyn, 2006). The prototype of the load taper philosophy is the Exeter stem (Stryker, Newburny, UK) designed by Ling and Lee in 1969 and characterized by a collarless polished double taper design (Fowler *et al.*, 1988) (Fig. 6.14). Other examples of this design include the collarless polished taper (Zimmer, Inc., Warsaw, IN, USA), and the C-stem (DePuy Orthopaedics, Warsaw, IN, USA).

In the composite-beam concept, the stem is not intended to subside so it needs to be rigidly bounded by the cement. The shape-closed design has features that transfer a large portion of the axial load directly to the cement. These features can be collars, ridges or profiles. An anatomic design is also considered a shape-closed design feature. These features contribute to the mechanical stability of the implant as well as a roughened surface. An example of this design is the Lubinus SPII stem (Link-Waldemar, Hamburg, Germany), which has an anatomical shape, longitudinal profiles, a matte surface finish, a collar and is made of cobalt–chromium; these design parameters promote the philosophy of maximal mechanical stability of the stem in the cement mantle, even if the stem debonds from the cement mantle. This philosophy correlates well with the small migration rates of this

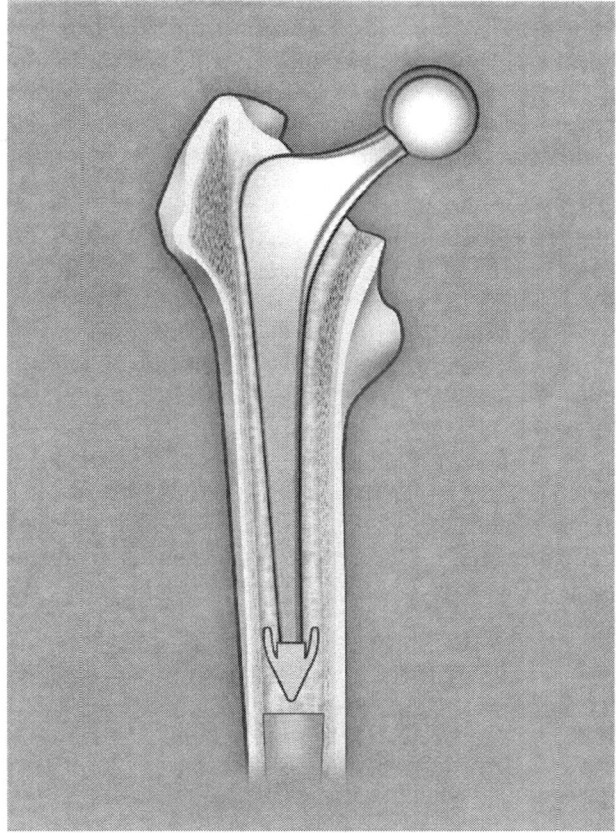

6.14 Exeter stem with distal centralizer used to facilitate subsidence (modified from http://www.exeterhip.co.uk/ex_pag_op-tech-trauma-stem.htm).

stem (Karrholm *et al.*, 2000). Cemented fixation of femoral stem arthroplasty remains the standard of care in elderly patients (Khanuja *et al.*, 2011) or when femoral cortex is thin or osteoporotic (Dorr *et al.*, 1990).

Cementless femoral components

Cementless fixation design principles have evolved since the first outcomes were reported in 1979 (Lord and Bancel, 1983). Various femoral stem geometries are currently in use, but the aim of each design is to obtain initial stability and osseous contact.

Initially, cementless stems were classified as straight or curved according to their shape; both engaged the femur in the metaphysis and in distal part.

Today, stems are often referred to by their geometry, length, location, characteristics of the porous-coated surface as well as according to the site of primary fixation and preservation of the bone. Here, we distinguish different types of stems based on their geometry, which is a modification of the six categories of classification described by Khanuja *et al.* (2011).

- *Type 1*. This category is characterized by a single-wedge design in order to engage the metaphyseal cortical bone in one plane: medial to lateral. The prostheses is flat and thin in the anterior–posterior plane and tapers distally. The coating is typically on the proximal one-third to five-eighths of the implant. With standard implants, primary stability is obtained by wedge fixation in the medial–lateral plane and three-point fixation along the stem length. For preparation, no distal reaming is necessary (Fig. 6.15).
- *Type 2*. Type 2 stems are typified by a double-wedge or metaphyseal-filling design. They are wider than single-wedge stems in the anterior–posterior plane according to their double proximal cortical contact (medial–lateral and anterior–posterior plane). The distal portion may be

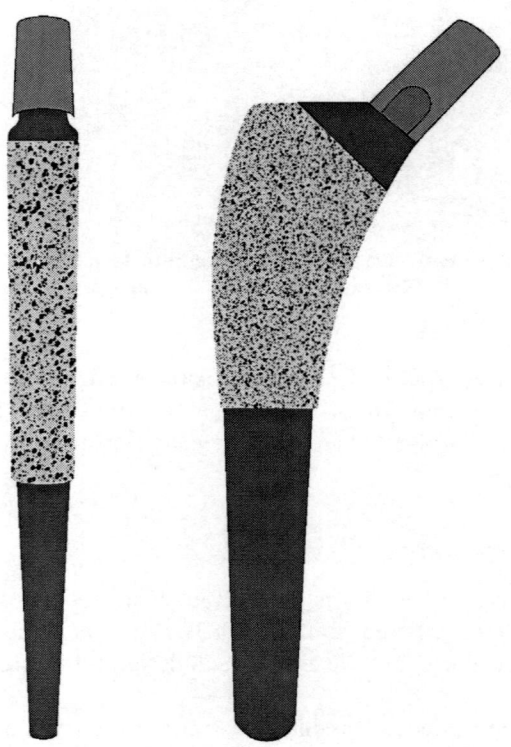

6.15 Single-wedge femoral stem (modified from Khanuja *et al.*, 2011).

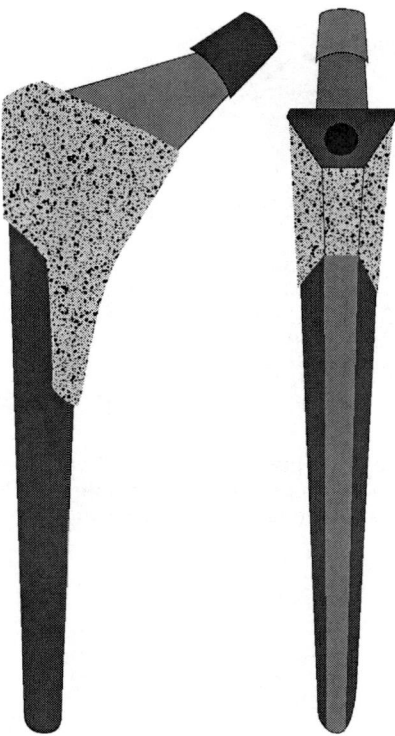

6.16 Double-wedge femoral stem (modified from Khanuja *et al.*, 2011).

tapered or rounded for canal fill. Normally, distal femoral reaming and proximal broaching are necessary during preparation (Fig. 6.16).

- *Type 3*. Type 3 prostheses include several designs, all of which have a long taper stem in both the medial–lateral and the anterior–posterior plane. Some are rounded conical designs grit-blasted across the length (Fig. 6.17(a)) or characterized by a rectangular, tapered, conical stem (Fig. 6.17(b)). Others have just a conical tapered design with longitudinally raised splines that provide rotational stability (Fig. 6.17(c)). Finally, the collarless three-plane tapered design is characterized by a three-dimensional wedge-shaped taper (Fig. 6.17(d)). The prosthesis is tapered in the anterior–posterior and medial–lateral plane as well as along its length. Typically, accentuated ribs in the proximal region are present, whereas the distal part of the stem has a round conical form.
- *Type 4*. This design is characterized by contact with cortical bone in the diaphysis along its entire length, and basically has a cylindrical shape and a proximal collar. The majority of these prostheses are coated with an ingrowth surface. A proximal collar enhances axial stability and

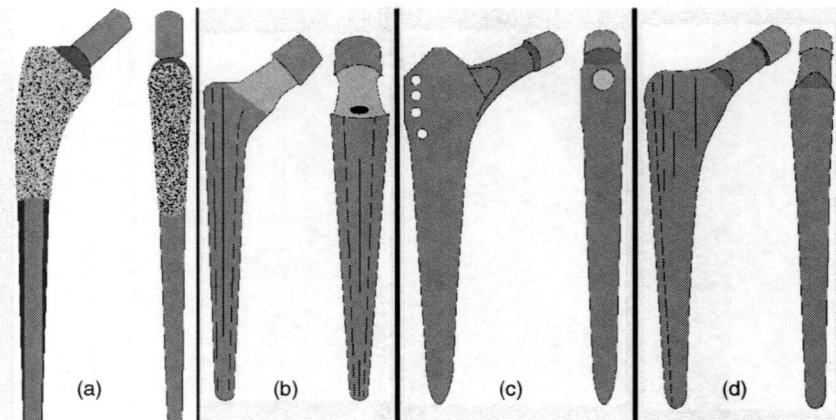

6.17 Stems with more than one plane taper: (a) conical grit-blasted design; (b) conical design with longitudinal raised splines; (c) rectangular design; (d) three-plane tapered design (modified from Khanuja *et al.*, 2011).

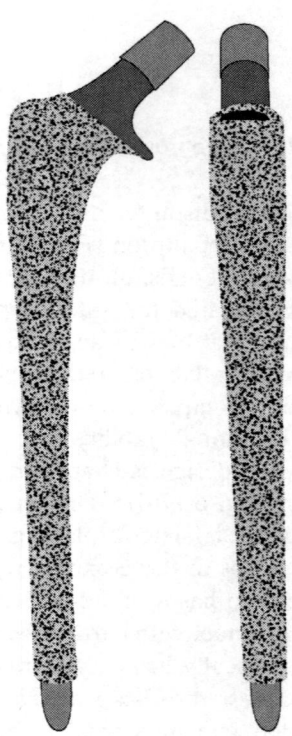

6.18 Cylindrical stems (modified from Khanuja *et al.*, 2011).

Orthopaedic implant materials and design 163

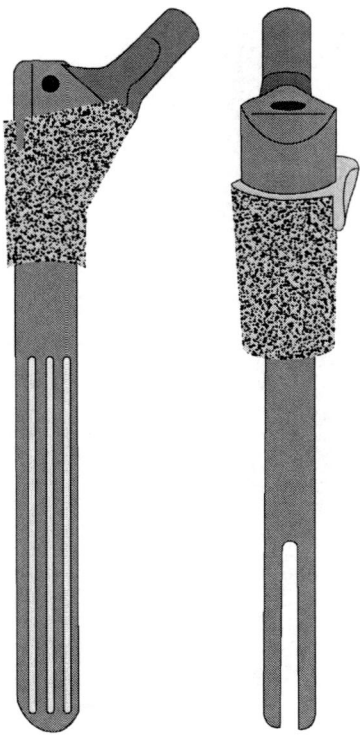

6.19 Full-modular stems (modified from Khanuja *et al.*, 2011).

transmits forces to the calcar. Preparation requires distal reaming and proximal broaching (Fig. 6.18).

- *Type 5.* Modular designs allow independent preparation and separate components for the metaphysis and diaphysis. Preparation involves diaphyseal reaming for the stem to obtain cortical contact, and the metaphysis and calcar are machined over the distal stem or stem trial with special milling (Fig. 6.19).
- *Type 6.* These prostheses are curved anatomic stems that match the proximal femoral endosteal geometry. They are wider proximally, both laterally and posteriorly. In the lateral plane, they bow posteriorly in the metaphysis and anteriorly in the diaphysis. These stems have anteversion of the neck and are produced for the right or left femur. Distally, they are either tapered or cylindrical. Stability is achieved through metaphyseal fill and the distal curve. Preparation, consisting of distal reaming and metaphyseal broaching, is less forgiving because of the close match of the shape of the prosthesis to the femoral canal (Fig. 6.20).
- *Type 7.* Short femoral stems, also called metaphyseal stems, are

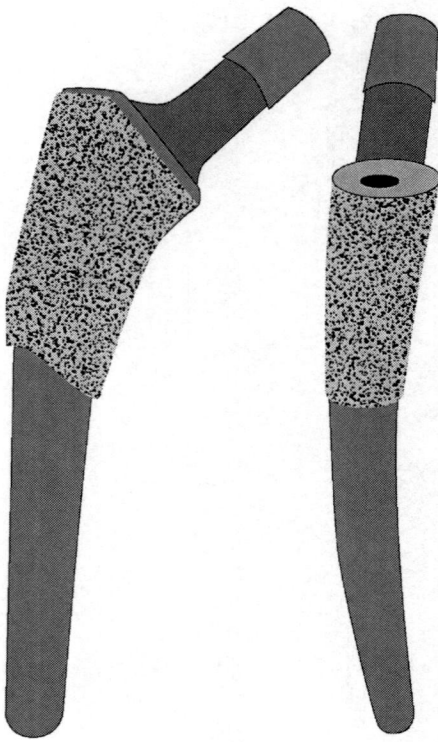

6.20 Curved anatomical stems (modified from Khanuja *et al.*, 2011).

frequently recommended for young and active patients, as they are potential candidates for subsequent revision arthroplasty. They are characterized by a multi-point cortical fixation supported by cancellous bone compression in the metaphyseal area. There are two main groups of short stems, those that are neck-preserving and those that do not preserve the femoral neck.

In non-neck-preserving stems, preparation is accomplished with a straightforward broaching of the canal without reamer use: short stems are bone-conserving. The straight double taper leans on the calcar while the implant tip acts like an implantation guide aligning itself in the proximal diaphyseal cavity. They violate less femoral bone stock, providing more favorable conditions should a revision be required (Fig. 6.21(a)).

The concept of a femoral neck-preserving hip replacement was introduced in the mid-1990s (Pipino and Molfetta, 1993). Preservation of the neck retains the trabecular systems of the metaphyseal cancellous bone, and thus allows for a more physiological load distribution along the diaphysis and the greater trochanter. Retention of the neck further permits an increased bone ingrowth, probably due to the protection of blood supply. Preparation consists of just metaphyseal broaching without distal reaming (Fig. 6.21 (b)).

6.4.3 Resurfacing hip prostheses

The concept of hip resurfacing is not new. Old and modern designs have evolved directly from the original mold arthroplasty introduced by Smith-Petersen in 1948 (Smith-Petersen, 1948). The first total resurfacing arthroplasty was developed by Charnley in the early 1950s using a Teflon-on-Teflon bearing, which was associated with early failure for both necrosis of the femoral head and poor wear characteristic of the material used (Charnley, 1961). Cemented hip resurfacing using polyethylene acetabular components and metal femoral components was carried out in 1971 by Paltrinieri and Trentani (Trentani and Vaccarino, 1978) in Italy (Fig. 6.22)

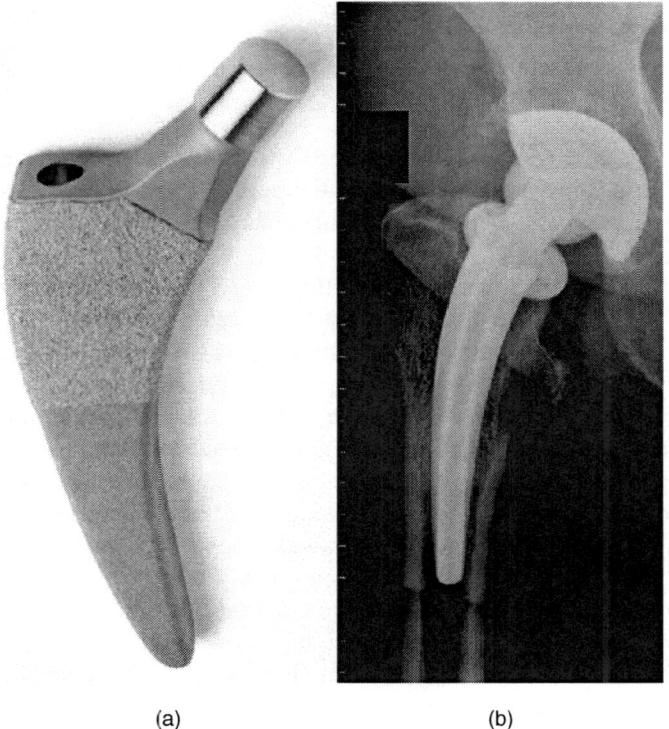

(a)   (b)

6.21 (a) Non-neck-preserving short femoral stem (Fitmore prosthesis, courtesy of Zimmer, Warsaw, IN, USA). (b) Neck-preserving short femoral stem.

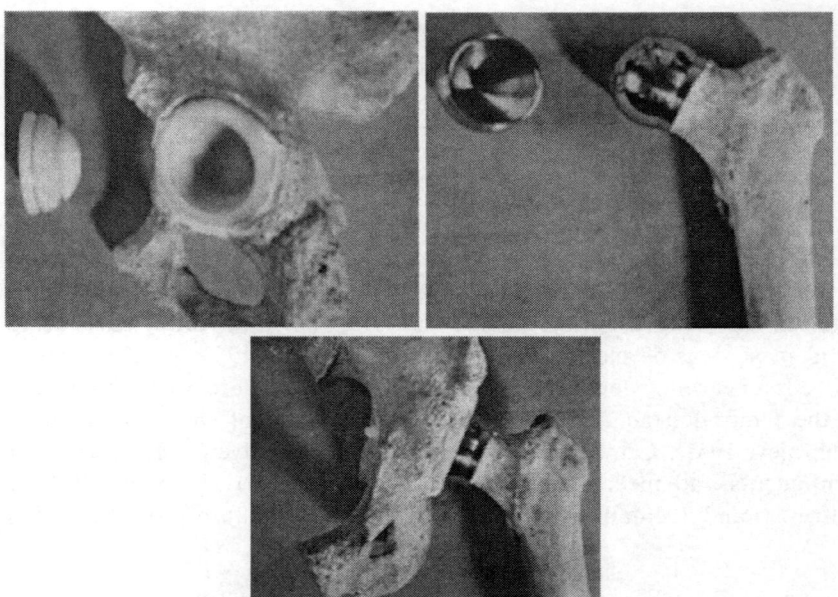

6.22 Paltrinieri–Trentani resurfacing hip prosthesis (courtesy of Paolo Trentani MD and Federico Trentani MD).

and some years later by Freeman (1978) in the UK and Wagner (1978) in Germany. The European experience followed the development in the USA of several cemented resurfacing designs (Amstutz *et al.*, 1977; Capello *et al.*, 1978).

In 1983, Amstutz developed the first cementless resurfacing arthroplasty with a titanium alloy femoral component, a modular acetabular component with polyethylene liners and a pure titanium mesh porous backing (Amstutz, 1991). In 1989, Buechel and Pappas introduced a cementless resurfacing system with a modular acetabular component and a titanium nitride ceramic-coated titanium alloy femoral component (Buechel, 1990).

The results in the first generation of hip resurfacing were disappointing and the procedure was largely abandoned by the mid-1980s. The principal mode of failure of the first generation of metal-on-polyethylene (MoP) resurfacings was attributed to accelerated wear and production of large volumes of biologically active particulate debris, leading to bone loss and implant loosening, due to the large diameter of the femoral component combined with thin polyethylene cups or liners. Retrieval studies have not confirmed whether resurfacing of the femoral head leads to avascular necrosis. The femoral neck fractures observed at that time were correlated to a combination of osteolysis of the femoral neck and intraoperative neck notching. The final complication was often a consequence of the valgus positioning of the implant, which was recommended to reduce the tension and shear stresses across the head–neck junction (Freeman et al., 1978).

The development of metal-on-metal (MoM) bearings with improved fluid film lubrication was the most important factor in the re-emergence of hip resurfacing as a concept. MoM hip resurfacing with a cementless, porous or hydroxyapatite-coated, non-modular socket in combination with a cemented, stemmed femoral component was reintroduced into clinical practice in the 1990s (Schmalzried et al., 1994).

In 1988 Weber introduced a cementless system in which the acetabular component was a titanium alloy shell with a Metasul inlay (Metasul is a high-carbon-containing Co–Cr alloy) and a two-layer femoral component (Weber, 1996). The first design was screwed onto the reamed femoral head, but because of insertion difficulties, a press-fit version was developed. Only small numbers of the Weber MoM resurfacings were used and no long-term results are available. At around the same time, in the UK, McMinn et al. (1996) developed a hip resurfacing based on a cast Co–Cr alloy thread, introducing the next generation of this surgery. After a phase where both cementless and cemented components were used with not excellent results, all contemporary main systems have in common cementless fixation of the acetabular component and cemented fixation of the femoral component. Another common characteristic is a bearing made from a high-carbon-containing Co–Cr alloy.

Short-term clinical follow-up reports of MoM hip resurfacing arthroplasties have been encouraging (Daniel et al., 2004); femoral neck fractures (Amstutz et al., 2004a) and femoral loosening (Amstutz et al., 2004b) are the most prevalent causes of failure, up to 5.6% and 2.3% respectively. However, these reports are mainly from the designer centers (Amstutz et al., 2004a; Treacy et al., 2005). Long-term data from other sources are still lacking so it is not possible to determine whether the results are less reproducible than those of THA or identify specific failure modes or prognosticators for early failure.

However according to the data, it is possible to identify three prognostic factors that differ in resurfacing arthroplasty and THA: gender, age and surgical indication. Male patients had a lower risk of revision of resurfacing arthroplasty than females irrespective of age: the 5-year CRR for females was 2.5 times higher than that of males. In addition, within gender, head sizes of 50 mm or greater were associated with a lower ($p < 0.001$) risk of revision at 5 years, which is comparable to the cumulative risk of revision of THA (Table 6.2). Age was found to be another important prognosticator, with males aged under 65 years having slightly better results at 5 years with resurfacing arthroplasty than with THA. In females, however, a dramatic increase in revision rate was seen in patients aged between 55 and 64 years, indicating that females should be age 55 years or younger at the time of

Table 6.2 Overview of the failure modes of resurfacing arthroplasties reported in three main national joint replacement registers

Failure mode	England and Wales	Sweden	Australia
PP fracture	44%	31%	41%
Aseptic loosening	20%	31%	NA
Pain	23%	NA	NA
Instability	4%	NA	NA
Osteolysis	4%	NA	NA
Technical issues	NA	14%	NA
Other (infection included)	12%	23%	NA

PP, periprosthetic fracture; NA, not available.

surgery (Prosser *et al.*, 2010). Concerns remain with the long-term biological effects of elevated metal ion levels found in all patients with MoM bearings *in situ* (Savarino *et al.*, 2006).

6.5 Future trends

Biological resurfacing of the joint with engineered tissue is at present no more than a theoretical possibility. Total joint replacement will therefore remain the treatment of choice for arthritis of the hip and knee for the foreseeable future.

Total hip and knee prosthetic components of various materials and a multitude of designs are currently available. Properly selected and correctly implanted, components of almost any design can be expected to yield satisfactory results in a high percentage of patients. Nevertheless, no implant design is appropriate for every patient and therefore general knowledge of the characteristics of the available implants is essential to gain better results. Furthermore, patients' expectations after joint replacement have changed. Today, quality of life issues, which sometimes include high-activity recreational interests, define their aspirations. For these reasons, designers and clinicians are oriented towards two directions:

- sparing surgery;
- material advancement that can reduce bearing wear rates in order to decrease morbidity and the risks associated with revision surgery related to wear particles.

In the last few years, improvements in operative techniques and instrumentation have allowed surgeons to perform joint replacement through smaller incisions than previously used. Several techniques have been described, for hip and knee, with or without computer or fluoroscopic guidance. Customized instrumentation, including smaller retractors with extended handles, angulated reamers and implant introducers, especially for hip surgery, has been produced and may be beneficial in avoiding excessive trauma or traction of soft tissues. Nevertheless, most of the implants used are the same as used previously. The need to use dedicated systems has become apparent in hip surgery, where several bone-conserving designs have appeared in recent years, and changes have been done recently for knee designs. With further follow-up, the utility of these designs and the improvements that they may bring over previous designs may become apparent.

Highly cross-linked polyethylene remains the preferred choice in THA. Although cross-linking is highly beneficial from the perspective of wear resistance, it comes at the price of less molecular mobility, lower material ductility, and reduced fatigue and fracture resistance due to the cross-linking of the molecular chains. For these reasons, new types of polyethylene have been developed, such as X3 (Stryker Orthopedics, Mahwah, NJ, USA) and ArCom XL and E-Poly (Biomet Orthopedics, Warsaw, IN, USA). The intent of these second-generation materials is to reduce the potential for material oxidation in the long term while preserving the bulk mechanical properties necessary to use cross-linked polyethylene in higher stress applications, such as thin acetabular liners and stabilized knee designs.

6.6 Sources of further information and advice

As sources of further information consultation of the Arthroplasty Registers is useful. They are powerful instruments with which to assess the performance of arthroplasty procedures and have been major sources in scientific discussions. The worldwide development of Arthroplasty Registers can be traced back to initiatives in Scandinavia in 1975 with the Knee Register and then in 1979 with the introduction of the Hip Register. According to the Efort Society, at present there are almost 30 national registers, along with the European Arthroplasty Register (EAR) coordinating center, a voluntary cooperation of national arthroplasty registers. EAR (www.ear.efort.org) supports the development of national projects in a supranational cooperation (Table 6.3).

For detailed reviews of alumina materials used in orthopaedics, the reader is referred to previous review articles (e.g. Hannouche *et al.*, 2005). Several excellent reviews summarizing the properties of zirconia ceramic biomaterials have also recently been published (Cales, 2000; Clarke *et al.*, 2003).

6.7 Acknowledgments

We would like to thank Luigi Lena and Carlo Piovani (Rizzoli Orthopaedic Institute) for their valuable help with the creation or processing of all images

Table 6.3 Some existing hip and knee joint arthroplasty registers

Register	Notes	Website
Sweden (Knee) 1975	Active nationwide	www.jru.orthop.gu.se
Sweden (Hip) 1979	Active nationwide	www.jru.orthop.gu.se
Finland 1980	Active nationwide	www.nam.fi/english/publications/
Norway 1987	Active nationwide	www.haukeland.no/nrl/
Denmark (Hip) 1995	Active nationwide	www.dhr.dk/ENGLISH.htm
Denmark (Knee) 1997	Active nationwide	www.dshk.org/DKR-frame.htm
New Zealand 1998	Active nationwide	www.cdhb.govt.nz/njr/
Hungary 1998	Active incomprehensive	www.ortopedtarsasag.hu
Australia 1999	Active nationwide	www.dmac.adelaide.edu.au/aoanjrr/
Canada 2000	Active nationwide	http://secure.cihi.ca/cihiweb/dispPage.jsp?cw_page=services_cjrr_e
Czech Republic 2001	Active incomprehensive	www.ksrzis.cz/Pages/171-NRKN-National-Register-of-Joint-Replacements.html
Romania 2001	Active nationwide	www.rne.ro/site/Default.aspx
Slovakia 2002	Active nationwide	https://sar.mfn.sk/
Austria 2002	Active pilot phase (about 30% coverage; comprehensive of the province of Tyrol)	www.biqg.org
England and Wales 2003	Active nationwide	www.njrcentre.org.uk
France 2006	Pilot phase	www.sofcot.fr/10-registre-national/registre-national.asp
Portugal 2006	Pilot phase	www.rpa.spot.pt/?lang=en-GB
Italy 2006	Regional registers	https://ripo.cineca.it/
Switzerland 2008	Pilot phase	www.siris-implant.ch/index.php?id=51&L=1
European Arthroplasty Register (EAR)		www.ear.efort.org/
National Joint Registry		www-new.njrcentre.org.uk/njrcentre/Default.aspx

in this chapter. The authors did not receive any external funding or grants in support of their research or in the preparation of this work.

6.8 References

Abdeen AR, Collen SB and Vince KG (2010) Fifteen-year to 19-year follow-up of the Insall–Burstein-1 total knee arthroplasty. *J Arthroplasty*, 25, 173–178.

Abernethy PJ, Robinson CM and Fowler RM (1996) Fracture of the metal tibial tray after Kinematic total knee replacement. A common cause of early aseptic failure. *J Bone Joint Surg Br* 78, 220–225.

Albrektsson T, Branemark PI, Hansson HA and Lindstrom J. (1981) Osseointegrated titanium implants. Requirements for ensuring a long-lasting, direct bone-to-implant anchorage in man. *Acta Orthop Scand*. 52, 55–70.

Alvarado J, Maldonado R, Marxuach J and Otero R. (2003) Biomechanics of hip and knee prostheses. *Applications of Engineering Mechanics in Medicine*. GED, University of Puerto Rico Mayaguez, pp. 1–20.

Amstutz HC (1991) Surface replacement arthroplasty. In: Amstutz HC, editor. *Hip Arthroplasty*. New York, NY, Churchill Livingstone, pp. 295–333.

Amstutz HC, Clarke IC, Cristie J, *et al*. (1977) Total hip articular replacement by internal eccentric shells. *Clin Orthop*, 128, 261–84.

Amstutz HC, Campbell PA and Le Duff MJ (2004a) Fracture of the neck of the femur after surface arthroplasty of the hip. *J Bone Joint Surg Am*, 86A, 1874–7.

Amstutz HC, Ma SM, Jinnah RH and Mai L (2004b) Revision of aseptic loose total hip arthroplasties. *Clin Orthop Relat Res*, 420, 2–9.

Bader R, Bergschmidt P, Fritsche A, Ansorge S, Thomas P and Mittelmeier W (2008) Alternative materials and solutions in total knee arthroplasty for patients with metal allergy. *Orthopäde*, 37, 136–142.

Bahraminasa M and Jahan A (2011) Material selection for femoral component of total knee replacement using comprehensive VIKOR. *Mater Design*, 32, 4471–7.

Bal BS, Khandkar A, Lakshmin Arayanan R, Clarke I, Hoffman AA and Rahman MN (2009) Fabrication and testing of silicon nitride bearings in total hip arthroplasty winner of the 2007 'HAP' PAUL award. *J Arthroplasty*, 24, 110–6.

Bell CJ, Walker PG and Blunn GW (1998) The effect of oxidation on delamination of UHMWPE tibial components. *J Arthroplasty*, 13, 280–90.

Bizot P, Nizard R, Lerouge S, Prudhommeaux F and Sedel L (2000) Ceramic/ceramic total hip arthroplasty. *J Orthop Sci*, 5, 622–7.

Black J (1992) *Biological Performance of Materials: Fundamentals of Biocompatibility*, 2nd edn. New York, NY, Marcel Dekker.

Bleobaum RD, Beeks D and Dorr L (1994) Complications with hydroxyapatite particulate separation in total hip arthroplasty. *Clin Orthop*, 298, 19–26.

Bobyn JD, Pilliar RM, Cameron HV and Weatherly GC (1980) The optimum pore size for the fixation of porous surfaced metal implants by the ingrowth of bone. *Clin Orthop*, 150, 263–70.

Bobyn JD, Stackpool GJ, Hacking SA, Tanzer M, Krtgier JJ. (1999) Characteristics of bone ingrowth and interface mechanics of a new porous tantalum biomaterial. *J Bone Joint Surg Br*, 81, 907–14.

Boehler M, Plenk Jr H. Salzer M (2000) Alumina ceramic bearings for hip endoprostheses: the Austrian experiences. *Clin Orthop Relat Res*, 379, 85–93.

Boss JH, Shajrawi I, Dekel S and Mendes DG (1993) The bone cement interface: histological observations on the interface of cemented arthroplasties within the immediate and late phases. *J Biomater Sci Polym Ed*, 5, 221–30.

Bourne RB, Barrack R, Rorabeck CH, Salehi A and Good V (2005) Arthroplasty options for the young patient: Oxinium on cross-linked polyethylene. *Clin Orthop Relat Res*, 441, 159–67.

Boutin P (1971) Alumina and its use in surgery of the hip. Experimental study. *Presse Med*, 79, 639–40.

Boutin P (1972) Total arthroplasty of the hip by fritted aluminum prosthesis.

Experimental study and 1st clinical applications. *Rev Chir Orthop Repar Appar Mot*, 58, 229–46.

Brand MG, Daley RJ, Ewald FC and Scott RD (1989) Tibial tray augmentation with modular metal wedges for tibial bone stock deficiency. *Clin Orthop Relat Res*, 248, 71–79.

Brooks PJ, Walker PS and Scott RD (1984) Tibial component fixation in deficient tibial bone stock. *Clin Orthop Relat Res*, 184, 302–8.

Bruijn JD, Seelen JL, Feenstra RM, *et al*. (1995) Failure of the Mecring screw-ring acetabular compon total hip arthroplasty. *J Bone Joint Surg Am*, 77A, 760–6.

Buechel FF (1990) Resurfacing total hip replacement for avascular necrosis in young patients: durability, revision options and future technology. *Presentation at 6th Annual Current Concepts in Joint Replacement Symposium, Orlando, FL*.

Buechel FF and Pappas MJ (1986) The New Jersey Low-Contact-Stress Knee Replacement System: biomechanical rationale and review of the first 123 cemented cases. *Arch Orthop Trauma Surg*, 105, 197–204.

Bureau MN (2005) Biomimetic polymer composites for orthopedic implants. *Proceedings of 3rd International Symposium on Advanced Biomaterials/Biomechanics, Montreal, Quebec*.

Burstein GT, Hutchings IM, and Sasaki K (2000) Electrochemically induced annealing of stainless steel surfaces. *Nature*, 407, 885–7.

Cales B (2000) Zirconia as a sliding material: histologic, laboratory, and clinical data. *Clin Orthop*, 379, 94–112.

Capello WN, Ireland PH, Tramell TR, *et al*. (1978) Conservative total hip arthroplasty: a procedure to conserve bone stock. Part I and Part II. *Clin Orthop*, 134, 59–74.

Carter DR (1983) Finite element analysis of a metal backed acetabular component. In: Hungerford DS, editor. *The Hip: Proceedings of the 11th Open Scientific Meeting of the Hip Society*. St Louis, CV Mosby, pp. 216–39.

Charnley JC (1961) Arthroplasty of the hip: a new operation. *Lancet*, 1, 1129–32.

Charnley J (1970) The reaction of bone to self-curing acrylic cement: a long-term histological study in man. *J Bone Joint Surg Br*, 52, 340–53.

Clarke IC, Manaka M, Green DD, Williams P, Pezzotti G, Kim YH, *et al*. (2003) Current status of zirconia used in total hip implants. *J Bone Joint Surg Am*, 85A (Suppl 4), 73–84.

Cook SD, Thomas KA, and Haddad Jr RJ (1988) Histologic analysis of retrieved human porous coated total joint components. *Clin Orthop*, 234, 90–101.

Cuckler JM, Bearcroft J and Asgian CM (1995) Femoral head technologies to reduce polyethylene wear in total hip arthroplasty. *Clin Orthop*, 317, 57–63.

Dalla Pria P (2007) Evolution and new application of the alumina ceramics in joint replacement. *Eur J Orthop Surg Traumatol*, 17, 253–256.

Dalstra M, Huisks R and Van Erning L (1995) Development and validation of a three-dimensional finite element model of the pelvic bone. *J Biomech Eng*, 117, 272–8.

Daniel J, Pynsent PB and McMinn DJ (2004) Metal-on-metal resurfacing of the hip in patients under the age of 55 years with osteoarthritis. *J Bone Joint Surg Br*, 86, 177–84.

Delaunay CP and Kapandji AI (1998) Survivorship of rough-surfaced threaded

acetabular cups: 382 conse primary Zweymuller cups followed for 0.2–12 years. *Acta Orthop Scand*, 69, 379–83.
Della Valle CJ, Berger RA, Shott S, et al. (2004) Primary total hip arthroplasty with a porous-coated acetabular component. A concise follow-up of a previous report. *J Bone Joint Surg Am*, 86A, 1217–22.
Dorr LD, Abstaz M, Gruen TA, Saberi MT and Doerzbacher JF (1990) Anatomic porous replacement hip arthroplasty: first 100 consecutive cases. *Semin Arthroplasty*, 1, 77–86.
Engh CA, Griffin WL and Marx CL (1990) Cementless acetabular components. *J Bone Joint Surg*, 72B, 53–59.
Engh CA, Hopper RH and Engh Jr CA (2004) Long-term porous-coated cup survivorship using spikes, screws, and press-fitting for initial fixation. *J Arthroplasty*, 19, 54–60.
Fowler JL, Gie GA, Lee JC and Ling RSM (1988) Experience with the Exeter total hip replacement since 1970. *Orthop Clin North Am*, 19, 477–89.
Fox GM, McBeath AA and Heiner JP (1994) Hip replacement with a threaded acetabular cup: a follow-up study. *J Bone Joint Surg Br*, 76A, 195–201.
Freeman MAR (1978) Some anatomical and mechanical considerations relevant to the surface replacement of the femoral head. *Clin Orthop*, 134, 19–24.
Freeman MAR, Cameron HU and Brown GC (1978) Cemented double cup arthroplasty of the hip. *Clin Orthop*, 134, 45–52.
Gonzalez, Della Valle A, Zoppi A, Peterson MGE, et al. (2004) Clinical and radiographic results associated with a modern, cementless modular cup design in total hip arthroplasty. *J Bone Joint Surg Am*, 86, 1998–2004.
Goodfellow J (1992) One step forward, two steps back. Knee prostheses. *J Bone Joint Surg Br*, 74B, 1–2.
Hannouche D, Hamadouche M, Nizard R, Bizot P, Meunier A and Sedel L (2005) Ceramics in total hip replacement. *Clin Orthop Relat Res*, 430, 62–71.
Hansen D and Jensen JS (1990) Prechilling and vacuum mixing not suitable for all bone cements. *J Arthroplasty*, 5, 287–90.
Hey-Groves EW (1927) Some contributions to the reconstructive surgery of the hip. *Br J Surgery* 14, 486–517.
Hood RW, Wright TM and Burstein AH (1983) Retrieval analysis of total knee prostheses: a method and its application to 48 total condylar prostheses. *J Biomed Mater Res*, 17, 829–42.
Hungerford DS, Kenna RV and Krackow KA (1982) The porous-coated anatomic total knee. *Orthop Clin North Am*, 13, 103–22.
Insall J, Ranawat CS, Scott WN and Walker P (1976) Total condylar knee replacement: preliminary report. *Clin Orthop Relat Res*, 120, 149–54.
Jafari SM, Bender B, Coyle C, Parvizi J, Sharkey PF and Hozach WJ (2010) Do tantalum and titanium cups show similar results in revision hip arthroplasty? *Clin Orthop Relat Res*, 468, 459–65.
Jazrawi LM, Bogner E, Della Valle CJ, Chen FS, Pak KI, Stuchin SA, et al. (1999) Wear rates of ceramic-on-ceramic bearing surfaces in total hip implants: a 12-year follow-up study. *J Arthroplasty*, 14, 781–7.
Judet J and Judet R (1950) The use of an artificial femoral head for arthroplasty of the hip joint. *J Bone Joint Surg Br*, 32B, 166–73.
Karrholm J, Nivbrant B, Thanner J, Anderberg C, Borlin N, Herberts P and

Malchau H (2000) Radiossterometric evaluation of hip implant design and surface finish. *Scientific Exhibition, AAOS, Orlando, FL.*

Khanuja HS, Vakil JJ, Goddard MS and Mont MA (2011) Cementless femoral fixation in total hip arthroplasty. *J Bone Joint Surg Am* 93, 500–9.

Kircher J, Bergschmidt P, Bader R, Kluess D, Besser-Mahuzir E, Leder A, Mittelmeier W (2007) The importance of wear couples for younger endoprosthesis patients. *Orthopäde*, 36, 337–46.

Klika AK, Murray TG, Darwiche H and Barsoum WK (2007) Options for acetabular fixation surfaces. *J Long Term Eff Med Implants*, 17, 187–92.

Lachiewicz PR, Suh PB and Gilbert JA (1989) *In vitro* initial fixation of porous coated acetabular total hip components: a biomechanical comparative study. *J Arthroplasty*, 4, 201–50.

Lancaster JG, Dowson D, Isaac GH and Fisher J (1997) The wear of ultra-high molecular weight polyethylene sliding on metallic and ceramic counterfaces representative of current femoral surfaces in joint replacement. *Proc Inst Mech Eng H*, 211, 17–24.

Langer G. (2002) Ceramic tibial plateau of the 70s. Bioceramics in joint arthroplasty. *Proceedings of the 7th International BIOLOX Symposium. Stuttgart, Thieme*, pp. 128–30.

Levine BR, Sporer S, Poggie RA, Della Valle CJ and Jacobs JJ (2006) Experimental and clinical performance of porous tantalum in orthopedic surgery. *Biomaterials*, 27, 4671–81.

Levine B, Sporer S, Della Valle CJ, Jacobs JJ and Paprosky W (2007) Porous tantalum in reconstructive surgery of the knee: a review. *J Knee Surg*, 20, 185–94.

Li MG, Zhou ZK, Wood DJ, Rohrl SM, Ioppolo JL and Nivbrant B (2006) Low wear with high-crosslinked polyethylene especially in combination with oxinium heads. A RSA evaluation. *Trans Orthop Res Soc*, 31, 643.

Li S and Burstein AH (1994) Current concepts review. Ultra high molecular weight polyethylene. *J Bone Joint Surg Am*, 76, 1080–90.

Lord G and Bancel P (1983) The madreporic cementless total hip arthroplasty: new experimental data a seven-year clinical follow-up study. *Clin Orthop*, 176, 67–76.

Majima T, Yasuda K, Tago H, Aoki Y and Minami A (2008) Clinical results of posterior cruciate ligament retaining TKA with alumina ceramic condylar prosthesis: comparison to Co–Cr alloy prosthesis. *Knee Surg Sports Trauma Arthrosc*, 16, 152–6.

Malchau H, Wang YX, Karrholm J, *et al.* (1997) Scandinavian multicenter porous coated anatomic tota arthroplasty study: clinical and radiographic results with 7- to 10-year follow-up evaluation. *J Arthroplasty*, 12, 133–48.

McKee GK and Watson-Farrar J (1966) Replacement of osteoarthritic hips by the McKee–Farrar prosthesis. *J Bone Joint Surg Br*, 48B, 245–59.

McKellop H, Shen FW, Lu B, *et al.* (1999) Development of an extremely wear-resistant ultra high molecular weight polyethylene for total hip replacements. *J Orthop Res*, 17, 157–67.

McMinn D, Treacy R, Lin K, *et al.* (1996) Metal-on-metal surface replacement of the hip. *Clin Orthop*, 329, S89–98.

Miyazaki T, Kim HM, Miyaji F, Kokubo T, Kato H and Nakamura T (2000)

Bioactive tantalum metal prepared by naoh treatment. *J Biomed Mater Res*, 50, 35–42.

Moore AT. (1952) Metal hip joint: a new self-locking Vitallium prosthesis. *South Med J*, 45, 1015–9.

Morlock M, Nassutt R, Wimmer MA and Schneider E (2002) Influence of resting periods on friction in artificial hip joint articulations. In: Garino JP, Willmann G, editors. *Bioceramics in Joint Arthroplasty, Proceedings of the 7th International BIOLOX Symposium*. Stuttgart, Thieme, pp. 6–20.

Morscher EW (1992) Current status of acetabular fixation in primary total hip arthroplasty. *Clin Orthop Relat Res*, 274, 172–93.

Moursi AM, Winnard AV, Winnard PL, Lannutti JL and Seghi RR (2002) Enhanced osteoblast response to a polymethylmethacrylate–hydroxyapatite composite. *Biomaterials*, 23, 133–44.

Muller ME (1970) Total hip protheses. *Clin Orthop*, 72, 46–68.

Muratoglu OK, Bradgon CR, O'Connor D, *et al.* (2001) A novel method of cross-linking ultra-high-molecular-weight polyethylene to improve wear, reduce oxidation, and retain mechanical properties. *J Arthroplasty*, 16, 149–60.

Muratoglu OK, Bradgon CR, O'Connor D, *et al.* (2003) Unified wear model for highly crosslinked ultra-high molecular weight polyethylenes (UHMWPE). *Biomaterials*, 20, 1463–70.

Nevelos AB, Evans PA, Harrison P and Rainforth M (1993) Examination of alumina ceramic components from total hip arthroplasties. *Proc Inst Mech Eng H*, 207, 155–62.

Nissen KI (1952) The Judet arthroplasty of the hip via Gibson's lateral approach. *Postgrad Med J*, 28, 412–23.

Oonishi H, Aono M, Murata N and Kushitani S (1992) Alumina versus polyethylene in total knee arthroplasty. *Clin Orthop*, 282, 95–104.

Oonishi H, Kim SC, Kyomoto M, Iwamoto M, Masuda S and Ueno M (2006) Ceramic total knee arthroplasty: advanced clinical experiences of 26 years. *Semin Arthroplasty*, 17, 134–40.

Peters CL and Miller MD (2007) The cementless acetabular component. In: Callaghan JJ, Rosenberg AG, Rubash HE, editors. *The Adult Hip*, 2nd edn. Pennsylvania, PA, Lippincott Williams & Wilkins, pp. 946–68.

Pipino F and Molfetta L (1993) Femoral neck preservation in total hip replacement. *Ital J Orthop Traumatol*, 19, 5–12.

Prosser GH, Yates PJ, Wood DJ, Graves SE, De Steiger RN and Miller LN (2010) Outcome of primary resurfacing hip replacement: evaluation of risk factors for early revision. *Acta Orthop*, 81, 66–71.

Pupparo F and Engh CA (1991) Comparison of porous-threaded and smooth-threaded acetabular components of identical design: two- to four-year results. *Clin Orthop*, 271, 201–6.

Rack R and Pfaff HG (2001) *Bioceramics in Joint Arthroplasty*. Stuttgart, Thieme.

Rajadhyaksha AD, Brotea C, Cheung Y, Kuhn C, Ramakrishnan and Zelicof SB. (2009) Five-year comparative study of highly cross-linked (crossfire) and traditional polyethylene. *J Arthroplasty*, 24, 161–7.

Reeves EA, Barton DC, Fitzpatrick DC and Fisher J (2000) Comparison of gas plasma and gamma irradiation in air sterilization on the delamination wear of the ultra-high molecular weight polyethylene used in knee replacements. *Proc Inst Mech Eng*, 214, 249–55.

Reina R, Rodriguez JA, Rasquinha VJ, *et al.* (2005) Fixation and osteolysis in plasma-sprayed hemispherical cups with hybrid total hip replacement: 5- to 11-year results. *Annual AAOS Meeting*, Washington, DC.

Ring PA (1968) Complete replacement arthroplasty of the hip by the Ring prosthesis. *J Bone Joint Surg Br*, 50B, 720–31.

Robinson RP (2005) The early innovators of today's resurfacing condylar knees. *J Arthroplasty*, 20, 2–26.

Rodriguez JA (2006) Acetabular fixation options: notes from the other side. *J Arthroplasty*, 21, 93–6.

Savarino L, Greco M, Cenni E, Cavasini L, Rotini R, Baldini N and Giuni A. (2006) Differences in ion release after ceramic-on-ceramic and metal-on-metal total hip replacement. Medium-term follow-up. *J Bone Joint Surg Br*, 88, 472–6.

Scheerlinck T and Casteleyn PP (2006) The design features of cemented femoral hip implants. *J Bone Joint Surg Br*, 88, 1409–18.

Schmalzried TP, Buttman D, Grecula M and Amstzut HC (1994) The relationship between the design, position, and articular wear of acetabular components inserted without cement and the development of pelvic osteolysis. *J Bone Joint Surg Am* 76, 677–88.

Scott RD (1982) Duopatellar total knee replacement: The Brigham experience. *Orthop Clin North Am*, 13, 89–102.

Sheth NP, Lemetowski P, Hunter G and Garino JP (2008) Clinical applications of oxidized zirconium. *J Surg Orthop Adv*, 17, 17–26.

Shimko DA, Shimko VF, Sander EA, Dickson KF and Nauman EA (2005) Effect of porosity on the fluid flow characteristics and mechanical properties of tantalum scaffolds. *J Biomed Mater Res B Appl Biomater*, 73, 315–24.

Sledge CB and Ewald FC (1979) Total knee arthroplasty experience at the Robert Breck Brigham Hospital. *Clin Orthop Relat Res*, 145, 78–84.

Smith-Petersen MN (1948) Evolution of mould arthroplasty of the hip joint. *J Bone Joint Surg Br*, 30, 59–75.

Stephen LI (1999) Ultra-high-molecula-weight polyethylene, the weak link. In: *Revision Total Knee Arthroplasty*. Philadelphia, PA, Lippincott-Raven, pp. 45–6.

Stiehl JB, Macmillan E and Skrade DA (1991) Mechanical stability of porous-coated acetabular components in total hip arthroplasty. *J Arthroplasty*, 6, 295–300.

Thompson FR (1952) Vitallium intramedullary hip prosthesis – preliminary report. *NY State J Med*, 52, 3011–20.

Treacy RB, McBryde CW and Pynsent PB (2005) Birmingham hip resurfacing arthroplasty. A minimum follow-up of five years. *J Bone Joint Surg Br*, 87, 167–70.

Trentani C and Vaccarino F (1978) The Paltrinieri–Trentani hip joint resurface arthroplasty. *Clin Orthop*, 134, 36–40.

Vallo CI, Montemartini PE, Fanovich MA, Porto Lopez JM and Cuadrado TR (1999) Polymethylmethacrylate–based bone cement modified with hydroxyapatite. *J Biomed Res*, 48, 150–8.

Vince KG, Insall JN and Kelly MA (1989) The total condylar prosthesis. 10- to 12-year results of a cemented knee replacement. *J Bone Joint Surg Br*, 71, 793–7.

Wagner H (1978) Surface replacement arthroplasty of the hip. *Clin Orthop*, 134, 102–30.
Weber BG (1996) Experience with the Metasul total hip bearing system. *Clin Orthop* 329S, S69–77.
Wiles PW (1958) The surgery of the osteoarthritic hip. *Br J Surgery*, 45, 488–97.
Wright TM, Rimnac CM, Faris PM and Bansal M (1988) Analysis of surface damage in retrieved carbon fiber-reinforced and plain polyethylene tibial components from posterior stabilized total knee replacement. *J Bone Joint Surg Am*, 70A, 1312–19.
Yasuda K (2004) Long-term clinical results of cruciate-retaining total knee arthroplasty using the alumina ceramic condylar prosthesis [abstract]. *Scientific Exhibit No. SE035, AAOS Meeting, San Francisco.*
Zardiackas LD, Parsell DE, Dillon LD, Mitchell DW, Nunnery LA and Poggie R (2001) Structure, metallurgy, and mechanical properties of a porous tantalum foam. *J Biomed Mater Res*, 58, 180–7.
Zhang Y, Ahn PB, Fitzpatrick DC, Heiner AD, Poggie RA and Brown TD (1999) Interfacial frictional behavior: cancellous bone, cortical bone, and a novel porous tantalum biomaterial. *J Musculoskeletal Res*, 3, 245–51.

7
Materials used for hip and knee implants

E. KAIVOSOJA, Helsinki University Central Hospital, Finland,
V.-M. TIAINEN, Orton Orthopaedic Hospital of the Invalid Foundation, Finland,
Y. TAKAKUBO, Helsinki University Central Hospital, Finland and Yamagata University School of Medicine, Japan,
B. RAJCHEL, Polish Academy of Sciences, Poland,
J. SOBIECKI, Warsaw University of Technology, Poland,
Y. T. KONTTINEN, Helsinki University Central Hospital, Finland, Orton Orthopaedic Hospital of the Invalid Foundation, Finland and COXA Hospital for Joint Replacement, Finland and
M. TAKAGI, Yamagata University School of Medicine, Japan

Abstract: The biomaterials used in hip and knee implants aim to maximise beneficial mechanical properties (e.g. wear resistance and fatigue strength), minimise material deterioration (e.g. corrosion and degradation) and enable the long-term integration of the implant into the musculoskeletal system. The major aim is to optimise the rate and quality of bone apposition and minimise the rate of wear, corrosion or other degradation products and the adverse tissue responses to them. This chapter discusses the evolution of materials used in hip and knee implants and the internal/surface treatments used to improve the properties of the implants.

Key words: hip prosthesis, knee prosthesis, osseointegration.

7.1 Introduction

Arthroplasties using ivory implants were performed in the 1890s (Gluck, 1890). Later, attempts were made using metal spacers and acrylate hinges (Macintosh, 1966; Walldius, 1996). The modern concept of low-friction hip arthroplasty was developed in the 1970s using polyethylene in the cup, stainless steel in the femoral head and stem, and polymethyl methacrylate (PMMA) as bone cement (Charnley, 1960, 1979). Charnley's total hip arthroplasty (THA) has a long and well-established record with long-term survival in more than 90% of patients over 60 years of age (Berry *et al.*, 2002; Della Valle, 2004; Wroblewski *et al.*, 2007). Many ways have been tried to improve implants, but the risk for their revision has remained unchanged in long-term follow-up (Hailer *et al.*, 2010; Robertsson, 2010). It would be very useful to be able to develop permanent arthroplasty implants as soon as possible, because increased numbers of total hip and knee arthroplasties are expected to be performed in the world in the future (Kurtz *et al.*, 2011).

7.2 Polymer evolution and internal/surface treatments

Polymers are formed by primary covalent linkage of small molecular size monomers to usually high molecular weight compounds. Polymers have been used for hip and knee implants for over 50 years: PMMA as bone cement since 1958 and ultra-high molecular weight polyethylene (UHMWPE) as cups since 1962. These two polymers are still universally used for hip and knee implants. More recently, growing interest in the development of isoelastic hip stems, with stiffness comparable to that of bone, has led to the introduction of polyaromatic polymers, such as poly (aryl-ether-ether-ketone) (PEEK). The properties of these polymers are presented in Table 7.1.

Table 7.1 Typical average physical properties of polymers used in hip and knee implants

	UHMWPE	HXLPE	PEEK[1] Unfilled	PEEK[2] 30% (w/w) C	PEEK[3] 68% (v/v) C	PMMA
Specific gravity	0.93	0.93	1.3	1.4	1.6	1.1
Flexural modulus (GPa)	0.8–1.6	0.876	4	20	135	1.5–4.1
Tensile strength (MPa)	39–48	56.7	94	170	>2000	29–49
Tensile elongation (%)	350–525	267	30–40	1–2	1	1–2

[1] Optima LT1
[2] Chopped carbon fibre reinforced (LT1CA30)
[3] Continuous carbon fibre reinforced (Endolign)
Note: adapted from Kurtz and Devine (2007) and Wang *et al.* (2008).

7.2.1 Polyethylene, UHMWPE and highly cross-linked polyethylene

The introduction of an UHMWPE cup, paired to the already then well-documented stainless steel stem with articulating head, took place in November 1962 and began the modern era of artificial joints. UHMWPE has been fundamental in the facilitation of excellent long-term results in total joint arthroplasties. Its biocompatibility in bulk format and its good material performance compared to, for example, polytetrafluoroethylene (superior wear resistance along with high fracture toughness) laid grounds for its extensive use. Today, UHMWPE remains the most widely used interposition material (tibial plateau) in total knee replacements and the most frequently used acetabular cup bearing in total hip replacements.

Polyethylene is derived from ethane monomers ($CH_2 = CH_2$), which are polymerised into high molecular weight form using the Ziegler process. The polymerisation process results in a powder that can be moulded or extruded into the desired shape. Polyethylene can be classified into subcategories defined by molecular weight – low-density polyethylene (LDPE), linear low-density polyethylene (LLDPE), high-density polyethylene (HDPE) and (UHMWPE), which in part defines its density, casting properties, wear resistance, oxidisation, colour and elasticity, and the degree of cross-linking in the polymer chains. The polyethylenes used in orthopaedics are UHMWPE and highly cross-linked polyethylene (HXLPE).

The critical factor in biocompatibility of polyethylene is the balance between suitable mechanical properties and degradation resistance. Wear debris has been widely discussed in the literature and it seems that the chemistry of the polymer has relatively little influence on foreign body inflammation, but the most relevant factors are the rate, volume and number of wear debris release (Goodman, 2005) and the physical form and dimensions of the wear particles (Ren *et al.*, 2003). Although many attempts have been made to improve polyethylene, those to reduce the wear rate, principally through cross-linking and sterilisation, have been the most clinically relevant (McKellop *et al.*, 2000). It is also possible that the host response could be at least marginally modulated pharmacologically, through the use of vitamins (antioxidants) for example. Due to their different geometries, the wear mechanism in knee prostheses is different from that of the hip and, consequently, the dominant issues also include material fatigue, delamination and fracture, particularly in those component designs that require the use of very thin polyethylene implants at least in some regions.

Ethylene oxide (EtO) sterilisation was originally used for sterilisation of UHMWPE. However, EtO sterilisation does not cause any cross-linking and therefore osteolysis remains an issue. In addition, unexpected oxidation in the bulk of EtO sterilised acetabular cups has been described (Costa *et al.*, 2005). Nowadays, sterilisation is usually done using gas plasma, gamma irradiation in nitrogen or EtO.

Radiation sterilisation at doses between 25 and 40 kGy was later found to be a cost-effective strategy for UHMWPE sterilisation. One further advantage of this technique is that the radiation improves wear resistance due to cross-linking of some of the molecular chains in the amorphous region of the material. Gamma radiation breaks polymer chains, inducing supplementary cross-linking. Unfortunately, this process also generates free radicals leading to material oxidation when it comes in contact with atmospheric oxygen. This eventually leads to material degradation, with lowering of molecular weight and impairment of mechanical properties. To limit this drawback, irradiation is now performed in an inert gas atmosphere (e.g. in nitrogen, argon or helium) or in a vacuum, followed by hermetic packaging in aluminium foil or polymer barrier containers. However, even with these precautions, oxidation continues *in vivo* after implantation (Kurtz *et al.*, 2006), so that delamination is delayed but not avoided.

Because cross-linking was found to improve wear resistance, the first generation of HXLPE was produced using somewhat higher gamma irradiation (50–100 kGy) or high-energy beta irradiation (electron beam) (Santavirta *et al.*, 2003). Gamma irradiation is an inexpensive and widely available method, which penetrates polyethylene very well but is relatively slow so that sterilisation of one batch can take hours. Electron beam sterilisation takes only a few minutes but an accelerator is needed so access to it is limited. Unfortunately, irradiation leads to the formation of alkyl free radicals, which induce an oxidation process (Gomez-Barrena *et al.*, 2008).

Post-treatment by annealing and/or remelting of HXLPE is performed to control the residual free alkyl radicals after cross-linking irradiation of the first-generation HXLPEs. Annealing is performed below the melting transition temperature of the polymer (around 137°C) and remelting above this temperature. Neither method significantly modifies the cross-linking density introduced by irradiation. Remelting stabilises the polymer better against oxidation, whereas annealing is not as effective. Both methods introduce changes in the microstructure, particularly in the crystallinity and the lamellar size, which are more pronounced after remelting than after annealing (Medel *et al.*, 2007). This negatively influences the capability of the implant to absorb energy before fracture (toughness) and even its fatigue resistance. Indeed, a large reduction in HXLPE toughness has been observed compared with non-irradiated material (Medel *et al.*, 2007). Consequently, material fracture is a risk, particularly in areas where the component thickness is thin due to design requisites. Significant research efforts have been made to secure a better post-treatment that would eliminate free radicals while maintaining the key mechanical properties.

Clinical results regarding the wear performance of first-generation HXLPE are now in the mid-term follow-up phase and indicate a common trend of wear rate decrease (38 to 95%) compared with conventional UHMWPE in a 4- to 8-year follow-up period (Calvert et al., 2009; Dorr et al., 2005; Engh et al., 2006; Geerdink et al., 2006, 2009; McCalden et al., 2009; Olyslaegers et al., 2008; Rajadhyaksha et al., 2009).

In spite of improved wear performance of HXLPE, clinical failures have been noticed in series, in which thinner HXLPE components have been used, as a result of rim cracking (Longevity®) due to relatively vertical cup alignment (Tower et al., 2007) and extended lip failure (Marathon®) by femoral neck impingement (Duffy et al., 2009).

Second-generation HXLPEs are being developed using different approaches to control the radicals and to improve oxidative stability. One of the approaches is to use three sequential 30 kGy irradiation steps, followed by annealing at 130°C for 8 hours. The aim is to maintain mechanical properties of annealed HXLPEs and to improve the oxidative resistance by reduction of the radicals in each cycle. This procedure can reduce free radical load to 1% when compared with conventional UHMWPE (Dumbleton et al., 2006; Wang et al., 2008).

Another strategy to decrease oxidative potential while maintaining mechanical properties is the use of antioxidants, like alpha-tocopherol (vitamin E) or nitroxide (RRNO) scavengers. Vitamin E can be blended with the resin before moulding or can diffuse into consolidated material as a result of doping. In the former method, the efficiency of cross-linking is decreased during irradiation; in the latter, it is difficult to control the concentration and distribution of the antioxidant. Both techniques introduce vitamin E only at trace concentrations, in a dose range under 500 ppm (Oral et al., 2005). Consequently, the wear resistance should be maintained while the microstructural changes and impaired mechanical properties generated during thermal treatments should be avoided. The near future promises market penetration of these second-generation HXLPE materials and evaluations of their clinical performance. The results of ongoing study demonstrate that the small amount of penetration into a liner doped with E vitamin occurring during the early period (0.04 ± 0.02 mm at 2 years), likely to be due to creep of the material, is low relative to that reported for non-vitamin E stabilised HXLPE (0.1 mm) (Greene et al., 2010).

HXLPE and antioxidant treatment were introduced in 1998 and the sterilisation methods have been improved due to problems related to wear debris, fatigue damage, osteolysis and aseptic loosening (Goodman, 2005; McKellop et al., 2000; Oral et al., 2005). These problems are caused by multiple factors, including the type of polyethylene resin, the manufacturing process, the degree of thermal stabilisation, sterilisation technique, the size of the femoral head, the alignment of the components, and patient's age, gender, diagnosis, body weight and activity level (Jacobs et al., 2007). Polyethylene wear from tibial and patellar components was a major cause of revision total knee arthroplasty (TKA), but since the introduction of HXLPE the results of TKA have improved in a similar fashion to those of THA (Wang et al., 2008). Although the use of second-generation HXLPE subjected to three doses of radiation, antioxidants or surface modifications to reduce free radicals has become widespread, information on its clinical performance is still limited and somewhat controversial (Jacobs et al., 2007; Schroder et al., 2011; Wang et al., 2008). The endurance of UHWPE should be improved even further to reach better long-term results (Hailer et al., 2010; Robertsson, 2010).

It is important to note that the type of resin used in the production of polyethylene can affect implant performance. First-generation HXLPE, mainly composed of GUR 1050 resin, has been most widely used for hips but not so much for knees, probably due to wear problems (Meding et al., 2011). In second-generation HXLPE, GUR 1020 is used in X3 (Stryker) for hips and knees (Kester et al., 2007) and Arcom with vitamin E (E-poly) has also been used both for hips and knees (Kurtz et al., 2009; Ridley and Jahan, 2009).

Surface modifications by ion implantation (e. g. nitrogen) or coating (see Section 7.4.2) aim to increase hardness and produce more resistant surfaces. Another nano-scale modification uses photo-induced radical polymerisation to graft 2-methacryloyloxyethyl phosphorylcholine polymer onto a polyethylene surface (Moro et al., 2010). New innovations to improve mechanical properties include composite materials, in which multi-wall carbon nanotubes are used as a reinforcing component. However, the biocompatibility of nanotubes needs to be confirmed and the effect of carbon nanotubes on metal wear and ion release should be investigated.

Even though not all the problems related to polyethylene have been solved, the current clinical use of UHMWPE is well motivated based on its tribologic and mechanical properties, the ease of moulding or machine-tooling it to any final component design, its shock absorbing properties, tolerance to edge loading, forgiveness for mild malalignment and relatively low price. Innovation will help to further improve both the material and polyethylene implant design so it is expected to continue to compete with alternative bearings and the somewhat different problems associated with their use.

7.2.2 Poly (aryl-ether-ether-ketone) PEEK

Interest in the development of isoelastic hip stems and fracture fixation plates with stiffness comparable to that of bone led up to the introduction of polyaromatic polymers. PEEK was commercialised for industry in the 1980s and, since confirmation of its biocompatibility two decades ago, it has been increasingly employed as a biomaterial for orthopaedic, trauma and spinal implants. PEEK consists of a backbone of aromatic rings linked to each other by ketone and ether groups. The chemical structure confers stability at high temperatures exceeding 300°C, resistance to chemical- and radiation-induced damage, compatibility with many reinforcing agents (such as glass and carbon fibres) and better strength than many metals. The elastic modulus of polyaromatic polymers (3–4 GPa without any reinforcing agents) can be tailored to match that of the cortical bone (18 GPa) or titanium alloys (110 GPa) by the production of carbon fibre reinforced composites with varying fibre length and orientation. Since April 1998, PEEK has been commercially available as a biomaterial for implants (Invibio Ltd, Thornton Cleveleys, UK).

The resonance-stabilised chemical structure of PEEK results in delocalisation of higher orbital electrons along the entire macromolecule, making PEEK extremely unreactive and resistant to chemical and thermal degradation. PEEK displays remarkable resistance to gamma and electron beam radiation. The free radicals generated during irradiation of PEEK decay rapidly, presumably due to recombination reactions enabled by the mobility of electrons along the molecular chain (Kurtz and Devine, 2007). Although PEEK itself is not susceptible to hydrolysis, concerns have been raised that the interface between the polymer and reinforcements, such as carbon fibres, may be vulnerable to fluid environments *in vivo* (Meyer *et al.*, 1994).

The inert chemical structure of PEEK in part explains its biocompatibility. Numerous studies on systemic toxicity and intracutaneous and intramuscular implantation have shown no adverse effects. Concern has been raised about the inertness of PEEK and limited osseointegration with bone. Efforts have been made to improve the bone–PEEK implant interface contact by producing composites with hydroxyapatite (HA), by Ti or HA coating, and by creating porous PEEK nets to allow bone ingrowth. Surface modification of PEEK can also be produced by wet chemistry (Noiset *et al.*, 1999, 2000) and by plasma treatment (Briem *et al.*, 2005; Schröder *et al.*, 2002). PEEK–HA composites are often made by injection moulding (Abu Bakar *et al.*, 2003a, 2003b, 2003c; Tang *et al.*, 2004), but sintering has also been used for this purpose (Yu, 2005).

Commercially available PEEK hip stems have been coated with HA by thermal plasma spray coating. Alternative implants are produced by plasma spraying with titanium, followed by thermal plasma coating with HA (see Sections 7.3.5 and 7.4.3). The objective of dual coating with titanium and HA is to ensure bone apposition with the biocompatible titanium implant surface after HA has been resorbed *in vivo*.

Several polymers have been evaluated for use in isoelastic femoral stems over the past 50 years, but PEEK has proven to be the only one with the required combination of mechanical properties, biocompatibility, manufacturability and consistent availability. Long-term clinical data are awaited to determine whether composite PEEK stems will provide extended implant life-in-service, but it will still take years before these novel approaches can be reliably compared with their historical predecessors with a long track record.

Mid-term results have been reported for the Epoch hip stem system (Versys®, Zimmer, Warsaw, IN, USA). The Epoch stem is a three-part composite consisting of a forged cobalt–chromium alloy inner core, an intermediate layer of PEEK resin and an outer bone in-growth layer of commercially pure titanium fibre metal. PEEK is thus an attractive material for use in arthroplasty bearing surfaces and resurfacing cups, but long-term results are needed (Kurtz and Devine, 2007).

7.2.3 Poly(methylmethacrylate) PMMA

The primary functions of relatively biocompatible PMMA-based bone cement are to secure orthopaedic implants to bone and act as an intermediate interface layer in the transfer of micromotion and mechanical loads from implant to bone. PMMA was first used as bone cement to secure a femoral component in 1958 (Charnley, 1960) and an acetabular component in 1961 (McKee and Watson-Farrar, 1966). By this method, a more natural anatomic position of the acetabular cup could be achieved in relation to the pelvic bone than by fixation with pelvic screws. PMMA ('Plexiglas') based bone cements are composed of two ready-made components; both components are chlorophyll-coloured to make the transparent PMMA more easily visible to the naked eye and easier to handle. The powder component of the final mixture contains pre-polymerised PMMA powder and co-polymers to modulate the physical properties of the cement, a toluidine initiator and a radio-opacifier (barium sulphate or zirconium dioxide) for better radiological imaging. In addition, many bone cements contain antibiotics, such as gentamicin, because it seems that this, combined with the use of prophylactic antibiotics, such as cephalosporins or vancomycin, diminishes deep implant-related infections (Jämsen *et al.*, 2010). Antibiotic-impregnated bone cement has been also used as a spacer, and contains higher concentrations of antibiotics than the cement used for regular implant fixation. This improves the success rate of two-stage revisions by diminishing recurrent implant-related infections (Hsieh et al., 2004; Ivarsson et al., 1994). The second component contains liquid MMA monomers, a stabiliser to prevent premature polymerisation and an accelerator to speed up polymerisation and minimise the release of potentially harmful and toxic MMA monomers from bone cement elsewhere into the body.

Bone cements are available as low-, medium- or high-viscosity brands, which differ in the length of the waiting, working and hardening phases during setting (cement curing). The idea is that use of an appropriate cementing technique can effectively fill the void between the implant and its bone bed. Bone cement was first applied by hand packing, but second-generation (intramedullary cement plug, a cement gun and pulsatile lavage) or third-generation (pressurisation of the cement, reduction of its porosity by centrifuge and pre-coating of the critical implant–bone interface with PMMA) cementing techniques are now more commonly used. Bone cement anchors the implant rapidly to bone without any biological osseointegrating processes. Cement penetrates into the cancellous bone and locks onto small surface irregularities on the implant. Shrinkage of the cement during curing also locks the cement onto the cement-facing surface of the device. Although PMMA bone cements have proven their usefulness in hip, knee and other artificial joint applications, it osseointegrates poorly and can even disturb bone healing and remodelling through its exotermic and genuinely inert properties. Tissue necrosis may be caused through heat production during curing. Primary mechanical instability may lead to the formation of an implant capsule, a synovial membrane-like interface membrane and subsequent aseptic loosening (El-Warrak et al., 2004b, 2004a). Despite all these potential and largey theoretical concerns, PMMA is still the most frequently used polymer bone cement (Hailer et al., 2010; Robertsson, 2010). Surgeons have to try to achieve mastery of cement use in arthroplasty due to its challenging biomechanical properties and the cardiovascular risks associated with its use (Crout et al., 1979).

Alternative methods for implant fixation have been developed (see Sections 7.3.5 and 7.4.3) and the use of bone cement in hip replacements has declined. However, bone cement is still routinely used in total knee replacements because it has been found that cemented total knees perform better than uncemented knees. In hip replacements, cement is also commonly used in elderly patients with severe osteoporosis because it allows rapid remobilisation of the patient after surgery. Younger, more physically active patients have a higher risk that a cemented implant may become loose.

Table 7.2 Typical average physical properties of metals used in hip and knee implants

	AISI 316L	CPTi	Ti-6Al-4V	CoCrMo
Density (g/cm^3)	7.9	4.5	4.43	7.8
Yield strength (MPa)	205–310	483	830	455
Tensile strength (MPa)	515–620	550	930	600–1795
Elastic modulus (GPa)	200	105	110	200–230
Hardness HV (MPa)	1500–3100	2400–2700	3000–3400	3000
Corrosion potential (mV)[1]	−400	−90 to −630	−180 to −510	−390

[1]The lower the corrosion resistance, the lower is this E_{corr} value
Note: adapted from Konttinen *et al.* (2008) and Katti *et al.* (2008).

7.3 Metal evolution and internal/surface treatments to use *in vivo*

At the moment the optimal balance of mechanical properties with metallic components of knee and hip implants is best achieved with either titanium (Ti) alloys or cobalt–chromium (CoCr) based alloys, which have largely replaced stainless steel due to their better corrosion resistance and lower stiffness. Table 7.2 presents the mechanical properties of metal alloys used for hip and knee implants. The major characteristic that controls the host response to these alloys is the rate of ion release and formation of degradation products. No specific biocompatibility characteristics are dependent on the alloying elements in Ti or CoCr alloys or, with the exceptions of rare idiosyncratic hypersensitivity responses (Williams, 2008). The precise chemical composition of Ti or CoCr alloys has little influence on the rate of the appositional bone formation or the strength of the bone attachment (Puleo and Thomas, 2006), but Ti alloys give stronger and faster attachment to bone than CoCr alloys (Jinno *et al.*, 1998). This is in contrast to the surface texture (surface roughness and/or porosity), which influence the bone response (Lossdörfer *et al.*, 2004; Puleo and Thomas, 2006). Production methods and micro-granularity modify the mechanical properties of metal alloys used in joint replacements. Metal alloys are generally cast, wrought or forged.

A cast alloy is manufactured by pouring or pressing liquid material into a mould, which contains a hollow cavity of the desired shape, where the liquid material is allowed to solidify. The casting process produces large grains and metallurgical imperfections, so that cast metals have lower mechanical properties than wrought or forged alloys. However, investment casting is regularly used in the manufacturing of orthopaedic implants because it provides an efficient way of producing near net shape parts out of materials that are difficult to produce by machining. Heat treatments can be used to modulate the microstructure and improve the mechanical properties of cast parts.

Wrought alloys are mechanically worked after casting by rolling, drawing or forging. For medical implants, a commonly used processing method is forging, which utilises the ductility of metals. In forging, heat and compressive force are applied to metal so that it, via plastic deformation, obtains the desired strength and shape. Forging requires sophisticated presses and complicated tools, which makes it expensive.

Section 7.3.4 further discusses material treatments that can be utilised to improve the mechanical properties of metallic alloys in implants and Sections 7.3.5 and 7.4.3 discuss the material treatment methods that can enhance the integration of bone to an implant.

7.3.1 Stainless steel

Stainless steel implants are superior to other implants in terms of fatigue strength, but are susceptible to corrosion and have a relatively low biocompatibility (Amstutz, 1990). In addition, steel presents a technical hitch in magnetic resonance imaging (Naraghi and White, 2006). The steel used in joint replacements is typically a low carbon (0.03%) austenitic steel containing 17–19% chromium (Cr), 14–16% nickel (Ni) and 2.3–4.2% molybdenum (Mo) as major constituents. Cr protects steel against corrosion as the surface of such Cr-containing steel produces a thin and relatively durable passivating oxide layer (enriched with Cr oxide), whereas Mo improves the corrosion resistance of the grain boundaries. Ni improves corrosion resistance by stabilising the austenitic (α-iron) face centred cubic phase microstructure of steel (FeCr steels are ferritic or γ-iron).

AISI 316L stainless steel (i.e. surgical steel) has relatively good corrosion resistance but, compared with CoCr and Ti alloys, it is sensitive to crevice and pit corrosion. Consequently, steel implants should not have porous surfaces as a large surface area increases leaching of implant components and additives.

Steel, with its 200 GPa modulus of elasticity, is approximately ten times stiffer than cortical bone. Some surgical metal alloys have an elastic modulus closer to that of cortical bone but, generally, metal implants are stiffer than bone. Due to this modulus mismatch, the implant shields part of the bone it is attached to from mechanical loading, whereas some other parts of the bone are subjected to a load that is heavier than normal – the stress distribution within the bone is thus changed. Living bone must be under a certain amount of loading to remodel and stay healthy. Unloaded or overloaded bone undergoes biological changes, which lead to bone resorption and weakening and deterioration of the implant–bone interface. Use of bone cement as an interface decreases this stress shield effect, because the elastic modulus of the cement, which forms a cement mantle interface, is much lower than that of the steel alloy. Due to the sensitivity of surgical steel to crevice and pit corrosion, porous metallic coatings cannot be used to improve bone bonding. This can be overcome by the use of porous ceramic coatings, which enhance the bone bonding of stainless steel devices (see Section 7.4.3).

Regular AISI 316L has a relatively good yield point in traction, 200–250 MPa. Forged stainless steel has a lower fatigue strength than other implant alloys. Production defects and improper design increase the risk of fatigue fracture; that is, a fracture based on repeated cyclic stress below the ultimate stress level. Metal implants usually fracture due to fatigue rather than mechanical overloading. The advantage of stainless steel over CoCr and Ti alloys is its greater ductility and easier machining. Due to femoral component fractures in early implant designs, stainless steel is no longer used routinely. From the perspective of erosion and fatigue life, stainless steel is inferior to other implant alloys.

7.3.2 Titanium and its alloys

Ti alloys are widely used for the manufacture of orthopaedic implants. The main types of Ti alloys in use are commercially pure titanium (CPTi), Ti-6Al-4V and TiAlNb. Ti alloys are biocompatible and have a relatively low modulus of elasticity and a high resistance to fatigue and corrosion (Kohn and Ducheyne, 1992; Willert et al., 1996). The wear resistance of titanium is not so good, but can be improved by eloxation (Eloxalverfahren, oxidation treatment), ion implantation, TiN coating (see Sections 7.3.4 and 7.4.2) and alloying.

Ti alloys have better corrosion resistance than Co-based materials and surgical steel. A thin oxide (TiO_2, titania) layer spontaneously forms on the surface of Ti-based implants and protects them against corrosion. In addition to TiO_2, the passive layer contains oxides of the other elemental constituents of the alloy (López et al., 2001; Marciniak 2002); for example, the passive layer formed on the Ti-7Nb-6Al alloy contains Ti oxide, aluminium (Al) oxide and small amounts of niobium (Nb) oxide, whereas the oxide layer formed on the Ti-13Nb-13Zr and Ti-15Zr-4Nb alloys contains Ti oxide, zirconium (Zr) oxide and small amounts of Nb oxide (López et al., 2001). The passive layers containing oxides of Zr and Nb are more resistant to corrosion than those with oxides of Al, vanadium (V) or Mo, and dissolve in the physiological fluids more slowly (Marciniak, 2002). Wear may damage this protective native oxide layer, but it is rapidly reproduced in repassivation. If mechanical chafing is continuous, this process produces so much oxide that the peri-implant tissues gradually turn black, but the biological effects of this metallosis are usually harmless although it can cause necrosis in periprosthetic tissue.

Ti exists in two different allotropic forms. The low-temperature α-form has a close packed hexagonal crystal structure with an axial (c/a) ratio of 1.587 at room temperature. The β-form has a body centred cubic structure and is stable above 882.5°C. The presence of V in Ti–Al alloy tends to lead to the formation of an α–β two-phase system at room temperature. The exact composition and thermal history controls the phase distribution and morphology of the alloy and hence determines the resulting properties. Ti-6Al-4V implants are generally classified by one of the three forming methods (cast, wrought or forged).

Cast alloys have a metallurgically stable homogeneous structure. They have a coarse acicular α–β structure with thick β grain boundaries. Wrought Ti-6Al-4V alloy has no β grain boundaries and has a high strength. A forged alloy has a fine-grained α-structure with a dispersion of varying β-phases. A final annealing treatment is often given to the alloy to obtain a stable microstructure without significantly altering its properties. Forged alloys typically have the highest strength of these alloys. All Ti-6Al-4V castings are hot isostatic pressed to ensure structural integrity. One of the major benefits of Ti alloys is that the elastic modulus of Ti-6Al-4V is 110 GPa, which is only half that of surgical stainless steel or Co-based alloys although still five times that of cortical bone. This leads to more physiological stress distribution in the peri-implant bone. Cement is used as an intermediate layer to improve the stress distribution of steel and Co-based implants, but is not necessary when Ti implants are used. To guarantee cementless fixation of Ti by bone in growth and micromechanical interlocking, porous-coated implants are often used (see Sections 7.3.5 and 7.4.3). Peri-implant bone around cementless stems is more resistant to osteolysis and mechanical failure than bone around cemented stems (Emerson *et al.*, 2002; Head *et al.*, 1995; Laupacis *et al.*, 2002).

Ti implants have an advantage in terms of their modularity and flexibility compared with implants made from other materials. However, Ti femoral stems in early designs failed, largely because the flexibility of the femoral stem increased stresses in the proximal cement layers (Huiskes, 1993; Niinimaki *et al.*, 1994) and the crevice corrosion between the stem and cement was problematic (Thomas *et al.*, 2004; Willert *et al.*, 1996). Recently, new Ti alloys containing Zr and Nb have been developed, for example Ti-13Zr-13Nb. These alloys have a high strength and low elastic modulus (65–80 GPa). NiTi shape memory alloy (Nitinol) implants can be deformed but return to their original shapes upon heating.

7.3.3 Cobalt-based alloys

Co-based alloys are the most used materials in arthroplastic implants because of their strength, resistance to stress fatigue and low incidence of stem fractures (Robertsson, 2007). Co-based alloys usually contain 30–60% Co and approximately 20–30% Cr. The main types of CoCr alloys are CoCr Mo alloy (which is usually used to cast products) and CoNiCrMo (which is generally wrought by hot forging). The castable CoCrMo alloy has been used for many decades whereas the wrought CoNiCrMo alloy is a relative newcomer. Cr is added to improve corrosion resistance and Mo is added to decrease grain size and thus improve mechanical properties (e.g. strength). In addition, these alloys can also contain other minor elements, such as wolfram (tungsten, W), iron (Fe), manganese (Mn) and silicon (Si).

CoCr alloys are highly resistant to corrosion although, as with all highly alloyed metals, they are susceptible subjected to galvanic corrosion in the body environment. Surgical steel should not be used in contact with CoCr implants, because the relatively poor corrosion resistance of steel leads to rapid galvanic corrosion. Ti alloys and CoCr alloys can be used together because they both have a relatively good corrosion resistance.

Co-based alloys are relatively stiff, having an elastic modulus of 200–300 GPa. Like steel implants, due to the stiffness mismatch between the alloy and cortical bone, bone cements are used to fix CoCr implants to bone. CoCr alloys have also been used in a cementless fashion with variable success (Section 7.3.5).

The microstructure of cast CoCr is a coarse Co–FCC (face centred cubic) dendritic matrix with the presence of a secondary phase such as $Mo_{23}C_6$ carbides, which are precipitated at grain boundaries and interdendritic points during cooling (Chiba et al., 2007). These precipitates form the main strengthening mechanism in these types of alloys.

Wrought CoCrMo has a microstructure very different from that of cast CoCrMo. This material typically has much smaller grains (1–5 μm) that are more spherical (i.e. have a more equal diameter in all directions) (Wimmer et al., 2001). Dispersed carbides and the small grain size make these alloys very strong and wear resistant.

Although both the wrought CoNiCrMo alloy and the cast CoCrMo alloy have similar abrasive wear properties, CoNiCrMo is not recommended for the bearing surface of joint prostheses because of its poor frictional properties in contact with CoNiCrMo itself or other materials. The superior fatigue and ultimate tensile strength of the wrought CoNiCrMo alloy make it suitable for such applications, which require long service without fracture or stress fatigue, e.g. the stems of hip joint prostheses.

7.3.4 Material treatment to improve mechanical properties

Several material treatments are used to improve the mechanical properties of metallic alloys. For example, wear resistance can be improved by plasma electrolytic oxidation and ion implantation or by the use of coatings with special elemental composition and nanostructure. In particular, the mechanical and biological properties of metallic prosthesis parts can be improved by a covering with a thin protective layer (Cui and Luo, 1999). Carbon-based coatings are frequently used for this purpose (Section 7.4.2).

Plasma electrolytic oxidation is an electrochemical surface treatment process that can be used to grow oxide layers on various metals. It is similar to anodising (the implant is held in a dilute alkaline electrolyte and a current is passed through it), but it employs higher potentials than anodising so that discharges occur and the resulting plasma modifies the structure of the oxide layer. This technique can be used to produce thicker oxide coatings (tens or hundreds of micrometres) than conventional anodising. The oxide coating forms a hard and continuous barrier that protects against wear and corrosion.

Ion implantation is a process in which ions of a selected material are accelerated in an electrical field and entered into the surface layer of another solid material. Ion implantation is used to modify the surface structure and elemental composition of materials at low temperature. It can be used to improve hardness, wear resistance, corrosion resistance, toughness and bioreactivity. Orthopaedic prostheses for hips and knees composed of Ti and CoCr alloys are among the most successful commercial applications of ion implantation used to improve wear resistance. A ten to hundred fold wear reduction can be achieved by implantation of nitrogen ions into these alloys (Hirvonen and Sartwell, 1994). Implantation of iridium improves the corrosion resistance of Ti-6Al-4V (Buchanan *et al.*, 1987) and the implantation of carbon or nitrogen ions is frequently used to increase the surface hardness of medical alloys and steels.

Glow discharge assisted nitriding applied to the surface of a Ti alloy produces a nitrided layer that increases the corrosion resistance of the alloy. When placed in a NaCl solution, both non-nitrided and nitrided samples show good corrosion resistance; however in a very aggressive environment (5% HCl) non-nitrided samples undergo serious corrosion whereas those that are nitrided appear to be resistant. This can be attributed to the chemical neutrality of the nitrides formed in the nitrided layer (Rossi *et al.*, 2003). Polarisation potential and resistance measured in a Hank solution was found to be highest in Ti-6Al-7Nb and Ti-5Al-2Nb-1Ta alloys, whereas the repassivation region was the smallest in samples nitrided at a high temperature 900°C. Moreover, in samples nitrided at 900°C, the capacitance of the interface layer (the boundary between the metal and the surrounding environment) was decreased and the resistance to the flow of electric charges increased compared with those measured in non-nitrided samples. This indicates that a stable nitrided layer has formed on the surface of the Ti-6Al-7Nb and Ti-5Al-2Nb-1Ta alloys (Gokul Lakshmi et al., 2003, 2004). In samples nitrided at a lower temperature 750°C, the corrosion potential decreased and, after about 27 days of the test, local corroded centres, formed due to damage to the nitrided layer, could be observed. This can be explained in terms of the thickness of the layer formed at this temperature, (it is thinner) and the corrosion resistance of the ε-TiN nitride (which constitutes the outer zone of the TiN + Ti$_2$N + αTi(N) layer formed at this reduced temperature) being lower than that of the δ-TiN nitride that forms at the higher temperature (Rossi et al., 2003).

As reported elsewhere, the diffusion-type Ti(CN) layer formed in the outer zone of the nitrided layer increases the corrosion resistance of titanium (tests were conducted in 0.5 M NaCl (Czarnowska et al., 1999; Fleszar et al., 2000; Sobiecki et al., 2001; Wierzchoń and Fleszar, 1997) and in Dulbecco incubation solution (Czarnowska et al., 1999)).

Oxynitriding of Ti alloys slightly decreases corrosion resistance because of the formation of TiO$_2$ oxide phase, which is hard but brittle, in the near-surface zone of the surface layer (Sobiecki and Wierzchoń, 2005; Wierzchoń and Fleszar, 1997). Due to the specific conditions under which the nitrided layer is oxidised, the TiN surface becomes very favourable for the nucleation of calcium phosphates. This suggests that the oxynitriding treatment of Ti alloys may facilitate the formation of phosphates or even HA on the surface of the so-treated Ti alloy implant (Piscanec et al., 2004).

Another important parameter for the biomedical properties of metallic materials is their resistance to frictional wear. Fine scraps of the material, abraded due to friction, that come into contact with human cells and tissues can induce inflammatory states (Cukrowska et al., 2004; Czarnowska et al., 2005). Unfortunately, Ti alloys have poor tribological properties and heat treatment and plastic deformation treatments do not always ensure sufficiently advantageous surface properties. This is why surface engineering techniques are increasingly used to prolong the in-service life of products made of Ti and its alloys intended for exploitation under frictional wear conditions (Czarnowska et al., 2000; Meletis, 2002; Wierzchoń and Fleszar, 1997).

Selection of a suitable surface treatment for a given product is quite difficult because various wear mechanisms operate simultaneously. This is why various surface treatments intended to improve the wear resistance of titanium alloys have been developed, from chemical and electro-chemical deposition of metals, through thermal spraying, physical vapour deposition (PVD) techniques, anodic oxidation and mechanical treatments to glow discharge assisted treatments (Czarnowska et al., 2000; Meletis, 2002;

Rolinski et al., 1998; Wierzchoń and Fleszar, 1997) and ion implantation and pulsed laser deposition (PLD) techniques (Dawei et al., 1993; Hutchings, 1985; Li et al., 1981; Nath et al., 1991; Raveh et al., 1993; Vardiman and Kant, 1982).

Particularly good prospects of increasing the wear resistance of Ti alloys are offered by glow discharge assisted nitriding, oxynitriding and, especially carbonitriding (Czarnowska et al., 2000; Meletis, 2002; Rolinski et al.,1998). Noda et al. (1996) report on plasma carbonitriding of Ti-33.5Al-1Nb-0.5Cr-0.5Si carried out at a temperature of 900°C in a methane + argon atmosphere; this yielded a 3 µm, Ti-2Al-C layer with a hardness of 8.52 GPa. Kim et al. (2003) give information concerning plasma carburising of Ti-6Al-4V, which improved performance properties of the alloy such as hardness and frictional wear resistance.

7.3.5 Porous coatings to improve bone bonding

Porous coatings have been used for cementless implants produced of Ti, CoCr and other biomaterials since the 1970s. Because PMMA cement is a bioinert material, the fixation of cemented implants depends on the strength of the micro-interlocking between the bone and the cement (El-Warrak et al., 2004b). Cementless implants with porous coatings are thought to be superior to cement implants in osteophilicity, which contributes to the bone in growth into the interface of coated implants (Froimson et al., 2007).

Surface finish determines the overall osseointegration potential (Sotereanos et al., 1995). Porous coated metal implants have been extensively used to promote bone in growth. Pore size (e.g. 50–400 µm), pore interconnectivity (e.g. 75–150 µm), particle interconnectivity, volume fraction porosity (e.g. 30–40% for spherical beads) and the area coated (e.g. proximal part of the implant) are important for cementless fixation. Ceramic coatings can be used to allow direct chemical bonding (see Section 7.4.3).

Ti alloys have osteoinductive properties, which makes them the material of choice for cementless fixation. In Europe, one of the most popular cementless Ti alloy devices is the Zweymuller implant (Variall®, Zimmer, SL Plus®, Plus Orthopaedics), which is showing excellent survivorship of 96–99% for stems at 10 years (Grübl et al., 2002; Traulsen et al., 2001). In some recent publications, a titanium alloy stem (Corail®, DePuy, Warsaw, IN, USA) and anatomic hip (Zimmer, Warsaw, IN, USA) showed no cases of aseptic loosening after an average of 11.5 and 10 years of follow-up, respectively, with no distal osteolysis and no thigh pain in the former (Archibeck et al., 2001; Froimson et al., 2007). However, the long-term results of cementless THA were inferior to those of cemented THA, mainly because of the poor performance of cementless cups (Hailer et al., 2010).

According to register studies from the Nordic countries, cemented implants were used in almost all TKAs (Robertsson, 2010).

To some extent, CoCr alloys can be used without bone cement. Cumulative probability of survival reached 96% at 12 years for patients of aged over 60 years. Osteolysis was, however, seen in 40% of cases (including patients younger than 60) at 10 year follow-up (Engh, 1998). Some systems have reached nearly 100% and 95% survivorship after 12–15 years of follow up (Kawamura *et al.*, 2001; Pellegrini *et al.*, 1998). Some methods used to produce porous metallic coatings are now briefly described.

- *Sintering.* Coatings can be produced by placing powder or fibres on the implant surface, followed by heating at temperatures sufficient to lead to adherence of the coating material to the implant surface (gravity sintering). For example, spherical beads of CoCr can be gravity sintered onto CoCr-based implants at temperatures reaching 90–95% of the melting point of the alloy. High-temperature sintering can impair the mechanical properties of metal implants and lead to low bond strength between coating and implant.
- *Diffusion bonding.* This is a process somewhat similar to sintering but, due to the application of pressure, it can be done at relatively low temperatures, 65–75% of the melting point. Microstructural changes that occur during gravity sintering of beads can thus be avoided. Diffusion involves the migration of atoms across the joint, due to concentration gradients. The CoCrMo fibre metal pad can be bonded to its substrate using a diffusion bonding process. Ti wire- and fibre-made coatings are used on Ti-6Al-4V implants. These coatings have very high pore volumes, up to approximately 65–70% (Davis, 2003).
- *Thermal spraying.* This technique is a coating processes in which melted (or heated) materials are sprayed onto a surface. The coating precursor is heated by electrical (plasma or arc) or chemical means (combustion flame). Thermal spraying can provide thick coatings (approximate thickness range is from 20 µm to several millimetres). The method enables high deposition rates and is economical. Thermal spraying is a line of sight technique, i.e. it is extremely difficult to coat undercuts and other complex surface features using thermal spraying. The method requires high temperatures, which tend to induce decomposition, and rapid cooling, which produces amorphous coatings (Sun *et al.*, 2001).
- *Plasma spraying.* This method is a type of thermal spraying that utilises partially melted metal powder or wire, which is injected into the plasma and accelerated towards the substrate. The plasma-sprayed coatings form irregular surfaces with very little interconnected porosity throughout the thickness of the coating. One of the most common applications is plasma spraying of CPTi onto Ti-6Al-4V implants,

although CoCrMo alloy can also be plasma sprayed onto CoCr implants. The porosity of the coating varies with thickness of the coating and pore sizes in the range 20–200 μm can be obtained in this process.
- *Electron beam deposition.* This is a form of physical vapour deposition in which the target is bombarded with an electron beam under high vacuum and the additive is normally brought under the beam spot as metal wire. This technique produces a dense, uniform film on any substrate at low temperatures. Ti has been coated on CoCr or PEEK surfaces using electron beam deposition (Han et al., 2009, 2010).

Trabecular Metal™ implants are porous tantalum (Ta) implants fabricated using vapour deposition techniques to create a metallic strut similar to trabecular bone. The bone-like properties contribute to extensive bone ingrowth. An animal study of transcortical implants demonstrated that new bone grew rapidly into the porous Ta implant (Bobyn et al., 1999). Furthermore, marked bone ingrowth has been observed at the time of revisions of these types of implants (Klein et al., 2008; Sanchez Marquez et al., 2009). As bone ingrowth is supposed to be related to lengthened life in-service, this sort of implant could help to diminish revisions performed for aseptic loosening. After a 2-years follow-up, Ta tibial implants appeared to maintain tibial bone mineral density at the same level as in the nonoperated contralateral limb and better than in historical controls (Harrison et al., 2010). The long-term survival rates of this implant have not yet been clinically confirmed.

Alkali- and heat-treated titanium can improve osseointegration of the cup and the stem (Nishiguchi et al., 2003). Clinical result at 4.8 years show improved survivorship of porous-coated titanium implants with alkali and heat treatment (Kawanabe et al., 2009).

7.4 Ceramic evolution and internal/surface treatments to use *in vivo*

Ceramic materials are utilised in joint replacements for two different purposes – as bearing surfaces or as coatings to improve bone bonding. The wear rates of metal-on-metal and metal-on-polyethylene bearings are often relatively high. Oxide ceramics are formed when a metal reacts with oxygen and releases a great amount of energy. Thus, these compounds are in a very low state of energy, i.e. they are chemically inert. Inert oxide ceramics are hard and wear-resistant and therefore minimise particle-induced osteolysis. Ceramics can be used for the fabrication of prosthetic devices or their parts, but ceramic materials such as titanium nitride (TiN) and diamond-like carbon (DLC) can also be utilised as coatings to improve the surface properties of bearing surfaces. Some ceramic coatings are osteoinductive and can be used to improve bone bonding (Ducheyne and Qiu, 1999; Geesink and Hoefnagels, 1995; Tanzer et al., 2004).

7.4.1 Ceramics as bearing surfaces

Inert oxide ceramics can be used as bearing surfaces, because their hardness improves wear resistance and minimises wear-debris-induced osteolysis. The extremely low wear rate of ceramic-on-ceramic bearings, their biocompatibility and the sparsity of allergic reactions to ceramic compounds compared with metal implants make ceramics an interesting choice for articulating joint replacement materials (Wang et al., 2003). However, the weak fracture toughness (brittleness) and low bending strength have caused concerns about ceramics used in joint replacement. Several studies have reported fractures (Boutin et al., 1988, Habermann et al., 2006; Piconi and Maccauro, 1999; Weisse et al., 2003). Control of the microstructure and manufacturing methods can reduce the incidence of fractures. Ceramic components are manufactured from powder, usually by sintering or hot isostatic pressing. The fracture toughness of a ceramic decreases in proportion to the size and number of material defects and the occurrence of such defects can be reduced by decreasing the porosity of the ceramic and by using a smaller grain size. Improved homogeneity of ceramic microstructure increases its toughness, i.e. its ability to absorb energy and plastically deform without fracturing (Ostrowski and Rödel, 1999).

Alumina (Al_2O_3) was the first ceramic material to be used in total hip arthroplasty in 1970 (Boutin, 1972) and in partial knee replacement in 1972 (Langer, 2002). Its low surface free energy and extremely low surface roughness yield excellent wear and friction properties.

Alumina parts are fabricated from high-purity alumina (around 99.7%) with a small percentage of magnesium oxide (MgO). MgO is introduced during sintering of the alumina, because this additive prevents the increase of alumina grain size during the sintering process. This allows a more homogenous and denser microstructure – characteristics that correlate positively with mechanical properties such as strength and wear resistance. An increase in average grain size to $>7\,\mu m$ decreases the mechanical properties by about 20%. International standards specify that alumina used in orthopaedic applications should have a grain size $<7\,\mu m$ (Hulbert, 1993). The high elastic modulus of oxide ceramics limits their use: the elastic modulus of medical-grade alumina ($>99.7\%$ Al_2O_3) is 15–55 times higher than that of cortical bone and 760–7600 times higher than that of cancellous bone (Hulbert, 1993).

One disadvantage of alumina is its brittleness and low tensile strength, leading to a relatively low fracture toughness. A number of femoral head component and ceramic cup fractures have demonstrated this disadvantage compared with the ductile metallic components used in total hip replacements. However, if a relatively thin ceramic coating (such as DLC) is used, implant deformation can be avoided even if catastrophic failure occurs. Complications encountered with ceramics are often connected to the ceramic–bone interface and the insufficient osseous integration of ceramic materials (Hannouche *et al.*, 2005). In addition, due to the only moderate flexural (bending) strength and toughness of alumina, the diameter of most femoral heads produced from alumina has been limited to 32 mm. This size of femoral head limits the post-operative range of motion and increases the risk of dislocation/luxation.

Zirconia was introduced in the 1980s to counter problems with the relatively low fracture toughness of alumina. This oxide ceramic has a biphasic tetragonal and monoclinic polycrystalline structure, with a bending strength almost twice that of alumina. The tetragonal phase of pure zirconia is in an unstable state and must therefore be stabilised, with yttrium for example. However, owing to the instability of its biphasic structure, zirconia undergoes an undesirable ageing process. The phase transition from the metastable tetragonal phase into the stable monoclinic phase results in a volume increase of around 3–4%. Therefore, ageing of zirconia may result in surface roughening. However, this same phase transformation can be beneficial when zirconia is under stress. The stress concentrates at a crack tip, which can cause the tetragonal phase to convert to monoclinic. This phase transition, known as transformation toughening, can put the crack into compression, retarding its growth, and enhance the fracture toughness. Zirconia has been used for femoral heads against polyethylene in hip replacements, but almina femoral heads have been found to produce less wear (Liang *et al.*, 2007).

Composite ceramic materials combine the stability of alumina with the better fracture toughness of zirconia (Merkert, 2003; Rack and Pfaff, 2000). Zirconia-toughened alumina (ZTA) has been used in mechanical applica-

Table 7.3 Typical average physical properties of ceramics used in hip and knee implants

	Alumina (Biolox® forte)	Zirconia (Y-TZP)	Composite (Biolox® delta)
Density (g/cm³)	3980	6040	4365
Grain size (μm)			
Flexural strength (MPa)	580	1050	1150
Hardness	2300 HV 0.5	1250 HV 0.5	1975 HV 1
Poisson's ratio	0.23	0.3	0.22
Young's modulus (GPa)	380	210	350

Note: adapted from Rack and Pfaff (2000).

tions for over 20 years but its use as a biomaterial is relatively new. For instance, the Biolox® delta ceramic, introduced in 2000, consists of an alumina matrix enforced with zirconia grains and strontium platelets. This ceramic contains about 75% alumina, the remainder is zirconium, strontium, yttrium or chromium oxides. Currently, a 36 mm size femoral head is available (Clarke et al., 2003). The high performance of composite oxide ceramics is encouraging further studies on their use in total hip and knee arthroplasties. Table 7.3 compares the mechanical properties of alumina, zirconia and composite ceramic implants used as bearing surfaces.

7.4.2 Ceramic coatings to improve wear resistance

TiN and DLC are extremely hard ceramic materials applied as thin coatings to harden and protect sliding surfaces. TiN and DLC coatings can be deposited by chemical and physical vapour deposition methods, the former also by thermal spraying. In addition to TiN, other multi-elemental coatings (e.g. CN, TiC, CrN) are also frequently used to optimalise the mechanical, chemical and biological properties of prostheses (Cui and Luo, 1999; Diesselberg, 2004). Coating methods are as follows.

- *Chemical vapour deposition* (CVD) is usually defined as deposition of a solid material from the vapour phase onto a (usually) heated substrate as a result of numerous chemical reactions.
- *Physical vapour deposition* (PVD) is a vacuum deposition method used to deposit thin films by the condensation of a vaporised or ionised gas (plasma) of a material onto various surfaces.
- *Ion beam sputter deposition* (IBSD) is a PVD method of forming complex coatings with very good adhesion to the substrate. Coatings are formed from atoms and ions sputtered by beam of heavy ions from auxiliary material. The elemental composition of the coating is a function of the elemental composition of the sputtered material.
- *Ion beam assisted deposition* (IBAD) is a PVD method for the formation of very complex coatings with excellent adhesion to the substrate. IBAD is frequently applied as IBSD with an additional beam of ions: the dynamically formed coating is bombarded by additional ('assisted') ions and this technique can be used to enter ions of reactive elements into coatings. The additional beam of ions is also helpful in the control of growth processes.

TiN coating forms a hard and corrosion-resistant layer with good wear properties. The properties of the coating are dependent on its microstructure, stoichiometry and thickness. TiN typically has a microstructure of columnar grains. When deposited using CVD techniques these columns grow in a shared, so-called preferred direction (Echigoyaa et al., 1991). PVD results in columnar orientation in the direction of coating growth (Burnett and Rickerby, 1988). Orientation of the columnar TiN grain affects the properties of the coating (Abadias, 2008; Azushimaa *et al.*, 2008; Yeh *et al.*, 2008). The TiN coatings initially produced were susceptible to delamination and failure, which raised concerns about all coatings (Harman *et al.*, 1997; Raimondi and Pietrabissa, 2000). Poor adhesion, low resilience to third-body wear and the adverse effects of coating debris on counterface wear stimulated research into alternative coatings. One initial problem was non-uniform Ti droplet size – removal of larger droplets can leave a void in the coating and smaller asperities can delaminate and create voids. Better control of the deposition improved the coating and modern TiN coating continues to be the major hip joint coating solution available on the market.

Diamond is the hardest material known to man (with a Vickers hardness value of ~85 GPa versus 23 GPa for aluminium oxide and 3 GPa for surgical steel). It is so hard that attempts to measure its hardness accurately have produced a range of results rather than one specific value. Diamond is also chemically inert. Therefore, the mechanical and chemical loads produced in the body cannot cause any significant diamond wear. A material that emits neither chemical nor mechanical wear products cannot by itself provoke any harmful tissue reactions; it is thus biocompatible in this respect. This hypothesis has proven correct in all research conducted thus far. Diamond has also a coefficient of friction so low that it is close to that of healthy human joints (Anttila *et al.*, 1999). This is beneficial because a low sliding resistance of the bearing surfaces of artificial joints minimises the transmission of friction-related stresses and strains into peri-implant support structures, reducing the risk of strain-induced osteolysis and implant detachment. Therefore, diamond would seem to be an interesting material to be considered in artificial hip and knee implants.

Diamond occurs in its natural form only as sparse and small crystals and therefore its applications are mainly limited to decorative jewellery and industrial cutting and grinding. The first attempts to synthesise diamond were based on the idea of squeezing carbon in a way that mimics the formation of natural diamonds in the earth's crust. This method has advanced into an industrial scale to produce small monocrystalline and polycrystalline diamonds for abrasives. However, a joint implant would require a relatively large, uniform and smooth bearing surface. The development of methods that allow deposition of DLC coatings for such purposes began in the mid-1980s and since then numerous variants of DLC and PVD-based processes have been developed (Robertson, 2002).

In a typical CVD coating system of DLC, a low-pressure carbon containing gas is ionised in a process chamber using for example, microwaves, an arc discharge or hot filaments. Under these conditions, hydrogen acts as a precursor for crystalline formation, allowing the formation of the coating. To obtain acceptable yield the substrate has to be very hot (~ 800°C), which limits the choice of substrate material and can cause adhesion problems. The films produced are polycrystalline and contain a variable amount of hydrogen. Although individual crystals can be as hard as natural diamond the crystallinity can also be a shortcoming (Field, 1992; Robertson, 2002).

In a crystal, individual atoms are organised into a regular pattern so that the basic structural unit, the lattice unit cell, is repeated side by side throughout the entire volume of the crystal. In such a close-packed system, atoms are close to each other (i.e. the bonds between them are short and consequently very strong). However, the lattice system – by definition – can be divided into adjacent planes of atoms. In a crystalline material these lattice planes provide a crack propagation route across the material. Therefore, a single crystal diamond can be cleaved into smaller pieces simply by using a sharp steel knife and a small amount of force – provided that the cleaving force is applied in the proper lattice plane orientation. Catastrophic failure across lattice planes also explains, as with the covalent bonds in ceramics, their hard but brittle nature (Callister, 1994).

This same phenomenon can happen on a microscopic scale on a polycrystalline film but, because the system consists of countless tiny crystals, there are no distinct cleavage planes across the whole material. Instead, a crack must travel across multiple randomly oriented crystals, which makes the crack propagation route more complex and toughens the material. On the other hand, the grain boundaries between individual crystals are normally weaker than the crystals themselves and provide another route for crack propagation. These grain boundaries can also serve as corrosion channels, compromising the interface between the coating and the substrate. Increasing the number of grains by decreasing their relative size within the coating by altering the process parameters or by making the coating thicker makes the corrosion route longer and more complex. A polycrystalline coating can also be rough and may require polishing if used as a bearing surface. The aforementioned limitations may be the reason why no medical applications of DLC coatings deposited with CVD are commercially available at the moment.

In a PVD system, carbon-containing material is transformed into ionised gas (plasma) using an electric arc discharge or a laser in a vacuum chamber. This plasma is then accelerated and/or steered towards the substrate and if the energy of the plasma ions is right, an amorphous carbon coating rich in diamond bonds is formed. Although the nominal plasma temperature can be higher than that of the sun, the substrate remains near room temperature. The resulting coating can have almost the same amount of diamond bonds as natural diamond but lacks all the long-term structural order of crystalline materials. If of good quality, it also possesses hardness and chemical inertness as similar to those of natural diamond. This material is sometimes called amorphous diamond (AD) although some scientists think that this name is contradictory and unorthodox and should only be used as descriptive term, if at all (Robertson, 2002). Due to the amorphous structure, there are no lattice planes to serve as crack propagation routes.

If pure graphite is used as the source material and the resulting material has a very high content (> 50%) of diamond bonds compared with graphite bonds (a high sp3/sp2 ratio), the material produced is called tetrahedral amorphous carbon (ta-C) (McKenzie, 1996). If the source material contains hydrogen (e.g. methane), the material produced is called hydrogenated tetrahedral amorphous carbon (ta-C:H) (Weiler et al., 1994). If the source material is a gas, there are no micro-particles emanating from the source cathode and no filtering is required. Most commonly, the source material is solid high-purity graphite and the source ionisation process also produces a significant number of graphite particles that have to be filtered out with baffles and/or a magnetic filter. Despite the filtering, there are practically always some graphite particles in the coating (Anttila, 1989). These particles can induce pinholes that serve as corrosion pathways, but this problem can be avoided by using corrosion-resistant intermediate layers or simply by increasing coating thickness (Anttila et al., 1997, 1999; Kiuru et al., 2003; Lappalainen et al., 1998). Graphite, being a solid lubricant, can also have a positive effect.

One adverse side effect of this deposition process is the internal compressive tension of the coating, which increases with coating thickness and can eventually exceed the force of adhesion of the coating to the substrate causing the coating to peel off. Normally, this effect is explained by interstitial sub-plantation of carbon atoms into the coating and it was, for a very long time, the limiting factor for the extensive use of ta-C as a protective coating. It was believed that high-quality ta-C coatings cannot be deposited thicker than 500 nm. This problem can be overcome by a proper choice of substrate and by using a high-energy plasma. In this way, ion mixing produces an adhesion layer rich in carbides that, together with the relaxation effects provided by suitably soft substrate, guarantees high adhesion and allows deposition of thick (> 10 μm) coatings (Anttila et al., 1997).

In the mid-1990s there was a significant amount of research aiming to diminish the wear of UHMWPE counterparts by coating the metal sliding surfaces with a thin layer of low-friction and low-stiction DLC material. Although laboratory investigations indicated a tenfold improvement in wear resistance (Santavirta et al., 1999) these benefits can be lost because of third-body impingement-induced wear and because of changes in lubrication conditions if realistic sliding geometry is used so that the lubricant is changed from saltwater to serum (Saikko et al., 2001; Scholes et al., 2000).

The only attempt to commercialise this approach was done in Switzerland by Implant Design AG with the Diamond Rota Gliding™ knee. Unfortunately, the DLC coating had poor adhesion and was rapidly worn out and delaminated. The rough gliding surface and third-body wear caused excessive wear of the UHMWPE counterface. This trial might have been successful if a properly produced and tested DLC coating had been used but, unfortunately, the required pre-clinical tests had not been conducted and permission to sell and install the product had not been sought. These problems led to premature revisions and in July 2001 the Swiss Federal Office of Public Health (SFOPH) banned the use of the implant. This and all the bad publicity led to the bankruptcy of the company, leaving as its only legacy a warning example of how poorly tested products should never be used (Hauert, 2003).

The introduction of thick ta-C coatings and the use of DLC on DLC as the sliding pair have proven to provide a more permanent solution than DLC-coated metal sliding on UHMWPE (Anttila et al., 1997). Advanced biomechanical hip simulator test results have been published on implants with thick ta-C coating on both sliding surfaces; the coatings diminished wear by a factor of one million when compared with commercially available hip implants (Lappalainen et al., 2003).

The behaviour of DLC on the implant–bone interface needs further investigation. It can be hypothesised that, being an extremely biocompatible material, diamond does not provoke any osteolysis (Aspenberg et al., 1996) but it does not provide a strong attachment interface either. This hypothesis is supported, at least partially, by the easy detachment of DLC-coated bone screws (Koistinen et al., 2005). The failures of the Diamond Rota Gliding knee also indicated that the residual coating on the bone interface could have caused inadequate bone ingrowth (Hauert, 2003). However, this conclusion comes from an uncontrolled and unauthorised experiment and therefore provides only anecdotal evidence. Nevertheless, if this hypothesis is true, some other material, such as Ta (as in, for example, Trabecular Metal®), may have to be used in order to guarantee that osseointegration lasts as long as the DLC-coated sliding surface.

A recent variation of ta-C is DLC polymer hybrid (DLC-p-h) coatings. The deposition process is similar to the graphite-based method filtered pulsed arc discharge (FPAD) process used for the production of high-quality ta-C. For DLC-p-h, the cathode and the process parameters are manipulated so that the carbon plasma and evaporated polymer oligomers are mixed and form a hybrid of amorphous DLC and polymer. By using anti-soiling additive polymers such as polytetrafluoroethylene (PTFE, commonly known as Teflon®) or polydimethylsiloxane (PDMS), one can produce DLC-PTFE-h and DLC-PDMS-h coatings that are reasonably hard (the same order of magnitude as aluminium oxide) and that are oleophobic and hydrophobic (Anttila *et al.*, 2003; Kiuru *et al.*, 2003). These coatings have been studied for their anti-microbial properties, which could provide a way to avoid painful implant infections (Calzado-Martín *et al.*, 2010).

To date, at least one allotropic form of carbon, pyrolytic carbon, is used in commercial medical applications as a material for artificial heart valves. This allotrope of carbon is close to graphite and hence its mechanical properties are not sufficient for hip and knee implants.

7.4.3 Bioactive ceramics and glasses as coatings to improve bone bonding

The need to improve the rate and amount of osseointegration of an implant in bone led to the introduction of osteoconductive surface chemistry and osteoinductive biomodulators on or in implants.

Calcium phosphate materials and bioglass ceramics have osteophilic characteristics, which make them interesting candidates for orthopaedic applications. However, because of their undesirable mechanical properties (e.g. brittleness, low strength and low fracture toughness) their application in load-bearing applications is limited. They have been studied as coatings on metallic alloys and ceramics such as zirconia and alumina. The metallic or oxide ceramic prosthesis carries the load and the glass coating improves bone ongrowth ingrowth. These bioactive materials develop an adherent interface with tissues that resist substantial mechanical forces. Various techniques have been explored to find a suitable coating method. Of these, plasma spraying, dip coating and electrophoretic deposition are described later.

Bioactive glasses were first noted in 1969 when Hench discovered that bone can chemically bond to a certain glass type of glass (Hench and Paschall, 1973). Bioglasses are mainly composed of SiO_4^{4-} but they can also contain oxides of calcium, sodium and phosphate in various compositions (Hench, 1991). The most important property of a bioactive glass is its controlled solubility, which enables bonding of tissue to the surface of the glass. Bioactive glass reacts with tissues via many phases and forms different surface layers over time (Hench and Andersson, 1999). Its worst disadvantages are mechanical weakness and low fracture stiffness, due to the two-dimensional amorphic glass-net structure. Glass has high-pressure strength, but low tensile strength. The coating is often prepared using glass powder that is burnt/melted/sintered onto the surface of the metal (Hench and Andersson, 1999).

The most common calcium phosphate ceramics are tricalciumphosphate (TCP, $Ca_3(PO_4)_2$) and hydroxyapatite (HA, $(Ca_{10}(PO_4)_6OH)_2$). Of all the calcium phosphate coatings, HA coatings have been most widely used in hip arthroplasty. HA has a similar chemical composition to the mineral fraction of bone. 70% of the weight and 50% of the volume of bone is HA (Shors and Holmes, 1999). HA is able to fill the gaps between bone and implant and stimulates bone ingrowth. However, HA can also lead to osteolysis when it is exposed to bone marrow and soft tissues (Bloebaum and Dupont, 1993). HA wear debris is thought to be the main cause for implant failure and its phagocytosis stimulates the release of pro-inflamatory and bone-resorption stimulating cytokines (Chow, 1988). Subsequently, these products have been held responsible for (granulomatous) inflammation, disturbance in bone remodelling and peri-implant osteolysis.

Plasma spraying of apatite onto metallic materials is widely used to produce a surface apatite layer. Coatings deposited by this method have relatively sharp interfaces (Wen *et al.*, 2000; Yan *et al.*, 2003). The low interface bonding strength to implant combined with the low toughness of the sprayed HA layer may result in fracture of the apatite coating under relatively low stress. To overcome this weakness, ion beam mixing has been used to produce apatite with a high interface bonding strength.

Ion beam mixing is a process used to adhere two or more layers, especially a substrate and a deposited surface layer. The process involves bombarding layered samples with appropriate doses of ion radiation to promote mixing at the interface. Ion beam mixing is often used to prepare electrical junctions, especially between non-equilibrium or metastable alloys and intermetallic compounds. Ion implantation equipment can be used to achieve ion beam mixing. This method produces 0.05–1.3 μm thick coatings with high adhesive strength. Its drawback is that it is an expensive line of sight technique (i.e. coating of complex surfaces is difficult).

Ion implantation of calcium and phosphorus has been used to improve the bone bonding of metallic implants. In addition, to induce strong bonding between the apatite film and the substrate, calcium ions are implanted during ion beam mixing process (Yoshinari *et al.*, 1994).

The sol-gel process, also known as chemical solution deposition, is a wet-chemical technique widely used primarily for the fabrication of materials from a chemical solution (or sol) that acts as the precursor to an integrated network (or gel) of particles. Coating less than 1 μm thick can be produced even on implants with complex shapes and at low processing temperatures.

Electrophoretic deposition is a process in which colloidal particles suspended in a liquid medium migrate under the influence of an electric field (electrophoresis) and are deposited onto an electrode. The method can be used to produce 0.1–2 mm thick uniform coatings rapidly, even on complex substrates. Unfortunately, it is difficult to produce crack-free coatings and the method requires sintering temperatures; these high temperatures can impair the mechanical properties of metal implants and lead to low bond strength and impurity of the HA.

Electrochemical treatment is commonly used to form an apatite layer on a metallic implant. Through an electrochemical process, carbonate-containing apatite with a desirable morphology can be precipitated on a substrate.

Biomimetic coating is an approach in which metal implants are immersed in simulated body fluids at a physiologic temperature and pH. HA coating then grows on the surface of the implant. HA coatings produced with this method have a high purity and bioactivity. It is possible to incorporate bone growth stimulating factors into the forming HA surface layer. However, it takes a long time to produce coatings of reasonable thickness using this method. Due to the low solubility of HA and the requirement of a continuous replenishment of HA to maintain the supersaturated state necessary for apatite crystal growth, this operation is extremely difficult and may lead to local precipitation or uneven coatings (Xie and Luan, 2008).

7.5 Conclusion

The modern concept of low-friction hip arthroplasty was developed in the 1970s. This chapter has discussed the evolution of materials used in hip and knee implants and the internal/surface treatments that are used to improve the properties of implants. These treatments aim to maximise beneficial mechanical properties, minimise material deterioration and enable long-term integration of the implant into the musculoskeletal system. However, despite the many attempts to improve implants, the risk for their revision has remained unchanged in long-term follow-up. New developments in permanent arthroplasty implants are therefore needed as soon as possible. This is critically important, as increased numbers of total hip and knee arthroplasties will be performed all over the world in the future.

7.6 References

Abadias, G. 2008, "Stress and preferred orientation in nitride-based PVD coatings," *Surf Coating Tech and*, 202(11): 2223–35, DOI: 10.1016/j.surfcoat.2007.08.029.

Abu Bakar, M.S., Cheang, P. and Khor, K.A. 2003a, "Tensile properties and microstructural analysis of spheroidized hydroxyapatite–poly (etheretherketone) biocomposites", *Mater Sci Eng A*, 345(1–2): 55–63, DOI: 10.1016/S0921-5093(02)00289-7.

Abu Bakar, M.S., Cheang, P. and Khor, K.A. 2003b, "Mechanical properties of injection molded hydroxyapatite-polyetheretherketone biocomposites", *Comp Sci Tech*, 63(3–4): 421–5, DOI: 10.1016/S0266-3538(02)00230-0.

Abu Bakar, M.S., Cheng, M.H.W., Tang, S.M., Yu, S.C., Liao, K., Tan, C.T., Khor, K.A. and Cheang, P. 2003c, "Tensile properties, tension–tension fatigue and biological response of polyetheretherketone–hydroxyapatite composites for

load-bearing orthopedic implants", *Biomaterials*, 24(13): 2245–50, DOI: 10.1016/S0142-9612(03)00028-0.
Amstutz, H.C. 1990, "Stem fracture incidence in Trapezoidal-28 stainless steel hip arthroplasty", *Clins Orthop Relat Res*, 1990(256): 105–14.
Anttila, A. 1989, Ion-beam induced diamond-like carbon coating. In *Structure–Property Relationships in Surface-Modified Ceramics, NATO ASI Series*, eds. R. Kossowsky, C.J. McHargue and W.O. Hofer. Dordrecht, Kluwer 17D: 455.
Anttila, A., Lappalainen, R., Tiainen, V.M. and Hakovirta, M. 1997, "Superior attachment of high-quality hydrogen-free amorphous diamond films to solid material", *Adv Mater*, 9(15): 1161, DOI: 0.1002/adma.19970091507.
Anttila, A., Lappalainen, R., Heinonen, H., Santavirta, S. and Konttinen, Y.T. 1999, "Superiority of diamondlike carbon coating on articulating surfaces of artificial hip joints", *New Diamond Front Carb Tech*, 9(4): 283–8.
Anttila, A., Tiainen, V, Kiuru, M., Alakoski, E. and Arstila, K. 2003, "Preparation of diamond-like carbon polymer hybrid films using filtered pulsed arc discharge method", *Surf Eng*, 19(6): 425–8, DOI: 10.1179/026708403225006195.
Archibeck, M.J., Berger, R.A., Jacobs, J.J., Quigley, L.R., Gitelis, S., Rosenberg, A. G. and Galante, J.O. 2001, "Second-generation cementless total hip arthroplasty–Eight to eleven–year results", *J Bone Joint Surg Am*, 83A(11): 1666–73.
Aspenberg, P., Anttila, A., Konttinen, Y.T., Lappalainen, R., Goodman, S.B., Nordsletten, L. and Santavirta, S. 1996, "Benign response to particles of diamond and SiC: bone chamber studies of new joint replacement coating materials in rabbits", *Biomaterials*, 17(8): 807–12, DOI: 10.1016/0142-9612(96)81418-9.
Azushimaa, A., Tannoa, Y., Iwataa, H. and Aokib, K. 2008, "Coefficients of friction of TiN coatings with preferred grain orientations under dry condition", *Wear*, 265(7–8): 1017–22, DOI: 10.1016/j.wear.2008.02.019.
Berry, D.J., Harmsen, W.S., Cabanela, M.E. and Morrey, B.F. 2002, "Twenty-five-year survivorship of two thousand consecutive primary Charnley total hip replacements: Factors affecting survivorship of acetabular and femoral components", *J Bone Joint Surg Br A*, 84A(2): 171–7.
Bloebaum, R.D. and Dupont, J.A. 1993, "Osteolysis from a press-fit hydroxyapatite-coated implant. A case study", *J Arthroplasty*, 8(2): 195–202, DOI: 10.1016/S0883-5403(09)80013-2.
Bobyn, J.D., Stackpool, G.J., Hacking, S.A., Tanzer, M. and Krygier, J.J. 1999, "Characteristics of bone ingrowth and interface mechanics of a new porous tantalum biomaterial", *J Bone Joint Surg Br*, 81(5): 907–14.
Boutin, P. 1972, "Total arthroplasty of the hip by fritted aluminum prosthesis. Experimental study and 1st clinical applications. Arthroplastie totale de la hanche par prothèse en alumine frittée. Etude expérimentale et premières applications cliniques", *Rev Chir Orthop Repara l'appar Moteur*, 58(3): 229–46.
Boutin, P., Christel, P., Dorlot, J.M., Meunier, A., de Roquancourt, A., Blanquaert, D., Herman, S., Sedel, L. and Witvoet, J. 1988, "The use of dense alumina alumina ceramic combination in total hip-replacement", *J Biomed Mater Res*, 22(12): 1203–32, DOI: 10.1002/jbm.820221210.
Briem, D., Strametz, S., Schröoder, K., Meenen, N.M., Lehmann, W., Linhart, W., Ohl, A. and Rueger, J.M. 2005, "Response of primary fibroblasts and

osteoblasts to plasma treated polyetheretherketone (PEEK) surfaces", *J Mater Sci Mater Med*, 16(7): 671–7, DOI: 10.1007/s10856-005-2539-z.

Buchanan, R.A., Rigney, E.D. and Williams, J.M. 1987, "Ion implantation of surgical Ti-6Al-4V for improved resistance to wear-accelerated corrosion", *J Biomed Mater Res*, 21(3): 355–66.

Burnett, P.J. and Rickerby, D.S. 1988, "The erosion behaviour of TiN coatings on steels", *J Mater Sci*, 23(7): 2429–43, DOI: 10.1007/BF01111900.

Callister, W.D.J. 1994, *Materials Science and Engineering: An Introduction*. Chichester, Wiley.

Calvert, G.T., Devane, P.A., Fielden, J., Adams, K. and Horne, J.G. 2009, "A double-blind, prospective, randomized controlled trial comparing highly cross-linked and conventional polyethylene in primary total hip arthroplasty", *J Arthroplasty*, 24(4): 505–10, DOI: 10.1016/j.arth.2008.02.011.

Calzado-Martín, A., Saldaña, L., Korhonen, H., Soininen, A., Kinnari, T.J., Gómez-Barrena, E., Tiainen, V.M., Lappalainen, R., Munuera, L.K., Y.T. and Vilaboa, N. 2010, "Interactions of human bone cells with diamond-like carbon polymer hybrid coatings", *Acta Biomater*, 6(8): 3325–38, DOI:doi:10.1016/j.actbio.2010.02.048.

Charnley, J. 1960, "Anchorage of the femoral head prosthesis to the shaft of the femur", *J Bone Joint Surg Br*, 42B: 28–30.

Charnley, J. 1979, *Low Friction Arthroplasty of the Hip: Theory and Practice*. Berlin, Springer.

Chiba, A., Kumagai, K., Nomura, N. and Miyakawa, S. 2007, "Pin-on-disk wear behavior in a like-on-like configuration in a biological environment of high carbon cast and low carbon forged Co-29Cr-6Mo alloys", *Acta Mater*, 55 (4): 1309–18, DOI: 10.1016/j.actamat.2006.10.005.

Chow, L.C. 1988, "Calcium phosphate materials: reactor response", *Adv Dent Res*, 2 (1): 181–6, DOI: 10.1177/08959374880020011201.

Clarke, I.C., Manaka, M., Green, D.D., Williams, P., Pezzotti, G., Kim, Y.-., Ries, M., Sugano, N., Sedel, L., Delauney, C., Nissan, B.B., Donaldson, T. and Gustafson, G.A. 2003, "Current status of zirconia used in total hip implants", *J Bone Joint Surg Am*, 85A: 73–84.

Costa, L., Jacobson, K., Bracco, P. and del Prever, E.M.B. 2005, "Oxidation of orthopaedic UHMWPE", *Biomaterials*, 26(3): 347–8, DOI: 10.1016/S0142-9612 (01)00288-5.

Crout, D.H.G., Corkill, J.A., James, M.L. and Ling, R.S.M. 1979, "Methylmethacrylate metabolism in man. The hydrolysis of methylmethacrylate to methacrylic acid during total hip replacement", *Clin Orthop Relat Res*, 141: 90–5.

Cui, F.Z. and Luo, Z.S. 1999, "Biomaterials modification by ion-beam processing", *Surf Coating Tech*, 112(1–3): 278–285.

Cukrowska, B., Sowinska, A., Zajaczkowska, A., Sobiecki, J., Wierzchon, T. and Czarnowska, E. 2004, "Cytokine secretion during in vitro cellular interaction with titanium alloy and nitrided surface layers produced under glow discharge conditions", *Ann Transplant*, 9(Suppl. 1A): 7.

Czarnowska, E., Wierzcho, T. and Maranda-Niedbaøa, A. 1999, "Properties of the surface layers on titanium alloy and their biocompatibility in *in vitro* tests", *J Mater Process Technol*, S92–93: 190–4, DOI: 10.1016/S0924-0136(99)00228-9.

Czarnowska, E., Wierzchoń, T., Maranda-Niedbaøa, A. and Karczmarewicz, E. 2000, "Improvement of titanium alloy for biomedical applications by nitriding and carbonitriding processes under glow discharge conditions", *J Mater Sci Mater Med*, 11(2): 73–81, DOI: 10.1023/A:1008980631780.

Czarnowska, E., Sowinska, A., Cukrowska, B., Sobiecki, J.R. and Wierzchon, T. 2005. "Response of human osteoblast-like cells and fibroblasts to titanium alloy nitrided under glow discharge conditions" *Mater Sci Forum*, 475–475: 2415–8, DOI: 10.1023/A:1008980631780.

Davis, J.R. 2003, Coatings. In *Handbook of Materials for Medical Devices*, ed. J.R. Davis. Materials Park, OH, ASM International, pp. 179–94.

Dawei, Z., Xinping, Z., Weicheng, Y. and Zhongguang, W. 1993, "Improvement in fatigue lifetime of Ti-6A1-4V alloy by boron implantation", *Surf Coat Tech*, 58 (2): 119–123, DOI: 10.1016/0257-8972(93)90182-N.

Della Valle, C.J. 2004, "Primary total hip arthroplasty with a flanged, cemented all-polyethylene acetabular component: evaluation at a minimum of 20 years", *J Arthroplastym*, 19(1): 23–6.

Diesselberg, M., Stock, H.R. and Mayr, P. 2004, "Corrosion protection of magnetron sputtered TIN coatings deposited on high strength aluminium alloys", *Surf Coat Tech*, 177–118: 399–403.

Dorr, L.D., Wan, Z., Shahrdar, C., Sirianni, L., Boutary, M. and Yun, A. 2005, "Clinical performance of a Durasul highly cross-linked polyethylene acetabular liner for total hip arthroplasty at five years", *J Bone Joint Surg Am*, 87(8): 1816–21, DOI: 10.2106/JBJS.D.01915.

Ducheyne, P. and Qiu, Q. 1999, "Bioactive ceramics: the effect of surface reactivity on bone formation and bone cell function", *Biomaterials*, 20(23–24): 2287–303, DOI: 10.1016/S0142-9612(99)00181-7.

Duffy, G.P., Wannomae, K.K., Rowell, S.L. and Muratoglu, O.K. 2009, "Fracture of a cross-linked polyethylene liner due to impingement", *J Arthroplasty*, 24(1): 158e1–e3, DOI: 10.1016/j.arth.2008.02.006.

Dumbleton, J.H., D'Antonio, J.A., Manley, M.T., Capello, W.N. and Wang, A. 2006, "The basis for a second-generation highly cross-linked UHMWPE", *Clin Orthop Relat Res*, 453: 265–71, DOI: 10.1097/01.blo.0000238856.61862.7d.

Echigoyaa, J., Liua, X.T., Imamurab, A. and Takatsub, S. 1991, "Transmission electron microscopy studies of growth and interface structure of chemically vapour deposited TiC and TiN films on WC–Co alloy subsrates", *Thin Solid Films*, 198(1–2): 293–300, DOI: 10.1016/0040-6090(91)90347-Z.

El-Warrak, A., Olmstead, M., Apelt, D., Deiss, F., Noetzli, H., Zlinsky, K., Hilbe, M., Bertschar-Wolfsberger, R., Johnson, A.L., Auer, J. and Von Rechenberg, B. 2004a, "An animal model for interface tissue formation in cemented hip replacements", *Vet Surg*, 33(5): 495–504, DOI: 10.1111/j.1532-950X.2004.04064.x.

El-Warrak, A.O., Olmstead, M., Schneider, R., Meinel, L., Bettschart-Wolfisberger, R., Akens, M.K., Auer, J. and von Rechenberg, B. 2004b, "An experimental animal model of aseptic loosening of hip prostheses in sheep to study early biochemical changes at the interface membrane", *BMC Musculoskel Disord*, 6: 7, DOI: 10.1186/1471-2474-5-7.

Emerson Jr., R.H., Head, W.C., Emerson, C.B., Rosenfeldt, W. and Higgins, L.L. 2002, "A comparison of cemented and cementless titanium femoral components used for primary total hip arthroplasty: A radiographic and survivorship study", *J Arthroplasty*, 17(5): 584–91, DOI: 10.1054/arth.2002.32696.

Engh, C.A. 1998, The anatomic medullary locking prosthesis. In *Total Hip Artroplasty Outcomes*, eds. G.A.M. Finerman, F.J. Dorey, P. Grigoris and H. A. McKellop. Kidlington, Churchill–Livingstone, pp. 117–39.

Engh Jr., C.A., Stepniewski, A.S., Ginn, S.D., Beykirch, S.E., Sychterz-Terefenko, C., Hopper Jr., R.H. and Engh, C.A. 2006, "A Randomized Prospective Evaluation of Outcomes After Total Hip Arthroplasty Using Cross-linked Marathon and Non-cross-linked Enduron Polyethylene Liners", *J Arthroplasty*, 21(6): 17–25, DOI: 10.1016/j.arth.2006.05.002.

Field, J.E. 1992, *The Properties of Natural and Synthetic Diamond*. London, Academic.

Fleszar, A., Wierzcho, T., Kim, S.K. and Sobiecki, J.R. 2000, "Properties of surface layers produced on the Ti–6Al–3Mo–2Cr titanium alloy under glow discharge conditions", *Surf Coat Tech*, 131(1–3): 62–5, DOI: 10.1016/S0257-8972(00) 00760-X.

Froimson, M.I., Garino, J., Machenaud, A. and Vidalain, J.P. 2007, "Minimum 10-year results of a tapered, titanium, hydroxyapatite-coated hip stem", *J Arthroplasty*, 22(1): 1–7, DOI: 10.1016/j.arth.2006.03.003.

Geerdink, C.H., Grimm, B., Ramakrishnan, R., Rondhuis, J., Verburg, A.J. and Tonino, A.J. 2006, "Crosslinked polyethylene compared to conventional polyethylene in total hip replacement: Pre-clinical evaluation, in-vitro testing and prospective clinical follow-up study", *Acta Orthop*, 77(5): 719–25, DOI: doi:10.1080/17453670610012890.

Geerdink, C.H., Grimm, B., Vencken, W., Heyligers, I.C. and Tonino, A.J. 2009, "Cross-linked compared with historical polyethylene in THA: an 8-year clinical study", *Clin Orthop Relat Res*, 467(4): 979–84, DOI: 10.1007/s11999-008-0628-2.

Geesink, R.G. and Hoefnagels, N.H. 1995, "Six-year results of hydroxyapatite-coated total hip replacement", *J Bone Joint Surg Br*, 77(4): 534–47.

Gluck, T. 1890, "Die invaginationsmetode der oste- und arthtoplastik", *Berl Klin Wschr*, 19: 732.

Gokul Lakshmi, S., Raman, V., Rajendran, N., Babi, M.A.K. and Arivuoli, D. 2003, "In vitro corrosion behaviour of plasma nitrided Ti–6Al–7Nb orthopaedic alloy in Hanks solution", *Sci Technol Adv Mater*, 4(5): 415–8, DOI: 10.1016/j.stam.2003.09.005.

Gokul Lakshmi, S., Tamilselvi, S., Rajendran, N., Babic, M.A.K. and Arivuoli, D. 2004, "Electrochemical behaviour and characterisation of plasma nitrided Ti–5Al–2Nb–1Ta orthopaedic alloy in Hanks solution", *Surf Coat Tech*, 182(2–3): 287–93, DOI: 10.1016/S0257-8972(03)00849-1.

Gomez-Barrena, E., Puertolas, J.A., Munuera, L. and Konttinen, Y.T. 2008, "Update on UHMWPE research: From the bench to the bedside", *Acta Orthop*, 79(6): 832–40, DOI: 10.1080/17453670810016939.

Goodman, S. 2005, "Wear particulate and osteolysis", *Orthop Clin North Am*, 36 (1): 41–8, DOI: 10.1016/j.ocl.2004.06.015.

Greene, M.E., Bragdon, C.R., Freiberg, A.A., Kwon, Y.M., Rubash, H.E. and Malchau, H. 2010, "RSA evaluation of wear of vitamin E stabilized highly cross-linked polyethylene", *American Association of Hip and Knee Surgeons, 20th Annual Meeting*, Texas, 5–7 Nov 2010.

Grübl, A., Chiari, C., Gruber, M., Kaider, A. and Gottsauner-Wolf, F. 2002, "Cementless total hip arthroplasty with a tapered, rectangular titanium stem and a threaded cup: a minimum ten-year follow-up", *J Bone Joint Surg Am*, 84A(3): 425–31.

Habermann, B., Ewald, W., Rauschmann, M., Zichner, L. and Kurth, A.A. 2006, "Fracture of ceramic heads in total hip replacement", *Arch Orthop Trauma Surg*, 126(7): 464–70, DOI: 10.1007/BF00434107.

Hailer, N.P., Garellick, G. and Kärrholm, J. 2010, "Uncemented and cemented primary total hip arthroplasty in the Swedish Hip Arthroplasty Register: Evaluation of 170,413 operations", *Acta Orthop*, 81(1): 34–41, DOI: 10.3109/17453671003685400.

Han, C.M., Kim, H.E., Kim, Y.S. and Han, S.K. 2009, "Enhanced biocompatibility of Co-Cr implant material by Ti coating and micro-arc oxidation", *J Biomed Mater Res B*, 90(1): 165–70, DOI: 10.1002/jbm.b.31270.

Han, C.M., Lee, E.J., Kim, H.E., Koh, Y.H., Kim, K.N., Ha, Y. and Kuh, S.U. 2010, "The electron beam deposition of titanium on polyetheretherketone (PEEK) and the resulting enhanced biological properties", *Biomaterials*, 31 (13): 3465–70, DOI: 10.1016/j.biomaterials.2009.12.030.

Hannouche, D., Hamadouche, M., Nizard, R., Bizot, P., Meunier, A. and Sedel, L. 2005, "Ceramics in total hip replacement", *Clin Orthop Relat Res*, (430): 62–71, DOI: 10.1097/01.blo.0000149996.91974.83.

Harman, M.K., Banks, S.A. and Hodge, W.A. 1997, "Wear analysis of a retrieved hip implant with titanium nitride coating", *J Arthroplasty*, 12(8): 938–45, DOI: 10.1016/S0883-5403(97)90164-9.

Harrison, A.K., Gioe, T.J., Simonelli, C., Tatman, P.J. and Schoeller, M.C. 2010, "Do porous tantalum implants help preserve bone? Evaluation of tibial bone density surrounding tantalum tibial implants in TKA", *Clin Orthop Relat Res*, 468(10): 2739–45, DOI: 10.1007/s11999-009-1222-y.

Hauert, R. 2003, "A review of modified DLC coatings for biological applications", *Diamond Relat Mater*, 12(3–7): 583–9, DOI: 10.1016/S0925-9635(03)00081-5.

Head, W.C., Bauk, D.J. and Emerson Jr., R.H. 1995, "Titanium as the material of choice for cementless femoral components in total hip arthroplasty", *Clin Orthop Relat Res*, 311: 85–90.

Hench, L.L. 1991, "Bioceramics: from concept to clinic", *J Am Ceram Soc*, 74 (7): 1487–510, DOI: 10.1111/j.1151-2916.1991.tb07132.x.

Hench, L.L. and Andersson, Ä.O. 1999, Bioactive glasses. In *An Introduction to Bioceramics*, eds. L.L. Hench and J. Wilson, second edn. Singapore, World Scientific, pp. 41–62.

Hench, L.L. and Paschall, H.A. 1973, "Direct chemical bond of bioactive glass-ceramic materials to bone and muscle", *J Biomed Mater Res*, 7(3): 25–42, DOI: 10.1002/jbm.820070304.

Hirvonen, J.K. and Sartwell, B.D. 1994, Ion implantation. In *Surface Engineering*, Vol 5. Warrendale, PA, ASM International, pp. 604–610.

Hsieh, P.H., Shih, C.H., Chang, Y.H., Lee, M.S., Shih, H.N., Yang, W.E. 2004, "Two-stage revision hip arthroplasty for infection: comparison between the interim use of antibiotic-loaded cement beads and a spacer prosthesis", *J Bone Joint Surg Am*, 86A (9): 1989–97.

Huiskes, R. 1993, "Failed innovation in total hip replacement. Diagnosis and proposals for a cure", *Acta Orthop Scand*, 64(6): 699–716.

Hulbert, S.F. 1993, The use of alumina and zirconia in surgical implant. In *An Introduction to Bioceramics*, eds. L.L. Hench and J. Wilson, second edn. Singapore, World Scientific, pp. 25–40.

Hutchings, R. 1985, "The subsurface microstructure of nitrogen-implanted metals", *Mater Sci Eng*, 69(1): 129–138, DOI: 10.1016/0025-5416(85)90383-0.

Ivarsson, I., Wahlström, O., Djerf, K., Jacobsson, S.A. 1994, "Revision of infected hip replacement: Two-stage procedure with a temporary gentamicin spacer", *Acta Orthop Scand*, 65(1): 7–8.

Jacobs, C.A., Christensen, C.P., Greenwald, A.S. and McKellop, H. 2007, "Clinical performance of highly cross-linked polyethylenes in total hip arthroplasty", *J Bone Joint Surg Am*, 89A(12): 2779–86, DOI: 10.2106/JBJS.G.00043.

Jämsen, E., Furnes, O., Engesaeter, L.B., Konttinen, Y.T., Odgaard, A., Stefánsdóttir, A. and Lidgren, L. 2010, "Prevention of deep infection in joint replacement surgery A review", *Acta Orthop*, 81(6): 660–6, DOI: 10.3109/17453674.2010.537805.

Jinno, T., Goldberg, V.M., Davy, D. and Stevenson, S. 1998, "Osseointegration of surface-blasted implants made of titanium alloy and cobalt-chromium alloy in a rabbit intramedullary model", *J Biomed Mater Res A*, 42(1): 20–29, DOI: 10.1002/(SICI)1097-4636(199810)42:1<20::AID-JBM4>3.0.CO;2-Q.

Katti, K.S., Verma, D. and Katti, D.R. 2008, Materials for joint replacement. In *Joint Replacement Technology*, ed. P.A. Revell. Cambridege, Woodhead, pp. 81–104.

Kawamura, H., Dunbar, M.J., Murray, P., Bourne, R.B. and Rorabeck, C.H. 2001, "The porous coated anatomic total hip replacement. A ten to fourteen-year follow-up study of a cementless total hip arthroplasty", *J Bone Joint Surg Am*, 83A(9): 1333–8.

Kawanabe, K., Ise, K., Goto, K., Akiyama, H., Nakamura, T., Kaneuji, A., Sugimori, T. and Matsumoto, T. 2009, "A new cementless total hip arthroplasty with bioactive titanium porous-coating by alkaline and heat treatment: average 4.8-year results", *J Biomed Mater Res Bed Mater Res B*, 90(1): 476–81, DOI: 10.1002/jbm.b.31309.

Kester, M.A., Herrera, L., Wang, A. and Essner, A. 2007, "Knee bearing technology. Where is technology taking us?", *J Arthroplasty*, 22(7): 16–20, DOI: 10.1016/j.arth.2007.05.012.

Kim, T.S., Park, Y.G. and Wey, M.Y. 2003, "Characterization of Ti-6Al-4V alloy modified by plasma carburizing process", *Mater Sci Eng A*, 361(1–2): 275–80, DOI: 10.1016/S0921-5093(03)00559-8.

Kiuru, M., Alakoski, E., Tiainen, V. Lappalainen, R. and Anttila, A. 2003, "Tantalum as a buffer layer in diamond-like carbon coated artificial hip joints", *J Biomed Mater Res B Appl Biomater*, 66(1): 425–8, DOI: 10.1002/jbm.b.10029.

Klein, G.R., Levine, H.B. and Hartzband, M.A. 2008, "Removal of a Well-Fixed Trabecular Metal Monoblock Tibial Component", *J Arthroplasty*, 23(4): 619–22, DOI: 10.1016/j.arth.2007.05.004.

Kohn, D.H. and Ducheyne, P. 1992, Materials for bone and joint replacement. In

Materials Science and Technology: Medical and Dental Materials, ed. D.F. Williams. Weinheim, VCH, pp. 31–109.

Koistinen, A., Santavirta, S.S., Kröger, H. and Lappalainen, R. 2005, "Effect of bone mineral density and amorphous diamond coatings on insertion torque of bone screws", *Biomaterials*, 26(28): 5687–94, DOI: 10.1016/j.biomaterials.2005.02.003.

Konttinen, Y.T., Miloševˇ, I., Trebše, R., Rantanen, P., Linden, R., Tiainen, V.M. and Virtanen, S. 2008, Metals for joint replacement. In *Joint Replacement Technology*, ed. P.A. Revell. Cambridge, Woodhead, pp. 115–62.

Kurtz, S.M. and Devine, J.N. 2007, "PEEK biomaterials in trauma, orthopedic, and spinal implants", *Biomaterials*, 28(32): 4845–69, DOI: 10.1016/j.biomaterials.2007.07.013.

Kurtz, S.M., Hozack, W.J., Purtill, J.J., Marcolongo, M., Kraay, M.J., Goldberg, V.M., Sharkey, P.F., Parvizi, J., Rimnac, C.M. and Edidin, A.A. 2006, "2006 Otto Aufranc award paper: Significance of in vivo degradation for polyethylene in total hip arthroplasty", *Clin Orthop Relat Res*, 453: 47–57, DOI: 10.1097/01.blo.0000246547.18187.0b.

Kurtz, S.M., Dumbleton, J., Siskey, R.S., Wang, A. and Manley, M. 2009, "Trace concentrations of vitamin E protect radiation crosslinked UHMWPE from oxidative degradation", *J Biomed Mater Res A*, 90(2): 549–63, DOI: 10.1002/jbm.a.32122.

Kurtz, S.M., Ong, K.L., Lau, E., Widmer, M., Maravic, M., Gómez-Barrena, E., de Fátima, d.P., Manno, V., Torre, M., Walter, W.L., de Steiger, R., Geesink, R.G.T., Peltola, M. and Röder, C. 2011, "International survey of primary and revision total knee replacement", *Int Orthop*, 35(12): 1786–89, DOI: 10.1007/s00264-011-1235-5.

Langer, G. 2002, Ceramic tibial plateau of the 70s ceramics for total knee replacement: status and options. In *Bioceramics in Joint Arthroplasty*, eds. J.P. Garino and G. Willmann. Stuttgart, Thieme, pp. 128–130.

Lappalainen, R., Heiskanen, H., Anttila, A. and Santavirta, S. 1998, "Some relevant issues related to the use of amorphous diamond coatings for medical applications", *Diamond Relat Mater*, 7(2–5): 482–5, DOI: 10.1016/S0925-9635(98)80003-4.

Lappalainen, R., Selenius, M., Anttila, A., Konttinen, Y.T. and Santavirta, S.S. 2003, "Reduction of wear in total hip replacement prostheses by amorphous diamond coatings", *J Biomed Mater Res B: Appl Biomater*, 66B(1): 410–3, DOI: 10.1002/jbm.b.10026.

Laupacis, A., Bourne, R., Rorabeck, C., Feeny, D., Tugwell, P. and Wong, C. 2002, "Comparison of total hip arthroplasty performed with and without cement. A randomized trial", *J Bone Joint Surg Am*, 84(10):1823–8.

Li, H.T., Liu, P.S., Chang, S.C., Lü, H.C., Wang, H.H. and Tao, K. 1981, "Some experimental studies on metal implantation", *Nucl Instrum Methods*, 182–183:915–7, DOI: 10.1016/0029-554X(81)90821-1.

Liang, B., Kawanabe, K., Ise, K., Iida, H. and Nakamura, T. 2007, "Polyethylene wear against alumina and zirconia heads in cemented total hip arthroplasty", *J Arthroplasty*, 22(2): 251–7, DOI: 10.1016/j.arth.2006.03.004.

López, M.F., Gutiérrez, A. and Jiménez, J.A. 2001, "Surface characterization of new non-toxic titanium alloys for use as biomaterials", *Surf Sci*, 482–485: 300–5, DOI: 10.1016/S0039-6028(00)01005-0.

Lossdörfer, S., Schwartz, Z., Wang, L., Lohmann, C.H., Turner, J.D., Wieland, M., Cochran, D.L. and Boyan, B.D. 2004, "Microrough implant surface topographies increase osteogenesis by reducing osteoclast formation and activity", *J Biomed Mater Res A*, 70(3): 361–9, DOI: 10.1002/jbm.a.30025.

Macintosh, D.L. 1966, "Athroplasty of the knee in rheumatoid arthritis", *J Bone Joint Surg Br*, 48: 179.

Marciniak, J. 2002, *Biomaterials*. Gliwice, Silesian University of Technology.

McCalden, R.W., MacDonald, S.J., Rorabeck, C.H., Bourne, R.B., Chess, D.G. and Charron, K.D. 2009, "Wear rate of highly cross-linked polyethylene in total hip arthroplasty: A randomized controlled trial", *J Bone Joint Surg Am*, 91(4): 773–82, DOI: 10.2106/JBJS.H.00244.

McKee, G.K. and Watson-Farrar, J. 1966, "Replacement of arthritic hips by the McKee–Farrar prosthesis", *J Bone Joint Surg Br*, 48(2): 245–59.

McKellop, H., Shen, F.W., Lu, B., Campbell, P. and Salovey, R. 2000, "Effect of sterilization method and other modifications on the wear resistance of acetabular cups made of ultra-high molecular weight polyethylene. A hip-simulator study", *J Bone Joint Surg Am*, 82A(12): 1708–25.

McKenzie, D.R. 1996, "Tetrahedral bonding in amorphous carbon", *Rep Prog Phys*, 59(12): 1611–64, DOI: 10.1088/0034-4885/59/12/002.

Medel, F.J., Pena, P., Cegonino, J., Gomez-Barrena, E. and Puertolas, J.A. 2007, "Comparative fatigue behavior and toughness of remelted and annealed highly crosslinked polyethylenes", *J Biomed Mater Res B*, 83(2): 380–90, DOI: 10.1002/jbm.b.30807.

Meding, J.B., Keating, M.E. and Davis, K.E. 2011, "Acetabular UHMWPE survival and wear changes with different manufacturing techniques", *Clin Orthop Relat Res*, 469(2): 405–1, DOI: 10.1007/s11999-010-1571-6.

Meletis, E.I. 2002, "Intensified plasma-assisted processing: science and engineering", *Surf Coat Tech*, 149(2–3): 95–113, DOI: 10.1016/S0257-8972(01)01441-4.

Merkert, P. 2003, 'Next generation ceramic bearings'. In *Ceramics in Orthopaedics 8th BIOLOX® Symposium Proceedings*, eds. H. Zipplel and M. Dietrich. Darmstadt, Steinkopff. pp. 123–5.

Meyer, M.R., Friedman, R.J., Del, JS., S and Latour Jr., R.A. 1994, "Long-term durability of the interface in FRP composites after exposure to simulated physiologic saline environments", *J Biomed Mater Res*, 28(10): 1221–31, DOI: 10.1002/jbm.820281012.

Moro, T., Takatori, Y., Kyomoto, M., Ishihara, K., Saiga, K., Nakamura, K. and Kawaguchi, H. 2010, "Surface grafting of biocompatible phospholipid polymer MPC provides wear resistance of tibial polyethylene insert in artificial knee joints", *Osteo Cart*, 18(9): 1174–82, DOI: 10.1016/j.joca.2010.05.019.

Naraghi, A.M. and White, L.M. 2006, "Magnetic resonance imaging of joint replacements", *Semin Musculoskelet Radiol*, 10(1): 98–106 DOI: 10.1055/s-2006-934220.

Nath, V.C., Sood, D.K. and Manory, R.R. 1991, "Ultramicrohardness and microstructure of Ti-6 wt.%Al-4 wt.%V alloy nitrided by ion implantation", *Surf Coat Tech*, 49(1–3): 510–3, DOI: 10.1016/0257-8972(91)90109-A.

Niinimaki, T., Puranen, J. and Jalovaara, P. 1994, "Total hip arthroplasty using isoelastic femoral stems. A seven- to nine-year follow-up in 108 patients", *J Bone Joint Surg Br*, 76B(3): 413–8.

Nishiguchi, S., Fujibayashi, S., Kim, H.-., Kokubo, T. and Nakamura, T. 2003, "Biology of alkali- and heat-treated titanium implants", *J Biomed Mater Res A*, 67(1): 26–35, DOI: 10.1002/jbm.a.10540.

Noda, T., Okabe, M. and Isobe, S. 1996, "Hard surfacing of TiAl intermetallic compound by plasma carburization", *Mater Sci Eng A*, 213(1–2): 157–161, DOI: 10.1016/0921-5093(96)10248-3.

Noiset, O., Schneider, Y. and Marchand-Brynaert, J. 1999, "Fibronectin adsorption or/and covalent grafting on chemically modified PEEK film surfaces", *J Biomed Sci Polym Ed*, 10(6): 657–77, DOI: 10.1163/156856299X00865.

Noiset, O., Schneider, Y.J. and Marchand-Brynaert, J. 2000, "Adhesion and growth of CaCo2 cells on surface-modified PEEK substrata", *J Biomed Sci Polym Ed*, 11(7): 767–86, DOI: 10.1163/156856200744002.

Olyslaegers, C., Defoort, K., Simon, J.P. and Vandenberghe, L. 2008, "Wear in conventional and highly cross-linked polyethylene cups: a 5-year follow-up study", *J Arthroplasty*, 23(4): 489–94, DOI: 10.1016/j.arth.2007.02.013.

Oral, E., Greenbaum, E.S., Malhi, A.S., Harris, W.H. and Muratoglu, O.K. 2005, "Characterization of irradiated blends of α-tocopherol and UHMWPE", *Biomaterials*, 26(33): 6657–63, DOI: 10.1016/j.biomaterials.2005.04.026.

Ostrowski, T. and Rödel, J. 1999, "Evolution of mechanical properties of porous alumina during free sintering and hot pressing", *J Am Ceram Soc*, 82: 3080–6 DOI: 10.1111/j.1151-2916.1999.tb02206.x.

Pellegrini, V.D., Olcott, C.W. and McCollister, E.C. 1998, The Tri-lock femoral systems. In *Total Hip Artroplasty Outcomes*, eds. Finerman, G.A.M., Dorey, F. J., Grigoris, P. and McKellop, H.A. Kidlington, Churchill – Livingstone, pp. 181–93.

Piconi, C. and Maccauro, G. 1999, "Zirconia as a ceramic biomaterial", *Biomaterials*, 20(1): 1–25, DOI: 10.1016/S0142-9612(98)00010-6.

Piscanec, S., Colombi Ciacchi, L., Vesselli, E., Comelli, G., Sbaizero, O., Meriani, S. and De Vita, A. 2004, "Bioactivity of TiN-coated titanium implants", *Acta Mater*, 52(5): 1237–45, DOI: 10.1016/j.actamat.2003.11.020.

Puleo, D.A. and Thomas, M.V. 2006, "Implant surfaces", *Dent Clin North Am*, 50 (3): 323–38, DOI: 10.1016/j.cden.2006.03.001.

Rack, R. and Pfaff, H.G. 2000, A new ceramic material for orhopaedics. *Bioceramics in Hip Joint Replacement: Proceedings*, eds. G. Willmann and K. Zweymüller. Stuttgart, Thieme, pp. 141–5.

Raimondi, M.T. and Pietrabissa, R. 2000, "The in-vivo wear performance of prosthetic femoral heads with titanium nitride coating", *Biomaterials*, 21 (9): 907–13, DOI: 10.1016/S0142-9612(99)00246-X.

Rajadhyaksha, A.D., Brotea, C., Cheung, Y., Kuhn, C., Ramakrishnan, R. and Zelicof, S.B. 2009, "Five-year comparative study of highly cross-linked (crossfire) and traditional polyethylene", *J Arthroplasty*, 24(2): 161–7, DOI: 10.1016/j.arth.2007.09.015.

Raveh, A., Bussiba, A., Bettelheim, A. and Katz, Y. 1993, "Plasma-nitrided α–β Ti alloy: layer characterization and mechanical properties modification", *Surf Coat Tech*, 57(1): 19–29, DOI: 10.1016/0257-8972(93)90332-I.

Ren, W., Yang, S.Y., Fang, H.W., Hsu, S. and Wooley, P.H. 2003, "Distinct gene expression of receptor activator of nuclear factor-kappaB and rank ligand in the inflammatory response to variant morphologies of UHMWPE particles", *Biomaterials*, 24(26): 4819–26, DOI: 10.1016/S0142-9612(03)00384-3.

Ridley, M.D. and Jahan, M.S. 2009, "Effects of packaging environments on free radicals in γ-irradiated UHMWPE resin powder blend with vitamin E", *J Biomed Mater Res A*, 88(4): 1097–103, DOI: 10.1002/jbm.a.32042.

Robertson, J. 2002, "Diamond-like amorphous carbon", *Mater Sci Eng R*, 37(4–6): 129–281, DOI: 10.1016/S0927-796X(02)00005-0.

Robertsson, O. 2007, "Knee arthroplasty registers", *J Bone Joint Surg Br*, 89(1): 1–4, DOI: 10.1302/0301-620X.89B1.18327.

Robertsson, O. 2010, "Knee arthroplasty in Denmark, Norway and Sweden", *Acta Orthop*, 81(1): 82–9, DOI: 10.3109/17453671003685442.

Rolinski, E., Sharp, G., Cowgill, D.F. and Peterman, D.J. 1998, "Ion nitriding of titanium alpha plus beta alloy for fusion reactor applications", *J Nucl Mater*, 252(3): 200–8, DOI: 10.1016/S0022-3115(97)00325-5.

Rossi, S., Fedrizzi, L., Bacci, T. and Pradelli, G. 2003, "Corrosion behaviour of glow discharge nitrided titanium alloys", *Corros Sci*, 45(3): 511–29, DOI: 10.1016/S0010-938X(02)00139-7.

Saikko, V., Ahlroos, T., Calonius, O. and Keränen, J. 2001, "Wear simulation of total hip prostheses with polyethylene against CoCr, alumina and diamond-like carbon", *Biomaterials*, 22(12): 1507–14, DOI: 10.1016/S0142-9612(00)00306-9.

Sanchez Marquez, J.M., Del Sel, N., Leali, A. and González, D.V. 2009, "Case reports: Tantalum debris dispersion during revision of a tibial component for TKA", *Clin Orthop Relat Res*, 467(4): 1107–10, DOI: 10.1007/s11999-008-0586-8.

Santavirta, S., Böhler, M., Harris, W.H., Konttinen, Y.T., Lappalainen, R., Muratoglu, O., Rieker, C. and Salzer, M. 2003, "Alternative materials to improve total hip replacement tribology", *Acta Orthop Scand*, 74(4): 380–88.

Santavirta, S.S., Lappalainen, R., Pekko, P., Anttila, A. and Konttinen, Y.T. 1999, "The counterface, surface smoothness, tolerances, and coatings in total joint prostheses", *Clin Orthop*, 369: 92–102.

Scholes, S.C., Unsworth, A. and Goldsmith, A.A.J. 2000, "A frictional study of total hip joint replacements", *Phys Med Biol*, 45(12): 3721–35, DOI: 10.1088/0031-9155/45/12/315.

Schroder, D.T., Kelly, N.H., Wright, T.M. and Parks, M.L. 2011, "Retrieved highly crosslinked UHMWPE acetabular liners have similar wear damage as conventional UHMWPE", *Clin Orthop Relat Res*, 469(2): 387–94, DOI: 10.1007/s11999-010-1552-9.

Schröder, K., Meyer-Plath, A., Keller, D. and Ohl, A. 2002, "On the applicability of plasma assisted chemical micropatterning to different polymeric biomaterials", *Plasmas Polym*, 7(2): 103–25, DOI: 10.1023/A:1016239302194.

Shors, E.C. and Holmes, R.E. 1999, Porous hydroxiapatite In *An Introduction to Bioceramic*, eds. L.L. Hench and J. Wilson, second edn. Singapore, World Scientific, pp. 181–98.

Sobiecki, J.R. and Wierzchoń, T. 2005, "Glow discharge assisted oxynitriding of the binary Ti6Al2Cr2Mo titanium alloy", *Vacuum*, 79(3–4): 203–8, DOI: 10.1016/j.vacuum.2005.03.008.

Sobiecki, J.R., Wierzchoń, T. and Rudnicki, J. 2001, "The influence of glow discharge nitriding, oxynitriding and carbonitriding on surface modification of Ti-1Al-1Mn titanium alloy", *Vacuum*, 64(1): 41–6, DOI: 10.1016/S0042-207X (01)00373-6.

Sotereanos, N.G., Engh, C.A., Glassman, A.H., Macalino, G.E. and Engh Jr., C.A. 1995, "Cementless femoral components should be made from cobalt chrome", *Clin Orthop Relat Res*, 313: 146–53.

Sun, L., Berndt, C.C., Gross, K.A. and Kucuk, A. 2001, "Material fundamentals and clinical performance of plasma-sprayed hydroxyapatite coatings", *J Biomed Mater Res*, 58(5): 570–92, DOI: 10.1002/jbm.1056.

Tang, S.M., Cheanga, P., AbuBakarb, M.S., Khorc, K.A. and Liao, K. 2004, "Tension–tension fatigue behavior of hydroxyapatite reinforced polyetheretherketone composites", *Int J Fatigue*, 26(1): 49–57, DOI: 10.1016/S0142-1123(03)00080-X.

Tanzer, M., Gollish, J., Leighton, R., Orrell, K., Giacchino, A., Welsh, P., Shea, B. and Wells, G. 2004, "The effect of adjuvant calcium phosphate coating on a porous-coated femoral stem", *Clin Orthop Relat Res*, 424: 153–60, DOI: 10.1097/01.blo.0000128282.05708.9a.

Thomas, S.R., Shukla, D. and Latham, P.D. 2004, "Corrosion of cemented titanium femoral stems", *J Bone Joint Surg Br*, 86(7): 974–8, DOI: 10.1302/0301-620X.86B7.14812.

Tower, S.S., Currier, J.H., Currier, B.H., Lyford, K.A., Van Citters, D.W. and Mayor, M.B. 2007, "Rim cracking of the cross-linked longevity polyethylene acetabular liner after total hip arthroplasty", *J Bone Joint Surg Am*, 89 (10): 2212–7, DOI: 10.2106/JBJS.F.00758.

Traulsen, F.C., Hassenpflug, J. and Hahne, H.J. 2001, "Long-term results with cement-free total hip prostheses (Zweymuller)", *Z Orthop Ihre Grenzgeb*, 129 (3): 206–11.

Vardiman, R.G. and Kant, R.A. 1982, "The improvement of fatigue life in Ti-6Al-4V by ion implantation", *J Appl Phys*, 53(1): 690–4, DOI: 10.1063/1.329977.

Walldius, B. 1996, "Arthroplasty of the knee using an endoprosthesis", *Clin Orthop*, 331: 4–10.

Wang, A., Dumbleton, J.H., Manley, M.T. and Sekerian, P. 2003, Role of ceramic components in the era of crosslinked polyethylene for THR. In *Bioceramics in Joint Arthroplasty*, eds. H. Zippel and M. Dietrich. Berlin, Steinkopff pp. 49–62.

Wang, A., Yau, S. Essner, A., Herrera, L., Manley, M. and Dumbleton, J. 2008, "A highly crosslinked UHMWPE for CR and PS total knee arthroplasties", *J Arthroplasty*, 23(4): 559–66, DOI: 10.1016/j.arth.2007.05.007.

Weiler, M., Sattel, S., Jung, K., Ehrhardt, H., Veerasamy, V.S. and Robertson, J. 1994, "Highly tetrahedral, diamond-like amorphous hydrogenated carbon prepared from a plasma beam source", *Appl Phys Lett*, 64(21): 2797–9, DOI: 10.1063/1.111428.

Weisse, B., Zahner, M., Weber, W. and Rieger, W. 2003, "Improvement of the reliability of ceramic hip joint implants", *J Biomech*, 36(11): 1633–9, DOI: 10.1016/S0021-9290(03)00186-6.

Wen, J., Leng, Y., Chen, J. and Zhang, C. 2000, "Chemical gradient in plasma-sprayed HA coatings", *Biomaterials*, 21(13): 1339–43, DOI: 10.1016/S0142-9612 (99)00273-2.

Wierzchoń, T. and Fleszar, A. 1997, "Properties of surface layers on titanium alloy produced by thermo-chemical treatments under glow discharge conditions", *Surf Coat Tech*, 96(2–3): 205–9, DOI: 10.1016/S0257-8972(97)00113-8.

Willert, H.-., Brobäck, L.-., Buchhorn, G.H., Jensen, P.H., Köster, G., Lang, I., Ochsner, P. and Schenk, R. 1996, "Crevice corrosion of cemented titanium alloy stems in total hip replacements", *Clin Orthop Relat Res*, 333: 51–75.

Williams, D.F. 2008, "On the mechanisms of biocompatibility", *Biomaterials*, 29 (20): 2941–53, DOI: 10.1016/j.biomaterials.2008.04.023.

Wimmer, M.A., Loos, J., Nassutt, R., Heitkemper, M. and Fischer, A. 2001, "The acting wear mechanisms on metal-on-metal hip joint bearings: in vitro results", *Wear*, 250(1–12): 129–39, DOI: 10.1016/S0043-1648(01)00654-8.

Wroblewski, B.M., Siney, P.D. and Fleming, P.A. 2007, "Charnley low-friction arthroplasty: Survival patterns to 38 years", *J Bone Joint Surg Br*, 89(8): 1015–8, DOI: 10.1302/0301-620X.89B8.18387.

Xie, J. and Luan, B.L. 2008, "Formation of hydroxyapatite coating using novel chemo-biomimetic method", *J Mater Sci Mater Med*, 19(10): 3211–20, DOI: 10.1007/s10856-008-3451-0.

Yan, L., Leng , Y. and Weng, L.T. 2003, "Characterization of chemical inhomogeneity in plasma-sprayed hydroxyapatite coatings", *Biomaterials*, 24 (15): 2585–92, DOI: 10.1016/S0142-9612(03)00061-9.

Yeh, T.S., Wu, J.M. and Hu, L.J. 2008, "The properties of TiN thin films deposited by pulsed direct current magnetron sputtering", *Thin Solid Films*, 516 (21): 7294–8, DOI: 10.1016/j.tsf.2008.01.001.

Yoshinari, M., Ohtsuka, Y. and Derand, T. 1994, "Thin hydroxyapatite coating produced by the ion beam dynamic mixing method", *Biomaterials*, 15(7): 529–35, DOI: 10.1016/0142-9612(94)90019-1.

Yu, S. 2005, "In vitro apatite formation and its growth kinetics on hydroxyapatite/polyetheretherketone biocomposites", *Biomaterials*, 26(15): 2343–52, DOI: 10.1016/j.biomaterials.2004.07.028.

Part II
Wear phenomena

8
Wear phenomena of ultra-high molecular weight polyethylene (UHMWPE) joints

C. CHO, The University of Kitakyushu, Japan,
T. MURAKAMI and Y. SAWAE, Kyushu University, Japan

Abstract: This chapter discusses wear phenomena of ultra-high molecular weight polyethylene (UHMWPE) in artificial joints. The importance of wear in artificial joints, lubrication modes in artificial joints as UHMWPE-on-hard and improving methods for wear reduction of UHMWPE are reviewed. Wear phenomena of UHMWPE artificial knee joints are discussed with reference to the wear characteristics of retrieved artificial knee joints, together with an experimental study on the delamination mechanism of UHMWPE, macroscopic contact analysis between the femoral component and tibial insert, and microscopic contact analysis between surface asperities and tibial inserts.

Key words: ultra-high molecular weight polyethylene (UHMWPE), wear phenomenon, artificial joints, contact analysis.

8.1 Introduction

Ultra-high molecular weight polyethylene (UHMWPE) is widely used for articulating components in various joint prostheses, such as hip, knee, ankle and other joints. The mechanical functions and durability of different joints change according to geometric designs and severity of operating conditions, which affect the types of wear and failures. Mixed or boundary lubrication modes are typically dominant in artificial joints composed of UHMWPE and anti-corrosive metal or bioinert ceramics. Wear of UHMWPE is therefore an important phenomenon in various joint prostheses. Effective methods for wear reduction are discussed, including pre-treatment for clinical use – particularly cross-linking, addition of vitamin E and surface grafting treatments for UHMWPE – and improvement of articulating counterface materials. The wear phenomenon of UHMWPE in artificial knee joints is described in detail in Section 8.2.

8.1.1 Importance of wear in artificial joints

Healthy, natural synovial joints can maintain very low friction and low wear, even under high load where hip and knee joints bear several times a person's bodyweight such as during walking, stair-climbing and running. In contrast, joints that are diseased due to osteoarthritis, rheumatoid arthritis and other arthritic diseases which cause disability of movement and severe pain may require replacement with superior artificial joints in order to relieve pain and enable the accomplishment of normal daily activities. Successful clinical application of total hip replacement was achieved by Sir John Charnley in 1962, using an UHMWPE acetabular cup against a stainless steel femoral head, which significantly reduced the wear of the polymeric component (Charnley, 1979). By using UHMWPE, Charnley overcame the excessive wear problems associated with polytetrafluoroethylene (PTFE) cups. This accomplishment promoted the clinical application of UHMWPE as a mating material against metallic or ceramic components in other artificial joints, such as knees, ankles, shoulders and elbows. Total joint arthroplasty thus became a reliable medical treatment. However, serious problems of joint loosening occurred in certain cases and it was noted that tissue reaction to an excessive release of wear particles was the main cause (Willert and Semlitsch, 1977). In particular, small polyethylene particles of sub-micrometer size appear to strongly affect the biological reaction of macrophages, causing production of cytokines such as TNF-α and precursors of osteoclasts. Activated osteoclasts resorb the bone, leading to osteolysis and joint loosening (Ingham and Fisher, 2005). The most important prevention against biological reaction is therefore to minimize production of wear debris.

To reduce various kinds of wear failures of UHMWPE components, the predominant wear mechanisms (such as adhesive, abrasive and/or fatigue wear) should first be identified. Subsequently, effective strategies for reducing those wear failures should be found. Strategies for reducing adhesive wear should consider not only improvement of the wear resistance of UHMWPE, but also the influence of transfer film formation, adsorbed film formation and bonding action by active molecules in lubricants. For abrasive wear, it is necessary to modify surface protrusions of the harder mating material and prevent the intervention of hard particles such as wear debris and bone cement between the rubbing surfaces. Delamination is a catastrophic surface fatigue failure, often observed in knee prostheses. This is a complicated mechanism in which repeated severe loading and sliding processes are accompanied by crack formation and propagation. The morphology, size, number and properties of wear particles change depending on wear modes. Reduction of UHMWPE wear and suppression of biological reaction to wear debris are therefore important in improving the longevity of joint prostheses.

As alternate clinical treatments, hard-on-hard hip prostheses have been tried, such as metal-on-metal, ceramic-on-ceramic and ceramic-on-metal. The superiority in wear resistance of rubbing materials and improvement of lubricating fluid film formation resulted in remarkable reduction of wear (Issac *et al.*, 2006). However, in certain cases, there are still unsolved problems: the harmful influences of metallic ions and small debris particles; stripe wear of ceramics; squeaking of ceramic-on-ceramic; breakage of ceramic components. Compliant artificial cartilage, used either as a solid elastomeric layer or compliant hydrogel, is another possible alternative. These compliant rubbing materials are expected to improve the lubrication mechanism with thicker fluid film formation and additional effects, but further studies on durability are required before they are ready for clinical application.

8.1.2 Lubrication modes in artificial joints as UHMWPE-on-hard

As with other rubbing surfaces, the extent of wear depends on the lubrication mode employed. The lubrication modes in total hip replacements were examined by studying frictional behaviors in simulator testing (Scholes *et al.*, 2000). In a Stribeck analysis, the frictional behaviors plotted against the parameter of (viscosity × sliding speed)/(load/(femoral head radius)) showed a decrease in friction as this parameter increased, for aqueous solutions of carboxy methyl cellulose of different viscosities, which is indicative of a mixed lubrication regime. Furthermore, the estimated minimum film thickness of less than 0.1 μm, based on the elastohydrodynamic theory for low elastic modulus materials, demonstrated the mixed lubrication mode for UHMWPE-on-hard hip joints. It is pointed out that, under these thin film conditions, the adsorbed films with proteins and other constituents in synovial fluid can enhance the friction level in simulator tests using bovine serum as lubricant.

Fluid film formation in knee prostheses with different geometrical congruities was examined using the electric resistance method in a knee joint simulator, in which the UHMWPE surface was given conductive properties by coating it with platinum or gold (Murakami *et al.*, 1993). The extent of fluid film formation was evaluated by the degree of separation, which is defined as the ratio of measured voltage to an applied voltage of 100 mV (a degree of separation of 1, indicates full separation; degree of separation of 0 indicates local intimate contact). This value depends on the electric resistance value R_p in parallel to rubbing specimens. Silicone oils of

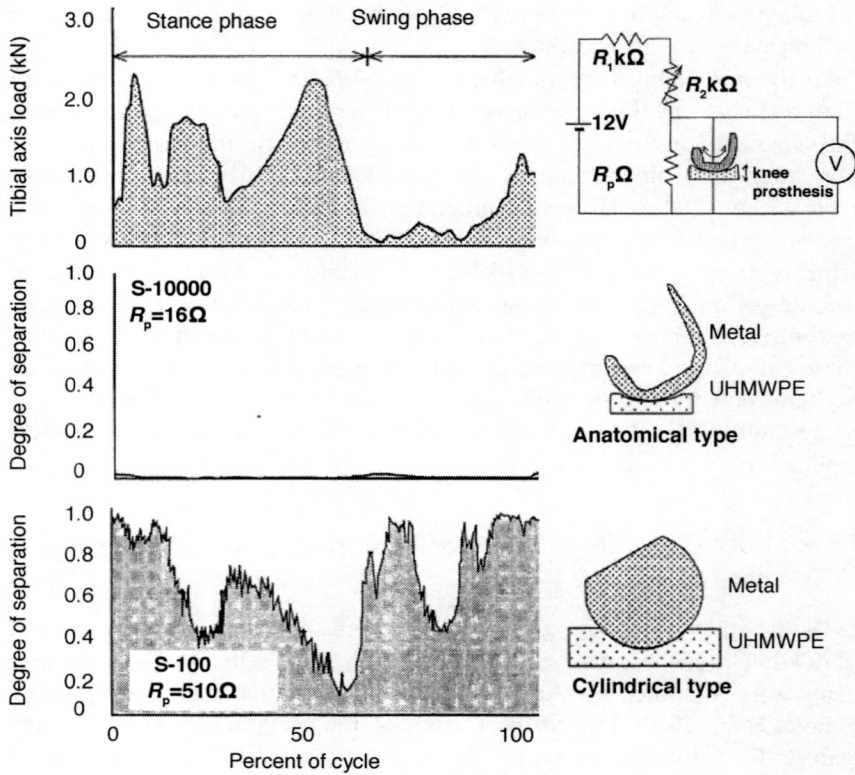

8.1 Evaluation of fluid film formation in knee prostheses during walking motion (Murakami *et al.*, 1993).

different viscosities (S-1 to S-10000, where the numeral represents the kinetic viscosity (measured in mm^2/s) at 25°C) have been used as lubricants. The changes in fluid film formation during walking are shown in Fig. 8.1 for an anatomical design (Okayama University Mark II) and a cylindrical knee prosthesis (radius of metallic femoral component is 30 mm and radial clearance is 0.3 mm). Very little fluid film formed in the anatomical knee prosthesis even with very viscous lubricants (S-10000) and low R_p condition. In contrast, in the cylindrical knee prosthesis with better geometrical congruity, considerable fluid film is formed, even during the loading stance phase, with medium viscosity lubricant S-100 of about 0.1 Pa s and $R_p = 510\ \Omega$. However, when lower viscosity lubricants similar to the human joint were used, significant direct contact between rubbing surfaces occurred, particularly during the stance phase.

It is difficult to expect the possibility of effective fluid film lubrication in artificial joints composed of UHMWPE and a hard material. Effective strategies for wear reduction are thus required.

8.1.3 Improving methods for wear reduction of UHMWPE

As a polymeric material, UHMWPE has good wear resistance and low friction properties. However, the linear wear level of traditional UHMWPE in most total hip prostheses is reported to be 0.05 – 0.30 mm/year (Semlitsch and Willert, 1997), producing significant wear debris. The reduction of wear, and subsequent minimization of wear debris, has therefore been the focus of much investigation.

Various techniques for improving the wear resistance of UHMWPE have been tried. Raising the molecular weight and suppressing oxidation degradation both proved effective. However, reinforcing the material with carbon fiber (Poly-II) had disastrous consequences in terms of wear, as did increasing its crystallinity (Hylamer).

Cross-linking of polyethylene

In 1970, Oonishi *et al.* tried to improve wear resistance in polyethylene by irradiating it with 1000 kGy gamma radiation and confirmed that durability and length of clinical use improved (Oonishi *et al.*, 1998a, 1998b). In modern products, gamma radiation treatments of 50–100 kGy are commonly used in order to achieve high levels of cross-linking and sterilization.

Multi-directional wear tests, involving a two-arc friction path lubricated with diluted bovine serum, showed that increasing radiation levels (and hence increasing the number of cross-links) resulted in a corresponding reduction in wear (Sawano *et al.*, 2005). Indeed, various laboratory studies have shown that wear decreases in proportion to the amount of cross-linking in UHMWPE (Williams *et al.*, 2007). UHMWPE subjected to gamma radiation doses above 200 kGy has shown no detectable wear in hip simulator studies (Oonishi *et al.*, 2004). However, higher levels cause reduction in elongation and tensile strength. It is therefore important to identify and select optimum levels of irradiation. For example, 50–200 kGy provides durability under secure conditions and adequate mechanical properties. Furthermore, although less wear occurs in cross-linked polyethylene compared with non-cross-linked polyethylene, its higher sensitivity under adverse wear conditions and the higher biological reactivity of smaller particles of wear debris may affect the longevity of hip prostheses.

Addition of vitamin E

Since the remarkable effect of adding vitamin E to UHMWPE in order to prevent fatigue cracks was discovered by Tomita *et al.* (1999), the consequences of vitamin E addition have merited investigation worldwide. In a sliding fatigue test at a multi-directional locus in two parallel lines, gamma-irradiated polyethylene demonstrated high rates of flaking-like destruction, while gamma-irradiated polyethylene containing vitamin E exhibited no subsurface crack formation or flaking-like destruction. It has been suggested that the presence of vitamin E reduces crack propagation due to reduced hardness at the grain boundary.

The main constituent of vitamin E, α-tocopherol, is usually added to provide oxidation resistance and fatigue wear resistance. Vitamin E is an effective chain-breaking antioxidant, consisting of tocopherols and tocotrienols. Vitamin E is about 90% α-tocopherol, and it is usually α-tocopherol that is added to UHMWPE (Oral and Muratoglu, 2009).

Two methods are used to incorporate vitamin E into UHMWPE. One is to blend vitamin E with UHMWPE powder prior to consolidation and the other is the diffusion of vitamin E into UHMWPE following radiation cross-linking. In the latter, the cross-linking efficiency is not adversely affected, but in the former the presence of vitamin E during irradiation can reduce the cross-linking efficiency. Wear reduction is not the only advantage of adding vitamin E to UHMWPE. Reduced numbers of inflammatory cytokines in cells cultured in the presence of wear debris from vitamin E blended UHMWPE have also been reported (Teramura *et al.*, 2009).

Polymeric brush treatment

To reduce wear and prevent bone-resorptive responses to wear particles in total hip prostheses, the effects of graft polymerization of biocompatible phospholipids polymer 2-methacryloyloxyethyl phosphorylcholine (MPC) onto UHMWPE surface were evaluated by Moro *et al.* (2004). The grafting of MPC onto a polyethylene hip acetabular liner was performed by a photoinduced polymerization technique, producing a covalent bond between the MPC and the polyethylene liner. Grafting MPC onto UHMWPE increased its hydrophilicity. A comparison of the wear behaviors (in a hip joint simulator) of traditional and cross-linked UHMWPE and cross-linked UHMWPE with grafted MPC is shown in Fig. 8.2. The MPC grafting lowered the amount of wear significantly accompanied with reducing friction. Furthermore, the osteoclastic bone resorption induced by subperiosteal injection of particles onto mouse calvariae was eliminated by the MPC grafting on particles. MPC grafting is therefore effective in preventing periprosthetic osteolysis.

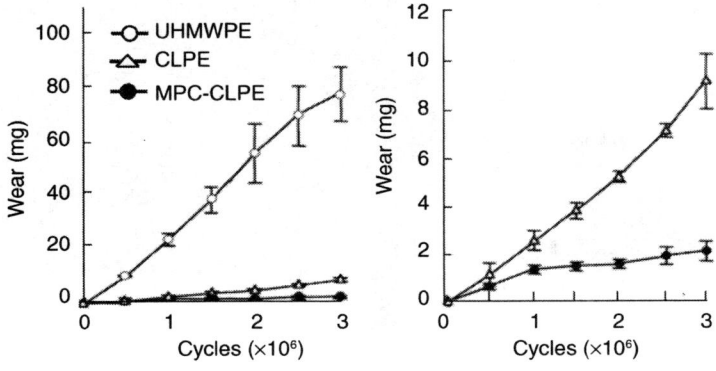

8.2 Improvement of wear properties with MPC grafting treatment onto cross-linked UHMWPE (CLPE) (Moro *et al.*, 2004).

Improvement of articulating mating material

Wear of UHMWPE depends on the counterface material and its properties. Alumina, a ceramic material, reduces wear by approximately 50% compared with metallic mating materials (Semlitsch and Willert, 1997). The superior surface finish and geometry without extrusion, together with the wear-resistant and hydrophilic properties of the ceramic itself, appear to be effective in reducing wear in clinical usage. However, similar wear occurs in both types in very highly cross-linked polyethylene (Oonishi *et al.*, 1998a). Appropriate modification of metallic surfaces is expected to improve the wear properties of UWMWPE.

8.2 Wear phenomena of UHMWPE knee joints

Preventing wear of UHMWPE components in knee joint arthroplasty is an important task. To achieve this, it is important to analyze retrieved specimens in order to establish a direct comparison with the results from *in vitro* wear tests and/or finite-element analyses. The retrieval, experimental and analytical studies in this section will contribute to a better understanding of the wear mechanism of UHMWPE.

8.2.1 The wear characteristics of retrieved artificial knee joints

The wear characteristics of UHMWPE tibial inserts and their counterparts (metallic femoral components) of five retrieved artificial knee joints were examined in a retrieval study by Cho *et al.* (2001, 2007, 2009, 2010). The

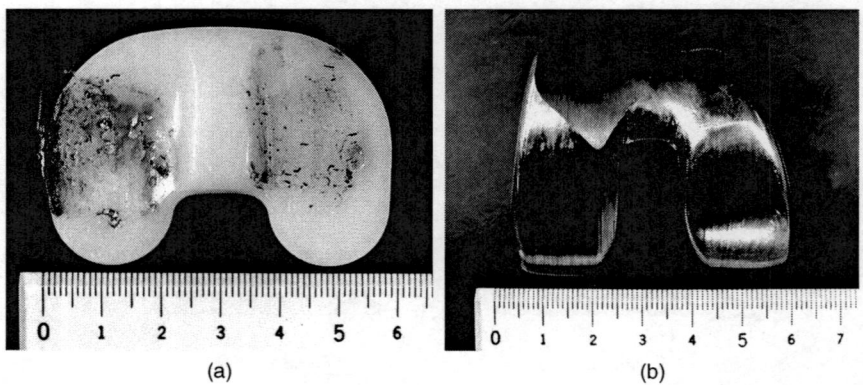

8.3 Components of a retrieved MG I type knee joint (right side, 114 months *in vivo*): (a) UHMWPE tibial insert; (b) femoral component (Cho *et al.*, 2005, 2007, 2010).

designs included four Miller–Galante I (MG I) type porous total knee systems (Zimmer Inc., USA) and one Press-Fit Condylar (PFC) type total knee system (Johnson & Johnson Co., USA). The retrieved artificial knee joints had an average *in vivo* duration of 120.4 months (74 to 149 months). Two examples of the retrieved tibial inserts and their counterparts are shown in Fig. 8.3 (MG I type) (Cho *et al.*, 2005) and Fig. 8.4 (PFC type) (Cho *et al.*, 2002). Examples of laser micrographs of the worn surface and the surface profile (along the straight white line shown in each image) of the retrieved tibial inserts are shown in Fig. 8.5 (Cho *et al.*, 2001, 2009).

In the case of the MG I type, the medial side of the retrieved tibial inserts demonstrated more excessive wear and plastic deformation than the lateral

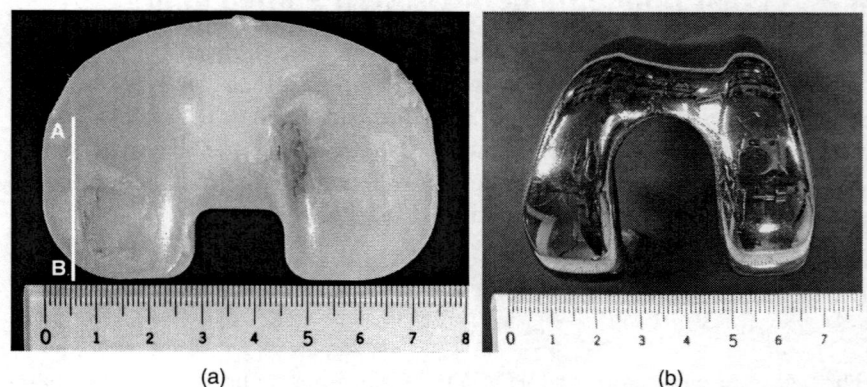

8.4 Components of a retrieved PFC type knee joint (left side, 74 months *in vivo*): (a) UHMWPE tibial insert; (b) femoral component (Cho *et al.*, 2002, 2007, 2010).

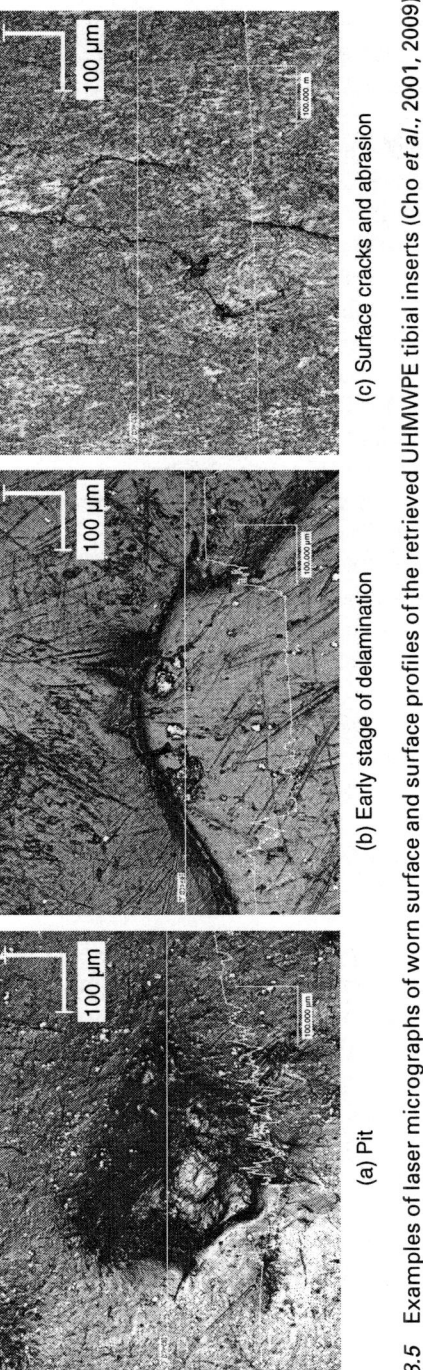

8.5 Examples of laser micrographs of worn surface and surface profiles of the retrieved UHMWPE tibial inserts (Cho *et al.*, 2001, 2009).

side, as shown in Fig. 8.3(a). Predominant wear patterns in these retrieved MG I type tibial inserts were delamination, pitting and abrasion. Furthermore, surface cracks and fine scratches caused by interposition of third-body metallic wear particles were also observed, as shown in Figs 8.5(a) and 8.5(b). In particular, on the metallic femoral components of some retrieved MG I type knee joints, excessive metallic wear due to direct contact between the femoral component and the patellar metal base as a result of the failure of the polyethylene of the metal-backed patellar component was observed. In such cases, very excessive wear due to surface roughness of the metallic components and interposition of third-body metallic wear particles occurs both in the femoral component and in the tibial insert. Fig. 8.3(b) (Cho *et al.*, 2007, 2010) shows such an example of the retrieved MG I type femoral components. In the medial and lateral condyle of this case, a number of microscopic scratches were observed. It is thought that microscopic surface asperities, caused by surface damage such as scratches, generate microscopic wear and contribute to increasing and/or accelerating wear of the UHMWPE tibial insert.

In the case of the PFC type, the retrieved tibial insert shown in Fig. 8.4(a) demonstrated relatively slight delamination and abrasion as compared with those of MG I type, as shown in Fig. 8.5(c). It appears that the primary reasons for the low wear are the higher degree of conformity between the femoral component and the tibial insert, and the thick polyethylene patellar component with non-use of the patellar metal base, rather than the shortest *in vivo* duration. Non-destructive cross-section testing of the retrieved PFC type tibial insert shown in Fig. 8.4(a) was performed using a micro-focus X-ray CT apparatus. The X-ray CT image of the retrieved PFC type tibial insert at line A–B is shown in Fig. 8.6 (Cho *et al.*, 2001, 2002, 2004, 2009). Subsurface cracks were observed about 1 mm below the surface of the tibial insert.

The predominant wear patterns of the retrieved UHMWPE tibial inserts in this study were delamination, pitting, abrasion, scratching and plastic deformation. Delamination due to fusion defects was also observed in the retrieved tibial inserts. On the whole, the medial side of the tibial inserts, the thinner inserts and those with lower surface conformity had a tendency to show severe wear and high plastic deformation. These wear characteristics are similar to examination results in other retrieval studies (Engh *et al.*, 1992; Kurtz, 2009a; Landy and Walker, 1988). In particular, delamination and pitting are most frequently reported for simulator-tested and retrieved polyethylene tibial inserts (Cho *et al.*, 2001; Currier *et al.*, 1998; Engh *et al.*, 1992; Kurtz, 2009a; Landy and Walker, 1988; Walker *et al.*, 1996). The consensus is that both surface failures result from fatigue, with delamination being caused when subsurface cracks continue to propagate in a tangential

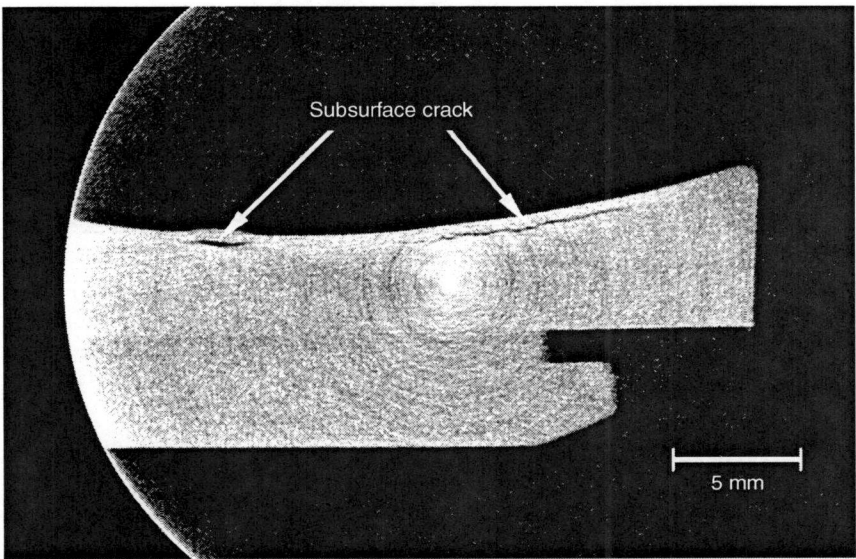

8.6 X-ray CT image of the retrieved PFC type UHMWPE tibial insert including subsurface cracks (Cho *et al.*, 2001, 2002, 2004, 2009).

path relative to the surface and pitting being caused by cracks that emanate at the surface and then propagate into the tibial insert (Lewis, 1997).

8.2.2 An experimental study on the delamination mechanism of UHMWPE

Severe delamination, which is one of the fatigue wear patterns, is frequently observed on the worn surface of the UHMWPE tibial inserts, especially in retrieved anatomically designed artificial knee joints. The contact stresses in the polyethylene tibial insert of such joints are generally higher than the yield stress of the material during normal gait. The fatigue wear that causes subsurface cracks in the polyethylene tibial insert and the generation of wear particles as delamination type is thought to result from repeated plastic deformation owing to the high contact stresses. In the experimental study of Cho *et al.* (2006a, 2006b), accelerated fatigue wear tests of the UHMWPE tibial inserts were performed using a knee joint simulator. The wear characteristics of each worn tibial insert were observed in order to investigate the delamination mechanism of the tibial insert in the artificial knee joint. A delamination mechanism of the UHMWPE tibial insert was proposed based on this experimental study.

In the fatigue wear tests, a 60 mm diameter sphere made of stainless steel (SUS316, JIS) was used as the femoral component. UHMWPE disk specimens (5 mm thick and 80 mm diameter) were used as the tibial inserts. Distilled water and diluted bovine serum solution were used as lubricants and the wear tests were performed in a temperature-controlled container at 37°C (body temperature).

The test conditions, such as flexion–extension motion of the femoral component and tibial axis load, were simplified in order to reproduce *in vivo* fatigue wear phenomena of the UHMWPE tibial insert in a short period of time. The femoral component was allowed to rotate about its axis of the flexion shaft but this flexion–extension motion was controlled with simplified flexion motion (0–60°) in the form of half-sine wave of frequency 1 Hz. The tibial insert was allowed to translate in the anterior–posterior direction and the displacement was also controlled in order to set the slip ratio (s). The wear tests were performed with three slip ratios ($s = 0$, pure rolling; $s = 0.5$, rolling and sliding; $s = 1$, pure sliding) with a constant tibial axis load of 2 kN.

Under lubrication with distilled water, delamination was observed in all three slip ratios. The higher slip ratios had a tendency to show earlier delamination and a higher wear rate. The wear rates increased significantly after delamination. On the contrary, under lubrication with bovine serum solution, delamination was not observed until one million cycles had been performed. The wear rates were lower than those for lubrication with distilled water. In these fatigue wear tests, delamination occurred only when distilled water was used as a lubricant. Figure 8.7 (Cho *et al.*, 2006a, 2006b) shows the change in the rubbing surface of the tibial insert with test cycle (in distilled water; $s = 0.5$). A characteristic change in the rubbing surface was not observed until 260,000 cycles, as shown in Fig. 8.7(a). However, the generation of a surface bulge was observed at the center of the rubbing surface of the tibial insert after 350,000 cycles, as shown in Fig. 8.7(b). This portion of the surface bulge caused large-scale delamination at the macroscopic level after 600,000 cycles, as shown in Fig. 8.7(c). Figure 8.8 (Cho *et al.*, 2006b) depicts the worn surface of the tibial insert, showing severe delamination and polyethylene wear debris after 690,000 cycles (in distilled water; $s = 0.5$).

The experimental results obtained in this study shed light on the process of delamination in UHMWPE, as shown in Fig. 8.9 (Cho *et al.*, 2006a, 2006b). In the early stages (Fig. 8.9(a)), the maximum plastic strain, which occurs below the surface of the tibial insert, increases with every pass of the femoral component under cyclic loading and/or motion. If this accumulated residual plastic strain reaches the ductile limit of the polyethylene, microcracks will form in the subsurface of the tibial insert. These microcracks can then propagate in a tangential path relative to the surface, because the maximum shear stress occurs in the subsurface. The upper polyethylene layer, above the subsurface crack, is extended in a direction

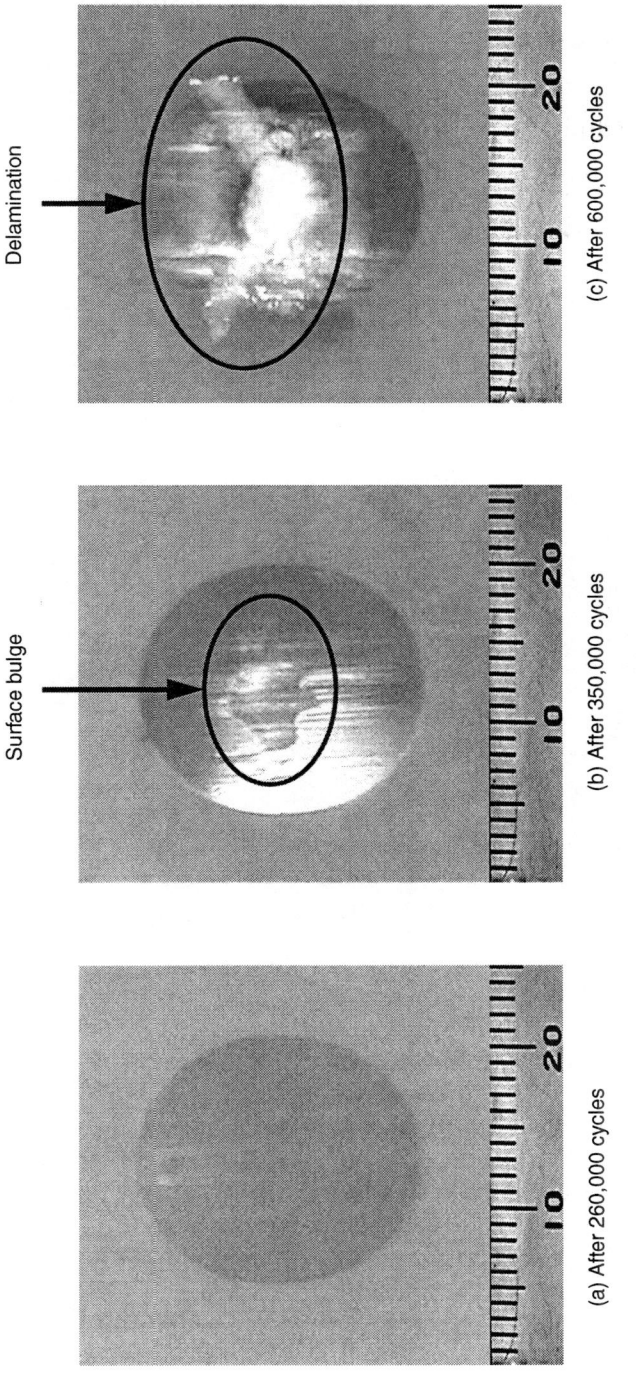

8.7 Change in rubbing surface of the UHMWPE tibial insert with test cycle (Cho et al., 2006a, 2006b).

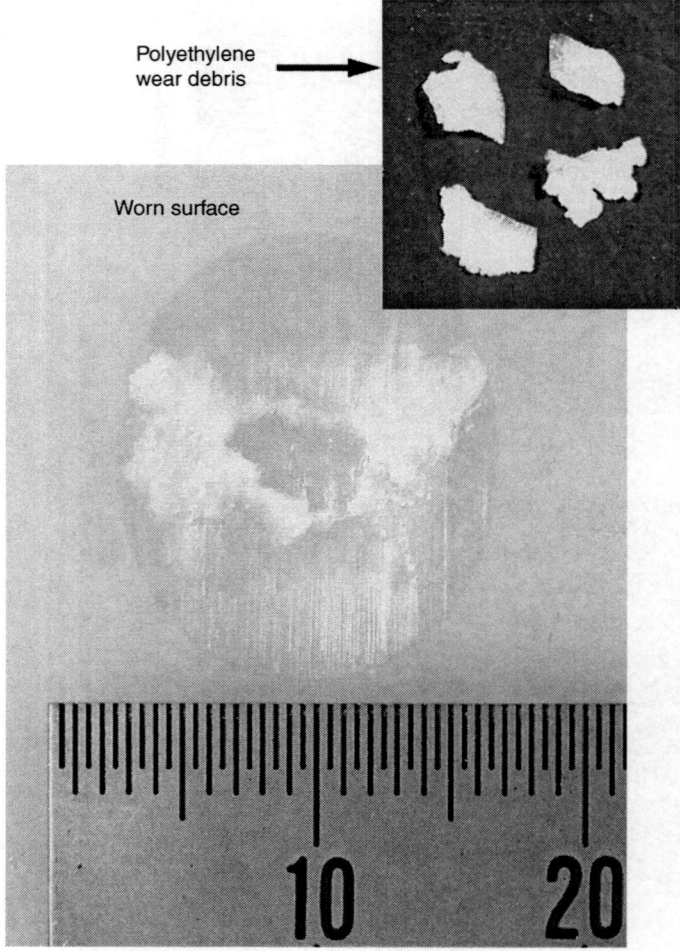

8.8 Worn surface of the UHMWPE tibial insert showing severe delamination (Cho *et al.*, 2006b).

parallel to the surface by repeated plastic deformation under cyclic loading and/or motion.

In the middle stage (Fig. 8.9(b)), the subsurface crack is propagated towards the surface and then the extended upper layer of polyethylene forms the surface bulge. It is thought that the degree of extension in the early stage determines the surface bulge at this stage. In the terminal stage (Fig. 8.9(c)), the subsurface crack reaches the surface, causing portions of the surface bulge to delaminate.

The results of this experimental study suggest that repeated plastic deformation on and below the surface of an UHMWPE tibial insert initiates

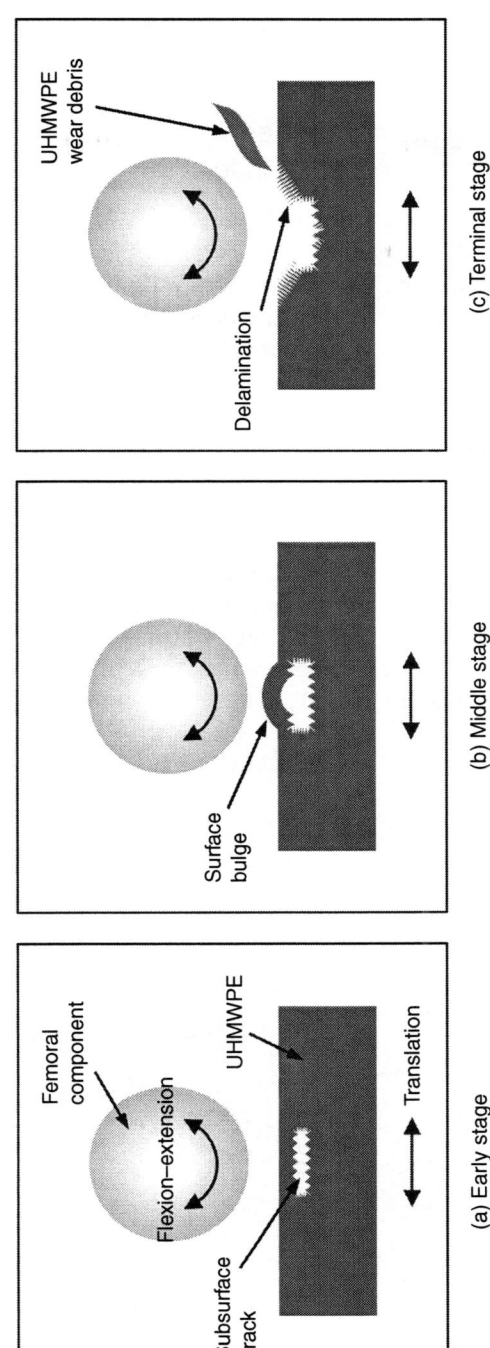

8.9 Schematic illustration of delamination process in an UHMWPE tibial insert (Cho et al., 2006a, 2006b).

subsurface cracks, generating surface bulges and eventually leading to delamination.

8.2.3 Macroscopic contact analysis between femoral component and tibial insert

A macroscopic analytical study (Cho *et al.*, 2002, 2004, 2009) was carried out to investigate the fatigue wear mechanism of an UHMWPE tibial insert. Elasto-plastic contact analysis of the UHMWPE tibial insert based on three-dimensional (3D) geometric measurement from a retrieved artificial knee joint was performed using a finite-element model (FEM) in order to investigate plastic deformation behavior in the tibial insert.

The UHMWPE tibial insert and the metallic femoral component of a retrieved PFC type total knee system (Johnson & Johnson Co., USA) (as shown in Fig. 8.4) were used to produce a 3D FEM of the retrieved artificial knee joint. On the basis of geometrical measurements from the tibial insert and the femoral component of the retrieved PFC type knee joint, the 3D FEM of the joint shown in Fig. 8.10 was constructed (Cho *et al.*, 2002).

The UHMWPE tibial insert shown in Fig. 8.4(a) was assumed to be an elasto-plastic body with a Poisson's ratio of 0.4. It was also assumed that the bottom surface of the tibial insert was entirely fixed to the rigid metallic tibial tray. The contacting metallic femoral component shown in Fig. 8.4(b)

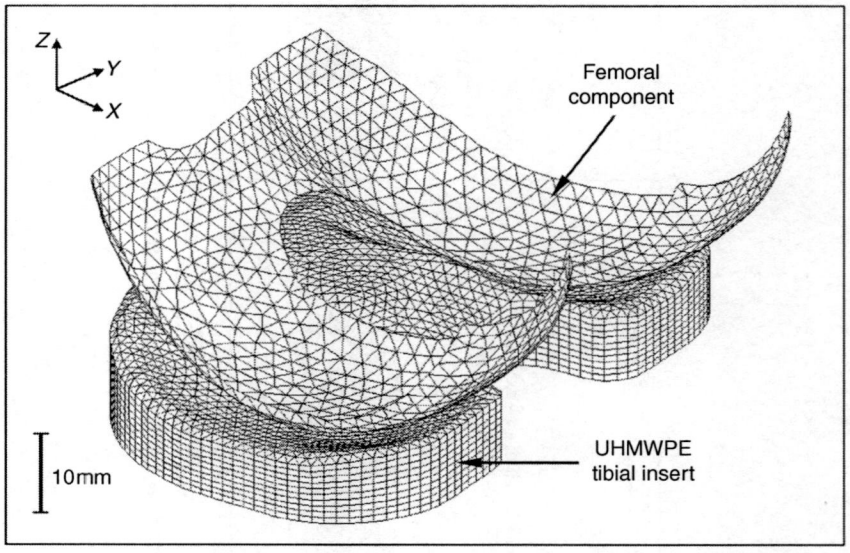

8.10 Three-dimensional FEM of the retrieved PFC type knee joint used in the analysis (Cho *et al.*, 2002).

(Cho et al., 2007, 2010) was assumed to be a rigid body. The contact between the femoral component and the tibial insert was simulated as a rigid body (the metallic femoral component) deforming a soft elasto-plastic body (the UHMWPE tibial insert). Only the static contact condition between the femoral component and the tibial insert in the standing position was considered in this FEM; the femoral component was simply pressed into the tibial insert with a constant normal load of 2 kN (approximately three times the patient's body weight). The coefficient of friction between the femoral component and the tibial insert was assumed to be 0.1. The elasto-plastic material model (a simplified true stress–strain curve) of UHMWPE, established in a previous study performed by the authors (Cho et al., 2002, 2004), was used as the FEM of the UHMWPE tibial insert. The linear elastic modulus and the yield stress of UHMWPE were 498 MPa and 13.3 MPa respectively.

The contact stress distribution and plastic deformation behavior in cross-sections of the tibial insert were investigated and the results of one such analysis are shown in Fig. 8.11 (Cho et al., 2002). The figure shows the contour plots of the cross-section that underwent maximum contact stress (von Mises equivalent stress) and the equivalent plastic strain in the lateral side of the tibial insert. This analysis is concerned with static contact between the femoral component and the tibial insert in a retrieved PFC type knee joint, based on geometrical measurements at the macroscopic level. It was found that high contact stresses, which exceed the yield stress of UHMWPE, and considerable plastic strains occurred below the surface of the tibial insert. The maximum plastic strain in the tibial insert occurred at approximately 1 mm below the surface of the lateral side. This depth corresponds closely to the location of subsurface cracks found in the lateral side of the retrieved PFC type UHMWPE tibial insert shown in Fig. 8.4(a) in the non-destructive cross-section observation, as shown in Fig. 8.6.

When the tibial insert shown in Fig. 8.4(a) was observed under a laser microscope, subsurface cracks that constitute the early stages of delamination were seen on the lateral side. Some of these subsurface areas of pre-delamination closely correspond to the location of the maximum plastic strain in this FEM analysis.

Considering the generation process of polyethylene wear particles, the maximum plastic strain, which occurs below the surface of the polyethylene tibial insert, will increase with every pass of the femoral component under cyclic loading and/or motion. Once the accumulated residual plastic strain reaches a certain value, i.e. the ductile limit of the polyethylene, microcracks will occur in the subsurface of the tibial insert (Reeves et al., 1998). These microcracks can then propagate at a high rate on a path tangential to the surface, because the maximum shear stress occurs in the subsurface, and

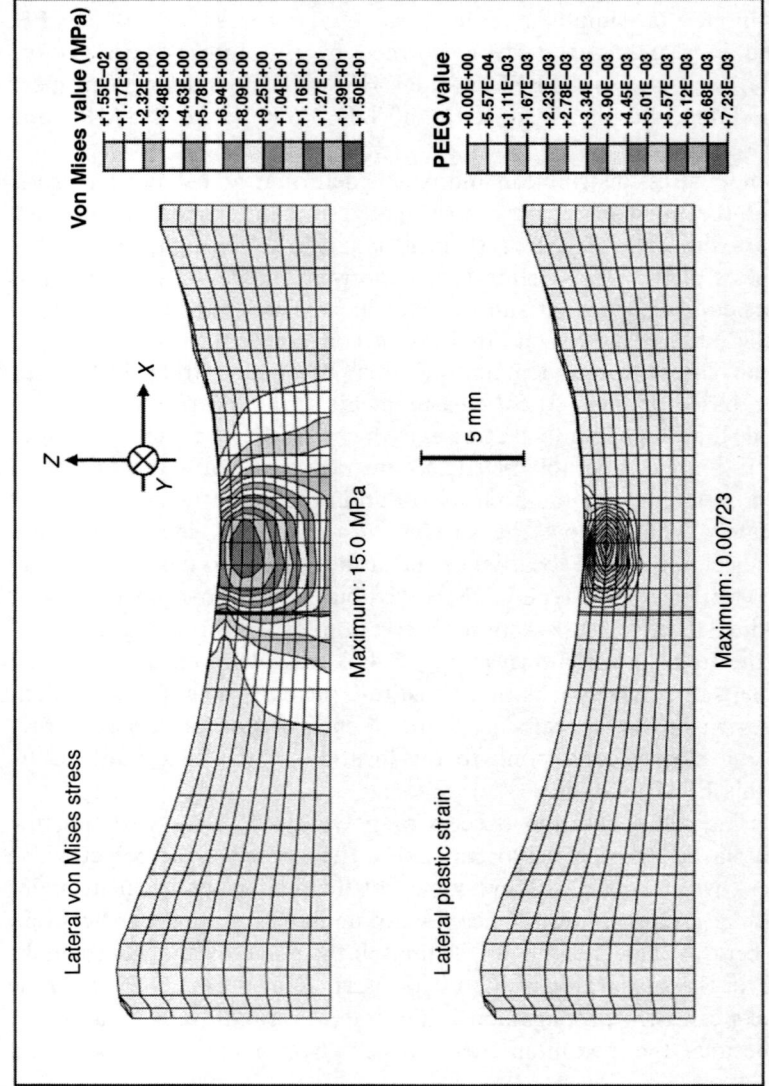

8.11 Contour plots of the von Mises stress and plastic strain in the PFC type UHMWPE tibial insert (Cho et al., 2002).

eventually result in delamination. Polyethylene wear particles are generated by this delamination.

8.2.4 Microscopic contact analysis between surface asperities and tibial insert

In studying the wear characteristics of the retrieved artificial knee joints, a number of microscopic scratches were observed on the metallic femoral components of the retrieved artificial knee joints, as shown in Fig. 8.3(b). Microscopic surface asperities caused by this surface damage affect the wear property of the UHMWPE tibial insert adversely.

The main purpose of the microscopic analytical study conducted by Cho et al. (2007, 2008, 2010) was to investigate the influence of microscopic surface asperities of damaged metallic femoral components on the wear of UHMWPE tibial inserts in retrieved artificial knee joints. For this purpose, 3D microscopic surface profile measurements were taken of the damaged surface of a retrieved metallic femoral component shown in Fig 8.3(b) using a laser microscope. The damaged femoral component surface was then reproduced using 3D computer-aided design (CAD) software in order to produce a 3D FEM of the microscopic surface asperities based on actual measurement data. Analyses of the elasto-plastic contact between the microscopic surface asperities and the UHMWPE tibial insert were also performed using the FEM. These analyses investigated the mechanical state (contact stress and plastic strain distributions), plastic deformation and microscopic wear behavior of the tibial insert caused by a microscopic surface asperity. In this study, asperity aspect ratio and asperity shape ratio were defined in order to represent the 3D shape of the asperity. The asperity aspect ratio was defined as the asperity height divided by the half-width; the asperity shape ratio was defined as the ratio of the minor axis to major axis of a cross-section perpendicular to the indentation direction of the asperity.

An example of a 3D FEM for one of the contact analyses performed in this study is shown in Fig. 8.12. The metallic surface asperity was assumed to be a rigid body. The UHMWPE tibial insert was assumed to be a semi-infinite elasto-plastic plate with a Poisson's ratio of 0.45. The bottom surface of the tibial insert was entirely fixed. The coefficient of friction between the asperity and the tibial insert surface was assumed to be 0.1. The contact between the asperity and the tibial insert was simulated as a rigid body (the metallic asperity) deforming a soft elasto-plastic plate (the UHMWPE tibial insert) by applying normal displacement to the asperity, which represents the indentation depth of the asperity.

An example of the results of a series of FEM contact analyses performed in this study is shown in Fig. 8.13 (Cho et al., 2008, 2010). From the results

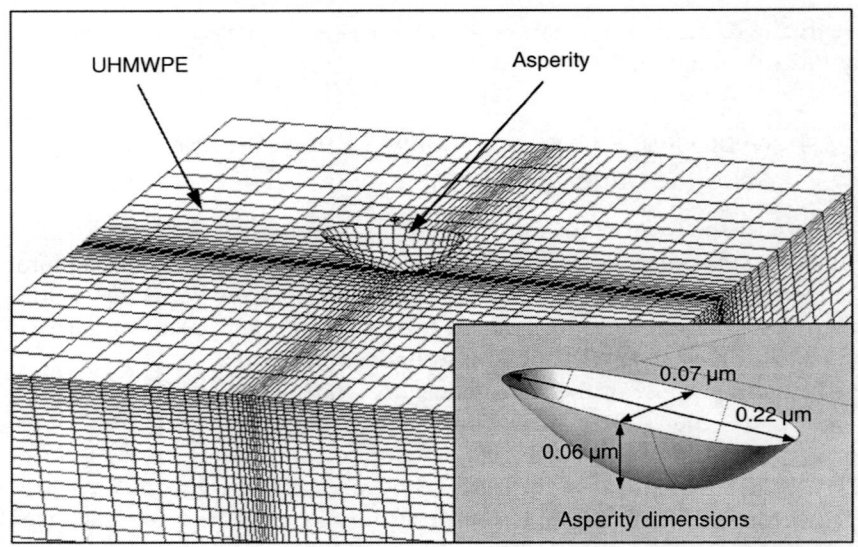

8.12 Three-dimensional FEM for one of the contact analyses (asperity height, 0.06 μm; length of major axis, 0.22 μm; length of minor axis, 0.07 μm; aspect ratio in major axis direction, 0.55; shape ratio, 0.32).

of this microscopic contact analysis, it was found that high contact stresses, exceeding the yield stress of UHMWPE, and considerable plastic strains occurred in the surface region of the tibial insert for even very small indentation depths as shown in Fig. 8.13. The generation regions of contact stress and plastic strain spread markedly with increasing indentation depth of the asperity. The maximum values of contact stress and plastic strain occurred just below the surface of the tibial insert, when the indentation depth was very small, after initial contact with the asperity. The locations of occurrence of these maximum values had a tendency to approach the surface of the tibial insert as the indentation depth increased and, finally, maximum contact stress and maximum plastic strain occurred on the surface of the tibial insert. This phenomenon is thought to be the cause of the generation of the microscopic surface scratches and cracks observed in the retrieved UHMWPE tibial insert in a previous retrieval study (Cho *et al.*, 2001, 2009). These surface scratches and cracks can propagate into the tibial insert and then pitting – a kind of fatigue wear – will eventually result. In general, pitting, which is the generation of small holes on the surface, is a typical failure type that occurs on the surface where rolling contact with sliding is repeated. In the case when there is surface failure of polyethylene in artificial joints, the generation of small holes caused by cracks that emanate at the surface and then propagate into polyethylene is called 'pitting'.

The influences of aspect ratio, shape ratio and indentation depth of the

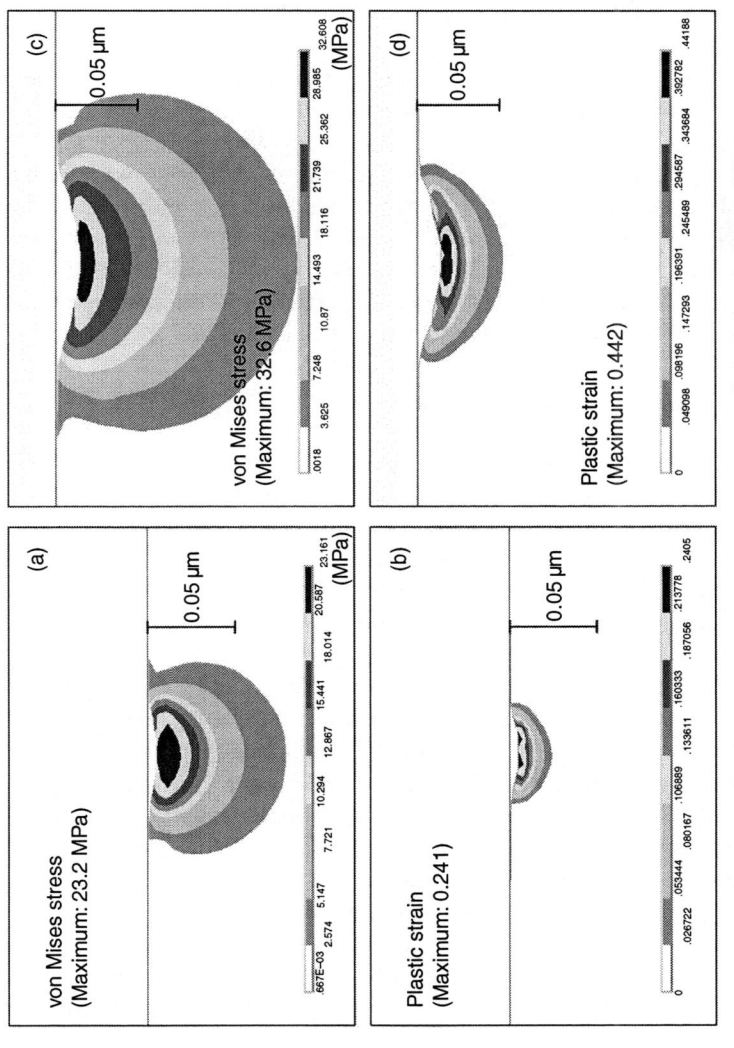

8.13 Contour plots of the von Mises stress and plastic strain in UHMWPE for different indentation depths (asperity height 0.06 μm; length of major axis, 0.22 μm; length of minor axis, 0.07 μm; aspect ratio in major axis direction, 0.55; shape ratio, 0.32) (Cho et al., 2008, 2010).

microscopic surface asperity were investigated. It was found that the maximum values of the contact stress and the plastic strain in the tibial insert, caused by contact with the surface asperity, increased non-linearly and markedly as the aspect ratio and indentation depth of the asperity increased, and had a tendency to increase with increasing the shape ratio of the asperity.

The results of this microscopic contact analysis suggest that the aspect ratio and the shape ratio, which represent the 3D shape of a microscopic surface asperity in a damaged metallic femoral component, together with its indentation depth, can significantly increase and/or accelerate wear of an UHMWPE tibial insert. Higher aspect ratios, shape ratios and indentation depths of microscopic surface asperities cause higher contact stresses and plastic strains in the surface region of a tibial insert. These are therefore significant factors influencing the microscopic failure and microscopic wear mechanism of UHMWPE tibial inserts in artificial knee joints.

8.3 Concluding remarks

UHMWPE possesses excellent material properties, making it particularly attractive for use in weight-bearing surfaces in total joint arthroplasty. However, wear of UHMWPE in the human body causes serious clinical and biomechanical reactions, restricting the longevity of artificial joints. A large number of studies (Kurtz, 2009b; Lewis, 1997; McGloughlin and Kavanagh, 2000) have been conducted to investigate the *in vivo* wear characteristics of UHMWPE and to improve the longevity of artificial joints.

Polyethylene components of artificial joints undergo unique and complex wear mechanisms in the human body, since the wear of prosthetic joint components is inevitably affected by both the characteristic multi-axial joint kinematics and the complicated chemical composition of the physiological environment. However, in the experimental and analytical studies reported in this chapter, discussions have been limited to the influences of simplified kinematic and environmental conditions on the wear of UHMWPE. It is well known that the multi-directional sliding motion associated with joint kinematics and protein and phospholipid concentrations relating to the joint environment play predominant roles in the UHMWPE wear mechanism (Sawae, 2009). Therefore, in order to evaluate the *in vivo* wear characteristics of UHMWPE exactly, it is necessary to consider the physiological factors relating to joint kinematics and the *in vivo* environment.

8.4 Acknowledgments

The authors gratefully acknowledge the receipt of retrieved knee prostheses from the Department of Orthopaedic Surgery, Graduate School of Medical

Sciences, Kyushu University, Japan. Figure 8.1 is reproduced from the book *Thin Films in Tribology* (edited by D. Dowson *et al.*, Elsevier, 1993, pp. 673–682 by Murakami *et al.*). Figure 8.2 is reproduced from *Nature Materials* (Vol. 3, 2004, pp. 829–836 by Moro *et al.*). Figures 8.3–8.11 and Figures 8.13 are reproduced from the *Japanese Journal of Clinical Biomechanics* (Vol. 22, 2001, pp. 169–173; Vol. 23, 2002, pp. 373–379; Vol. 26, 2005, pp. 319–325; Vol. 27, 2006, pp. 253–260; Vol. 28, 2007, pp. 247–254; Vol. 29, 2008, pp. 373–380; by Cho *et al.*); permission was granted by the Council of the Japanese Society for Clinical Biomechanics. For Figures 8.7 and 8.9, from *Proceedings of the Third Asia International Conference on Tribology* (Vol. 2, 2006, pp. 441–442 by Cho *et al.*); permission was granted by the Council of the Japanese Society of Tribologists. Figures 8.3(b), 8.4(b), 8.6 and 8.13 were adapted from the *Proceedings of the Institution of Mechanical Engineers, Part H: Journal of Engineering in Medicine* (Vol. 218, 2004, pp. 251–259; Vol. 224, 2010, pp. 515–529; by Cho *et al.*). Figures 8.3(a), 8.4 (a), 8.5(b), 8.5(c) and 7.6 were adapted from *Biomechanical Systems Technology: Muscular Skeletal Systems* (Ch. 8, 2009, pp. 245–277 by Cho *et al.*).

8.5 References

Charnley J (1979) *Low Friction Arthroplasty of the Hip*. Berlin, Springer.
Cho C H, Murakami T, Sawae Y, Miura H, Kawano T, Nagamine R, Urabe K, Matsuda S and Iwamoto Y (2001) Evaluation of wear in retrieved knee prostheses. *Japan J Clin Biomech*, 22, 169–73 (in Japanese).
Cho C H, Murakami T, Sawae Y, Sakai N, Miura H, Kawano T and Iwamoto Y (2002) Elasto-plastic contact analysis on fatigue wear behavior of UHMWPE tibial components. *Japan J Clin Biomech*, 23, 373–9 (in Japanese).
Cho C H, Murakami T, Sawae Y, Sakai N, Miura H, Kawano T and Iwamoto Y (2004) Elasto-plastic contact analysis of an ultra-high molecular weight polyethylene tibial component based on geometrical measurement from a retrieved knee prosthesis. *Proc Inst Mech Eng Part H: J Eng Med*, 218, 251–9.
Cho C H, Murakami T, Sawae Y, Miura H and Iwamoto Y (2005) An experimental study on the cold flow of UHMWPE tibial insert. *Japan J Clin Biomech*, 26, 319–25 (in Japanese).
Cho C H, Murakami T and Sawae Y (2006a) Experimental study on delamination mechanism of ultra-high molecular weight polyethylene in knee prostheses. *Proc. Third Asia Int Conf Tribology*, 2, 441–2.
Cho C H, Murakami T and Sawae Y (2006b) An experimental study on the delamination mechanism of UHMWPE for artificial joints. *Japan J. Clin Biomech*, 27, 253–60 (in Japanese).
Cho C H, Murakami T and Sawae Y (2007) Influence of microscopic surface asperity of metallic femoral component on the wear of ultra-high molecular weight polyethylene tibial insert. *Japan J Clin Biomech*, 28, 247–54 (in Japanese).
Cho C H, Murakami T and Sawae Y (2008) Contact analysis between microscopic

surface asperity of femoral component and ultra-high molecular weight polyethylene in total knee arthroplasty. *Japan J Clin Biomech*, 29, 373–80 (in Japanese).

Cho C H, Murakami T, Sawae Y, Sakai N, Miura H and Iwamoto Y (2009) Wear phenomena in knee prostheses and their finite element analyses. In *Biomechanical Systems Technology: Muscular Skeletal Systems*, ed Leondes C T. Singapore, World Scientific, pp. 245–77.

Cho C H, Murakami T and Sawae Y (2010) Influence of microscopic surface asperities on the wear of ultra-high molecular weight polyethylene in a knee prosthesis. *Proc Inst Mech Eng Part H: J. Eng Med.* 224, 515–29.

Currier J H, Duda J L, Sperling D K, Collier J P, Currier B H and Kennedy F E (1998) *In vitro* simulation of contact fatigue damage found in ultra-high molecular weight polyethylene components of knee prostheses. *Proc Inst Mech Eng Part H: J Eng Med*, 212, 293–302.

Engh G A, Dwyer K A and Hanes C K (1992) Polyethylene wear of metal-backed tibial component in total and unicompartmental knee prostheses. *J Bone and Joint Surg Br*, 74B, 9–17.

Ingham E and Fisher J (2005) The role of macrophages in osteolysis of total joint replacement. *Biomaterials*, 26, 1271–86.

Issac G H, Thompson J, Williams S and Fisher J (2006) Metal-on-metal bearings surfaces: materials, manufacture, design, optimization, and alternatives. *Proc Inst Mech Eng Part H: J Eng Med*, 220, 119–33.

Kurtz S M (2009a) The clinical performance of UHMWPE in knee replacements. In *UHMWPE Biomaterials Handbook, Second Edition: Ultra-High Molecular Weight Polyethylene in Total Joint Replacement and Medical Devices*, ed Kurtz S M. New York, Academic, pp. 97–116.

Kurtz S M (ed) (2009b) *UHMWPE Biomaterials Handbook, Second Edition: Ultra-High Molecular Weight Polyethylene in Total Joint Replacement and Medical Devices*. New York, Academic.

Landy M M and Walker P S (1988) Wear of ultra-high-molecular-weight polyethylene components of 90 retrieved knee prostheses. *J Arthroplasty*, 5, S73–S85.

Lewis G (1997) Polyethylene wear in total hip and knee arthroplasties. *J Biomed Mater Res (Appl Biomater)*, 38, 55–75.

McGloughlin T M and Kavanagh A G (2000) Wear of ultra-high molecular weight polyethylene (UHMWPE) in total knee prostheses: a review of key influences. *Proc Inst Mech Eng Part H: J Eng Med*, 214, 349–59.

Moro T, Takatori Y, Ishihara K, Konno T, Takigawa Y, Matsushita T, Chung U, Nakamura K and Kawaguchi H (2004) Surface grafting of artificial joints with a biocompatible polymer for preventing periprosthetic osteolysis. *Nat Mater*, 3, 829–36.

Murakami T, Ohtsuki N and Higaki H (1993) The adaptive multimode lubrication in knee prostheses with compliant layer during walking motion. In *Thin Films in Tribology*, ed Dowson D et al. New York, Elsevier, pp. 673–82.

Oonishi H, Tsuji E and Kim Y Y (1998a) Retrieved total hip prostheses. Part I: The effects of cup thickness, head sizes and fusion defects on wear. *J Mater Sci: Mater Med*, 9, 393–401.

Oonishi H, Tsuji E and Kim Y Y (1998b) Retrieved total hip prostheses. Part II: Wear behaviour and structural changes. *J Mater Sci: Mater Med*, 9, 575–81.

Oonishi H, Clarke I, Yamamoto K, Masaoka T, Fujisawa A and Masuda S (2004) Assessment of wear in extensively irradiated UHMWPE cups in simulator studies. *J Biomed Mater Res*, 68A, 52–60.

Oral E and Muratoglu O K (2009) Highly crosslinked UHMWPE doped with vitamin E. In *UHMWPE Biomaterials Handbook, Second Edition: Ultra-High Molecular Weight Polyethylene in Total Joint Replacement and Medical Devices*, ed Kurtz S M. New York, Academic, pp. 221–36.

Reeves E A, Barton D C, FitzPatrick D P and Fisher J (1998) A two-dimensional model of cyclic strain accumulation in ultra-high molecular weight polyethylene knee replacements. *Proc Inst Mech Eng Part H: J Eng Med*, 212, 189–98.

Sawae Y (2009) Effects of physiological factors on wear of UHMWPE for joint prosthesis. In *Polymer Tribology*, ed Sinha S K and Briscoe B J. London, Imperial College Press, pp. 195–226.

Sawano T, Murakami T and Sawae Y (2005) Evaluation of wear resistance of ultra-high molecular weight polyethylene for joint prostheses in the multi-directional pin-on-plate tester. In *Life Cycle Tribology*, ed Dowson D et al. New York, Elsevier, pp. 161–9.

Scholes S C, Unsworth A, Hall R M and Scott R (2000) The effects of material combination and lubricant on the friction of total hip prostheses. *Wear*, 241, 209–13.

Semlitsch M and Willert H G (1997) Clinical wear behaviour of ultra-high molecular weight polyethylene cups paired with metal and ceramic ball heads in comparison to metal-on-metal pairings of hip joint replacements. *Proc Inst Mech Eng Part H: J Eng Med*, 211, 73–88.

Teramura S, Russell S, Ingham E, Fisher J, Tomita N, Fujiwara K and Tipper J K (2009) Reduced biological response to wear particles from UHMWPE containing Vitamin E. *Proc. Annual Meeting ORS*, Poster 2377.

Tomita N, Kitakura T, Onmori N, Ikada Y and Aoyama E (1999) Prevention of fatigue cracks in ultrahigh molecular weight polyethylene joint components by the addition of vitamin E. *J Biomed Mater Res (Appl Biomater)*, 48, 474–78.

Walker P S, Blunn G W and Lilley P A (1996) Wear testing of materials and surfaces for total knee replacement. *J Biomed Mater Res (Appl Biomater)*, 33, 159–75.

Willert H J and Semlitsch M (1977) Reaction of the articular capsule to wear products of artificial joint prostheses. *J Biomed Mater Res*, 11, 157–64.

Williams P A, Yamamoto K, Masaoka T, Oonishi H and Clarke I (2007) highly crosslinked polyethylenes in hip replacements: Improved wear performance or paradox? *Tribology Trans*, 50, 277–90.

9
Wear phenomena of metal joints

N. DIOMIDIS, Ecole Polytechnique Fédérale de Lausanne, Switzerland

Abstract: The *in vivo* degradation of metal alloy implants is undesirable mainly for two reasons: it may decrease the structural integrity of the implant, and the release of degradation products, such as ions and particles, may elicit an adverse biological reaction in the host. Material loss from metallic implants results from electrochemical dissolution phenomena, wear or a synergistic combination of the two. Dissolution and wear are results of the chemical and mechanical reactivity of the metallic surface. Thus, the surface properties of metals and the interactions at the interface with the environment are the main criteria for the biocompatibility of metallic materials.

Key words: corrosion, wear, surface reactions, biotribocorrosion, fretting.

9.1 Alloys for orthopaedic implants

Metals and alloys are widely used as biomedical materials and are indispensable in the medical field due to their high strength, resistance to fracture, elasticity, formability and electrical conductivity. Metallic materials are essential for orthopaedic implants, bone fixators, artificial joints, etc., since they can substitute for the function of hard tissues in orthopaedics. Stents and stent grafts are placed at stenotic blood vessels for dilation. In dentistry, metals are used for restorations, orthodontic wires and dental implants (Hanawa, 2002). Important properties of an orthopaedic implant include long fatigue life, adequate strength, elastic modulus equivalent to that of bone and high biocompatibility. For artificial joints, which have to withstand forces more than four times the body weight and millions of cycles during their lifetime, wear and corrosion resistance are particularly essential properties.

Table 9.1 Chemical composition of common implant alloys

Alloy	ISO	Composition (wt %)
316L	5832-1	17–19 Cr, 13–15 Ni, 2.25–3.5 Mo, 0.03 C, 2.0 Mn, 0.50 Cu, 0.75 Si, bal. Fe
Co-28Cr-6Mo	5832-12	26–30.0 Cr, 5–7 Mo, 1.0 Ni, 1.0 Mn, 0.75 Fe, 0.05–0.25 C, bal. Co
Ti-6Al-4V	5832-3	5.5–6.75 Al, 3.4–4.5 V, 0.30 Fe, 0.20 O, bal. Ti
Ti-6Al-7Nb	5832-11	5.5–6.5 Al, 6.5–7.5 Nb, 0.25 Fe, 0.20 O, 0.50 Ta, bal. Ti

Source: Pilliar (2009).

9.1.1 Chemical composition

Three main families of metallic alloys are commonly used for arthroplasty: stainless steel, cobalt–chromium–molybdenum (CoCrMo) alloys and titanium (Ti)-based alloys. The chemical composition of various alloys used for the manufacture of implants is shown in Table 9.1.

Stainless steel has been widely used for the manufacture of fracture repair devices. It has also been used for making some joint replacement components such as femoral heads and cemented stems (Semlitsch and Willert, 1995), although its use in such applications is becoming less common. 316L stainless steel has an austenitic microstructure and low carbon content. This is done to avoid chromium depletion by the precipitation of chromium carbides at the grain boundaries and the risk of integranular corrosion.

CoCrMo alloys exist in low- and high-carbon variants. The considerable wear resistance of the high-C alloy is a result of the formation primarily of chromium carbides throughout the structure during solidification (Pilliar, 2009). CoCrMo alloys are commonly used for the manufacture of the femoral stem and ball and the acetabular cup in total hip replacements, as well as the femoral component in total knee replacements. CoCrMo implants can be coarse blasted or coated by a porous layer made from CoCrMo beads or hydroxyapatite, which acts as a bone interfacing surface, promoting bone ingrowth to achieve a secure implant-to-bone fixation without the use of acrylic bone cement.

Ti-6Al-4V has an $\alpha + \beta$ microstructure and is the most commonly used Ti alloy for load-bearing applications. Reports on the toxicity of vanadium (V) (Steinemann, 1980, 1985) led to the development of the $\alpha + \beta$ Ti-6Al-7Nb and Ti-5Al-2.5Fe alloys, which have grown in popularity in recent years. Ti-based alloys have low density, high fatigue resistance and elasticity, and excellent *in vivo* corrosion resistance. Their major drawback is poor wear resistance, which makes them unsuitable for articulating surfaces without surface modification. Increased wear resistance can be achieved by the formation of a very hard TiN coating on the surface (Rabbe *et al.*, 1994). Ti alloys are commonly used for the femoral stem and the liner of ultra-high molecular weight polyethylene (UHMWPE) acetabular caps for hip implants. The majority of cementless fixation stems are made from Ti-based alloys due to their osseointegration properties (Semlitsch and Willert, 1995). For such applications, a porous bioactive surface is created on the stem by grit blasting/shot peening combined with anodizing, sintering of particles, plasma spraying of powder, or compaction and vacuum sintering of titanium fibers (Wolner et al., 2006).

9.1.2 Mechanical properties

The mechanical properties of biomedical alloys and other materials they may interface with during arthroplasty are shown in Table 9.2. The considerable difference in elasticity between the alloys commonly used in manufacturing bone interfacing implants and the surrounding bone is noteworthy. This mechanical mismatch can lead to structural changes in bone tissue situated next to a metallic implant when the implant is securely fastened to the bone and is oriented with the length of the implant juxtaposing a significant length of bone (Pilliar, 2009). An example is a femoral stem inside a host femur. The metallic implant acts as a reinforcement bearing the major stresses, thereby stress shielding the host bone. Disuse atrophy and bone loss can result over time. In addition, considerably high stresses can develop in the bone at regions were force is transferred from the implant to the bone, like at the lower tip of the femoral stem.

Table 9.2 Mechanical properties of materials relevant to joint replacement

	Elastic modulus (GPa)	Yield strength (MPa)	Ultimate tensile strength (MPa)
316 L stainless steel	205	160–690	490–1350
CoCrMo	200–230	450–1175	655–1510
Ti-6Al-4V	110	860	930
Ti-6Al-7Nb	105	795	860
Ti-5Al-2.5Fe	110	820	900
Ti-12Mo-6Zr-2Fe (TMZF)	74–85	1000–1060	1060–1100
Ti-13Nb-13Zr	79–84	863–908	973–1037
Ti-35.5Nb-7.3Zr-5.7Ta (TNZT)	55–66	793	827
UHMWPE	0.5	15–20	
PMMA	0.3		
Alumina	350	300	
Zirconia	200		
Bone	10–30	120–150	
Articular cartilage	0.001–0.17		

Note: adapted from Pilliar (2009) and Long and Rack (1998).

As an attempt to reduce the elastic modulus of orthopaedic alloys, titanium alloys with β microstructure were developed. As shown in Table 9.2, TMZF and TiNbZr exhibit an elastic modulus of around 80 GPa (Diomidis et al., 2011a); TNZT alloys for orthopaedic applications have demonstrated an even lower elastic modulus, but one that is still higher than that of bone. The added benefit of using β stabilizing agents like niobium (Nb) and tantalum (Ta) is that they are incorporated and strengthen the spontaneously formed passive surface layer instead of being released into the environment like aluminum (Al) and vanadium (V). As a result, Ti, Nb, Zr (zirconium) and Ta have been classified among the most biocompatible metals (Steinemann, 1980).

9.2 Electrochemical aspects of corrosion

As soon as a metallic material is implanted in a biological environment, it starts to interact with the chemical species present, giving rise to phenomena such as general or localized corrosion. Corrosion is an irreversible interfacial reaction of a material with its environment, resulting in the loss of material or in the dissolution of some of the constituents of the environment into the material. In principle, such interactions disturb the natural equilibrium of the host organism by increasing the quantities of naturally occurring metals or introducing other metals that have no part in the biological cycle, which can lead to adverse biological reactions. As a result, the biocompatibility of metallic materials greatly depends on their corrosion resistance (Pilliar, 2009).

Corrosion results from the system consisting of an implant and its environment; as a result it is influenced by a wide variety of factors. Such factors include the metallic material itself (chemical composition, microstructure, surface condition), the chemical composition of the environment (pH, O_2 content, aggressive ions, adsorbing species), the prevailing physical parameters in the vicinity of the implant (temperature, flow conditions, electrical conductivity, stresses), and the design and construction of the implant (geometry, surrounding materials, presence of crevices). Changes in any of these variables can have an influence on the mode and rate of metal ion release.

9.2.1 Oxidation of metals

The corrosion of metals is due to an irreversible oxidation–reduction reaction between the metal and an oxidizing agent in the environment (Landolt, 2007). It involves an exchange of electrons between species and can be written in the form of partial reactions as follows.

Oxidation of an active metal with the release of ions:

$$M \rightarrow M^{n+} + ne^- \qquad [9.1]$$

Oxidation of a passive metal with the formation of oxide:

$$M + nH_2O \rightarrow MO_n + 2nH^+ + 2ne^- \qquad [9.2]$$

Reduction of an oxidizing agent (proton, dissolved oxygen or water) with the consumption of electrons:

$$2H^+ + 2e^- \rightarrow H_2 \qquad [9.3]$$

$$O_2 + 2H_2O + 4e^- \rightarrow 4OH^- \qquad [9.4]$$

$$H_2O + 2e^- \rightarrow 2OH^- + 2H^+ \qquad [9.5]$$

Whether a metal will corrode or not depends on thermodynamic driving forces. If the oxidation reaction of the metal releases energy, it will occur spontaneously. However, due to the exchange of charged species, separation of positive and negative charges takes place. Positive metal ions are released into solution, while negatively charged electrons remain in the metal and take part in the reduction of the oxidizing agent or other reactions. This gives rise to the formation of an electrical double layer across the metal–solution interface and creates an electrical potential difference between the metal and the solution. This potential is an indication of the reactivity of the metallic surface. Some noble metals, such as gold (Au) and platinum (Pt), have little or no tendency to oxidize in an aqueous environment and can therefore remain in metallic form indefinitely in the human body. The metals that are commonly used in orthopaedics, such as Ti, Co or Cr are thermodynamically more stable in their oxidized form.

The rate at which a metal will corrode involves kinetic barriers that physically limit the rate of the oxidation or reduction processes. In general, kinetic barriers to corrosion prevent migration of electrons and metal ions across the metal–solution interface. An example is the formation of a compact oxide film on a metallic surface, which shields the metal from the environment, leading to passivation and a decrease of the corrosion rate by several orders of magnitude. All the alloys used in orthopaedic applications owe their high corrosion resistance to such passive films. The rate of corrosion is associated with a flow of electrons, i.e. an electric current, which can be used as a measure of the reaction rate.

The evolution of the rate of surface reactions (current) with respect to the driving force for oxidation (potential) illustrates the different phenomena that can take place on the surface of a metal (Fig. 9.1). At potentials below

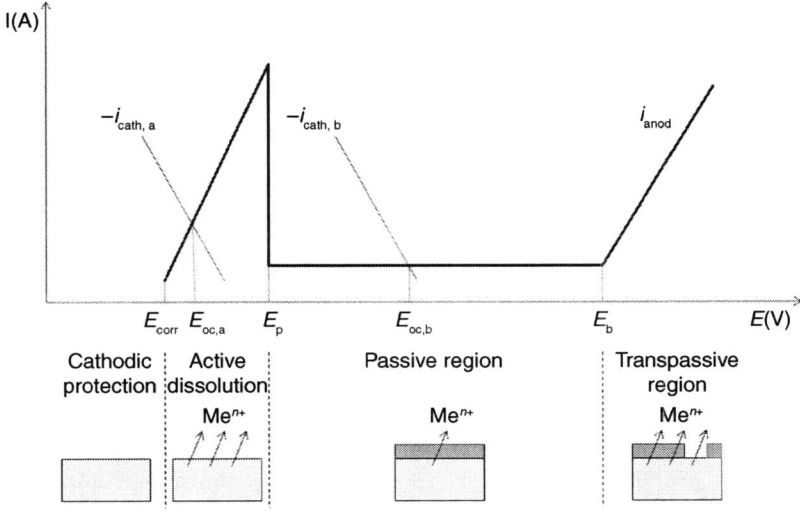

9.1 Schematic representation of a polarization curve of a passivating metal indicating the effect of the cathodic partial reaction on the equilibrium potential: E_{corr}, corrosion potential; E_p, passivation potential; E_b, breakdown potential; E_{oc}, open circuit potential.

the corrosion potential (E_{corr}), the metallic form is thermodynamically more stable and oxidation is suppressed. At potentials above E_{corr}, active dissolution of the metal occurs. The decrease of the current indicates that at the passivation potential (E_{pass}) an active to passive transition occurs where a protective passive film is formed and oxidation is blocked. At even higher potentials, a breakdown of the passive film and/or oxidation of water occur (E_b). When equilibrium is reached, the oxidation and reduction reactions occurring at the surface proceed at the same rate. Therefore, at steady state the electrical currents originating from each reaction have the same magnitude. The potential at which the steady state is reached depends as much on the reactivity of the metal as on the environment. A solution with low oxidizing tendency may shift the equilibrium potential (open circuit potential) at values coinciding with the area of active dissolution of the metal ($E_{oc,a}$). A solution with a higher oxidizing tendency can shift the equilibrium potential in the passive area of the metal ($E_{oc,b}$).

9.2.2 The corrosive environment of the human body

When a metallic prosthesis is implanted it comes into contact with body fluids, which can include blood, synovial and interstitial fluids. The typical composition of blood plasma is shown in Table 9.3. Critical to the

Table 9.3 Composition of human blood serum

Cations	mmol/l	Anions	mmol/l
Na^+	142	Cl^-	101
K^+	4	HCO_3^-	27
Ca^{2+}	5	HPO_4^{2-}	2
Mg^{2+}	2	SO_4^{2-}	1
Total	153	Total	131
		Organic acids	6
		Proteins	16

Source: Milošev (2011).

corrosivity of the body is the high concentration of chloride ions due to their ability to induce the breakdown of passive films. Other ions can also influence corrosion, either as accelerators or inhibitors. Body fluids contain amino acids, proteins and sugars which can absorb on the surface and affect interfacial reactions. Changes in the pH of body fluids are generally small because they are buffered solutions and the pH usually remains between 7.15 and 7.35. However, during the first post-operative weeks or due to inflammation or disease, the pH around the implant can drop to approximately 5.2, inducing a hundredfold increase in the H^+ concentration. The concentration of dissolved oxygen in serum is about one fourth of that in atmospheric air, leading to a slower regeneration of surface oxides. The action of macrophages can produce strong oxidizing agents such as active oxygen species (O_2^-) or peroxide (H_2O_2) in the vicinity of the implant (Hanawa, 2002). The normal body temperature of 37°C can increase the corrosion rate of materials compared with simulated tests done at room temperature.

For *in vitro* testing of materials, it is desirable to replicate the conditions in the human body as closely as possible. As a result, different kinds of simulated physiological solutions are used (Table 9.4). Biophysiological solutions are also used by the addition of various cell products such as

Table 9.4 Composition of physiological solutions used for *in vitro* testing of metallic biomaterials

Solution	Composition (g/l)
0.9% NaCl	9 NaCl
Hank's balanced salt solution	8 NaCl, 0.40 KCl, 0.35 NaHCO$_3$, 0.25 NaH$_2$PO$_4$.2H$_2$O, 0.06 Na$_2$HPO$_4$.2H$_2$O, 0.19 CaCl$_2$.2H$_2$O, 0.41 MgCl$_2$.6H$_2$O, 0.06 MgSO$_4$.7H$_2$O, 1 glucose, pH: 7.4
Ringer's solution	8.60 NaCl, 0.30 KCl, 0.33 CaCl$_2$.2H$_2$O, pH: 7.4

proteins or organic acids. Typical additives for *in vitro* testing of joint replacement materials are bovine serum albumin or hyaluronic acid.

9.3 Passivity and corrosion of implant alloys

9.3.1 Passive layers

The polarization curves of 316L stainless steel, Co-28Cr-6Mo, Ti-6Al-4V and Ti-6Al-7Nb alloys in physiological solution are shown in Fig. 9.2. On the surface of the alloys a passive film is spontaneously formed as evidenced by the absence of an active to passive transition (see Fig. 9.1). Stainless steel and CoCrMo exhibit similar behaviors with comparatively short passive regions, indicating a danger of transpassive dissolution at highly oxidizing environments. Passive films on titanium alloys are stable up to much higher potentials, indicating that passive films with different properties can be formed depending on the composition of the base alloy.

A variety of factors can influence a passive film's protective character; for example, its chemical composition, microstructure, thickness and presence of defects in the crystal lattice such as vacancies or impurities. In the case of

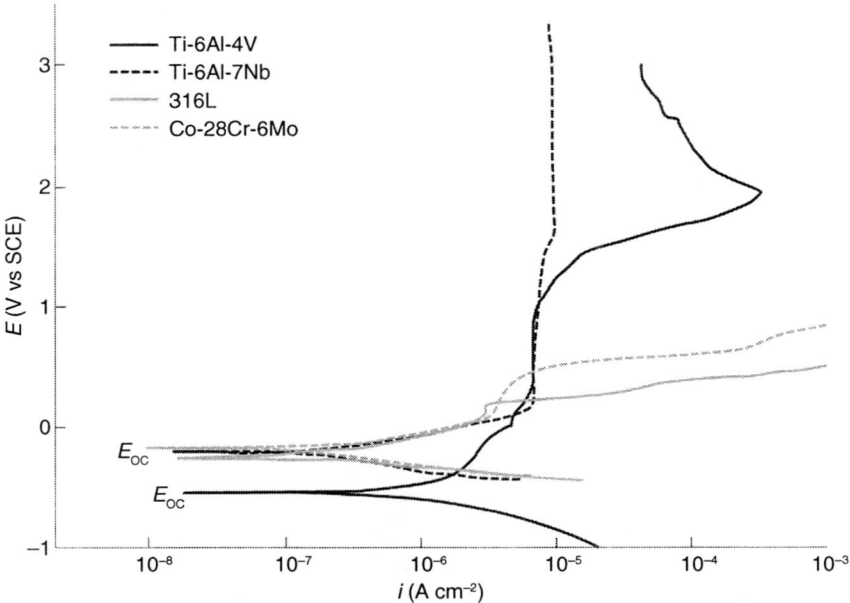

9.2 Potentiodynamic polarization curves for 316L stainless steel, Co-28Cr-6Mo, Ti-6Al-4V and Ti-6Al-7Nb alloys in Hank's solution. Adapted from Milošev (2011).

alloys, the passive layer is usually a mixed oxide of the alloying elements. Typically, the composition of the base alloy is not directly reflected in the composition of the oxide due to selective oxidation of some of the metallic constituents.

The passive film formed on austenitic stainless steel consists mainly of Cr_2O_3 containing smaller amounts of iron, nickel and molybdenum oxides and it has a thickness of 3–4 nm. Iron is enriched in the surface oxide, while Ni, Mo and manganese (Mn) are enriched in the alloy substrate just under the oxide (Hanawa, 2004). Chromium oxide is also the main constituent of the passive layer formed on CoCrMo alloys in Hank's solution with small contributions of CoO and MoO_3 (Milošev and Strehblow, 2003). The concentration of Cr and Mo is higher at the outer part of the layer, while Co is mainly present close to the metal–oxide interface. The thickness of the passive layer can range between 2.5 and 5.0 nm depending on the potential (Hanawa et al., 2001). When titanium is brought into contact with biological solutions, a TiO_2 film is formed. This film contains a small amount of TiO and Ti_2O_3 suboxides close to the metal–oxide interface. Passive films found on Ti alloys have a similar structure to those formed on pure titanium (Hanawa, 2004). Al_2O_3 is detected at the outer parts of the layer close to the oxide–solution interface on aluminum-containing alloys. V_2O_5 plays a smaller role in the formation of the passive layer, in contrast with Nb which is present mainly as Nb_2O_5 particularly at the outer parts of the layer near the oxide–solution interface (Milošev, 2011). Passive layers on Ti-based materials are in the range of 3 to 9 nm depending on potential (Milošev et al., 2000).

Apart from ion transport and dissolution through the film, passive layers in an aqueous environment undergo a continuous process of partial dissolution and reprecipitation on a microscopic scale (Fig. 9.3). Therefore, the composition of a passive layer changes according to its environment. As a result, the evolution of environmental conditions such as the electrolyte composition, concentration of oxidizing agents, exposure time and temperature can affect the nature and stability of passive films. Furthermore, passive layers in contact with aqueous solutions tend to be hydrated, as evidenced by the presence of OH^-, particularly in areas close to the layer–electrolyte interface.

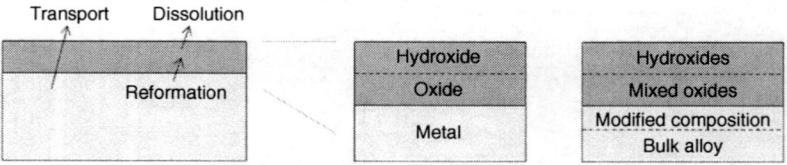

9.3 Schematic illustration of passive layers on metals and alloys.

9.3.2 Interaction with biomolecules

Interaction between passive layers on implanted metals and organic or inorganic constituents of biological fluids can lead to the formation of chemical species that deposit on the surface or form soluble complexes with metallic ions influencing the corrosion process. Calcium phosphate precipitates on passive layers on all orthopaedic alloys when immersed in physiological solutions and *in vivo* (Hanawa, 2004). Hydrated phosphate ions adsorb on the hydrated oxide surface, then calcium ions adsorb on the phosphate ions, eventually forming calcium phosphate.

Proteins are a primary constituent of the synovial fluid, while other organic components such as hyaluronic acid and lubricin are also present. Organic molecules present in body fluids are generally regarded as complexing agents forming soluble complexes with metal ions which can then migrate away from the metallic surface. Proteins can also adsorb on metals and oxides and become incorporated in surface layers. The effect of such molecules on the corrosion of implants appears to be specific for each metal/biomolecule couple. The corrosion of stainless steel and CoCrMo alloys is increased in the presence of proteins (Hanawa, 2004; Virtanen *et al.*, 2008), and the concentration of metal ions in the environment depends on the nature of the added protein (Minovič *et al.*, 2003). On the other hand, proteins are reported to have no effect or even increase the corrosion resistance of Ti-based alloys (Khan *et al.*, 1999; Williams *et al.*, 1988).

9.3.3 Ion release

Representative data of the corrosion rate of metallic implant alloys *in vivo* indicate a material loss of around 0.2 $\mu g\,cm^{-2}$ per day (Steinemann, 1980). For a typical hip joint replacement implant this is equivalent to 10–15 mg per year of metallic ions being released in the body of the host. With the naturally occurring amount of metals such as Co, Cr, Mo, Ni, Ti, Al and V in a 70 kg human ranging between 1 and 60 mg, it is evident that a considerable increase in the concentration of metal ions is expected in the presence of a corroding implant. Indeed, significantly elevated metal concentrations are found in the body fluids of patients with metallic hip implants (Okazaki and Gotoh, 2005).

316L stainless steel releases the largest amount of metal ions compared with the other orthopaedic alloys (Okazaki and Gotoh, 2005). Iron (Fe) ions are preferentially released with smaller contributions from Cr and Ni ions. CoCrMo alloys preferentially release Co with amounts of Cr and Mo of about one order of magnitude smaller. Furthermore, acidification of the environment tends to increase the total ion release from stainless steel and CoCrMo. All aluminum-containing Ti alloys release primarily Ti and Al ions. The cytotoxicity of vanadium, which is released from Ti-6Al-4V, has become an issue of concern. However, the total metal ion release from a TiZrNbTa alloy is considerably smaller, indicating an increased protective character of passive films consisting of valve metal oxides.

9.3.4 Corrosion mechanisms in orthopaedic implants

Apart from uniform corrosion, implanted metallic biomaterials may undergo localized corrosion, which can be triggered by material, environmental, design or stress factors.

Pitting corrosion

Pitting corrosion refers to a localized attack of a passive metal that leads to the development of small cavities. Due to its localized aspect, pitting corrosion damage can be quite important even if the total amount of dissolved material is small. Pitting requires the presence of aggressive ions (most often chloride ions) and an oxidizing agent such as dissolved oxygen. An electrochemical cell is formed between the growing pit and the passive area that surrounds it. The pit acts as an anode, where oxidation takes place, and the passive surface acts as the cathode where reduction of the oxidizing agent takes place. Due to the small anode–cathode surface area ratio, dissolution inside the pit is considerably accelerated. Stainless steel shows a higher susceptibility than CoCrMo- or Ti-based alloys. On the other hand, Ti alloys show a very high resistance to pitting and no pits are usually detected either *in vivo* or *in vitro* (Burstein *et al.*, 2005).

Crevice corrosion

Crevice corrosion is a localized phenomenon taking place inside crevices or other occluded areas where, due to geometric reasons, mass transport and replenishment of the electrolyte is hindered. In such areas, depletion of O_2, acidification of the electrolyte and the action of chlorides, can activate the passive surface and lead to increased dissolution rate. Stainless steel is the most susceptible of the orthopaedic alloys.

Other mechanisms

Other forms of corrosion acting on implant alloys include stress corrosion cracking and corrosion fatigue, which occur when residual, applied or cyclic mechanical stresses are acting on the metal. They involve the nucleation and propagation of cracks and can have a detrimental effect on the mechanical integrity of the implant. Galvanic corrosion takes place when two dissimilar metals are brought into electrical contact in a corrosive environment. The less noble metal will act as an anode and oxidize, while the more noble metal will be the cathode and be protected from corrosion. Due to the passive nature of implant alloys, galvanic corrosion of modular hip implants is avoided as long as the passive film remains intact. Wear-accelerated corrosion takes place when a relative motion between surfaces in contact leads to damage of the protective passive film.

9.4 Surface phenomena in biotribocorrosion

Biotribocorrosion is the surface degradation of metallic materials under relative motion in a biological environment. It is characterized by the interrelation between electrochemical and mechanical processes. Interactions between corrosion and wear are dependent on the kinematics and stresses in the contact area, the mechanical properties of surface films and base alloys, as well as the electrochemical reaction kinetics. Surface phenomena have been identified as critical to the degradation of metallic joint replacement implants (Iwabuchi *et al.*, 2007; Okazaki, 2002).

9.4.1 Tribological contacts in orthopaedic implants

Different materials can be in contact with metals in total hip replacement prostheses, as shown in Fig. 9.4. In a typical hip implant, metals may be in contact with ceramics, polymers, bone or other metals. The femoral stem is usually made of Ti-6Al-4V or CoCrMo and can be in contact with the bone of the femur or polymethylmethacrylate (PMMA) cement depending on the fixation method. In the case of a modular implant, the femoral stem will also be in contact with a ceramic or CoCrMo femoral ball. At the articulation, a CoCrMo ball can be in contact with a CoCrMo or UHMWPE acetabular cup. In the case of total knee replacement implants, a CoCrMo femoral component is in contact with a UHMWPE tibial component and PMMA cement (Semlitsch and Willert, 1995).

Depending on the amplitude of relative motion, different tribological contacts may be formed. At the femoral ball/acetabular cup articulation, large-amplitude relative motion (~40 mm) leads to sliding tribocorrosion phenomena. At rigid contacts, vibrations and small-amplitude motion (<100 µm) lead to fretting. Fretting corrosion occurs to some extent on all load-bearing metallic orthopaedic implants. In total hip and knee replacements fretting occurs at the stem–bone or the stem–cement interface, and at the interfaces of modular junctions between implant components. Fretting also occurs at areas of cyclic load-bearing contacts on screw–plate, bone–plate and screw–bone interfaces.

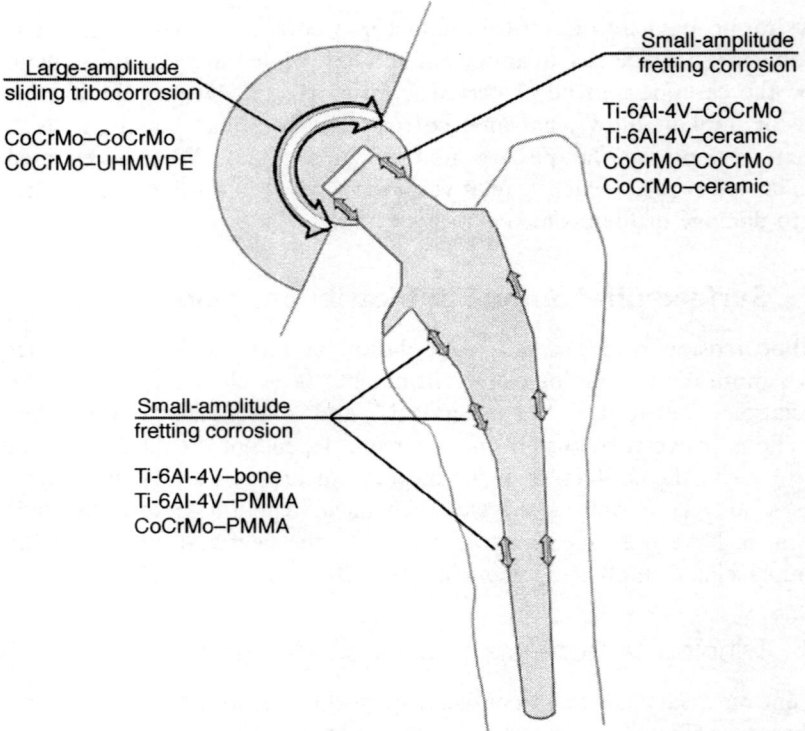

9.4 Interfacing materials and types of tribological contacts involving metals commonly found in a hip joint replacement implant.

9.4.2 Interactions between corrosion and wear

The common characteristic in all of the above-mentioned tribological contacts and material combinations is the important role of surface films spontaneously forming on metallic surfaces. On implant alloys, layers form the interface between the metallic surface and the biological environment, and their properties dictate the results of chemical and mechanical interactions. Once chemical and mechanical interactions are combined, biotribocorrosion results in the cyclic removal and regrowth of surface layers – a phenomenon closely linked to the biocompatibility of metallic implants (Wolner *et al.*, 2006). In this dynamic environment, an interrelation between chemical and mechanical processes arises (Fig. 9.5), which can be either synergistic or antagonistic (Celis *et al.*, 2006; Diomidis *et al.*, 2010).

In a tribological contact, the structure and composition of the native passive layer can be transformed by tribochemical interactions. When it reaches a critical thickness, the layer can spall off by surface fatigue, resulting in wear particles of metal oxides. Consequently, depassivated bare

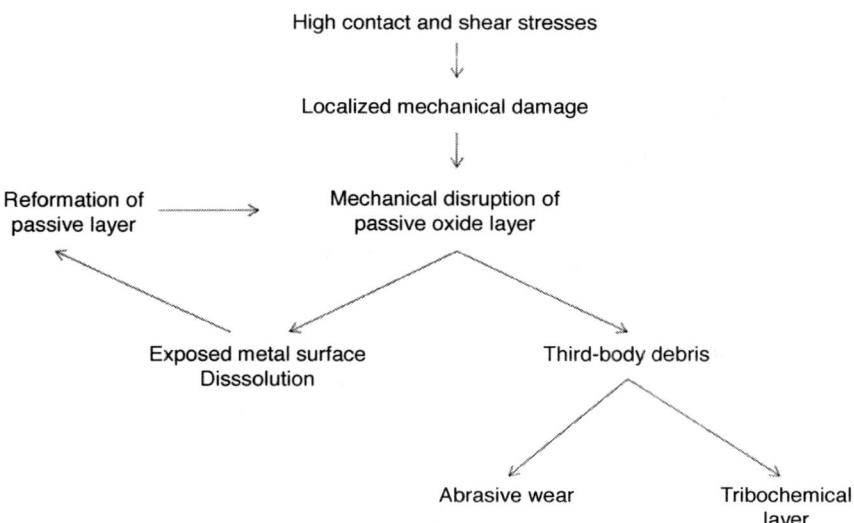

9.5 The sequence of events during biotribocorrosion of metallic implant alloys.

metal is exposed to the interfacial medium. The rate of depassivation depends mainly on the applied contact stress, i.e. more extensive depassivation occurs at elevated loads and increased sliding velocity. Due to the different oxidation tendencies of the exposed metal and the surrounding surface oxide, an electrochemical cell is formed. At that cell, the oxidation and reduction reactions are spatially separated. Oxidation takes place mainly at the metallic surface and the reduction reaction occurs at the surface of the layer. In most cases, the surface area of the layer is considerably larger than the surface area of the exposed metal. As a result, the oxidation reaction of the metal is accelerated. Oxidation of the metal produces dissolved metal ions that can interact with the environment and a fresh surface oxide, leading to repassivation. Biomolecules can react with the dissolved metal ions forming, for example, metal–protein complexes or deposits. Proteins can also adsorb on the metallic surface, become incorporated in the passive layer and affect the repassivation process. The acceleration of metal oxidation by mechanical action in the contact is termed wear accelerated corrosion (Fig. 9.6).

At either exposed areas or areas covered by a surface film, mechanical action can generate metallic wear particles by cyclic contact stresses. Due to the small size of such debris and their large surface area, they tend to react quickly, resulting in particles that have an oxide layer just at the surface or that are completely oxidized. Depending on their properties, particles in the contact can affect the wear of the material in different ways. Oxides tend to

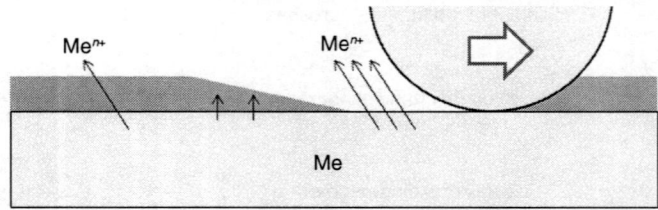

9.6 Schematic representation of wear-accelerated corrosion.

be harder than the parent metal, so oxide particles can induce three-body abrasion and accelerate mechanical wear. In other cases, particles can effectively roll between the surfaces and facilitate displacement or be compacted into wear-resistant surface films that decrease degradation of the surface by mechanical action.

9.4.3 Measuring corrosion–wear interactions

The mechanical integrity and wear performance of joint replacement implants is assessed by hip and knee simulators, aiming to recreate as closely as possible the three-dimensional load, motion patterns and chemical environment found *in vivo* (Affatato *et al.*, 2008). However, in order to study corrosion–wear interactions on metallic surfaces, triboelectrochemical techniques are used (Landolt *et al.*, 2001; Mathew *et al.*, 2009; Mischler, 2008; Ponthiaux *et al.*, 2004). The introduction of electrochemical measurements during sliding or fretting allows monitoring of the removal and regrowth of surface films. This is a critical point in the biocompatibility of metallic materials since surface layers are responsible for the release of the majority of ions and particles. In simulated biological fluids, electrochemical techniques offer the possibility to measure or control *in situ* the surface reactivity of metals (Mischler, 2008). These techniques are increasingly applied in biotribocorrosion studies because they allow an understanding of how wear affects the kinetics of corrosion reactions and the assessment of the influence of these reactions on the mechanical behavior of the contact (Diomidis *et al.*, 2011b).

Electrochemical testing can reveal the breakdown of layers by monitoring the potential between the metal and the solution (Fig. 9.7). Once the surface layers are removed by mechanical action, the reactivity of the exposed base metal is reflected in the shift of the potential to less noble values. The self-healing ability of passive surface films is evidenced by the increase of the potential once the mechanical perturbation ceases, indicative of restoration of the surface film. On the other hand, if a potential is externally imposed, the disruption of the surface layer and the accelerated oxidation of the exposed metal induce an increase in the oxidation current, which is linked to

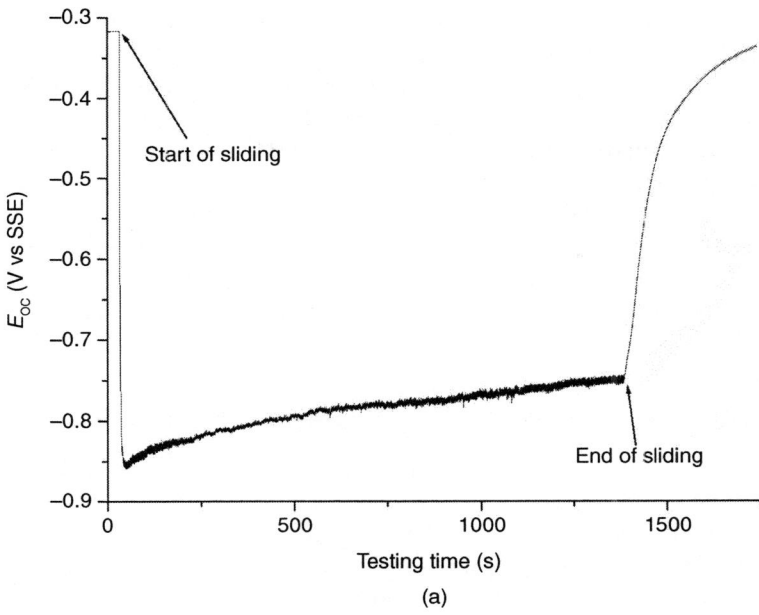

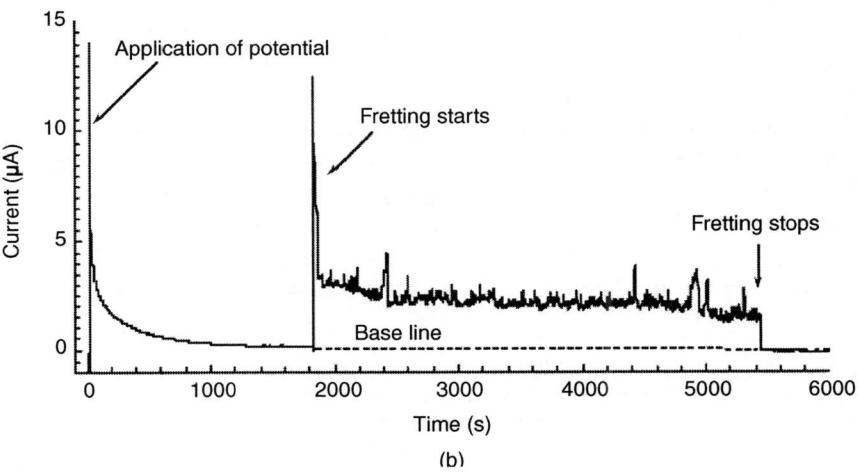

9.7 Measuring the removal and regrowth of surface layers.
(a) Evolution of the open circuit potential with time during sliding of 316L stainless steel (Diomidis *et al.*, 2010). (b) Evolution of the current during fretting of Ti-6Al-4V at a potential in the passive region (Barril *et al.*, 2004).

the amount of metal lost by corrosion. Other electrochemical techniques, such as electrochemical impedance spectroscopy, can quantify the electrochemical reactivity of surfaces and shed light on the charge transfer mechanism at the interface (Diomidis *et al.*, 2010). By combining such techniques with tribological testing in a physiological solution, determination of the material loss due to mechanical or corrosion-related processes can be achieved. An ASTM standard guide to determine the synergism between wear and corrosion exists (ASTM, 2001). Recently, a new experimental methodology has been proposed that is specifically aimed at studying the effect of surface layers on passive metals allowing quantification of their effect on corrosion–wear interactions (Diomidis *et al.*, 2010).

9.5 Tribocorrosion at the articulating interface

At the articulating surface, the large range of motion and the presence of pseudosynovial fluid lead to a lubricated sliding contact (Mattei *et al.*, 2011). Depending on the material couple, the roughness, and the design of the implant different lubrication regimes can arise. In the case of CoCrMo/UHMWPE implants, boundary lubrication prevails. In this regime, considerable asperity contacts exist, and as a result adsorbed surface layers on the contacting surfaces can significantly affect the friction and wear response (Gispert *et al.*, 2006). In the case of CoCrMo/CoCrMo implants, a mixed lubrication regime prevails. Under mixed lubrication, a partial separation of the surfaces takes place, a smaller number of asperity contacts exist which take up part of the applied load, with the rest taken up by the fluid. Typical surface, friction, and wear parameters of metal-on-metal and metal-on-polyethylene implants are shown in Table 9.5.

The importance of corrosion–wear interactions in the sliding articulation of CoCrMo hip implants has been widely acknowledged in *in vitro* (Igual

Table 9.5 Typical surface, friction and wear parameters of the articulation of implants involving a metallic component

	Metal-on-metal	Metal-on-polyethylene
Femoral head	CoCrMo	CoCrMo
R_a (μm)	0.005–0.025	0.005–0.025
Wear rate (μm/year)	5	1.5
Acetabular cup	CoCrMo	UHMWPE
R_a (μm)	0.01–0.025	0.1–2.5
Wear rate (μm/year)	5	1950
Lubrication regime	Mixed	Boundary
Coefficient of friction in bovine synovial fluid	0.25	0.05–0.10

Note: adapted from Long and Rack (1998) and Crockett *et al.* (2008).

Muñoz and Mischler, 2001; Sinnett-Jones *et al.*, 2005; Wimmer *et al.*, 2001; Yan *et al.*, 2006a, 2006b) and retrieval studies (Wimmer *et al.*, 2010). Debris and high contact stresses can damage and remove the protective surface layers at the majority of the contact area (Morita *et al.*, 1998; Yan *et al.*, 2009). As a result, an increase of oxidation rate of up to 20–60 times can occur due to wear-accelerated corrosion, and up to 30–40% of the total material loss can be attributed to corrosion-related processes (Yan *et al.*, 2007). Consequently, layer properties such as high mechanical resistance and high regrowth rate are important. High-carbon CoCrMo alloys (0.20–0.25%) are commonly reported to be more wear resistant than low-carbon alloys (0.10%) (Rieker *et al.*, 2004) and also exhibit limited wear-accelerated corrosion (Yan *et al.*, 2006b). However, the chemical composition of the environment can considerably affect the wear ranking of CoCrMo alloys, a critical point for pre-clinical evaluation of artificial joints through tests carried out in simulated body fluids that hardly reflect the *in vivo* chemistry of synovial fluids (Igual Muñoz and Mischler, 2001).

9.5.1 Metal-on-polyethylene implants

In metal-on-polyethylene (MoP) hip and knee implants, the vast majority of wear arises from the polyethylene. Although considerably smaller than polyethylene wear (Bufort and Goswami, 2004), wear of the metallic component of MoP implants also takes place (Jasty *et al.*, 1994; Poggie *et al.*, 1992; Wilches *et al.*, 2008). The wear of CoCrMo when sliding against UHMWPE proceeds mainly through three-body abrasion. Detached Mo-rich particles from the surface during sliding have been identified as an important cause of CoCrMo abrasion (Gispert *et al.*, 2006). Furthermore, particles of PMMA cement, bone, UHMWPE and metallic oxides and carbides arising from the surgery or from wear can be present in the articulating interface and in surrounding tissues. Even though considerable wear is mainly expected from particles that are harder than the alloy, bone and PMMA particles have been shown to cause abrasion of CoCrMo by ploughing (Que and Topoleski, 2000). Contact stresses and abrasion damage the passive film that protects the metal from corrosion, releasing oxide particles in the contact and inducing wear-accelerated corrosion (Okazaki, 2002). The surface roughness of the metallic component, which increases by abrasion, is critical to the wear rate of the polyethylene (Smith *et al.*, 1999). UHMWPE adheres to and tends to form transfer layers on CoCrMo counterfaces in water by interlamellar shear of the polymer (Galetz *et al.*, 2010). However, the formation of the transfer film depends on the tribological conditions, the presence of proteins (Crockett *et al.*, 2008) and the electrochemical conditions. Such transfer films have been shown to affect the friction coefficient and wear of the polymer, but their influence on the surface degradation mechanism of the metal is still unclear.

9.5.2 Metal-on-metal implants

A significant increase in the concentration of metals is found in patients with metal-on-metal (MoM) compared with MoP implants; this is indicative of the larger wear of the metal when sliding against a hard counterface. For CoCrMo–CoCrMo artificial hip joints, using a larger diameter femoral head and decreasing the clearance between the contacting surfaces induces a decrease in the wear volume. Different wear rates are found depending on the number of cycles *in vitro* or the years of implantation *in vivo*. Usually, a higher wear rate is found at the early stages (run-in phase) than at the later stages (steady-state wear), mainly due to the evolution of the surface chemistry and roughness (Catelas *et al.*, 2003).

The mechanisms responsible for the wear of CoCrMo have been identified as abrasion, surface fatigue and tribochemical reactions, both *in vivo* and *in vitro* (Wimmer *et al.*, 2003). Even though the articulation is a self-mated metallic contact, adhesion is not a prevailing wear mechanism, indicating that there is no direct metal–metal contact and underlining the important role of surface films. Surface fatigue by repeated loading leads to local delaminations and the formation of pits due to the detachment of metallic or carbide particles. The carbide–metal matrix interface is the weakest link in such events (Wimmer *et al.*, 2001). Foreign particles and particles originating from the degradation of the surface, such as fractured carbides, compacted wear debris and plastically deformed parts of the metal matrix, are present in the contact area. Such particles can abrade the metallic surface, forming grooves predominantly parallel to the sliding direction by microcutting and microploughing (Büscher *et al.*, 2005).

Tribochemical reactions between the contacting surfaces and the interfacial medium occur in the articulation of MoM implants, and the resulting surface layers have been identified both *in vitro* and *in vivo* (Wimmer *et al.*, 2003). Tribochemical reaction layers partly cover the surface of the contact and have an inhomogeneous thickness. They appear to be formed from compacted debris, and contain scratches, cracks and a surrounding rim of surface oxide (Fig. 9.8). The tribochemical films are characterized by increased oxygen, carbon and oxidized chromium content of about 100 nm thickness (Wimmer *et al.*, 2010). Calcium, phosphorus and nitrogen arising from the environment are also found in the tribochemical layer. The carbon has been linked to organic molecules from the synovial fluid, and the formation of organometallic compounds or the decomposition of proteins are possible sources. Such surface layers protect the metallic substrate from corrosion (Yan *et al.*, 2007), act as a solid lubricant to

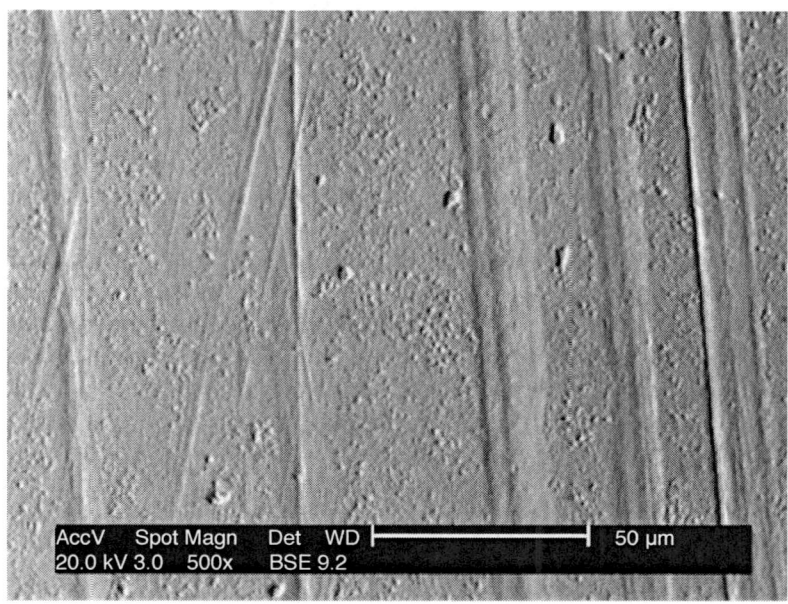

(a)

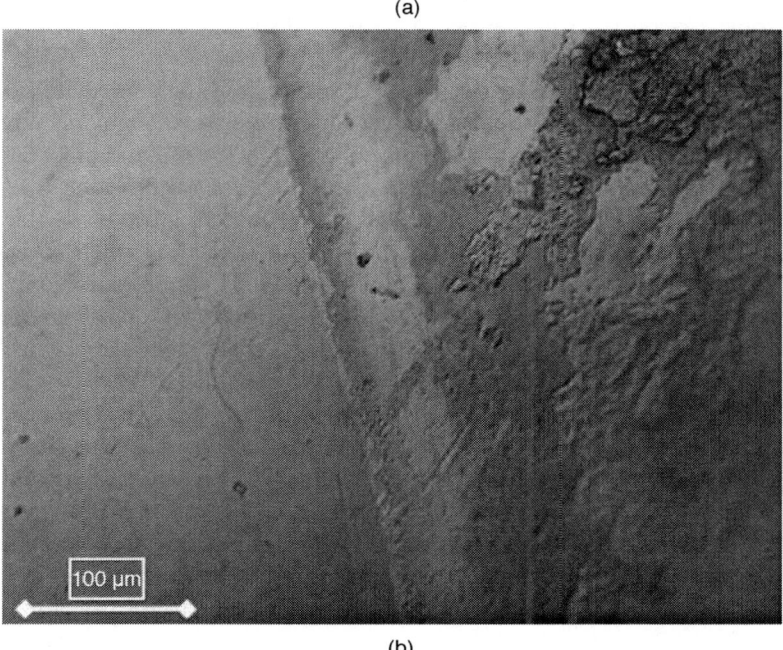

(b)

9.8 (a) Abrasion grooves and surface fatigue pits (Wimmer *et al.*, 2001) and (b) edge of the tribochemical reaction layer (Wimmer *et al.*, 2003) on CoCrMo hip joint prostheses.

decrease the coefficient of friction and protect the metal from wear (Wimmer et al., 2010). Strengthening such surface layers has been proposed as a possible strategy to decrease the wear of MoM hip implants.

Apart from the inclusion of carbon, the microstructure of the alloy in the immediate subsurface of the contact is also modified. A nanocrystalline microstructure is found arising from strain-induced phase transformations. This tribologically transformed area is found in the top 500 nm of the surface and is characterized by a grain size of 50–80 nm (Büscher et al., 2005). Such nanocrystals can assist in the convective transport of material in the top few nanometers of the surface, since they are known to rotate under high mechanical stresses. This mechanism of shear stress accommodation allows the surface to dissipate the frictional energy without particle release and thus decrease wear (Catelas et al., 2011). The mechanical mixing action can incorporate surface oxides and/or adsorbed proteins inside the alloy and explains the presence of carbon at depths of up to 200 nm. As a result, a complex structure forms from the metallic, organic and ceramic species found on the surface. Below the tribochemically transformed surface, stacking faults and strain-induced ε-martensite are found. Such bulk transformations most probably occur during forging of the prosthesis but some plastic deformation during use is also conceivable (Büscher et al., 2005).

The nanocrystalline structure of the surface and the immediate subsurface of the contact is of particular interest since this area is the main source of the wear debris. Up to 10^{14} particles sized less than 250 nm and most commonly close to 50 nm are released from a typical MoM prosthesis each year (Doorn et al., 1998). The size of the particles closely matches the size of the crystals in the tribochemically transformed area, indicating their origin. The particular characteristic of particles from MoM implants is their reactive nature and tendency to oxidize. Both *in vitro* and *in vivo*, particles are mostly round to oval but some needle-shaped particles have also been detected (Büscher et al., 2005; Catelas et al., 2011). Rounded particles appear to originate from the nanocrystalline subsurface, while needle-like particles could originate from the subsurface martensitic phase transformation (Büscher et al., 2005). Most particles consist of chromium oxides and only a small proportion are CoCrMo particles, indicating their predominantly superficial source. However, the chemical composition seems to depend on the size of the particle since bigger particles are metallic and crystalline, while smaller particles are amorphous oxides that can consist of Cr(III) and Cr(VI) (Ward et al., 2010). The alloy and the number of cycles can influence particle characteristics such as size, shape and chemical composition but the differences are rather small (Catelas et al., 2011).

9.6 Fretting corrosion

Whereas sliding occurs at articulating surfaces, fretting is usually found between surfaces that are intended to be fixed to each other. Fretting can lead to loosening of artificial joints, resulting in increased vibration and acceleration of wear. The correlation between the metal ion concentration in the environment and the fretting wear volume of metallic biomaterials has been established (Kovacs et al., 1992). Cyclic loading, which is often closely related to fretting displacement, can also lead to fatigue, the growth of cracks and even mechanical failure of the prosthesis. In the human body, it is probable that crack growth is also accelerated by the environment through corrosion fatigue (Maruyama, 2010).

A particular characteristic of fretting is that the elastic properties of the contacting materials can influence the fretting response. The higher the elasticity of the contacting materials, the larger the amount of applied stress will be accommodated by elastic deformation instead of relative motion and wear at the interface. Applied cyclic stresses can induce the nucleation and propagation of cracks. However, when fretting wear is considerable, the removal of superficial material where cracks nucleate can limit the effect of fatigue. An additional characteristic of fretting is the closed geometry of the contact zone. As a result of this, exchange of material between the contact area and the environment is obstructed. Wear debris can easily become entrapped and the behavior of these particles is critical since they act as a third body between the two contacting bodies. Additionally, replenishment of the electrolyte in the contact is difficult and local electrochemical conditions may differ from those in the bulk solution.

The interplay between mechanical and electrochemical interactions at the fretting contacts of orthopaedic implants has been widely reported (Barril et al., 2004; Gilbert and Jacobs, 1997; Iwabuchi et al., 2007; Kovacs et al., 1992; Mroczkowski et al., 2006). In a fretting contact, mechanical removal of the base alloy occurs through a plastically deformed area in the immediate subsurface of the contact zone. However, under fretting corrosion, about 50% of the total material loss of CoCrMo and Ti-6Al-4V can be ascribed to wear-accelerated corrosion. Cyclic compressive and shear stresses and fretting motion at the contact fracture the oxide film. Corrosion and wear particles in the contact induce abrasion and exacerbate the mechanical removal of material. Unprotected substrate is then exposed to the aqueous local environment, leading to a sequence of electrochemical reactions of ionic dissolution and repassivation, which continue with repeated loading. Due to the difficult replenishment of the electrolyte, the local environment in the contact becomes acidic and the chloride ion concentration increases. In addition, the solution becomes deaerated as available oxygen is consumed during repassivation. The process thus autoaccelerates, making the oxide film less resistant to fretting and corrosion. In the occluded spaces between modules and between the implant and bone or cement this gives rise to mechanically assisted crevice corrosion.

9.6.1 The neck–head junction of modular implants

In modular hip implants a cylindrical taper junction (Morse cone) exists between the femoral stem and the head. In certain designs, the neck is also modular and a second taper junction exists between the stem and neck (Viceconti et al., 1997). The presence of body fluids and the non-axial loading that induces bending micro-movements at the interface of the junctions between the modules induce the release of corrosion and wear products. Metal ion release from orthopaedic implants likely emanates from modular head–neck junctions rather than passive dissolution of the CoCrMo stems (Jacobs et al., 1998).

Numerous studies have reported on the failure in modular junctions (Kop and Swarts, 2009). However, other cases have found no damage, indicating that it can be avoided (Cook et al., 1994). Some of the factors promoting damage at the taper junction appear to be linked to the implantation procedure since assembly load, the presence of liquid in the bore (Mroczkowski et al., 2006) and good anchoring at the stem–bone interface (Cook et al., 1994) have been shown to affect it. Other parameters that affect the fretting corrosion at modular junctions include material combination, metallurgical factors, implantation time, rigidity of the neck and environment. The combination of materials is an important parameter since corrosion and wear are significantly more common in mixed alloy implants (Ti-6Al-4V–CoCrMo) compared with implants made from the same alloy (CoCrMo–CoCrMo) (Cook et al., 1994; Mroczkowski et al., 2006). This indicates that galvanic corrosion can occur due to passive film disruption and electrical contact between dissimilar alloys (Gilbert and Jacobs, 1997; Mroczkowski et al., 2006). Furthermore, increased fretting corrosion has been reported for CoCrMo–CoCrMo compared with CoCrMo–ZrO_2 junctions (Hallab et al., 2004).

Fretting, crevice and galvanic corrosion result in a large amount of corrosion products inside the junction, as well as around the entrance (Urban et al., 1997). The corrosion products from different designs of implants and different materials combinations, even when a ceramic head is used, are quite similar. Corrosion products inside the crevice form a thin layer of crystalline mixed oxides of Cr, Mo and Ti. The corrosion products found outside the entrance of the crevice can have a thickness of several millimeters and consist of amorphous hydrated chromium phosphate. Due to their position, chromium phosphate particles can easily migrate to

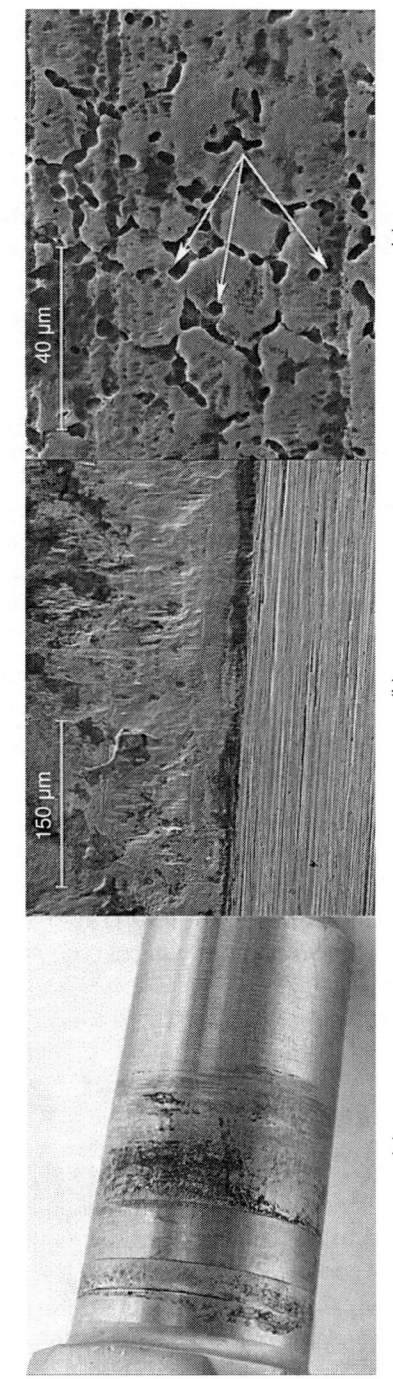

9.9 (a) Macrostructure of neck–stem taper. (b) SEM image of affected area. (c) Intergranular corrosion in the affected area (Kop and Swarts, 2009).

neighbouring areas and have been found in the surrounding tissue and at the articulating surface (Urban et al., 1997). Additionally, areas of surface irregularity with associated debris, pits, etch marks and fretting scars are found on the alloy surface as shown in Fig. 9.9. The affected area exhibits plastic deformation of the surface perpendicular to the original machining marks, indicative of fretting movement. A characteristic pattern of preferential dissolution occurs, indicating intergranular corrosion associated with the chromium carbide phase.

9.6.2 The stem fixation interface of cemented and uncemented implants

A large number of studies have been published comparing the effectiveness of cemented and uncemented femoral stem fixation with usually contradictory results. The use of uncemented fixation appears to have considerably increased in recent years in Japan (Yamada et al., 2009) even though a meta-analysis of the literature available in 2007 concluded that although the performance of uncemented fixation has improved over the years, it is still outperformed by cemented fixation (Morshed et al., 2007). The conflicting results could indicate the existence of a wide number of factors affecting the success of the stem–bone fixation, which could include implant design and materials selection.

Uncemented implants

Surface damage occurs on both well-fixed (Jasty et al., 1994) and loose (Maccauro et al., 2000) uncemented hip stems. Burnishing of the femoral stem against the bone and metal staining of tissues opposite the porous coatings were found on well-fixed stems. Fretting corrosion at the stem–bone interface is a source of particles that can migrate and increase three-body abrasive wear at the articulation. Fretting has been proposed as the main cause of corrosion on loose uncemented Ti alloy stems at points of increased contact stress such as the inferior part of the stem and particularly the tip.

Cemented implants

The femoral stem–bone cement interface, which functions as a transitional zone between two materials with significantly different mechanical properties, has consistently been regarded as a weak link in the total joint system. Retrieval studies have demonstrated that failed hip prostheses are always associated with debonding at this interface. Due to the unmatched strain

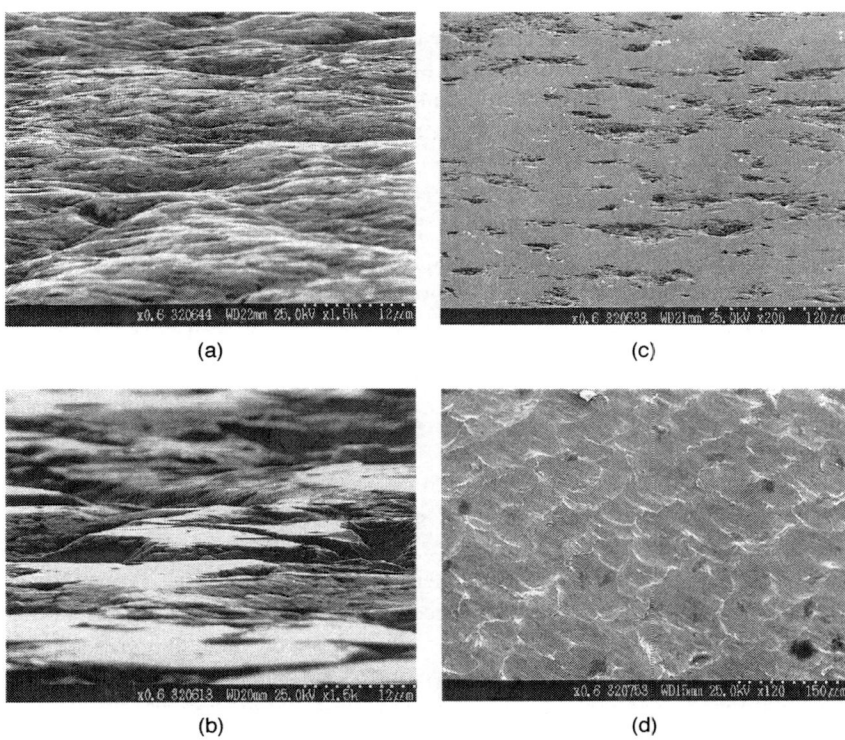

9.10 SEM images of retrieved femoral stems showing (a) an unworn matte stem, (b) an area of slight polishing wear of a matte stem, (c) an area of marked polishing wear of a matte stem and (d) a worn area of a polished stem (Howell *et al.*, 2004).

under physiological loading, the stem–cement interface experiences low-amplitude oscillatory micromotion and fretting *in vivo* (Zhang *et al.*, 2009a).

Loose stems exhibit significantly more wear than well-fixed stems due to the increased range of motion (Howell *et al.*, 2004). This results in the production of metal wear debris, damage to the cement leading to enlargement of the internal dimensions of the cement mantle and crevice corrosion. Different wear mechanisms are identified depending on the surface microstructure of the stem, but irrespective of the material (Fig. 9.10). In the case of matte stems, polishing wear at the tip of the asperities has been reported, leading to a progressively flatter surface and the formation of an interfacial membrane with high metal concentration in loose stems. In highly worn areas of loose matte stems, a surface microstructure similar to that obtained from slurry erosion is found, indicating the important aspect of the behavior of wear debris produced by fretting and trapped in the contact area (Howell *et al.*, 2004). In the case of polished stems, plastic deformation of the surface results in a structure consisting of elliptical pits orientated along the axis of the micro-motion and exhibiting retention of debris. A detailed study of the implant–cement interface (Blunt *et al.*, 2009; Zhang *et al.*, 2009a, 2009b) indicated that the structure of the cement and particularly the size of micropores in contact with the metal is a critical parameter in the initiation and propagation of fretting at the interface. Nevertheless, when the clinical consequences are considered, the modes of mass transport between the metallic surface and the biological environment through the bone cement are equally important to the wear.

9.7 Conclusions

The degradation of metal joints, which occurs through surface processes at the interface between the alloy and the environment, can considerably affect the biocompatibility of metallic materials. Surface layers form spontaneously on orthopaedic alloys and their properties determine the rate and outcome of corrosion and wear processes. The presence of surface layers creates an interrelation between electrochemical and mechanical phenomena. At the articulation, corrosion accelerated by wear leads to ion release. However, compacted corrosion products and subsurface deformation under applied stress in the contact transform the metal close to the interface and decrease wear. Modifying the alloy composition to strengthen such surface layers or applying hard and corrosion-resistant coatings can decrease the material loss. At fretting contacts, the disruption of surface films induces material loss through mechanically assisted crevice and galvanic corrosion. Developing alloys with an elasticity modulus similar to that of the surrounding bone will alleviate the mismatch between the contacting surfaces, decreasing stress shielding of the femur and micro-motions at the interface.

9.8 References

Affatato S, Spinelli M, Zavalloni M, Mazzega-Fabbro C and Viceconti M (2008) Tribology of total hip joint replacement: Current concepts in mechanical simulation. *Med Eng Phys*, 30, 1305–17.

ASTM (2001) ASTM standard G119: Standard guide for determining amount of synergism between wear and corrosion. In *Annual Book of ASTM Standards, Volume 03.02: Wear and Erosion, Metal Corrosion*.West Conshohocken, PA, ASTM.

Barril S, Mischler S and Landolt D (2004) Influence of fretting regimes on the tribocorrosion behavior of Ti6Al4V in 0.9 wt% sodium chloride solution. *Wear*, 256, 963–72.

Blunt L A, Zhang H, Barrans S M, Jiang X and Brown L T (2009) What results in fretting wear on polished femoral stems? *Tribol Int*, 42, 1605–14.

Bufort A and Goswami T (2004) Review of wear mechanisms in hip implants: Paper I – General. *Mater Des*, 25, 385–93.

Büscher R, Täger G, Dudzinski W, Gleising B, Wimmer M A and Fischer A (2005) Subsurface microstructure of metal-on-metal hip joints and its relationship to wear particle generation. *J Biomed Mater Res Part B*, 72B, 206–14.

Burstein G T, Liu C and Souto R M (2005) The effect of temperature on the nucleation of corrosion pits on titanium in Ringer's physiological solution. *Biomaterials*, 26, 245–56.

Catelas I, Bobyn J D, Medley J B, Krygier J J, Zukor D J and Huk O L (2003) Size, shape and composition of wear particles from metal–metal hip simulator testing: Effects of alloy and number of loading cycles. *J Biomed Mater Res Part A*, 67A, 312–27.

Catelas I, Wimmer M A and Utzschneider S (2011) Polyethylene and metal wear particles: characteristics and biological effects. *Semin Immunopathol*, 33, 257–71.

Celis J P, Ponthiaux P and Wenger F (2006) Tribo-corrosion of materials: interplay between chemical, electrochemical, and mechanical reactivity of surfaces. *Wear*, 261, 939–46.

Cook S D, Barrack R L and Clemow A J T (1994) Corrosion and wear at the modular interface of uncemented femoral stems. *J Bone Joint Surg Br*, 76B, 68–72.

Crockett R, Roba M, Naka M, Gasser B, Delfosse D, Frauchinger V and Spencer N D (2008) Friction, lubrication, and polymer transfer between UHMWPE and CoCrMo hip-implants materials: A fluorescence microscopy study. *J Biomed Mater Res Part A*, 89A, 1011–8.

Diomidis N, Celis J P, Ponthiaux P and Wenger F (2010) Tribocorrosion of stainless steel in sulphuric acid: identification of corrosion-wear components and effect of contact area. *Wear*, 269, 93–103.

Diomidis N, Mischler S, More N S, Roy M and Paul S N (2011a) Fretting-corrosion behavior of β titanium alloys in simulated synovial fluid. *Wear*, 271, 1093–102.

Diomidis N, Mischler S, More N S and Roy M (2011b) Triboelectrochemical characterization of metallic biomaterials for total joint replacement. *Acta Biomater*, doi:10.1016/j.actbio.2011.09.034.

Doorn P F, Campbell P A, Worrall J, Benya P D and McKellop H A (1998) Metal wear particle characterization from metal on metal total hip replacements: TEM study of periprosthetic tissues and isolated particles. *J Biomed Mater Res*, 42, 103–11.

Galetz M C, Seiferth S H, Theile B and Glatzel U (2010) Potential for adhesive wear in friction couples of UHMWPE running against oxidized zirconium, titanium nitride coatings, and cobalt chromium alloys. *J Biomed Mater Res Part B*, 93B, 468–75.

Gilbert J L and Jacobs J J (1997). The mechanical and electrochemical processes associated with taper fretting crevice corrosion: a review. In Marlowe D E, Parr J E and Mayor M B (eds) *STP1301 Modularity of Orthopaedic Implants*. West Conshohocken, PA, ASTM, pp. 45–59.

Gispert M P, Serro A P, Colaço R and Saramago B (2006) Friction and wear mechanisms in hip prostheses: comparison of joint materials behavior in different lubricants. *Wear*, 260, 149–58.

Hallab N J, Messina C, Skipor A and Jacobs J J (2004) Differences in the fretting corrosion of metal-metal and ceramic-metal modular junctions of total hip replacements. *J Orthop Res*, 22, 250–9.

Hanawa T (2002) Evaluation techniques of metallic biomaterials *in vitro*. *Sci Technol Adv Mater*, 3, 289–95.

Hanawa T (2004) Metal ion release from metal implants. *Mater Sci Eng C*, 24, 745–52.

Hanawa T, Hiromoto S and Asami K (2001) Characterization of the surface oxide film of a Co–Cr–Mo alloy after being located in quasi-biological environments using XPS. *Appl Surf Sci*, 183, 68–75.

Howell J R, Blunt L A, Doyle C, Hooper R M, Lee A J C and Ling R S M (2004) In vivo surface wear mechanisms of femoral components of cemented total hip anrthroplasties. *J Arthroplasty*, 19, 88–101.

Igual Muñoz A and Mischler S (2001) Effect of the environment on wear ranking and corrosion of biomedical CoCrMo alloys. *J Mater Sci, Mater Med*, 22, 437–50.

Iwabuchi A, Lee J W and Uchidate M (2007) Synergistic effect of fretting wear and sliding wear of Co-alloy and Ti-alloy in Hank's solution. *Wear*, 263, 492–500.

Jacobs J J, Skipor A K and Patterson L M (1998) Metal release in patients who have had a primary total hip arthroplasty: a prospective, controlled, longitudinal study *J Bone Joint Surg Am*, 80A, 1447–58.

Jasty M, Brandon C, Jiranek W, Chandler H, Maloney W and Harris W H (1994) Etiology of osteolysis around porous-coated cementless total hip arthroplasties. *Clin Orthop Relat Res*, 308, 111–26.

Khan M A, Williams R L and Williams D F (1999) The corrosion behavior of Ti-6Al-4V, Ti-6Al-7Nb and Ti-13Nb-13Zr in protein solution. *Biomaterials*, 20, 631–7.

Kop A M and Swarts E (2009) Corrosion of a hip stem with a modular neck taper junction, a retrieval study of 16 cases. *J Arthroplasty*, 24, 1019–23.

Kovacs P, Davidson J A and Daigle K (1992) Correlation between the metal ion concentration and the fretting wear volume of orthopaedic implant materials. In St. John K R (ed) *STP1144 Particulate Debris from Medical Implants, Mechanisms of Formation and Biological Consequences*. Philadelphia, PA, ASTM, pp. 160–76.

Landolt D (2007) *Corrosion and Surface Chemistry of Metals*. Lausanne, EPFL Press.

Landolt D, Mischler S and Stemp M (2001) Electrochemical method in tribocorrosion: a critical appraisal. *Electrochim Acta*, 46, 3913–29.

Long M and Rack H J (1998) Titanium alloys in total joint replacement – a materials science perspective. *Biomaterials*, 19, 1621–39.

Maccauro G, Piconi C, Pilloni L, Proietti L, De Santis V and De Santis E (2000) Surface analysis of a femoral stem after failed total hip replacement *Int Orthop*, 24, 231–3.

Maruyama N (2010) Fatigue and fretting fatigue behavior of metallic biomaterials *Mater Sci Forum*, 638–42, 618–23.

Mathew M T, Srinivasa Pai P, Pourzal R, Fischer A and Wimmer M A (2009)

Significance of tribocorrosion in biomedical applications: overview and current status. *Adv Tribol*, 2009, paper 250986.

Mattei L, Di Puccio F, Piccigallo B and Ciulli E (2011) Lubrication and wear modeling of artificial hip joints: a review. *Tribol Int*, 44, 532–49.

Milošev I (2011) Metallic materials for biomedical applications: Laboratory and clinical studies. *Pure Appl Chem*, 83, 309–24.

Milošev I and Strehblow H H (2003) The composition of the passive film formed on CoCrMo alloy in simulated physiological solution. *Electrochim Acta*, 48, 2767–74.

Milošev I, Metikoš-Hugović M and Strehblow H H (2000) Passive film on orthopaedic TiAlV alloy formed in physiological solution investigated by X-ray photoelectron spectroscopy. *Biomaterials*, 21, 2103–13.

Minovič A, Milošev I and Pihlar B (2003) The influence of complexing agent and proteins on the corrosion of stainless steels and their metallic components. *J Mater Sci Mater Med*, 14, 69–77.

Mischler S (2008) Triboelectrochemical techniques and interpretation methods in tribocorrosion: a comparative evaluation. *Tribol Int*, 41, 573–83.

Morita M, Inoue Y and Sasada T (1998) Biocompatibility of prosthetic joint materials (Part 1): Evaluation of passivation film damage on metal surface associated with sliding motion. *Japan J Tribol*, 43, 653–63.

Morshed S, Bozic K J, Ries M D, Malchau H and Colford J M Jr (2007) Comparison of cemented and uncemented fixation in total hip replacement. A meta analysis. *Acta Orthop*, 78, 315–26.

Mroczkowski M L, Hertzler J S, Humphrey S M, Johnson T and Blanchard C R (2006) Effect of impact assembly on the fretting corrosion of modular hip tapers. *J Orthop Res*, 24, 271–9.

Okazaki Y (2002) Effect of friction on the anodic polarization properties of metallic biomaterials. *Biomaterials*, 23, 2071–7.

Okazaki Y and Gotoh E (2005) Comparison of metal release from various metallic biomaterials *in vitro*. *Biomaterials*, 26, 11–21.

Pilliar R M (2009) Metallic Biomaterials In Narayan R (ed) *Biomedical Materials*. Dordrecht, Springer Science + Business Media, pp. 41–81.

Poggie R A, Wert J J, Mishra A K and Davidson J A (1992) Friction and wear of UHMWPE in sliding contact with Co–Cr, Ti-6Al-4V, and zirconia implant bearing surfaces. In Denton R and Keshavan M K (eds) *STP1145 Wear and Friction of Elastomers*, Baltimore, MD, ASTM, pp. 65–81.

Ponthiaux P, Wenger F, Drees D and Celis J P (2004) Electrochemical techniques for studying tribocorrosion processes. *Wear*, 256, 459–68.

Que L and Topoleski L D T (2000) Third-body wear of cobalt–chromium–molybdenum implant alloys initiated by bone and poly(methyl methacrylate) particles. *J Biomed Mater Res Part A*, 50, 322–30.

Rabbe L M, Rieu J, Lopez A and Combrade P (1994) Fretting deterioration of orthopedic implant materials: Search for solutions. *Clin Mater*, 15, 221–6.

Rieker C B, Schön R and Köttig P (2004) Development and validation of a second generation metal-on-metal bearing. *J Arthroplasty*, 19, 5–11.

Semlitsch M and Willert H G (1995) Implant materials for hip endoprostheses: old proofs and new trends. *Arch Orthop Trauma Surg*, 114, 61–7.

Sinnett-Jones P E, Wharton J A and Wood R J K (2005) Micro-abrasion-corrosion of a CoCrMo alloy in simulated artificial hip joint environments. *Wear*, 259, 898–909.

Smith S L, Elfick A P D and Unsworth A (1999) An evaluation of the tribological performance of zirconia and CoCrMo femoral heads. *J Mater Sci*, 34, 5159–62.

Steinemann S G (1980) Corrosion of surgical implants – *in vivo* and *in vitro* tests. In Winter G D, Leray J L and de Groot K (eds) *Evaluation of Biomaterials*, New York, Wiley, pp. 1–34.

Steinemann S G (1985) Corrosion of titanium and titanium alloys for surgical implants. In *Titanium'84 Science and Technology Vol. 2*. Munich, Deutsche Gesellschaft für Metallkunde EV, pp. 1373–9.

Urban R M, Jacobs J J, Gilbert J M, Rice S B, Jasty M, Bragdon C R and Galante J O (1997) Characterization of solid products of corrosion generated by modular head femoral stems of different designs and materials. In Marlowe D E, Parr J E and Mayor M B (eds) *STP1301 Modularity of Orthopaedic Implants*, West Conshohocken, PA, ASTM, pp. 33–44.

Viceconti M, Baleani M, Squarzoni S and Toni A (1997) Fretting wear in modular neck hip prosthesis. *J Biomed Mater Res*, 35, 207–16.

Virtanen S, Milošev I, Gomez-Barrena E, Trebše R, Salo J and Konttinen Y T (2008) Special modes of corrosion under physiological and simulated physiological conditions. *Acta Biomater*, 4, 468–76.

Ward M B, Brown A P, Cox A, Curry A and Denton J (2010) Microscopical analysis of synovial fluid wear debris from failing CoCr hip prostheses. *J Phys Conf Ser*, 241, 1–4.

Wilches L V, Uribe J A and Toro A (2008) Wear of materials used for artificial joints in total hip replacement. *Wear*, 265, 143–9.

Williams R L, Brown S A and Meritt K (1988) Electrochemical studies on the influence of proteins on the corrosion of implant alloys. *Biomaterials*, 9, 181–6.

Wimmer M A, Loos J, Nassutt R, Heitkemper M and Fischer A (2001) The acting wear mechanisms on metal-on-metal hip joint bearings: in vitro results. *Wear*, 250, 129–39.

Wimmer M A, Sprecher C, Hauert R, Täger G and Fischer A (2003) Tribochemical reaction on metal-on-metal hip joint bearings: A comparison between in-vitro and in-vivo results. *Wear*, 255, 1007–14.

Wimmer M A, Fischer A, Büscher R, Pourzal R, Sprecher C, Hauert R and Jacobs J J (2010) Wear mechanisms in metal-on-metal bearings: The importance of the tribochemical reaction layers. *J Orthop Res*, 28, 436–43.

Wolner C, Nauer G E, Trummer J, Putz V and Tschegg S (2006) Possible reasons for the unexpected bad biocompatibility of metal-on-metal hip implants. *Mater Sci Eng C*, 26, 34–40.

Yamada H, Yoshihara Y, Henmi O, Morita M, Shiromoto Y, Kawano T, Kanaji A, and o K, Nakagawa M, Kosaki N and Fukawa E (2009) Cementless total hip replacement: past, present, and future. *J Orthop Sci*, 14, 228–41.

Yan Y, Neville A, Dowson D and Williams S (2006a) Tribocorrosion in implants – assessing high carbon and low carbon Co–Cr–Mo alloys by in situ electrochemical measurements. *Tribol Int*, 39, 1509–17.

Yan Y, Neville A and Dowson D (2006b) Biotribocorrosion-an appraisal of the time dependence of wear and corrosion interactions: I. The role of corrosion. *J Phys D: Appl Phys*, 39, 3200–5.

Yan Y, Neville A and Dowson D (2007) Biotribocorrosion of CoCrMo orthopaedic implantmaterials – assessing the formation and effect of the biofilm. *Tribol Int*, 40, 1492–9.

Yan Y, Neville A, Dowson D, Williams S and Fisher J (2009) Effect of metallic nanoparticles on the biotribocorrosion of behaviour of metal-on-metal hip prostheses. *Wear*, 267, 683–8.

Zhang H, Brown L T, Blunt L A, Jiang X and Barrans S M (2009a) Understanding initiation and propagation of fretting wear on the femoral stem in total hip replacement. *Wear*, 266, 566–9.

Zhang H Y, Brown L, Barrans S, Blunt L and Jiang X Q (2009b) Investigation of the relative micromotion at the stem-cement interface in total hip replacement. *Proc Inst Mech Eng H*, 223, 955–64.

10
Wear phenomena of ceramic joints

S. AFFATATO, Istituto Ortopedico Rizzoli Italy and
P. TADDEI, Università di Bologna, Italy

Abstract: Ceramic materials offer a number of beneficial mechanical properties such as considerable hardness, good chemical resistance, high tensile strength and good fracture toughness. The use of ceramic-on-ceramic as bearing surfaces for hip joint prostheses has been reported to produce a lower wear rate than other material combinations in total hip arthroplasty. These advantages may increase the life expectancy of hip implants and improve the life of patients. To date, more than 2.5 million alumina femoral heads have been implanted. Material scientists have progressively improved the mechanical strength of alumina, leading to three subsequent generations of medical-grade alumina. A significant effort was devoted to the development of composites such as zirconia-toughened alumina, with the aim of combining the best characteristics of alumina and zirconia. This new class of composite material was introduced in 2004 and is known under the trade name of Biolox® delta. Biolox® delta has 10 years of clinical records in hip replacements and is beginning to be used in knee replacements. Improvements in material manufacturing have decreased the failure rate of second- and third-generation alumina. Retrieved alumina-on-alumina hip prostheses have revealed a small band of wear around the rim of acetabular cups, due to the microseparation phenomenon. Introducing microseparation into *in vitro* wear simulator tests, the wear rates, patterns and mechanisms observed *in vivo* may be successfully reproduced.

Key words: ceramic materials, alumina, zirconia, ZTA, Biolox® delta.

10.1 Introduction

Total hip replacement (THR) is one of the most successful surgical procedures with relatively few complications (Fisher *et al.*, 2006; Stea *et al.*, 2009). Although the polyethylene–metal coupling has been commonly used for THR, its lifetime is limited by loosening, due to biological response against polyethylene wear debris. To solve these critical problems, wear-reduction strategies have been developed with the aim of improving implant fixation and design and surgical methods. Thus, alternative bearing couplings, such as metal-on-metal and ceramic-on-ceramic have been championed for younger patients undergoing THR, at least by some investigators (Callaghan et al., 2008; Pattyn and De Smet, 2008). Alumina was selected as a biomaterial 40 years ago for its unsurpassed biological safety and stability in the living environment (Rose et al., 1980; Willmann, 1998).

Ceramic materials constitute a class of new engineering materials for wear-resistant applications under severe environments. Ceramics have also been defined the materials of the future since they derive from 'sand', which is about 25% of the earth's crust as compared to 1% for all metals (Hsu, 1996). Ceramics include a broad range of inorganic/non-metallic compositions; in most cases, these materials have been treated at a high temperature at some stage during manufacture (Ravaglioli and Krajewski, 1992). Ceramics are used in glass products, cements and plasters, some abrasive and cutting tool materials, various electrical insulation materials, porcelain and refractory coatings for metals, etc. (Higgins, 1994).

In recent years ceramic materials have been recognised as being increasingly important for their chemical and physical characteristics, and have progressively attracted interest in the biomedical field (Toni et al., 1995). Ceramic materials present excellent biocompatibility, good mechanical resistance (Boehler et al., 1994; Cuckler et al., 2004; Macchi and Willman, 2001; Toni et al., 2006), high wettability, significant wear reductions over traditional metal–polyethylene bearings (Affatato et al., 1999, 2001) and good properties at high temperatures where metals cannot be used (Costa et al., 1997; Toni et al., 1995).

The intrinsic properties of pure alumina limit its mechanical properties, especially toughness, and the improvement of medical-grade alumina is a task that was therefore actively pursued by ceramic manufacturers. Subsequent clinical outcomes revealed limitations of ceramic technology in THR, such as a possible higher incidence of bearing dislocation related to design constraints in alumina femoral heads and acetabular liners (Mai et al., 2008) and a finite risk of catastrophic failure of femoral heads *in vivo* (Cuckler et al., 2004; Rhoads et al., 2008). Of most concern, despite favourable *in vitro* wear testing of alumina bearings that showed virtually no bearing wear after 20 million hip simulator cycles (Shishido et al., 2003), clinical outcomes sometimes showed severe wear requiring revision surgery even at intermediate-term follow-up.

10.2 Developments in ceramic technology

Alumina and partially stabilized zirconia are currently in extensive use as constituents of prosthetic components for total hip and knee replacement (Fig. 10.1) in consequence of their high strength, wear resistance and stability, non-toxicity and biocompatibility *in vivo* (Li and Hastings, 1999; Willmann, 1998, 2000). Alumina ceramics have been widely used for their thermo-mechanical and tribologic properties: they show a very high hardness, wear resistance and chemical stability (Li and Hastings, 1999). Zirconia ceramics have been introduced into orthopaedics as an alternative to alumina (Derbyshire *et al.*, 1994); they have several advantages over other ceramic materials due to the transformation toughening mechanism operating in their microstructure (Piconi and Maccauro, 1999). Alumina is chemically more stable than zirconia but mechanically weaker; the phase changes (or transformation mechanism) in the latter produce a ceramic material with much higher strength and higher fracture toughness than alumina or other ceramics (Li and Hastings, 1999; Piconi and Maccauro, 1999).

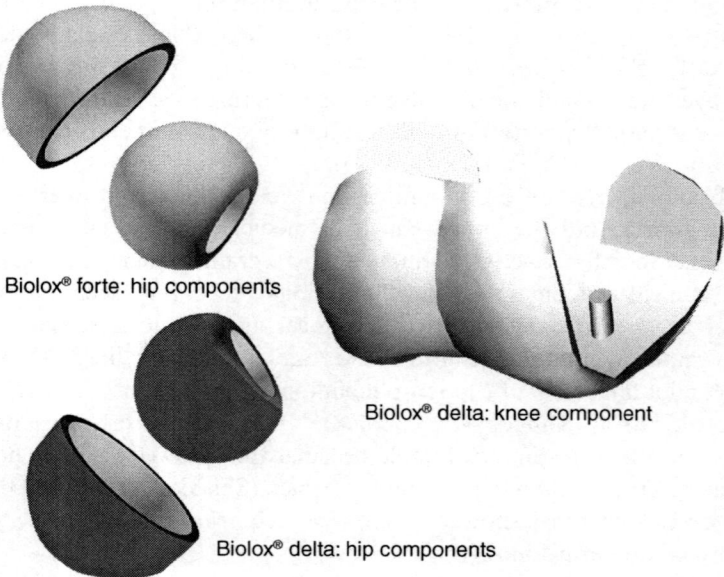

10.1 Hip and knee ceramic components made out of Biolox® forte and Biolox® delta.

10.2.1 Alumina

Alumina (aluminum oxide, Al_2O_3) is a highly inert material resistant to most corrosive environments. The alumina ceramic used in biomedical application is α-alumina, known as corundum. Single crystals of this material that occur in nature are known as ruby if containing Cr_2O_3 impurities.

The Al_2O_3 molecule is characterized by strong bonds, making it one of the most stable oxides and practically unaffected by galvanic reactions (absence of corrosion, absence of ion release from bulk materials and wear debris). These bonds also give alumina its chemical stability under adverse conditions such as strong acidic or alkaline environment at high temperatures.

The term high-purity alumina refers to materials that have a 97% minimal content of alumina. High-purity alumina (Table 10.1) has been being used in orthopaedics for THR since the 1970s (Boutin, 1972; Fruh et al., 1997) and could be called first-generation alumina. In 1974, alumina obtained from chemically purified and grounded corundum powders was introduced to the market as Biolox® (second-generation alumina) (Fig. 10.2). The so-called third-generation alumina, Biolox® forte, became commercially available in 1995; this material is composed of high-purity alumina (> 99.8 %) with a small percentage of magnesium oxide (MgO) added to prevent an increase in grain size of alumina during sintering. This strategy yielded a more homogenous and dense microstructure (Fig. 10.2) with improved mechanical characteristics (Table 10.1). The better surface finishing of Biolox® forte can also be demonstrated by photoluminescence measurements (Fig. 10.3); according to Schilling et al. (2002) a higher

Table 10.1 Characteristics of ceramic materials used in orthopaedic applications, as recommended by international guidelines

Property	ISO 6474-1[1]	Alumina (1970s)[2]	Biolox® (> 1974)[2]	Biolox® forte (> 1995)[2]	ZTA[3]	Biolox® delta (> 2004)[2]
Density (g/cm^3)	> 99.5	3.90	3.95	3.97	5.49	4.37
Bending strength (MPa)	> 400	465	500	631	1008	1384
Young modulus (GPa)	–	380	410	407	259	358
Fracture toughness (MPa m$^{1/2}$) K_{IC}	–	< 3.0	3.0	3.2	5.49	6.5
Hardness, HV1 (GPa)	–	< 20	20	20	15.3	19
Av. grain size (μm)	–	≤ 4.5	4	1.75	0.69	0.56

[1]ISO 6474-1:2010 Implants for surgery. Ceramic materials. Part 1: Ceramic materials based on high purity alumina.
[2]http://www.ceramtec.com/pdf/biolox_delta_en.pdf.
[3]Experimental values quoted by Centro Ceramico, Italy.

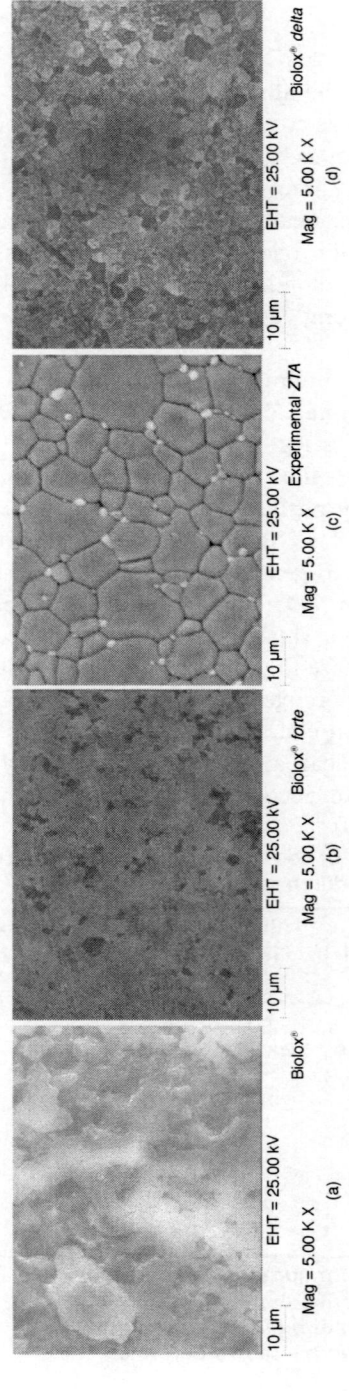

10.2 Microstructure of (a) Biolox®, (b) Biolox® forte, (c) ZTA and (d) Biolox® delta at SEM analysis.

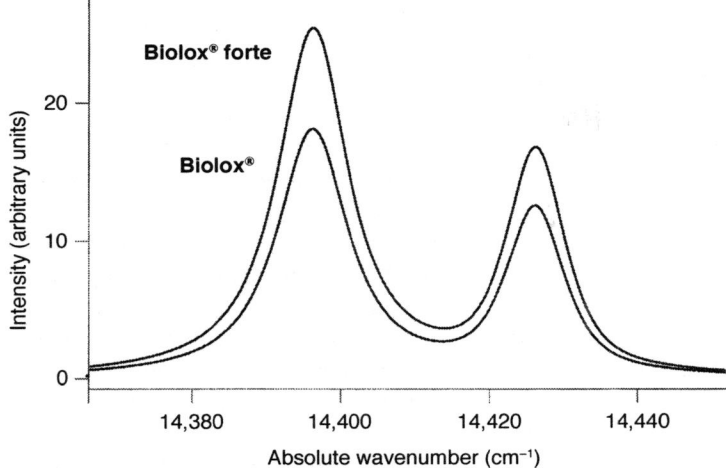

10.3 Fluorescence spectra of Biolox® and Biolox® forte. The two strong and sharp fluorescence bands at about 14,400 and 14,430 cm^{-1} are due to the radiative transitions of the Cr^{3+} ions, present as natural substitution impurities in alumina.

fluorescence intensity is indicative of a material with higher density and lower porosity.

Although clinical follow-up with current alumina ceramics is significant, it must be borne in mind that their use has been restricted so far to a limited number of designs of hip components in which mechanical loading is less demanding. For example, 22 mm heads are not currently manufactured using alumina, for reliability reasons. Alumina has proved a good material for femoral ball heads articulating against polyethylene acetabular cups or in alumina-on-alumina combinations, although the latter exhibit a significant increase of failure ratios. This is related to the modest mechanical properties of alumina: the material performs very well under compression, but is brittle under tension. As with many ceramics, alumina does not show room-temperature plastic deformation before fracture (e.g. no yield point in the stress–strain curve before fracture) and, once started, fractures progress very rapidly due to its low toughness (Piconi *et al.*, 2003).

10.2.2 Zirconia

Zirconia (zirconium dioxide, ZrO_2) was identified in 1789 by the German chemist Martin Heinrich Klaproth and was used for a long time as pigment for ceramics (Hench and Hethridge, 1975). Its good chemical and dimensional stability, mechanical strength and toughness, coupled with a Young's modulus comparable to that of stainless steel, attracted the attention of biomedical ceramic manufacturers and zirconia ceramics were introduced to the orthopaedic community in France and the USA in 1986. The early developments were focused on magnesia partially stabilized zirconia (Mg-PSZ); most of the subsequent efforts concentrated on yttria-stabilized tetragonal zirconia polycrystals (Y-TZP), formed by submicron-sized grains (0.3–0.5 μm) (Piconi et al., 2003).

In the 1990s, Y-TZP became a popular alternative to alumina as a structural ceramic because of its substantially higher fracture toughness and strength. The use of zirconia has opened the way towards new implant designs that were not possible with the more brittle alumina. Biomedical-grade zirconia has the best mechanical properties among single-phase oxide ceramics: this is as a consequence of phase conversion toughening, which increases the crack propagation resistance. The stress-induced phase transformation involves the transformation of metastable tetragonal grains to the monoclinic phase at the crack tip. This is accompanied by 3–4% volume expansion and induces compressive stresses that hinder crack propagation (Fig. 10.4). However, ring-on-disk tests demonstrated that the wear rate of zirconia articulating against itself was disastrous (Willmann

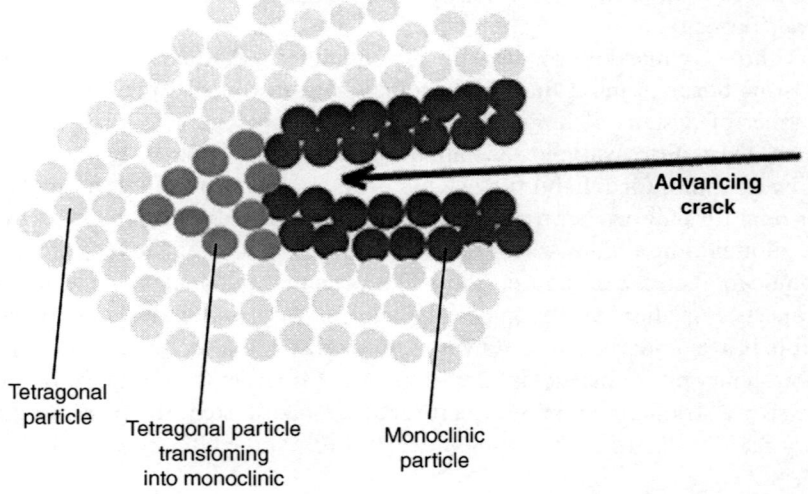

10.4 Phase conversion toughening mechanism in Y-TZP-based ceramics. The energy associated with an advancing crack is dissipated through the tetragonal to monoclinic phase transformation, which is accompanied by a 3–4% volume expansion able to hinder crack propagation.

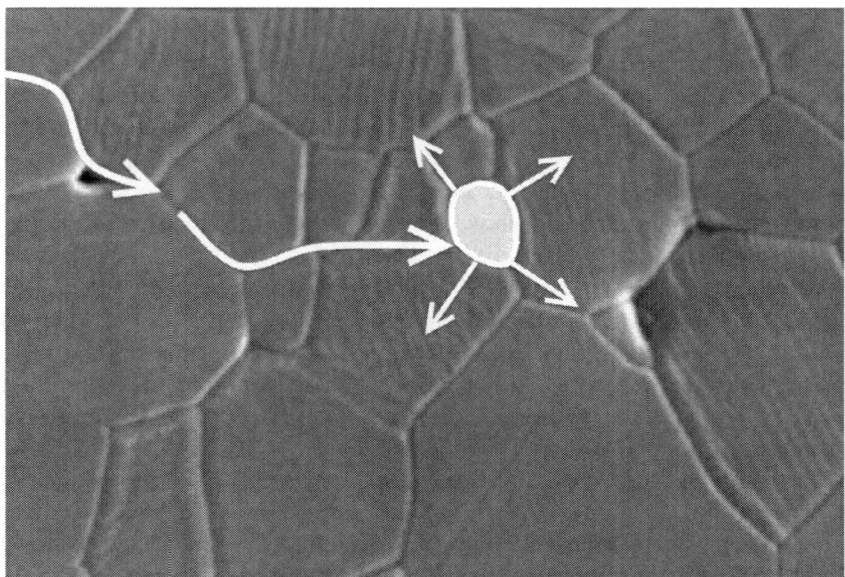

10.5 Phase conversion toughening mechanism in ZTA and Biolox® delta. If the leading edge of a micro-crack encounters a tetragonal zirconia particle, the crack energy causes a phase transformation, increasing the particle volume and closing the crack tip.

et al., 1996), indicating that TZP should not be used for acetabular cups. The low thermal shock resistance of zirconia is thought to be responsible for the extensive cracking and loss of material observed on its wear tracks; infact, if the zirconia is heated above a critical temperature due to friction, then the phase transformation starts with the consequent formation of cracks and worsening of mechanical properties. On the other hand, due to its metastability, zirconia is prone to ageing in the presence of water (Chevalier, 2006). Some clinical reports show that zirconia can exhibit progressive ageing degradation even under 'normal' situations, which limits its long-term stability (Chevalier *et al.*, 2007).

10.2.3 Zirconia-toughened alumina

Between 1975 and 1977, the development of zirconia-toughened alumina (ZTA) yielded materials with higher strength and toughness than alumina (Affatato *et al.*, 2006) (Table 10.1). This new class of composite ceramics derives from the insertion of zirconia (up to 25% wt) into an alumina matrix. The zirconia particles remain in the tetragonal phase due to the constraint exerted by the alumina matrix. The toughening of the material is due to the tetragonal to monoclinic transformation of the zirconia particles.

If the leading edge of a micro-crack encounters a tetragonal zirconia particle, the crack energy causes a phase transformation, increasing the particle volume and closing the crack tip (Fig. 10.5). Therefore, the transformation absorbs the energy of the crack and the strength of the ceramic increases. Alumina–zirconia micro-composites (with both alumina and zirconia grains in the micrometer range) are under development in the orthopaedic community and show improvement in mechanical properties and ageing resistance (De Aza et al., 2002; Deville et al., 2003; Willmann, 1998). New alumina–zirconia composites, with an alumina matrix in the micrometer range and nano-sized zirconia particles have been developed (Chevalier et al., 2005); they exhibit fracture resistance properties that have not yet been reached with oxide ceramics. These nano-composites should open the way to the development of nano-structured oxide ceramics in orthopaedics.

Biolox® delta (Dalla Pria and Burger, 2003; Macchi, 2004) represents the last generation of ceramics for orthopaedic applications. As already noted, zirconia possesses excellent strength and toughness, while alumina shows higher performance in terms of wear, chemical and hydrothermal stability. The Biolox® delta ceramic was developed with the aim of combining the best characteristics of both materials in order to obtain a composite material with good biocompatibility, high resistance to wear and good mechanical properties (i.e. toughness and strength, Table 10.1). To obtain these characteristics, nano-sized particles of tetragonal Y-TZP were uniformly distributed in an alumina matrix, with the phase conversion toughening mechanism already described (Fig. 10.5) A small amount of chromium oxide (Cr_2O_3) was then added to counterbalance the reduction of hardness caused by the introduction of zirconia. Finally, strontium oxide (SrO) was added to the material to form strontium aluminate ($SrAl_{12-x}Cr_xO_{19}$) platelets during the sintering process. Due to their size, these flat, elongated crystals prevent any cracks from advancing by dissipating crack energy (Fig. 10.6). In fact, when a crack reaches one of these crystals, it needs extra energy to go round it; in the absence of this energy, the crack does not propagate. The final product is a mixture of roughly 75% alumina, 25% zirconia and less than 1% chromium oxide and strontium oxide. As claimed by the manufacturer, Biolox® delta was introduced to avoid ageing phenomena. Pezzotti et al. (2008) showed that a Biolox® delta femoral head underwent a tetragonal to monoclinic transformation upon ageing in an autoclave operating at 121°C under a vapor pressure of 0.1 MPa (accelerated tests); this standard treatment was used to simulate the effect of environmental ageing in the human body. The data reported by these authors disagreed with previous studies that claimed that no phase change or minor variations were detected after environmental exposure to water vapor (Burger and Richter, 2001; Insley and Streicher, 2004).

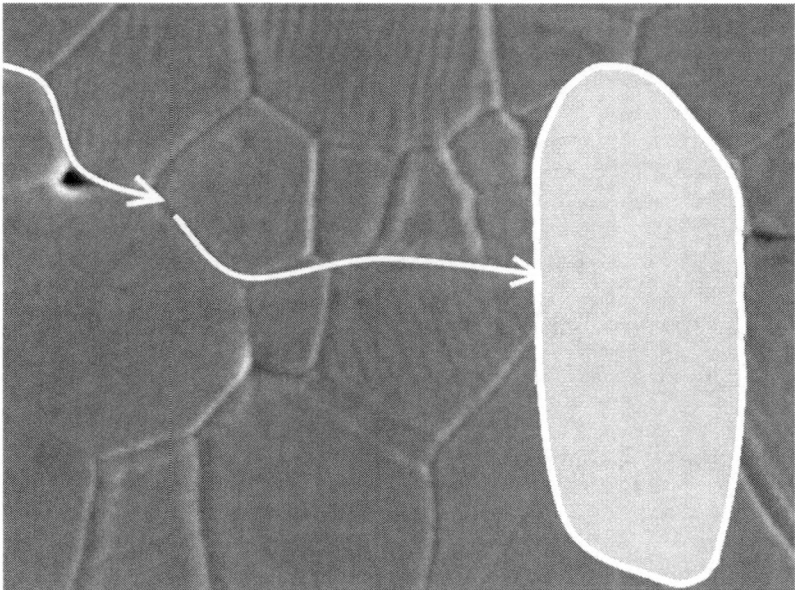

10.6 The strontium aluminate platelets in Biolox® delta prevent any cracks from advancing by dissipating crack energy. When the crack reaches one of these crystals, it needs extra energy to go round it; in the absence of this, the crack does not propagate.

Raman spectroscopy has been found to be particularly useful for detecting the occurrence of this phase transformation, since tetragonal and monoclinic zirconia are easily distinguishable through marker bands characteristic of each form (Dorn and Nickel, 2004; Pezzotti and Porporati, 2004). As shown in Fig. 10.7, the main bands characteristic of the tetragonal phase can be identified at 142, 265, 317 and 460 cm^{-1}, while the marker bands of the monoclinic phase are located at 178, 190, 339, 384 and 480 cm^{-1}. Quantitative methods have been developed to determine the amount of the monoclinic phase from the Raman spectrum (Katagiri *et al.*, 1988; Tabares and Anglada, 2010). Recent Raman studies on new and retrieved Biolox® delta femoral heads showed that a detectable amount of monoclinic zirconia was present in the as-received components and tended to increase upon wear (Fig. 10.7 and unpublished results). In the new component, presumably dating back to 2009, the monoclinic content was about 10 vol%, i.e. lower than that reported by Pezzotti *et al.* in 2008 (about 20 vol%). This would indicate an improvement in the material since its introduction to the market.

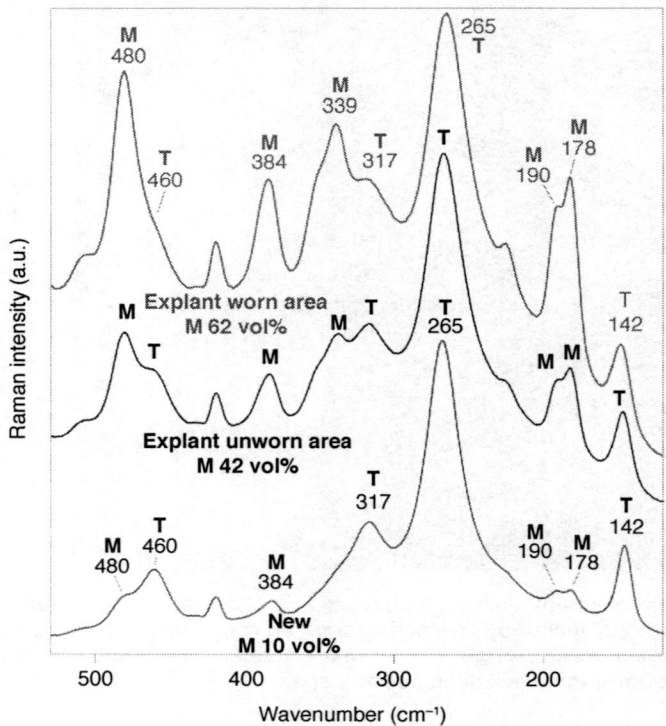

10.7 Micro-Raman spectra recorded on a new Biolox® delta femoral head (presumed dating back to 2009) as well as on the unworn and worn control areas of a retrieved Biolox® delta femoral head implanted in 2003. The bands prevalently due to monoclinic (M) and tetragonal (T) zirconia are indicated as well as the vol% of monoclinic zirconia, calculated according to the method of Katagiri *et al.* (1988).

10.3 Wear of ceramic components

One of the major problems in THR is osteolysis caused by polyethylene wear debris (Fisher *et al.*, 1999; Ingham and Fisher, 2000). The objective of material improvements is to develop wear couplings that reduce both the amount of polyethylene wear and the size of the wear particles. During the wear process, worn material is expelled from the contact between two surfaces in the form of debris. The wear products of hip implants can cause adverse tissue reactions, leading to massive bone loss around the implant and consequently loosening of the fixation (Brown and Clarke, 2006). Such aseptic loosening requires revision surgery, in which the failed prosthesis is replaced with a new one; this process is complicated, expensive and dangerous. Alumina ceramics are bioinert as bulk material and the wear particles also are biocompatible. The orthopaedic community demands that the failure rate of alumina femoral heads is minimized.

10.3.1 Wear in total hip replacements

Ceramic-on-ceramic articulations represent a satisfactory solution for reducing or eliminating polyethylene wear and its associated osteolysis. Several studies have reported improved wear properties and reduced osteolysis and ceramic fracture in short-term (Bierbaum et al., 2002) and long-term (Hamadouche et al., 2002; Huo et al., 1996; Lusty et al., 2007; Nizard et al., 2008; Yoo et al., 2005) follow-up with ceramic-on-ceramic couplings.

Materials scientists have substantially improved the mechanical strength of alumina. The improved mechanical properties have reduced overall wear rates of 28 mm heads in a hip simulator wear test from $1.84\,mm^3$ to $0.16\,mm^3$ per million cycles, going from alumina-on-alumina to alumina matrix composite (Lombardi et al., 2010). On the other hand, the wear rate of zirconia-on-zirconia couplings is too high to permit use in prosthetic joints. Murakami and Ohtsuki (1989) showed that this type of coupling wore about 5000 times more than alumina-on-alumina. Contradicting results have been reported for zirconia-on-UHMWPE couplings, probably due to the different characteristics (processing, finishing and roughness) of the materials used in the tests as well as to the different testing conditions.

While the US Food and Drug Administration (FDA) approved alumina-on-alumina (Biolox® forte) articulations in 2003 and alumina matrix composite (Biolox® delta) ceramic heads on polyethylene in 2005, the safety and effectiveness of Biolox® delta ceramic heads coupled with Biolox® forte liners are unknown (Lombardi et al., 2010).

The highest rate of component fracture, up to 0.14%, occurred mainly with early-generation alumina femoral heads during the first years of clinical use (Piconi and Maccauro, 1999). Second-generation ceramics showed improvements in the purification of alumina powder, leading to a smaller grain size. This, along with refined manufacturing, increased the density, resulting in a decrease in fracture rate to 0.014% (Lombardi et al., 2010; Tateiwa et al., 2008). Third-generation Biolox® forte fracture rates have been reduced to 0.004% (Lombardi et al., 2010; Tateiwa et al., 2008). In fact, at present, the fracture of alumina heads occurs very infrequently and is mainly due to a severe traumatic accident or technical error.

Knowledge of laboratory wear rate is an important aspect in the pre-clinical validation of prostheses and wear tests are conducted on materials and designs used in prosthetic hip implants to obtain quality control and acquire further knowledge about the tribological processes in joint prostheses. Joint simulator tests have been developed to simulate the biomechanics of human joints in controlled conditions. Results from simulator testing can provide confirmation of the material's performance for a given geometric design under a variety of operating conditions. Different simulator designs provide different wear results for different bearings, as shown in Fig. 10.8; as a consequence, it is not possible to compare the wear behaviour obtained with different simulator rigs even when testing the same prostheses. In any case, it must be noted that wear is a complex phenomenon and accurate reproduction of *in vivo* operating conditions requires knowledge of the role that each one of the factors involved plays in controlling wear.

As shown in Fig. 10.8, under 'ideal' conditions in the laboratory hip joint simulator, extremely low wear rates have been obtained for ceramic-on-ceramic hip prostheses (in the range of 0.01–0.1 mm^3 per million cycles). However, these wear rates are significantly lower than those obtained *in vivo*, typically 1–5 mm^3 per annum (Nevelos *et al.*, 1999). The need to reproduce clinically relevant wear rates *in vitro* has led to several studies

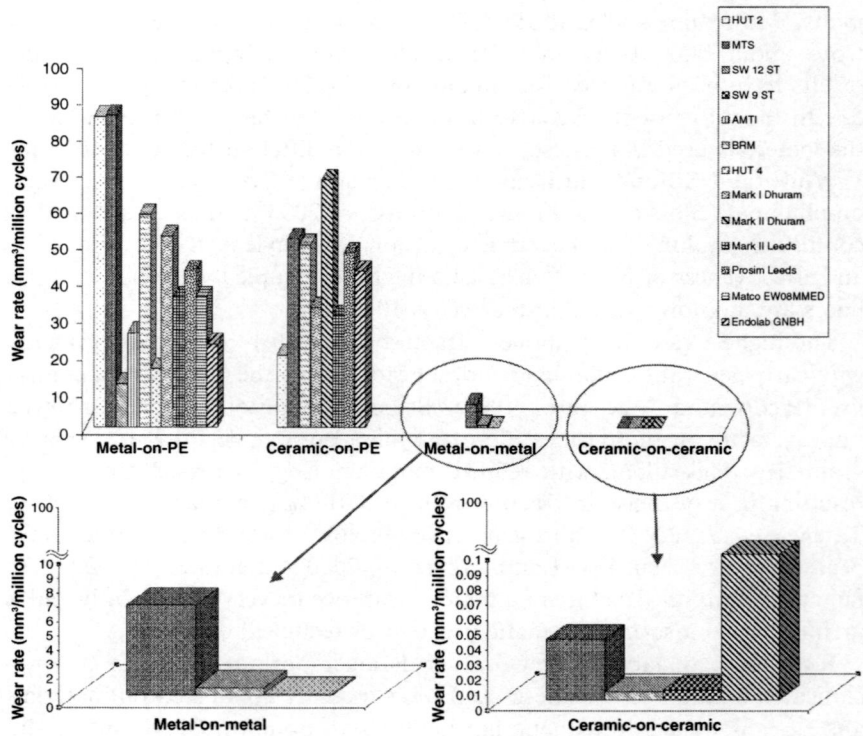

10.8 Volumetric wear data measured for different bearings on all worldwide hip joint simulators.

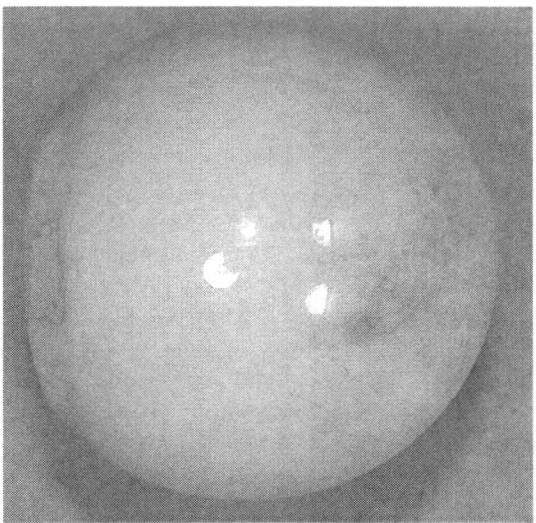

10.9 'Stripe' wear in a retrieved alumina hip femoral head.

investigating the influence of different factors (i.e. composition of lubricant, angle of inclination of the acetabular cup) on wear (Nevelos *et al.*, 1999, 2001).

Examination of retrieved alumina-on-alumina hip prostheses (manufactured after 1995) revealed a small band of wear ('stripe' wear, Fig. 10.9) around the rim of the acetabular cups (Nevelos *et al.*, 2000), similar to that found in retrieved first-generation alumina-on-alumina prostheses (Nevelos *et al.*, 1999). This phenomenon could be associated with the microseparation between the head and the cup: the femoral head and acetabular insert can separate during the swing phase of normal walking in the direction of the cup axis (Nevelos *et al.*, 2000) and the femoral head moves vertically (inferior and superior contact) until relocated in the cup (Mak *et al.*, 2002). This phenomenon is illustrated in Fig. 10.10. This microseparation mechanism could explain the initiation of stripe wear observed on retrieved ceramic-on-ceramic hip prostheses. Introducing microseparation into *in vitro* wear simulator studies, Nevelos and co-workers reproduced, for the first time, the wear rates, patterns and mechanisms observed *in vivo* (Nevelos *et al.*, 2000; Tipper *et al.*, 2002).

10.3.2 Wear in total knee replacements

In the field of total knee arthroplasty (TKA), ceramic materials were introduced by Langer in 1973 (Langer, 2002) in unicompartmental implants. Since then until the early 1980s, experience with ceramic TKA was almost

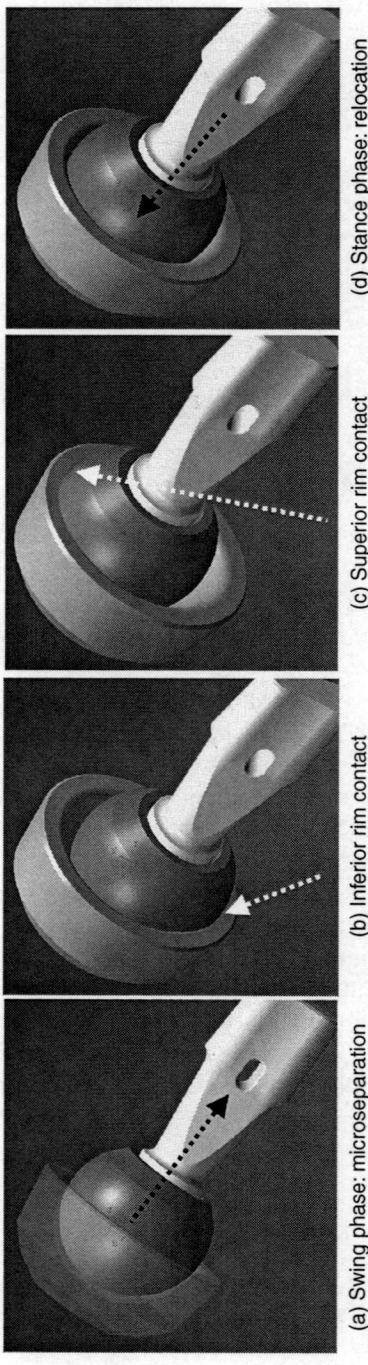

10.10 Schematization of the microseparation phenomenon.

exclusively in Japan (Akagi et al., 2000; Koshino et al., 2002). This was based on the use of alumina; prosthetic designs were either cruciate-retaining or posterior-stabilised and the coupling was always ceramic-on-polyethylene. The first implants were produced by Kyocera Corp. and performed by Oonishi et al. (2005).

The designs required in TKA (in particular for the femoral component) and the contact conditions need to be of an adequate size to avoid stress forces at the edges of the femoral resections (traction stress) and at the points of contact with the polyethylene (contact stress under the surface) (Benazzo et al., 2007). Alumina prostheses are therefore thicker than equivalent metal implants and thus require a larger bone resection. This problem was only partially resolved with the introduction of zirconia, while new designs have been made possible by the introduction of Biolox® delta (Dalla Pria and Burger, 2003). At the moment, only preliminary studies on Biolox® delta femoral components have been performed; they were carried out by CeramTec in collaboration with the Orthopaedic Institute of Rizzoli (Bologna, Italy) (Cristofolini et al., 2009). Wear results are under review and will be published soon.

10.4 References

Affatato, S., Testoni, M., Cacciari, G. L. and Toni, A. (1999) Mixed oxides prosthetic ceramic ball heads. Part 2: effect of the ZrO_2 fraction on the wear of ceramic on ceramic joints. *Biomaterials*, 20, 1925–9.

Affatato, S., Goldoni, M., Testoni, M. and Toni, A. (2001) Mixed oxides prosthetic ceramic ball heads. Part 3: effect of the ZrO_2 fraction on the wear of ceramic on ceramic hip joint prostheses. A long-term in vitro study. *Biomaterials*, 22, 717–23.

Affatato, S., Torrecillas, R., Taddei, P., Rocchi, M., Fagnano, C., Ciapetti, G. and Toni, A. (2006) Advanced nanocomposite materials for orthopaedic applications. I. A long-term in vitro wear study of zirconia-toughened alumina. *J Biomed Mater Res B Appl Biomater*, 78B, 76–82.

Akagi, M., Nakamura, T., Matsusue, Y., Ueo, T., Nishijyo, K. and Ohnishi, E. (2000) The bisurface total knee replacement: a unique design for flexion. Four-to-nine-year follow-up study. *J Bone Joint Surg Am*, 82, 1626–33.

Benazzo, F., Macchi, F., Rossi, S. and Dalla Pria, P. (2007) Ceramic total knee arthroplasty–an update. *Euro Musculoskel Rev*, 2, 59–62.

Bierbaum, B. E., Nairus, J., Kuesis, D., Morrison, J. C. and Ward, D. (2002) Ceramic-on-ceramic bearings in total hip arthroplasty. *Clin Orthop Relat Res*, 405, 158–63.

Boehler, M., Knahr, K., Plenk, H., Walter, A., Salzer, M. and Schreiber, V. (1994) Long-term results of uncemented alumina acetabular implants. *J Bone Joint Surg Br*, 76B, 53–9.

Boutin, P. (1972) Arthroplastie total de la hanche par prosthèse on alumina frittèe. *Rev Chir Orthop*, 58, 229–46.

Brown, S. S. and Clarke, I. C. (2006) A review of lubricant conditions for wear simulation in artificial hip joint replacements. *Trib Trans*, 49, 72–8.

Burger, W. and Richter, H. G. (2001) High strength and toughness alumina matrix composites by transformation toughening and 'in situ' platelet reinforcement (ZPTA)–the new generation of bioceramics. *Key Eng Mater*, 192–5, 545–8.

Callaghan, J. J., Cuckler, J. M., Huddleston, J. I. and Galante, J. O. (2008) How have alternative bearings (such as metal-on-metal, highly cross-linked polyethylene, and ceramic-on-ceramic) affected the prevention and treatment of osteolysis? *J Am Acad Orthop Surg*, 16, S33–S38.

Chevalier, J. (2006) What future for zirconia as a biomaterial? *Biomaterials*, 27, 535–43.

Chevalier, J., Deville, S., Fantozzi, G., Bartolomé, J. F., Pecharroman, C., Moya, J. S., Diaz, L. A. and Torrecillas, R. (2005) Nanostructured ceramic oxides with a slow crack growth resistance close to covalent materials. *Nanoletters*, 5, 1297–301.

Chevalier, J., Gremillard, L. and Deville, S. (2007) Low temperature degradation of zirconia and implications on biomedical implants. *Ann Rev Mater Res*, 37, 1–32.

Costa, H. L., Pandolfelli, V. C. and Biasoli de Mello, J. D. (1997) On the abrasive wear of zirconias. *Wear*, 203–4, 626–36.

Cristofolini, L., Affatato, S., Erani, P., Tigani, D. and Viceconti, M. (2009) Implant fixation in knee replacement: Preliminary in vitro comparison of ceramic and metal cemented femoral components. *The Knee*, 6, 101–8.

Cuckler, J. M., Moore, K. D., Lombardi, A. V. J., McPherson, E. and Emerson, R. (2004) Large versus small femoral heads in metal-on-metal total hip arthroplasty. *J Arthroplasty*, 19, 41–4.

Dalla Pria, P. and Burger, W. (2003) Una nuova ceramica per l'ortopedia: BIOLOX® Delta. *Riv Patol Appar Locom*, 2, 63–9.

De Aza, A. H., Chevalier, J., Fantozzi, G., Schehl, M. and Torrecillas, R. (2002) Crack growth resistance of alumina, zirconia and zirconia toughened alumina ceramics for joint prostheses. *Biomaterials*, 23, 937–45.

Derbyshire, B., Fisher, J., Dowson, D., Hardaker, C. and Brummitt, K. (1994) Comparative study of the wear of UHMWPE with zirconia ceramic and stainless steel femoral heads in artificial hip joints. *Med Eng Phys*, 16, 229–36.

Deville, S., Chevalier, J., Fantozzi, G., Bartolomé, J. F., Requena, J., Moya, J. S., Torrecillas, R. and Diaz, L. A. (2003) Low-temperature ageing of zirconia-toughened alumina ceramics and its implication in biomedical implants. *J Euro Ceram Soc*, 23, 2975–82.

Dorn, M. T. and Nickel, K. G. (2004) Zirconia ceramics: phase transitions and Raman microspectroscopy. In Gogotsi, Y. and Domnich, V. (eds) *High-pressure Surface Science and Engineering*. London, IOP Publishing Ltd, pp. 467–520.

Fisher, J., Ingham, E., Stone, M. H., Wroblewski, B. M., Besong, A. A., Tipper, J., Firkins, P., Minakawa, H., Matthews, J. B. and Green, T. (1999) Wear particle morphologies in artificial hip joints: particle size is critical in the response of macrophages. In Rieker, C., Windler, M. and Wyss, U. (eds) *Metasul–A Metal-on-Metal Bearing*. Bern, Hans Huber, pp. 121–4.

Fisher, J., Jin, Z., Tipper, J., Stone, M. and Ingham, E. (2006) Tribology of alternative bearings. *Clin Orthop Relat Res*, 453, 25–34.

Fruh, H. J., Willmann, G. and Pfaff, H. G. (1997) Wear characteristics of ceramic-on-ceramic for hip endoprostheses. *Biomaterials*, 18, 873–8.

Hamadouche, M., Boutin, P., Daussange, J., Bolander, M. E. and Sedel, L. (2002) Alumina-on-alumina total hip arthroplasty: a minimum 18.5 year follow-up study. *J Bone Joint Surg Am*, 84, 69–77.

Hench, L. L. and Hethridge, E. C. (1975) Biomaterials – the interfacial problem. *Adv Biomed Eng*, 5, 35–50.

Higgins, R. A. (1994) Ceramics and glasses. In Arnold, E. (ed) *Properties of Engineering Materials*. London. Edward Arnold, pp. 315–44.

Hsu, S. M. C. (1996) Ceramic wear maps. *Wear*, 200, 154–175.

Huo, M. H., Martin, R. P., Zatorski, L. E. and Keggi K, J. (1996) Ceramic total hip replacements done without cement: an average 9-year follow-up study. *Clin Orthop Relat Res*, 332, 143–50.

Ingham, E. and Fisher, J. (2000) Biological reactions to wear debris in total joint replacement. *Proc Inst Mech Eng, Part H: J Eng Med*, 214, 21–37.

Insley, G. M. and Streicher, R. M. (2004) Next generation ceramic based on zirconia toughened alumina for hip joint prostheses. *Key Eng Mater*, 192–195, 781–4.

Katagiri, G., Ishida, H., Ishitani, A. and Masaki, T. (1988) Direct determination by a Raman microprobe of the transformation zone size in Y_2O_3 containing tetragonal ZrO_2 polycrystals. *Adv Ceram*, 24A, 537–44.

Koshino, T., Okamoto, R., Takagi, T., Yamamoto, K. and Saito, T. (2002) Cemented ceramic YMCK total knee arthroplasty in patients with severe rheumatoid arthritis. *J Arthroplasty*, 17, 1009–15.

Langer, G. (2002) Ceramic tibial plateau of the 70s. *In Bioceramics in Joint Arthroplasty. 7th International BIOLOX® Symposium*. Stuttgart, Thieme, pp. 128–30.

Li, J. and Hastings, G. W. (1999) Oxide bioceramics: inert ceramic materials in medicine and dentistry. In Black, J. and Hastings, G. (eds) *Biomaterial Properties*. London, Chapman & Hall, pp. 340–53.

Lombardi JR, A. V., Berend, K. R., Seng, B. E., Clarke, I. C. and Adams, J. B. (2010) Delta ceramic-on-alumina ceramic articulation in primary THA. *Clin Orthop Relat Res*, 468, 367–4.

Lusty, P. J., Tai, C. C., Sew-Hoy, R. P., Walter, W. L., Walter, W. K. and Zicat, B. A. (2007) Third-generation alumina-on-alumina ceramic bearings in cementless total hip arthroplasty. *J Bone Joint Surg Am*, 89, 2676–83.

Macchi, F. (2004) Alumina ceramics in joint prostheses. *J Bone Joint Surg Br*, 87B, 187–8.

Macchi, F. and Willman, G. (2001) Allumina Biolox forte: evoluzione, stato dell'arte e affidabilità. *Lo Scalpello*, 15, 99–106.

Mai, K., Hardwick, M. E., Walker R. H., Copp, S. N., Ezzet, K. A. and Colwell, C. W. J. (2008) Early dislocation rate in ceramic-on-ceramic total hip arthroplasty. *HSS J*, 4, 10–3.

Mak, M. M., Besong, A. A., Jin, Z. M. and Fisher, J. (2002) Effect of microseparation on contact mechanics in ceramic-on-ceramic hip joint replacements. *Proc Inst Mech Eng Part H: J Eng Med*, 216, 403–8.

Murakami, T. and Ohtsuki, N. (1989) Friction and wear characteristics of sliding pairs of bioceramics and polyethylene. In Oonishi, H., Aoki, H. and Sawai, K. (eds) *Bioceramics*. Brentwood, MO, Ishiyaku EuroAmerica Inc., pp. 365–72.

Nevelos, J., Ingham, E., Doyle, C., Streicher, R., Nevelos, A., Walter, W. and Fisher, J. (2000) Microseparation of the centres of alumina–alumina artificial hip joints during simulator testing produces clinically relevant wear rates and patterns. *J Arthroplasty*, 15, 793–5.

Nevelos, J. E., Ingham, E., Doyle, C., Fisher, J. and Nevelos, A. B. (1999) Analysis of retrieved alumina ceramic components from Mittelmeier total hip prostheses. *Biomaterials*, 20, 1833–40.

Nevelos, J. E., Ingham, E., Doyle, C., Nevelos, A. B. and Fisher, J. (2001) The influence of acetabular cup angle on the wear of 'BIOLOX Forte' alumina ceramic bearing couples in a hip joint simulator. *J Mater Sci Mater Med*, 12, 141–4.

Nizard, R., Pourreyron, D., Raould, A., Hannouche, D. and Sedel, L. (2008) Alumina-on-alumina hip arthroplasty in patients younger than 30 years old. *Clin Orthop Relat Res*, 466, 317–23.

Oonishi, H., Kim, S. C., Kyomoto, M., Masuda, S., Asano, T. and Clarke, I. C. (2005) Change in UHMWPE properties of retrieved ceramic total knee prosthesis in clinical use for 23 years. *J Biomed Mater Res B Appl Biomater*, 74, 754–9.

Pattyn, C. and De Smet, K. A. (2008) Primary ceramic-on-ceramic total hip replacement versus metal-on-metal hip resurfacing in young active patients. *Orthopedics*, 31, 1078.

Pezzotti, G. and Porporati, A. A. (2004) Raman spectroscopic analysis of phase transformation and stress patterns in zirconia hip joints. *J Biomed Opt*, 9, 372–84.

Pezzotti, G., Yamada, K., Sakakura, S. and Pitto, R. P. (2008) Raman spectroscopic analysis of advanced ceramic composite for hip prosthesis. *J Am Ceram Soc*, 91, 1199–206.

Piconi, C. and Maccauro, G. (1999) Zirconia as a ceramic biomaterial. *Biomaterials*, 20, 1–25.

Piconi, C., Maccauro, G., Muratori, F. and Brach del Prever, E. (2003) Alumina and zirconia ceramics in joint replacements. *J Appl Biomater Biomech*, 1, 19–32.

Ravaglioli, A. and Krajewski, A. (1992) Materials for surgical use. In Hall, C. (ed) *Bioceramics: Materials, Properties, Applications*. London, Springer, pp. 100–96.

Rhoads, D. P., Baker, K. C., Israel, R. and Greene, P. W. (2008) Fracture of an alumina femoral head used in ceramic-on-ceramic total hip arthroplasty. *J Arthroplasty*, 23, 25–30.

Rose, R. M., Nusbaum, H. J., Schneider, H., Ries, M., Paul, I., Crugnola, A., Simon, S. R. and Radin, E. L. (1980) On the true wear rate of ultra high-molecular-weight polyethylene in the total hip prosthesis. *J Bone Joint Surg Am*, 62, 537–49.

Schilling, C. H., Garcia, V., Li, C. P. and Jakowiak, R. (2002) Luminescence imaging of surface cracks and surface-density gradients in alumina. *Am Ceram Soc Bull*, 81, 5–30.

Shishido, T., Clarke, I. C., Williams, P., Boehler, M., Asano, T., Shoji, H., Masaoka, T., Yamamoto, K. and Imakiire, A. (2003) Clinical and simulator wear study of alumina ceramic THR to 17 years and beyond. *J Biomed Mater Res B Appl Biomater*, 67, 638–47.

Stea, S., Bordini, B., De Clerico, M., Petropulacos, K. and Toni, A. (2009) First hip arthroplasty register in Italy: 55,000 cases and 7 year follow-up. *Int Orthop*, 33, 339–46.

Tabares, J. A. M. and Anglada, M. J. (2010) Quantitative analysis of monoclinic phase in 3Y-TZP by Raman spectroscopy. *J Am Ceram Soc*, 93, 1790–5.

Tateiwa, T., Clarke, I. C., Williams, P. A., Garino, J., Manaka, M., Shishido, T., Yamamoto, K. and Imakiire, A. (2008) Ceramic total hip arthroplasty in the United States: safety and risk issues revisited. *Am J Orthop*, 37, E26–E31.

Tipper, J. L., Hatton, A., Nevelos, J. E., Ingham, E., Doyle, C., Streicher, R., Nevelos, A. B. and Fisher, J. (2002) Alumina–alumina artificial hip joints. Part II: characterisation of the wear debris from in vitro hip joint simulations. *Biomaterials*, 23, 3441–8.

Toni, A., Terzi, S., Sudanese, A., Tabarroni, M., Zappoli, F. A., Stea, S. and Giunti, A. (1995) The use of ceramic in prosthetic hip surgery. The state of the art. *Chir Organi Mov*, 80, 13–25.

Toni, A., Traina, F., Stea, S., Sudanese, A., Visentin, M., Bordini, B. and Squarzoni, S. (2006) Early diagnosis of ceramic liner fracture. Guidelines based on a twelve-year clinical experience. *J Bone Joint Surg Am*, 88, 55–63.

Willmann, G. (1998) Ceramics for total hip replacement–what a surgeon should know. *Orthopedics*, 21, 173–7.

Willmann, G. (2000) The evolution of ceramics in total hip replacement. *Hip Int*, 10, 193–203.

Willmann, G., Fruh, H. J. and Pfaff, H. G. (1996) Wear characteristics of sliding pairs of zirconia (Y-TZP) for hip endoprostheses. *Biomaterials*, 17, 2157–62.

Yoo, J. J., Kim, Y. M., Yoon, K. S., Koo, K. H., Song, W. S. and Kim, H. J. (2005) Alumina-on-alumina total hip arthroplasty: a five-year minimum follow-up study. *J Bone Joint Surg Am*, 87, 530–5.

11
The influence of surgical techniques on implant wear

X. FLECHER, S. PARRATTE, J. M. AUBANIAC and
J. N. ARGENSON, Institut du Mouvement et de l'Appareil
Locomoteur, France

Abstract: Joint replacement is an extremely successful orthopaedic procedure, commonly resulting in pain relief and activity recovery. However, it is recognised that, in the longer term, polyethylene (PE) wear particles generated at the articulating surfaces lead to chronic inflammatory tissue reactions, osteolysis and loosening of the prostheses. PE wear is a multi-factorial phenomenon influenced by some patient-related factors, such as gender, age, activity level and weight. In hip arthroplasty, femoral head size and composition and PE quality and configuration are also related to wear. Surgical technique can also influence PE wear, because increased contact stress between the articular surfaces can be reduced by accurate component positioning. Regarding knee arthroplasty, many structural and design factors related to the PE bearing surface have been shown to affect the extent of wear that occurs over time (e.g. PE processing, manufacturing and sterilization methods). Selecting a well-designed component with minimal counter surface roughness is also important in minimizing the generation of PE wear debris and subsequent osteolysis. This chapter describes current knowledge of the influence of surgical technique on total hip and knee arthroplasty.

Key words: polyethylene wear, arthroplasty, hip, knee, surgical technique.

11.1 Introduction

Joint replacement is probably the most successful modern orthopaedic procedure; artificial joints commonly provide pain relief and result in activity recovery. Over the last 30 years, the majority of these prostheses have used clinically ultra-high molecular weight polyethylene (UHMWPE) as the bearing surface. These bearing surfaces are very effective and rarely wear out but it is now recognised that, in the longer term, micron and submicron UHMWPE wear particles generated at the articulating surfaces lead to chronic inflammatory tissue reactions, osteolysis and loosening of the prostheses.

Polyethylene (PE) wear is a multi-factorial phenomenon influenced by some patient-related factors, such as gender, age, activity level and weight.[1–4] In hip arthroplasty, femoral head size[5] and composition[6–8] and PE quality and configuration can also impact upon wear.[9, 10] Finally, surgical technique may influence PE wear, because increased contact stress between the articular surfaces can be reduced by accurate component positioning; the center of hip location,[11] the cup inclination[12] and the femoral offset have been noted as factors.[13, 14]

There are many structural and design factors relating to the PE bearing surface in knee arthroplasty that have been shown to affect the extent of wear that occurs over time. For instance, the processing, manufacturing and sterilization methods of polyethylene are all critical factors in determining its mechanical and wear-resistant properties. Selecting a well-designed component with minimal counter surface roughness is also important in minimizing the generation of PE wear debris and subsequent osteolysis. Finally, while the importance of restoring rotational alignment is well-known to avoid 'lift-off' of the condyles, and ligamentous balancing has been shown to influence stresses on the tibial tray, the influence of mechanical axis restoration on wear remains debated.

11.2 Hip arthroplasty

11.2.1 Acetabular side

During hip arthroplasty, the surgeon aims to choose the best cup orientation (inclination and anteversion) and position (hip center), as well as femoral positioning (offset, length and rotation). Correct acetabular orientation may reduce contact stresses.[15, 16] Orientation of the positioned cup is typically 45° relative to the horizontal plane and 20° anteverted.[17, 18] Adverse factors such as higher cup angles should be associated with greater amounts of linear wear. However, the literature is equivocal regarding the exact effect of acetabular orientation on linear and volumetric PE wear.[19–22]

Biomechanical considerations such as medialization of the acetabular cup have also been shown to be beneficial in decreasing wear rates.[23] Medialization of the cup would predictably have less effect on hip mechanics than lateralization of the femur. The moment arm extending from the midline of the body to the hip center is much larger than the moment arm from the hip center to the tip of the greater trochanter. Thus, the latter moment arm would be much more sensitive to changes in length. However, inadequate medialization of the hip center may modify long-term results[24, 25] and superior or lateral placement of the cup may increase the risk of loosening in both the femoral and the acetabular component, because joint loads are greater in the superior-lateral position than in the medial-inferior position.[26–30] This higher risk of aseptic loosening is both due to failure at the bone–implant acetabular interface and increase in wear. Conversely, restoring the normal hip center of rotation has provided good long-term results.[31–33] It allows the restoration of leg length and lever arm with an appropriate femoral offset, which contributes to a better function.[34, 35] Few studies have analyzed hip center restoration after total hip arthroplasty (THA).[35, 36] Eggli and Muller[37] reported a good precision for hip center planning, but they did not analyze whether the center was closely restored to the natural one before the hip was damaged by osteoarthritis. Sariali et al.[38] performed three-dimensional (3D) preoperative THA planning in 223 patients and showed that they precisely restored the proper hip center. However, to date, no study has specifically related the influence of hip center location to wear.

11.2.2 Femoral side

Among all the factors involved in acetabular cup or stem positioning, femoral offset is known to influence the results of THA.[39–41] This represents femoral lateralization and has been defined as the distance from the center of the femoral head to the femoral diaphysis axis.[42] Adequate femoral lateralization has been shown to enhance hip stability,[40] improve the range of motion and abductor strength,[43] and decrease contact force and thus polyethylene wear.[44] The degree of offset of the femoral prosthesis theoretically influences the mechanics of the hip after THA. An increased offset increases the moment arm of the abductor muscles. This reduces the abductor force required for normal gait and consequently reduces the force across the hip. Of course, this is a simplified interpretation of gait, because other muscles about the hip in addition to the abductors are active during walking.

Recent clinical studies demonstrated that an increase of femoral offset could significantly decrease wear,[44] while this increase could also cause early aseptic loosening of the femoral stem by increasing the bending moment.[45] It is unclear, however, how a surgeon should decide on the proper post-operative femoral offset value in THA, from a strict pre-operative reproduction to an 'ideal' value, based on clinical or biomechanical considerations.

To the authors' knowledge, very few studies have reported the influence of femoral offset on wear. Sakalkale et al.[44] reviewed 17 staged, bilateral THAs performed in 17 patients to compare side-to-side polyethylene wear. The implants used on both sides were similar except for implant offset: one hip in each patient was replaced using a femoral component having a standard implant offset, whereas the other side had a lateral offset implant. The only statistically different parameter between the sides was the femoral component offset. On the side with a standard femoral component, the mean prosthetic offset (determined by manufacturer's specifications) was 35.2 mm and the radiologic offset was 31.5 mm. All other parameters affecting polyethylene wear, such as period of follow-up, head size, head type, cup size, cup inclination, medialization of cup and patient-related factors were similar on both sides. The mean pre-operative radiographic offset of the femur was 38.8 mm. Regression analysis revealed that only femoral component offset and cup size correlated significantly with linear wear rate. On the side with a standard femoral component, the linear wear rate was 0.21 mm per year, whereas on the side with a lateralized femoral component, the linear wear rate was 0.10 mm per year. The differences in the linear wear rates were thus significant.

Lateralization of the femoral component in this series more closely restored pre-operative hip biomechanics and significantly decreased polyethylene wear. Patients with a lateral offset implant had an increase in femoral offset, as determined radiographically, by a mean of 8.6 mm; this led to a reduction in the linear polyethylene wear rate by 52.4% (linear wear rate of 0.10 mm per year versus a linear wear rate of 0.21 mm per year). However, the disadvantage of an increased offset is an increased bending moment on the implant. This could adversely increase the stress through the femoral prosthesis and lead to stem breakage. An increase in offset also could lead to increased stress at the bone–implant interface, which could cause loosening of the femoral component, or failure to achieve bone ingrowth.

However, in another study, Davey et al.[46] reported there was no significant increase in strain across the medial cement mantle of a femoral component with greater offset. While studying the effect of offset on uncemented THA, Wong et al.[47] concluded that, even if an increase in offset led to increased stress at the bone–implant interface, it did not affect the amount of bone ingrowth. Devane and Horne[48] studied the factors affecting PE wear in THA. They compared the ability of two different THAs to restore normal femoral offset. They then compared PE wear in the two groups. In the implant that restored femoral offset to within 1 mm of normal, there was no correlation between offset and wear. In the implant that reduced native femoral offset by an average of 7 mm, they observed a strong correlation between reducing femoral offset in the reconstructed THA and increased PE wear. They concluded that under-restoration of femoral offset leads to an increase in PE wear.[48]

Femoral anteversion may also theoretically affect wear, and the adequate value, pre-operative templating and intraoperative restitution are all unknown. Assuming an accepted normal value of femoral anteversion close to 15°,[41, 49] it was found that, using CT scan pre-operative analysis, great individual variation occurred, ranging from 2° to 80° in a previous study on a DDH (developmental dysplasia of the hip) patient[50] and from −22° to 85° in patients aged under 50 years.[51] Two-dimensional (2D) radiographic offset templating meets some limitations regarding the influence of anteversion on femoral offset measurement. In the case of the presence of hip deformity or contracture, femoral anteversion value may influence 2D femoral offset assessment, which can be underestimated.[52]

Sariali et al.[53] reported an analysis of 223-osteoarthritic hips using CT and a specific image processing software to determine 3D morphological data of the hip, focusing on femoral offset. Mean femoral offset was found to be 42.2 ± 5.1 mm, 2.2 mm greater than the 2D values reported in the literature. The femoral offset was found to be above 45 mm in 31% of patients and greater than 50 mm in 12%. The error associated with the use of conventional plane X-rays to measure femoral offset was found to be 3.5 ± 2.5 mm, with the X-ray technique generally underestimating the measure of femoral offset. The sum of acetabular and femoral anteversion was found to be out of the safe zone regarding dislocation risk in 47% of patients.

Furthermore, femoral anteversion cannot yet be accurately measured or reproduced. Differences of up to 22° between pre- and post-operative femoral anteversion have been measured.[54] Intraoperative tools to reproduce the femoral offset have been described,[55] while Sarin et al.[56] showed that inaccurate intraoperative femur positioning had an adverse effect on the precision of intraoperative femoral offset restoration. Moreover, with contemporary canal-filling press-fit stems, there is poor adjustability of stem position in the canal and therefore the canal anatomy determines stem version. Emerson[57] compared 64 hips studied with fluoroscopy to 46 non-arthritic and 41 arthritic hips studied with MRI for determining pre-operative and post-operative femoral version following THA. For the hips that had been operated upon, the mean anatomic hip version was less than the stem version: 18.9° versus 27.0°. The difference on average was 8.1° of increased anteversion (standard deviation, 7.4°). Both MRI series showed that the femoral neck was more anteverted on average than the femoral head, thereby explaining the operative findings.

Component positioning can influence impingement between the prosthetic neck and the liner, and is a factor that contributes to failure in total hip replacement (THR), causing instability and early wear. Its true frequency is unknown, but cup-retrieval series reported rates varying from 27 to 84%. Marchetti et al.[58] studied a series of 416 cups retrieved during revision for various reasons. Macroscopic examination looked for component impingement signs. Risk factors were investigated by uni- and multi-variate analyses in the 311 cases for which there were complete demographic data. In these 311 cases, removal was for aseptic loosening (131 cases), infection (43 cases), instability (56 cases), osteolysis (28 cases) or unexplained pain (48 cases). Impingement was found in 214 of the 416 cups (51.4%) and was severe (notch > 1 mm) in 130 (31.3%). In the sub-population of 311 cups, impingement was found in 184 cases (59.2%) and was severe in 109 (35%). Neither the duration of implant use nor cup diameter or frontal orientation emerged as risk factors. On univariate analysis, impingement was more frequently associated with revision for instability, young patient age at THR, global hip range of motion > 200° or use of an extended femoral head flange (or of an elevated anti-dislocation rim liner), and was more severe in the case of a head/neck ratio <2. On multi-variate analysis, only use of an extended head flange (RR 3.2) and revision for instability (RR 4.2) remained as independent risk factors for impingement.

It is hypothesized that a custom neck based on pre-operative 3D analysis may provide adequate femoral offset and version correction. The authors recently reported encouraging clinical and radiological results of THA with individual femoral 3D positioning in high-risk populations, such as osteoarthritis secondary to developmental dysplasia of the hip[50] or patients under 50,[51] with a survivorship respectively of 89.5% at 13 years and 96.1% at 10 years. However, no wear analysis was performed in these studies. With this same stem customized design associated to a hemispheric titanium press-fit cup, poor PE wear was found in an unpublished study of wear using Imagika system on 97 hips at the minimum follow-up of 10 years, with a mean linear annual wear of 0.09 ± 0.05 mm/per year. Our results compared favorably with average wear published with metal-backed cups. Woolson and Murphy[59] found a mean rate of 0.14 ± 0.09 mm (range 0–0.35 mm) per year in 80 Harris–Galante acetabular components at a mean follow-up of 68 months, whereas Devane et al.[43] reported a mean rate of linear wear of 0.15 mm/per year in 80 consecutive Harris–Galante I total hip arthroplasties at a mean follow-up of 5.78 ± 1.28 years. Eight hips (10%) had radiologic osteolysis around either the femoral or acetabular component.[43]

11.3 Knee arthroplasty

Once a problem primarily associated with THA, osteolysis has also now emerged as a significant problem in total knee arthroplasty (TKA). The development of osteolysis is often related to wear of the PE bearing surface, resulting in the production of biologically active particulate debris. Many structural and design factors related to the PE bearing surface have been shown to affect the extent of wear that occurs over time. For instance, the processing, manufacturing and sterilization methods of PE all are critical factors in determining its mechanical and wear-resistant properties. Cross-linking of PE bearing surfaces in TKA, however, may not demonstrate the same degree of improved resistance to wear as seen in THA. Optimization of PE bearing surface thickness, with a goal to insert at least 8 mm of PE, has been shown to minimize contact stresses and subsequent fatigue failure of total knee implants. Selecting a well-designed component with minimal counter surface roughness is also important in minimizing the generation of PE wear debris and subsequent osteolysis. Finally, proper surgical technique, including restoration of mechanical axis, rotational alignment and ligamentous balancing is critical to minimizing wear and maximizing the longevity of TKAs.

One long-held tenet of TKA is that, to promote implant durability, the overall post-operative limb alignment should be corrected to within $0° \pm 3°$ of the mechanical axis (as defined by the center of the femoral head and the center of the talus).[60] Finite-element analysis,[61] *in vitro* studies involving a knee simulator[62] and cadaver studies[63, 64] have supported the contention that a mechanical axis of $0° \pm 3°$ results in more favorable knee loading. A careful review of the available literature, however, suggests that the scientific clinical support for the widely held contention that a post-operative mechanical axis of $0° \pm 3°$ will improve implant survival following total knee arthroplasty is surprisingly weak.[65–70] Thus, given that a target of $0° \pm 3°$ is a relatively broad and generic target that does not account for patient-specific differences in gait dynamics, it is reasonable to ask whether hitting that broad, generic target provides a clinically meaningful improvement in decreasing wear after TKA.

Rotational alignement can lead to an abnormal 'lift-off' of the condyles, causing higher stress on the PE insert. Dennis *et al.*[71] carried out weight-bearing video radiological studies on 40 patients with a TKA in order to determine the presence and magnitude of femoral condylar lift-off. Half (20) had posterior-cruciate-retaining (PCR) and half (20) had posterior-cruciate-substituting (PS) prostheses. The selected patients had successful arthroplasties with no pain or instability. Each carried out successive weight-bearing knee bends to maximum flexion and the radiological video tapes were analysed using an interactive model-fitting technique. Femoral lift-off was seen at some increment of knee flexion in 75% of patients (PCR TKA 70%; PS TKA 80%). The mean values for lift-off were 1.2 mm with a PCR TKA and 1.4 mm with a PS TKA. Lift-off mostly occurred laterally with the PCR TKA, and both medially and laterally with the PS TKA. Separation between the femoral condyles and the articular surface of the tibia was recorded at 0°, 30°, 60° and 90° of flexion. Femoral condylar lift-off may contribute to eccentric PE wear, particularly in designs of TKA that have flatter condyles.

Ligamentous balancing is also a crucial part of TKA in order to ensure proper kinematics. Failure to do so may result in a limited range of motion, premature PE wear or patello-femoral tracking problems. Balancing in extension is dependent on the type and extent of correctional ligamentous release. Flexion balance is dependent on proper femoral rotation. There are two methods to determine femoral rotation. In the classic method, the knee is tensed in flexion after ligamentous release in extension. The anteroposterior cut then is made parallel to the cut tibial surface. Alternatively, the anteroposterior cut can be based on fixed femoral landmarks. Fehring[72] determined the variance between balancing the flexion gap with the classic method versus the technique of using fixed femoral landmarks to determine rotation. Using the classic method, 100 consecutive posterior-stabilized knee arthroplasties were performed and the resected posterior condyles in each case were measured. The difference between the resected condyles using the classic method was compared with the calculated difference of resected bone using bony landmarks to determine rotation. A variance analysis then was performed. Compared with classically balanced knees, rotational errors of at least 3° occurred in 45% of patients when rotation was determined from fixed bony landmarks. These patients had trapezoidal rather than rectangular flexion gaps. Such errors may have implications regarding PE wear, range of motion and long-term clinical results.

11.4 Conclusion

Long-term failure of joint arthroplasty is mainly related to wear and osteolysis. This is a multi-faceted problem that includes patient-related, implant, manufacturing and surgical factors. Surgical techniques have been widely studied, mainly in hip arthroplasty, which remains the most widely implanted joint arthroplasty. Biomechanics studies and the relationship between fundamental and clinical aspects are both necessary to further our understanding of how 3D individual reconstruction of joints can positively influence wear and thus increase longevity.

11.5 References

1. Bennett D, Humphreys L, O'Brien S, Kelly C, Orr J and Beverland DE (2008) Activity levels and polyethylene wear of patients 10 years post hip replacement. *Clin Biomech*, 23, 571–6.
2. Kobayashi S, Eftekhar NS and Terayama K (1997) Comparative study of total hip arthroplasty between younger and older patients. *Clin Orthop*, 339, 140–51.
3. Livermore J, Ilstrup D and Morrey B (1990) Effect of femoral head size on wear of the polyethylene acetabular component. *J Bone Joint Surg Am*, 72, 518–28.
4. Schmalzried TP and Huk OL (2004) Patient factors and wear in total hip arthroplasty. *Clin Orthop Relat Res*, 418, 94–7.
5. Lee PC, Shih CH, Chen WJ, Tu YK and Tai CL (1999) Early polyethylene wear

and osteolysis in cementless total hip arthroplasty: the influence of femoral head size and polyethylene thickness. *J Arthroplasty*, 14, 976–81.
6. Davidson JA (1993) Characteristics of metal and ceramic total hip bearing surfaces and their effect on longterm ultra high molecular weight polyethylene wear. *Clin Orthop*, 294, 361–78.
7. Saikko V, Paavolainen P and Slatis P (1993) Wear of the polyethylene acetabular cup: metallic and ceramic heads compared in a hip simulator. *Acta Orthop Scand*, 64, 391–402.
8. Tanaka K, Tamura J, Kawanabe K, Shimizu M and Nakamura T (2003) Effect of alumina femoral heads on polyethylene wear in cemented total hip arthroplasty. Old versus current alumina. *J Bone Joint Surg Br*, 85, 655–60.
9. Bankston AB, Cates H, Ritter MA, Keating EM and Faris PM (1995) Polyethylene wear in total hip arthroplasty. *Clin Orthop*, 317, 7–13.
10. Bragdon CR, Kwon YM, Geller JA, Greene ME, Freiberg AA, Harris WH and Malchau H (2007) Minimum 6-year followup of highly cross-linked polyethylene in THA. *Clin Orthop Relat Res*, 465, 122–7.
11. Karachalios T, Hartofilakidis G, Zacharakis N and Tsekoura M (1993) A 12- to 18-year radiographic follow-up study of Charnley low-friction arthroplasty. The role of the center of rotation. *Clin Orthop Relat Res*, 296, 140–7.
12. Kennedy JG, Rogers WB, Soffe KE, Sullivan RJ, Griffen DG and Sheean LJ (1998) Effect of acetabular component orientation on recurrent dislocation, pelvic osteolysis, polyethylene wear, and component migration. *J Arthroplasty*, 13, 530–4.
13. Ebied A, Hoad-Reddick DA and Raut V (2005) Medium-term results of the Charnley low-offset femoral stem. *J Bone Joint Surg Br*, 87, 916–20.
14. Sakalkale DP, Sharkey PF, Eng K, Hozack WJ and Rothman RH (2001) Effect of femoral component offset on polyethylene wear in total hip arthroplasty. *Clin Orthop Relat Res*, 388, 125–34.
15. Robinson RP, Simonian PT, Gradisar IM and Ching RP (1997) Joint motion and surface contact area related to component position in total hip arthroplasty. *J Bone Joint Surg Br*, 79, 140–6.
16. Rixrath E, Wendling-Mansuy S, Flecher X, Chabrand P and Argenson JN (2008) Design parameters dependences on contact stress distribution in gait and jogging phases after total hip arthroplasty. *J Biomechanics*, 41, 1137–42.
17. Lewinnek GE, Lewis JL, Tarr R, Compere CL and Zimmerman JR (1978) Dislocations after total hip-replacement arthroplasties. *J Bone Joint Surg Am*, 60, 217–20.
18. Nogler M, Kessler O, Prassl A, Donnelly B, Streicher R, Sledge JB and Krismer M (2004) Reduced variability of acetabular cup positioning with use of an imageless navigation system. *Clin Orthop Relat Res*, 426, 159–63.
19. Del Schutte H Jr, Lipman AJ, Bannar SM, Livermore JT, Ilstrup D and Morrey BF (1998) Effects of acetabular abduction on cup wear rates in total hip arthroplasty. *J Arthroplasty*, 13, 621–6.
20. Hirakawa K, Mitsugi N, Koshino T, Saito T, Hirasawa Y and Kubo T (2001) Effect of acetabular cup position and orientation in cemented total hip arthroplasty. *Clin Orthop Relat Res*, 388, 135–42.
21. Kligman M, Michael H and Roffman M (2002) The effect of abduction

differences between cup and contralateral acetabular angle on polyethylene component wear. *Orthopedics*, 25, 65–7.
22. Patil S, Bergula A, Chen PC, Colwell CW Jr and D'Lima DD (2003) Polyethylene wear and acetabular component orientation. *J Bone Joint Surg Am*, 85 (suppl 4), 56–63.
23. Karachalios T, Hartofilakidis G, Zacharakis N, *et al.* (1993) A 12 to 18 year radiographic follow-up study of Charnley low-friction arthroplasty: The role of the center of rotation. *Clin Orthop*, 296, 140–7.
24. Kennedy JG, Rogers WB, Soffe KE, *et al.* (1998) Effect of acetabular component orientation on recurrent dislocation, pelvic osteolysis, polyethylene wear, and component migration. *J Arthroplasty*, 13, 530–4.
25. McQueary FG and Johnston RC (1988) Coxarthrosis after congenital dysplasia. Treatment by total hip arthroplasty without acetabular bone-grafting. *J Bone Joint Surg Am*, 70, 1140–4.
26. Linde F and Jensen J (1988) Socket loosening in arthroplasty for congenital dislocation of the hip. *Acta Orthop Scand*, 59, 254–9.
27. Yoder SA, Brand RA, Pedersen DR, *et al.* (1988) Total hip acetabular component position affects component loosening rates. *Clin Orthop Relat Res*, 228, 79–83.
28. Jensen JS, Retpen JB and Arnoldi CC (1989) Arthroplasty for congenital hip dislocation. Techniques for acetabular reconstruction. *Acta Orthop Scand*, 60, 86–90.
29. Linde F, Jensen J and Pilgaard S (1988) Charnley arthroplasty in osteoarthritis secondary to congenital dislocation or subluxation of the hip. *Clin Orthop Relat Res*, 227, 164–70.
30. Doehring TC, Rubash HE, Shelley FJ, *et al.* (1996) Effect of superior and superolateral relocations of the hip center on hip joint forces. An experimental and analytical analysis. *J Arthroplasty*, 11, 693–7.
31. Yoder SA, Brand RA, Pedersen DR, *et al.* (1988) Total hip acetabular component position affects component loosening rates. *Clin Orthop Relat Res*, 228, 79–83.
32. Bozic KJ, Freiberg AA and Harris WH (2004) The high hip center. *Clin Orthop Relat Res*, 420, 101–5.
33. Cameron HU, Botsford DJ and Park YS (1996) Influence of the Crowe rating on the outcome of total hip arthroplasty in congenital hip dysplasia. *J Arthroplasty*, 11, 582–6.
34. Delp SL, Wixson RL, Komattu AV, *et al.* (1996) How superior placement of the joint center in hip arthroplasty affects the abductor muscles. *Clin Orthop Relat Res*, 328, 137–40.
35. Jerosch J, Steinbeck J, Stechmann J, *et al.* (1997) Influence of a high hip center on abductor muscle function. *Arch Orthop Trauma Surg*, 116, 385–9.
36. Lewinneck G, Lewis J, Tarr R, Compere C and Zimmerman J (1978) Dislocations after total hip-replacement arhroplasties. *J Bone Joint Surg Am*, 60, 217–24.
37. Eggli S and Muller M (1998) The value of pre-operative planning for total hip arthroplasty. *J Bone Joint Surg Br*, 80, 382–90.
38. Sariali E, Mouttet A, Pasquier G, Durante E and Catone Y (2009) Accuracy of

reconstruction of the hip using computerised three-dimensional pre-operative planning and a cementless modular neck stem. *J Bone Joint Surg Br*, 91, 333–40.
39. Bankston AB, Cates H, Ritter MA, Keating EM and Faris PM (1995) Polyethylene wear in total hip arthroplasty. *Clin Orthop*, 317, 7–13.
40. Fackler CD and Poss R (1980) Dislocation in total hip arthroplasties. *Clin Orthop Relat Res*, 151, 169–78.
41. Bontrager KC (2001) Proximal femur and pelvic girdle. In *Radiographic Positioning and Related Anatomy*, 5th edn London, Mosby.
42. Bourne RB and Rorabeck CH (2002) Soft tissue balancing: the hip. *J Arthroplasty*, 17 (Suppl 1), 17–22.
43. Devane PA, Horne JG and Martin K (1997) Three dimensional polyethylene wear of a press-fit titanium prosthesis: factors influencing generation of polyethylene debris. *J Arthroplasty*, 12, 256–66.
44. Sakalkale DP, Sharkey PF, Eng K, Hozack WJ and Rothman RH (2001) Effect of femoral component offset on polyethylene wear in total hip arthroplasty. *Clin Orthop Relat Res*, 388, 125–45.
45. Ramaniroka NA, Rakotomanana LR, Rubin PJ and Leyvraz P (2000) Noncemented total hip arthroplasty: influence of extra medullary parameters on initial implant stability and on bone–implant interface stresses. *Rev Clin Orthop Reparatrice Appar Mot*, 86, 590–7 (in French).
46. Davey JR, O'Connor DO, Burke DW, *et al.* (1993) Femoral component offset: its effect on strain in bonecement. *J Arthroplasty*, 8, 23–6.
47. Wong PKC, Otsuka NY, Davey JR, *et al.* (1993) The effect of femoral component offset in uncemented total hip arthroplasty. *Proceedings Canadian Orthopaedic Society, 48th Annual Meeting, June 18, Montreal, Quebec.*
48. Devane PA and Horne JG (1999) Assessment of polyethylene wear in total hip replacement. *Clin Orthop Relat Res*, (2001) 369, 59–72.
49. Breathnach AS (1965) *Frazer's Anatomy of the Human Skeleton*. London, Churchill.
50. Flecher X, Parratte S, Aubaniac JM and Argenson JN (2007) Three-dimensional custom-designed cementless femoral stem for osteoarthritis secondary to congenital dislocation of the hip. *J Bone Joint Surg Br*, 89, 1586–91.
51. Flecher X, Pearce O, Parratte S, Aubaniac JM and Argenson JN (2010) Custom cementless stem improves hip function in young patients at 15-year follow-up. *Clin Orthop Relat Res*, 468, 747–55.
52. Hananouchi T, Sugano N, Nakamura N, Nishii T, Miki H and Yamamura M (2007) Preoperative templating of femoral components on plain X-rays. Rotational evaluation with synthetic X-rays on ORTHODOC. *Arch Orthop Trauma Surg*, 127, 381–2.
53. Sariali E, Mouttet A, Pasquier G and Durante E (2009) Three-dimensional hip anatomy in osteoarthritis. Analysis of the femoral offset. *Arthroplasty*, 24, 990–7.
54. Schidlo C, Becker C and Jansson V (1999) Change in the CCD angle and the femoral anteversion angle by hip prosthesis implantation. *Z Orthop Grenzgeb*, 137, 259–64.
55. Bourne RB and Rorabeck CH (2002) Soft tissue balancing: the hip. *J Arthroplasty*, 17 (suppl 1), 17–22.

56. Sarin VK, Pratt WR and Bradley GW (2005) Accurate femur repositioning is critical during intraoperative total hip arthroplasty length and offset assessment. *J Arthroplasty*, 20, 887–91.
57. Emerson RH Jr (2012) Increased anteversion of press-fit femoral stems compared with anatomic femur. *Clin Orthop Relat Res*, 470, 477–81.
58. Marchetti E, Krantz N, Berton C, Bocquet D, Fouilleron N, Migaud H and Girard J (2011) Component impingement in total hip arthroplasty: frequency and risk factors. A continuous retrieval analysis series of 416 cup. *Orthop Trauma Surg Res*, online publication 4 March.
59. Woolson ST and Murphy M (1995) Wear of polyethylene of Harris–Galante acetabular components inserted without cement. *J Bone Joint Surg Am*, 77, 1311–4.
60. Jeffery RS, Morris RW and Denham RA (1991) Coronal alignment after total knee replacement. *J Bone Joint Surg Br*, 73, 709–14.
61. D'Lima DD, Chen PC and Colwell CW Jr (2001) Polyethylene contact stresses, articular congruity, and knee alignment. *Clin Orthop Relat Res*, 392, 232–8.
62. D'Lima DD, Hermida JC, Chen PC and Colwell CW Jr (2001) Polyethylene wear and variations in knee kinematics. *Clin Orthop Relat Res*, 392, 124–30.
63. Werner FW, Ayers DC, Maletsky LP and Rullkoetter PJ (2005) The effect of valgus/varus malalignment on load distribution in total knee replacements. *J Biomechanics*, 38, 349–55.
64. Green GV, Berend KR, Berend ME, Glisson RR and Vail TP (2002) The effects of varus tibial alignment on proximal tibial surface strain in total knee arthroplasty: the postero-medial hot spot. *J Arthroplasty*, 17, 1033–9.
65. Bargren JH, Blaha JD and Freeman MA (1983) Alignment in total knee arthroplasty. Correlated biomechanical and clinical observations. *Clin Orthop Relat Res*, 173, 178–83.
66. Lotke PA and Ecker ML (1977) Influence of positioning of prosthesis in total knee replacement. *J Bone Joint Surg Am*, 59, 77–9.
67. Hsu RW, Himeno S, Coventry MB and Chao EY (1990) Normal axial alignment of the lower extremity and load-bearing distribution at the knee. *Clin Orthop Relat Res*, 255, 215–27.
68. Ritter MA, Faris PM, Keating EM and Meding JB (1994) Postoperative alignment of total knee replacement. Its effect on survival. *Clin Orthop Relat Res*, 299, 153–6.
69. Hvid I and Nielsen S (1984) Total condylar knee arthroplasty. Prosthetic component positioning and radiolucent lines. *Acta Orthop Scand*, 55, 160–5.
70. Parratte S, Pagnano MW, Trousdale RT and Berry DJ (2010) Effect of postoperative mechanical axis alignment on the fifteen-year survival of modern, cemented total knee replacements. *J Bone Joint Surg Am*, 92, 2143–9.
71. Dennis DA, Komistek RD, Walker SA, Cheal EJ and Stiehl JB (2001) Femoral condylar lift-off *in vivo* in total knee arthroplasty. *J Bone Joint Surg Br*, 83, 33–9.
72. Fehring TK (2000) Rotational malalignment of the femoral component in total knee arthroplasty. *Clin Orthop Relat Res*, 380, 72–9.

12
Factors contributing to orthopaedic implant wear

L.C. JONES, Johns Hopkins University School of Medicine, USA,
A.K. TSAO, Sun Valley Orthopedic Surgeons, USA and
L.D.T. TOPOLESKI, University of Maryland,
Baltimore County, USA

Abstract: Implant wear can be a major factor limiting the long-term survivorship of a medical implant. Wear results in degradation of the implant surface, which can ultimately lead to the failure of the implant or an adverse response to the wear particles. To reduce the type, quantity and rate of wear, an understanding of the factors contributing to the wear process is needed. These factors can be categorized as implant-specific (materials, designs), manufacturing, surgical and patient-related. In reality, a number of factors are likely to occur simultaneously. The aim of this chapter is to characterize each of these factors.

Key words: patient factors, implant wear, surgical factors, implant design, implant manufacturing, implant materials.

12.1 Introduction

Orthopaedic implants are frequently used to achieve the primary goals of orthopaedic surgery: to alleviate pain and restore function of arthritic joints. Although total joint replacement is counted as one of the most successful surgical procedures, many of the reasons limiting the survivorship of the reconstructed joint are often implant-related. Approaches to extending the longevity of orthopaedic implants depend on our understanding of the factors that may ultimately compromise their survival. Over the past few decades, the primary causes of failure have been osteolysis, implant loosening and infection (Bauer and Schils, 1999; Jones and Hungerford, 1987; Kim et al., 2011; Wright and Goodman, 1996). Wear of the implant is associated with each of these conditions.

Materials scientists and mechanical engineers have studied the surfaces of orthopaedic implants to understand how they function *in situ*. Evaluating *in situ* wear and damage mechanisms on the surfaces of retrieved implants is difficult because they have likely been exposed to varying conditions and continuous degradation mechanisms over their lifetimes. For example, an implant that has minimal initial stability may become loose, for any number of reasons, and is then subject to more motion than an intact joint, thereby resulting in wear at the articulating surfaces. However, an implant that was initially stable, but subject to loading conditions exceeding the material strength of the component, will also generate wear debris. The aim of the following chapter is to describe various factors that have been shown to have an effect on the wear of orthopaedic implants.

12.1.1 Wear

Wear is defined as the 'loss of material in particulate form as a consequence of relative motion between two surfaces' (Hallab *et al.*, 2004). While historically this discussion has focused on the articulating surfaces of joint replacements, it may also include wear at the implant/bone interface or wear between two juxtaposed components such as screws and plates or heads and trunions.

Wear is generated by mechanical factors such as loading and the subsequent motions that occur, such as articulation of prosthetic components against each other or of an implant moving against the host bone. The mechanical factors can be qualitatively and quantitatively defined and characterized: the magnitude and duration of load; the magnitude of interface strain; direction of motion (compression, torsion, shear); frequency of motion (high and low frequency); and number and frequency of rest periods. In addition, the material characteristics of a surface, such as material properties and surface topography, will also be determining factors in the extent and severity of wear. There are obvious sources of motion such as activity (walking, running, stair climbing), but less obvious sources may also act to exacerbate wear (turning while sleeping, shifting while sitting, etc.). The amount of motion between interfaces and the loads experienced by articulating surfaces have been studied in detail by numerous investigators using computer modeling, cadaver specimens and transducers on patients (Burke *et al.*, 1991; Engh *et al.*, 1992a; Stern *et al.*, 1997).

Wear can be categorized as either two-body or three-body wear. Two-body wear is wear from the relative motion between two surfaces; a common everyday example is the articulation of sandpaper on wood. Two-body wear can occur when the two surfaces do not have identical material properties, as is seen with metal–polyethylene or metal–ceramic couples. However, it can also be observed between two similar materials when the friction is significant, particularly when the surface is inadequately lubricated. Three-body wear occurs when a third body, i.e. an abrasive particle, is introduced between two surfaces and causes damage to one or both of the surfaces; an everyday example is using abrasive cleanser on a countertop. With orthopaedic implants, the sources of the material may be the implant itself, generating particles from the surfaces, from particles of bone or polymethylmethacrylate (PMMA), or possibly from the cutting surfaces of the instrumentation generated during insertion of the component. With two-body and three-body wear, material is either removed, rearranged or transferred on one or more of the surfaces by different mechanisms.

Different types of wear have been identified and well characterized in orthopaedic biomaterials and will be only briefly described here. The three primary mechanisms are abrasion, adhesion and fatigue. Abrasive wear occurs between two surfaces with different levels of hardness. The morphology of the one surface (e.g. surface roughness or sharp edges of a third body) enables the harder surface to plow through the softer surface. The mechanism of third-body wear is often abrasion. In third-body wear, there are several potential sources of abrasive bodies including intraoperative debris (PMMA fragments, bone, debris from the instrumentation), impingement of the metal underlying worn-through polyethylene against metal from the opposing component, or fracture of the component, cement mantle, cerclage wires or screws. Adhesive wear, on the other hand, occurs when two materials in contact essentially form a weld that fractures off from one of the surfaces during continued motion and transfers to the second surface. This can result in the formation of a 'transfer film.' Fatigue wear can be defined as the surface wear associated with surface or subsurface fatigue of particles or layers of material. Examples include the formation of particles of metal carbides or the delamination of polyethylene.

Other terms have also been used to characterize the wear that can occur with orthopaedic implants. Fretting wear is used to describe the wear that occurs from small, oscillatory motion between two surfaces, usually of the order of micrometers. Erosive wear is caused by the impingement of particles of solid or liquid against the surface. Corrosive wear occurs when corrosive products are removed from the surface by a sliding of one surface over the other; new corrosive products can be formed and the process repeated. During the immediate post-operative period, any asperities on the surface resulting from the manufacturing processes are worn away; this is called the 'wearing-in period.'

In practice, a single type of wear rarely occurs in isolation; several different mechanisms may be operative. For example, surface fatigue can generate particles. Those particles may become abrasive third bodies to cause further damage through three-body wear. The presence of other failure mechanisms (delamination, corrosion, fracture) may actually accelerate the wear process and may eventually lead to implant failure.

The loss of material from the surface of an implant may occur on the molecular (e.g. transfer films) or macro (e.g. shards removed from delaminated polyethylene) scale. Histological examination of the tissues surrounding worn components have indicated a diversity of material compositions, sizes and shapes of wear debris (Freeman et al., 1969; Schmiedberg et al., 2007). It is difficult to actually estimate the extent of material loss into the surrounding tissue as the material may be either at the submicron level, as with polyethylene, or the ionic level, as with metals. Furthermore, particles generated at one site may migrate to other sites or be taken up by lymph nodes; metal ions may be taken up by other tissues, enter the blood stream or be excreted. Historically, it was assumed that only particles below 10 μm could be phagocytized and would then lead to osteolysis (Horowitz et al., 1988). Maximum phagocytosis appears to occur when the particles are 0.5 μm (Ishikawa et al., 1991). However, larger particles have been associated with foreign body giant cells and a process called 'frustrated phagocytosis' is capable of stimulating an inflammatory response (Gelb et al., 1994).

Wear is influenced by the material couple, friction, lubrication, contact area, surface finish and the loads to which the surfaces are subjected. When testing against a known material, different materials have been shown to have different wear rates (Firkins et al., 2001; Goldsmith et al., 2000; McKellop et al., 1981). In fact, it should be emphasized that articulation of any bearing or bearing surfaces involves at least three materials: surface A, surface B and the inter-bearing lubricant. Lubricants can be solids (e.g. graphite), liquid (e.g. oil or synovial fluid) or gas (e.g. air). The interaction between the lubricant and the surfaces can have an enormous impact on the wear of the surfaces. Ideally, the lubricant thickness should be great enough to completely separate the micro-asperities of the articulating surfaces. Ideal lubricants must remain between the two surfaces and reduce the coefficient of friction between the surfaces. Synovial fluid is an ideal lubricant for the natural joint, working through a complex interaction with the surface cartilage. It is not clear, however, that synovial fluid is the ideal lubricant for existing artificial joint surfaces. It may be possible to design artificial joint surfaces that are optimized to interact with natural joint fluids.

All of the types of wear described above have been observed in orthopaedic implants. Table 12.1 lists different types of implants and references to related concerns regarding wear.

12.1.2 Failure: implant or patient

The consequences of wear encompass everything from failure of the implant itself to adverse biological responses to wear debris leading to loss of fixation and osteolysis. Failure of the implant can occur with wear-through

Table 12.1 Types of wear for different orthopaedic implants

Implant	Reference
Hip	
Cemented	Isaac et al., 1992
	McKellop et al., 1996, 1999a
	Onsten et al., 1998
Uncemented	Garcia-Rey and Garcia-Cimbrelo, 2008
	Onsten et al., 1998
Backside wear	Barrack et al., 1997
	Krieg et al., 2009
	Yamaguchi et al., 1999
Impingement	Kligman et al., 2007
	Usrey et al., 2006
Metal-on-metal	Bolland et al., 2011
	Ebramzadeh et al., 2011
	Huber et al., 2010
	Matthies et al., 2011
	Willert et al., 1996
Knee	
Cemented	Noble et al., 2003
Uncemented	Noble et al., 2003
	Que and Topoleski, 1999
	Stulberg et al., 1988
	Tsao et al., 1993
	Wright et al., 1992
Backside wear	Billi et al., 2010
	Conditt et al., 2004a, 2004b, 2005
	Engh and Ammeen, 2004
	Harman et al., 2007
	Jayabalan et al., 2007
	Li et al., 2002
	Taki et al., 2004
Unicondylar	Harman et al., 2010
	Manson et al., 2010
Rotating or Mobile-bearing	Manson et al., 2010
	Willis-Owen et al., 2011
Post-impingement	Callaghan et al., 2002
	Dolan et al., 2011
	Li et al., 2005
PCL retaining or sacrificing	Hirakawa et al., 1999
Fusion defects	Wrona et al., 1994
Manufacturing techniques	Meding et al., 2011
Shoulder	
Shoulder replacements	Elmaraghy and Devereaux, 2008
	Hertel and Ballmer, 2003
	Hopkins et al., 2007
	Khan et al., 2008
	Matsen et al., 2008
	Nam et al., 2010a, 2010b

Table 12.1 (cont.)

Implant	Reference
	Nho *et al.*, 2009
	Scarlat and Matsen, 2001
Spine	
Dynesys-screws	Ianuzzi *et al.*, 2010
Total disk	Kurtz *et al.*, 2005, 2007
	Murtagh *et al.*, 2009
	Pitzen *et al.*, 2007
DIAM–interspinal implant	Jerosch and Moursi, 2008
Pedicle screws	Kim *et al.*, 2007
	Wang *et al.*, 1999
Rods	Villarraga *et al.*, 2006
Fracture fixation	
Dynamic hip screw plates	Shahgaldi and Compson, 2000
Plates-osteotomy	Mathieu *et al.*, 2008

of polyethylene resulting in exposure of the underlying metal in a modular component. This can then lead to impingement of the underlying metal with the metal of the corresponding couple. Uneven wear on one side of a joint replacement can lead to incongruencies in the geometry of the articulating surfaces and uneven loading of the component. Fracture of the implant can occur. With cement fixation, breakdown of the cement mantle with generation of cement particles can also have deleterious consequences. In addition to inciting an adverse tissue response at the implant–bone interface, PMMA particles can migrate to the articulating surfaces and cause third-body wear. With uncemented prostheses that rely on biologic fixation, the loss of the integrity of the porous coating can also have similar consequences regarding osteolysis and third-body wear.

The surface finish of the implant can change over time. As already mentioned, the wearing-in process can smooth out large asperities that might be initially present (Hallab *et al.*, 2004). Any material fatigue of the surface or subsurface and any abrasion that may have occurred may serve to roughen the articulating surface and increase the rate of wear. With metal components, motion of the implant may initiate a process of passivation and repassivation, enabling metal ions to leach into the surrounding tissues. There can also be changes in the geometry of the component due to creep, plastic deformation or wear (Hood *et al.*, 1983; Wright and Goodman, 1996).

Implantation biology is a dynamic process: the biologic response to the implant changes with increasing times of implantation. Initially, processes associated with wound healing and wear predominate. As the body responds to the physiological and biomechanical alterations associated with surgery and prosthetic implantation, bony remodeling may occur. For certain implant designs this may involve rounding off such as that seen at the calcar for many hip prostheses. If the implant is uncemented, ingrowth and ongrowth onto the porous surface may enable fixation and stabilization of the implant. Stress shielding, a potential adverse response, is associated with alterations in mechanical loading of the bone. Following Wolff's law, bone adapts to different loading conditions by either forming more (increased loading) or less (decreased loading) bone. This can be a consequence of implant design or fixation of the implant. Less is known about the adaptation of the implanted bone to bony changes associated with ageing or ongoing disease. One might expect that wear would be influenced by changes in gait with ongoing musculoskeletal disease – be it with other joints in the same leg, the contralateral leg or spine.

Much has been written about the adverse biologic responses associated with wear debris. Wear debris instigates a negative biologic reaction that may ultimately lead to a loss of implant stability associated with increased micromotion. Both *in vitro* and *in vivo* experiments have demonstrated that particles of the materials used with orthopaedic implants are capable of inciting inflammatory responses and may stimulate innate or acquired immune responses (Bauer and Schils, 1999; Caicedo *et al.*, 2010; Goodman *et al.*, 2009; Hallab and Jacobs, 2009). Clinically, the harbingers of an adverse response may include an increasingly thickened fibrous tissue membrane around the implant associated with progressive radiolucencies. Eventually, there is a corresponding loss of bone (osteolysis) and the implant fixation can be compromised. This process can become self-perpetuating. Once the component is loose, the osteolysis becomes more aggressive.

There is considerable debate regarding the exact mechanisms that are involved with osteolysis and whether it involves innate or acquired immune systems. Regardless of mechanism, the initial step in this process is the phagocytosis of the particles and activation of macrophages. Particles of 2–3 μm in size have been shown to be optimal for phagocytosis, although it is possible for larger particles to be internalized (Champion *et al.*, 2008). Attempts by phagocytes to break down the inorganic materials are largely ineffective, and the particles can be released back into the surrounding tissue to repeat the cycle. It is possible, as with particles of metal alloy, that the lysosomal contents can cause metal ion release from the surfaces of the particles.

The diversity of biological responses appears to run the gamut from mild, with encapsulation of the debris, to severe as with tumors (malignant or otherwise). This diversity likely reflects individual variability regarding non-specific and specific immune responses, as is seen with any exposure to microbes or foreign bodies. Non-specific responses, also called innate immunity, are primarily characterized by an inflammatory reaction involving leukocytes (associated with infection), macrophages and fibroblasts. If left unabated, this response can result in formation of a granuloma. Specific responses, also called acquired immunity, are in response to specific antigens on the surface of the inciting material. Of the four hypersensitivity reactions, Type IV hypersensitivity (also called delayed type or DTH), is a T-cell-mediated response involving antigen presenting cells (macrophages, dendritic cells), T lymphocytes (can be T-helper or T-cytotoxic cells) and specific cytokines or other co-stimulatory molecules. Tissue injury can occur through the responses of the surrounding cells to cytokines and other enzymes and molecules released into the surrounding milieu.

Variable responses may also reflect diverse sources of stimulation, such as particles from dissimilar materials (metal alloy, polymers, ceramics) or metal ions from different alloys.

Studies have shown that particles of PMMA or polyethylene can stimulate inflammatory reactions that are primarily characterized by the presence of macrophages and fibroblasts and the cytokines associated with innate immunity (Goodman, 2007). On the other hand, metal particles are capable of stimulating the innate or acquired immune systems. Recently, there has been concern over the observation of a significant adverse tissue response with metal-on-metal prostheses. This response has been called a pseudotumor or adverse local tissue reaction (ALTR) and characterized as aseptic, lymphocyte-dominated, vasculitis-associated lesions (Campbell *et al.*, 2010; Counsell *et al.*, 2008). While the severe form has been associated with metal-on-metal implants, this type of response has also been observed with metal-on-polyethylene implants (Campbell *et al.*, 2010; Fujishiro *et al.*, 2011).

Periprosthetic infection is also associated with osteolysis, loosening and the subsequent development of wear debris. The infection may also have an impact on wear-related biological responses. Wear debris provides another potential surface for bacterial adherence. Furthermore, wear particles and metal ions may alter the periprosthetic environment as well as the immune responses to infection (Au *et al.*, 2006, Goodman, 2007; Hosman *et al.*, 2010).

The numerous factors that have been shown to influence the wear of medical implants can be segregated into the following categories: implant-specific (material, implant design and manufacturing), surgical and patient-related. Of course, the reality is that several factors are often present simultaneously and there is likely to be an interaction between several of these variables.

12.2 Implant-specific factors – materials and design

12.2.1 General material considerations

The function of a material dictates which materials are appropriate to use for a specific implant. The function may be structural (e.g. femoral stem, plate), for an articulating surface (e.g. any total joint prosthesis), for an interface for fixation (e.g. biologic fixation), to stimulate bone apposition or growth (biologics, coatings) or be malleable (e.g. cages to contain graft). Material selection is governed by material and mechanical properties as well as biocompatibility considerations. Material properties relating to orthopaedic implants include chemical, electrical, biological, manufacturing, magnetic and radiological. Mechanical properties include tensile strength, stiffness, toughness, hardness, ductility and fatigue resistance. The biocompatibility of the material is important, and includes responses to the structurally intact material as well as its degradative products, and the response of the material to the biologic environment and reactions to the presence of the material. While the potential for toxic and carcinogenic effects of a material must be appreciated, we also must know whether it has the capacity to stimulate the innate or acquired immune responses or has any potential teratogenic effects. Decisions regarding material selection are made more complicated as many orthopaedic implants comprise multiple components made up of different materials.

Paramount to the decision making process is establishing how the material degrades under certain circumstances in a biologic environment and whether there are any biological consequences to these degradation products. While the materials used with medical implants are generally considered corrosion resistant, there are numerous reports in the literature of evidence of galvanic, pitting and crevice corrosion (Collier *et al.*, 1991; Cook *et al.*, 1994; Gilbert *et al.*, 1994). Furthermore, corrosion of wear particles created by other degradation mechanisms may also occur (Schmiedberg *et al.*, 2007; Shahgaldi *et al.*, 1995; Willert *et al.*, 1996). Grain size of the metals and ceramics used in orthopaedic implants affects the wear resistance – a smaller grain size results in greater wear resistance (Hallab *et al.*, 2004). The properties of the wear debris may also have an impact on their behavior as third-body abrasive particles (hardness, shape) and their ability to stimulate an inflammatory response.

When choosing a material, the type of biologic response to that material is taken into consideration. While one may want to select for a 'bioinert' material (i.e. a material that does not elicit a biologic response or interaction) it is unlikely that such a material exists (Black, 1992). In fact, one of the first biological responses is likely to be contact of the implant with blood and the adhesion of proteins to the surface of the material. The decision is really to select a material that does not stimulate an adverse biologic response. On the other hand, one may actually want to stimulate a specific biologic response such as osteointegration onto an implant surface. Selecting a material such as a ceramic or tantalum would then be of interest.

12.2.2 General design considerations

Implant design involves selection of materials, including materials for the bearing surfaces, type of implant fixation, how much of the anatomy is being restored and how closely the design mimics the anatomy and restores function, what sizes to create and whether it should be modular. Each of these design considerations can have an impact on the wear behavior of an implant.

For total joint implants, the anatomy must be taken into consideration in the design of the implant. For total knee replacements, design considerations include whether the implant is cruciate sacrificing or retaining, how the patella tracks along the trochlear groove and how much roll-back is permitted. For total hip replacements, implants can be straight anatomic stems. A more dramatic example is the reverse shoulder.

As undersizing or oversizing an implant can influence wear, maximizing the availability of implant sizes is important. With femoral stems, sizing includes proximal fit and flare. Design must take into account the fact that the geometry may be different for different sizes. Anthropometric measurements are also influenced by patient sex and race (Chin *et al.*, 2002; Low *et al.*, 2000; Uehara *et al.*, 2002). Extremes in patient size necessitate the use of custom prostheses; while these may mimic the anatomy of the patient, less is known about the impact of these one-off designs and the kinematics that can be achieved. Femoral head size can also have an effect on the long-term outcome of total hip replacement. Smaller femoral heads are associated with greater polyethylene wear (Hoeltzel *et al.*, 1989). Increasing the head size increases implant stability, reduces the rate of dislocation and increases the range of motion while decreasing the chance of impingement (Cinotti *et al.*, 2011; Lombardi *et al.*, 2011).

Modular implants allow for more customizing of the sizing with off-the-shelf prostheses. For example, the availability of different femoral head components permits adjustments to the head–neck ratio and different thicknesses of tibial components allow for adjustments in the joint line. Metal backing enables modularity of polyethylene components. This is good for both primary and revision procedures. With primary procedures, it allows for more choices (e.g. thickness, different designs of cups). With modular components, worn polyethylene can be removed and exchanged with new polyethylene – even exchanging conventional with cross-linked. Early studies have demonstrated that metal backing may result in decreased system and peak stresses (Harris, 1984; Lewis *et al.*, 1982). However, modularity has introduced its own set of problems. Crevice corrosion has been observed around the head–neck junction with some implants (Cook *et al.*, 1994; Goldberg *et al.*, 2002). Greater wear has been observed with thinner inserts and liners (Bartel *et al.*, 1986; Plante-Bordeneuve and Freeman, 1993; Weber and Morris, 1996); this may be related to the extent of deformation of the thinner polyethylene (Collier *et al.*, 2003). Motion between the non-articulating surface of the polyethylene and the metal component can lead to significant wear, also called backside wear (Kurtz *et al.*, 1998; Williams *et al.*, 1997). Complete failure of the locking mechanism can result in gross motion of the polyethylene liner and catastrophic failure (Cooke *et al.*, 2003). If there is wear-through, impingement of metal against metal can occur (Gonzalez Della Valle *et al.*, 2001; Stulberg *et al.*, 1988).

12.2.3 Function: material and design considerations

Structural

The mechanical strength of a material is a primary consideration for a variety of orthopaedic implants including femoral stems, plates and screws, rods and fixation screws. While most of these components are made from metals and metal alloys, ceramics and composites have also been used. Most metal implants have used either stainless steel, cobalt–chromium alloy or titanium alloy. More recently, zirconium (articulating surface) and tantalum (bone interface) have also been utilized. Contemporary implants have used ceramic femoral heads and some designs include ceramic-on-ceramic articulations. There has been increasing interest in the potential of composites that may allow for different design features not possible with conventional materials (Kurtz and Devine, 2007; Scotchford *et al.*, 2003).

Articulations

There has been a long history of different bearing couples for orthopaedic implants. The original designs included the interpositional 'mold arthroplasty' for hips made from glass developed by Smith-Petersen and the hinged metal-to-metal knee designed by Shiers (Hallab *et al.*, 2004; Shiers, 1959). Bearing couples have included metal-on-polyethylene, metal-on-metal, ceramic-on-metal, ceramic-on-polyethylene and ceramic-on-ceramic. The rationale for material choice is based upon the materials' strength, hardness, resistance to wear, resistance to scratching/notch sensitivity and friction moments (Davis, 2003).

Many articulating surfaces are made of cobalt–chromium–molybdenum

(CoCrMo) alloy. Early reports using titanium femoral heads indicated that it experienced significant wear (McGovern et al., 1996; Nasser et al., 1990). The strength, hardness and relative bioinertness of ceramics (alumina, zirconia) have made them excellent candidates for articulating surfaces. Early designs were particularly susceptible to cracking; improved manufacturing with improved clearances has led to the reintroduction of ceramic bearings. Various approaches have been undertaken to treat the surfaces of metal implants to improve their wear resistance. Nitrogen ion implantation (McKellop and Rostlund, 1990), diamond-like carbon film (Ozeki et al., 2010) and a polycrystalline diamond compact articulation surface have been used on articulating surfaces (http://www.orthopaediclist.com/products-details.asp? ProductID = 8172).

Metal-on-polyethylene
Following poor experience with Teflon® (polytetrafluoroethylene or PTFE), Sir Walter Charnley switched to high-density polyethylene as a bearing surface because of its better wear behavior (Charnley, 1972). The initial clinical experience was much improved and other manufacturers introduced their own version of metal-on-polyethylene prostheses. However, concerns with polyethylene wear began to surface in the late 1960s and early 1970s (Amstutz, 1969; Charnley and Halley, 1975). Wear could be inferred from eccentric alignment of components on X-ray and techniques were developed to estimate wear rates from sequential radiographs to follow patients over time.

The apprehension concerning polyethylene wear was amplified with the finding of submicron-sized wear particles identified using polarized light and with specific isolation and staining methods (Schmalzried et al., 1993). Clinical and laboratory studies now identified polyethylene wear particles as a primary factor contributing to osteolysis and loosening of total joint prostheses (Jacobs et al., 1994; McKellop et al., 1995).

In the late 1990s, various strategies were used to improve the wear properties of high molecular weight polyethylene. Using hot isostatic pressing, polyethylene could be formed with an extended chain crystallite morphology with thick lamellae and high crystallinity (Bellare and Kurtz, 2009). This resulted in a slightly higher yield and ultimate strength and significantly higher elastic modulus and creep resistance. Reports of high wear rates with this material, also called Hylamer®, led several surgeons to discontinue using implants with this type of polyethylene (Chmell et al., 1996; Ezzet, 1996).

Considerable research and development efforts have gone into creating highly cross-linked polyethylene (HXPE). Cross-linking of the polymer chains can be achieved through irradiation or chemical methods (peroxide or silane chemistry) (Kurtz et al., 1999). Compared with conventional polyethylene, HXPE has improved resistance to abrasive and adhesive wear (McKellop et al., 1999a; Muratoglu et al., 2002; Pruitt, 2005). As these are the primary wear mechanisms associated with hip implants, cross-linked polyethylene was first used for acetabular liners (McKellop et al., 1999b). The first-generation cross-linked polyethylene had reduced resistance to fatigue and crack propagation and inferior mechanical properties and was not believed to be a good material candidate for tibial trays, where wear is associated with fatigue of subsurface layers and delamination (McKellop et al., 1999b; Sobieraj and Rimnac, 2009). The evolution of HXPE has resulted in improvements in wear and fatigue resistance, although tibial trays have not been available in this material until recently (Popoola et al., 2010; Stoller et al., 2011). In a meta-analysis of clinical wear of polyethylene in total hip replacement, Kuzyk et al. (2011) reported linear wear rates ranging from 0.07 to 0.14 mm/year for conventional polyethylene as compared with 0.01 to 0.12 mm/year for cross-linked polyethylene. However, there remains cautious optimism regarding the longevity of HXPE with reports of wear; it is important to recognize that all HXPEs are not the same (Kurtz et al., 1999; MacDonald et al., 2011).

Sterilization by gamma irradiation was determined to decrease the wear resistance of polyethylene. Further discussion of approaches to address the issue is provided in Section 12.2.4.

In a study of 1287 knees implanted with Press-Fit Condylar total knee replacements with greater than 5-year follow-up, Fehring et al. (2004) explored several factors that could potentially have an impact on wear. They noted five variables associated with wear-related failure: patient age; patient gender; polyethylene sheet vendor; polyethylene finishing method; and polyethylene shelf life. Increased shelf age was a primary factor, with a dramatic difference between shelf ages of less than one year and more than one year. Regarding finishing methods, polycarbonate tumbling was better than machined without tumbling, which was better than wood tumbling.

Wear of a polyethylene implant is influenced by the thickness of the implant; this is because stress in the polyethylene insert depends on its thickness. With metal backing, early designs included relatively thin polyethylene inserts, and increased wear was observed with thinner inserts and liners (Engh et al., 1992b; Lee et al., 1999). Based on these findings, it is recommended that the minimal thickness of the UHMWPE should be greater than 8 mm (Weber and Morris, 1996; Wright and Goodman, 1996).

If the contact stresses exceed the yield stress of polyethylene, the consequence is increased surface wear (McNamara et al., 1994; Wright and Goodman, 1996). Several investigators have shown that a larger contact area, associated with higher conformity, results in lowering the contact and subsurface stresses (D'Lima et al., 2001; Sathasivam and Walker, 1994; Wright and Goodman, 1996). However, malalignment has a negative impact on high conforming designs (D'Lima et al., 2001). Mobile-bearing knee designs have built on this concept with their unconstrained rotation, greater articular conformity and minimized contact stresses (Vertullo et al., 2001). However, this has been tempered by concerns of backside wear.

Polyethylene is sensitive to edge loading, impingement and third-body wear. With total knee implants, edge loading is more commonly seen on the medial side (Currier et al., 2005). Impingement and fracture of the acetabular rim have also been noted (Schroder et al., 2011; Tower et al., 2007). Third-body wear has been observed in the polyethylene components for different joints (Matsen et al., 2007; Sychterz et al., 1999; Wasielewski et al., 1994).

Metal-on-metal
As an alternative to the traditional metal-on-polyethylene bearing surface, total hip and resurfacing hip prostheses have been designed with metal-on-metal articulating surfaces. Metal-on-metal implants are manufactured from cobalt–chromium alloy since it is the metal of choice (at this time) for bearing surfaces due to its material and mechanical properties. The clinical experience with early designs was compromised primarily as a consequence of inadequate manufacturing (Triclot, 2011). Improvements in manufacturing and design have led to the development of implants with better clearances and larger femoral heads. Metal-on-metal bearings have a distinct 'wear-in' or 'run-in' period with a high rate of wear during the first 2 years (Clarke et al., 2000; Sieber et al., 1999). In vitro and in vivo studies have demonstrated that high cup angle is associated with higher rates of wear (Hart et al., 2011; Williams et al., 2008). It is also important to have the proper head–neck offset in order to reduce the chance of impingement (Beaule et al., 2007).

Ceramics and articulations
Ceramics have been used as one of the components in the following bearing couples: ceramic-on-ceramic, ceramic-on-polyethylene and recently ceramic-on-metal. In total hip replacement, femoral heads made of alumina or zirconia have demonstrated very low rates of wear (Clarke et al., 2000; Smith and Unsworth, 2001). While laboratory studies indicated that the wear rate of polyethylene for ceramic-on-polyethylene implants was better than that for metal-on-polyethylene, the clinical results have been inconclusive (Jung and Kim, 2010). As with other hard-on-hard bearings, there is a 'wearing-in' period (Clarke et al., 2000). One of the primary factors contributing to the poor clinical results of the earlier designs was fracture, a consequence of the brittle nature of ceramics. Recent improvements in ceramic technology have included smaller grain size, more uniform distribution of grains, minimum porosity and an absence of

inclusions (Boutin *et al.*, 1988) and, consequently, fracture is now relatively uncommon (Hannouche *et al.*, 2003; Wright and Goodman, 2000). Similar to metal-on-metal bearings, impingement can be a concern regarding placement of the cup and head. Ceramics are now being used in total knee replacements, particularly for the femoral component.

Method of fixation

Orthopaedic implants can be fixed to bone with screws or with PMMA, also called bone cement. Alternatively, they can be press-fit into place or have surfaces that permit biologic ingrowth. For total joint arthroplasty, manufacturers have implant designs for both cement and biologic ingrowth prostheses so the choice is left up to surgeon preference.

Cement
Sir John Charnley first used PMMA to fix early total hip replacements to bone (Charnley, 1961). This resulted in a strong interface, immediate fixation and an implant that was able to load bear almost immediately. Clinical studies of cemented implants have established a satisfactory outcome over time, with reports of cement fixation lasting more than 20 years (Callaghan *et al.*, 2009; Caton and Prudhon, 2011). However, over the past several decades there have been a number of publications describing degeneration of the cement mantle resulting in particles of cement and associated with bone loss (Harris *et al.*, 1976; Ries *et al.*, 1994). The biological response to these particles was characterized by significant numbers of macrophages, inflammatory cytokines and degradative enzymes (Goldring *et al.*, 1983; Jasty *et al.*, 1992; Jones and Hungerford, 1987; Jones *et al.*, 1999, Lennox *et al.*, 1987). While initial studies focused on the material properties of the PMMA (such as mechanical strength and creep), inadequate cement technique was identified as the primary factor contributing to the breakdown of the cement interface. Poor mixing technique can result in the introduction of air bubbles on the one hand or undissolved PMMA powder on the other. Other technical concerns include introducing the cement onto an inadequately prepared surface or when it is too hardened or not hardened enough (Campbell *et al.*, 2009; Liu *et al.*, 2001). Analyses of retrieved failed implants have demonstrated thin cement mantles, uneven distribution of cement around the implant (including areas without cement), voids within the cement mantle and debonding of the cement from the implant surface (Clarke *et al.*, 2000; Hart *et al.*, 2011; McKellop *et al.*, 1999a, 1999b; Pruitt, 2005; Sieber *et al*, 1999; Williams *et al.*, 2008). Improvements in cement techniques have resulted in better clinical outcomes (Kim *et al.*, 2003; Okamoto *et al.*, 1997; Schmalzried and Harris, 1993). Technique modifications have included the use of cement

spacers and centralizers, vacuum mixing, centrifugation (Kim et al., 2003; Smith et al., 1998). One approach to improving the cement fixation is to precoat the stem with a layer of PMMA; the clinical results have been mixed as to whether this has had a significant impact on the survivorship (Ong et al., 2002).

Any loss of fixation can result in wear at the articulating surface as well as wear along the bone–implant interface. PMMA particles can act as third bodies to accelerate wear at these surfaces. The negative biologic response to PMMA particles leading to osteolysis and increased implant instability has been well documented (Goldring et al., 1986; Goodman et al., 1985; Jones and Hungerford, 1987; Jones et al., 2001).

Biologic ingrowth prostheses
With increasing concerns about cement fixation, implants with surfaces permitting biologic fixation were developed. Designs varied from beaded surfaces to meshes to roughened finishes (Hallab et al., 2004). The concept was that bone would grow into or onto the porous or textured surface, thereby fixing the implant in a three-dimensional interlock. Favorable initial to mid-term clinical outcomes were reported for many of the designs (Clarke et al., 2000; Sieber et al., 1999; Williams et al., 2008). However, because there is no immediate fixation, the outcomes of procedures using these prostheses are particularly sensitive to surgical technique and bone quality. Micromotion of the prostheses may prevent bone ingrowth (Sieber et al., 1999). While several studies have shown variable bony ingrowth with areas of substantial fibrous tissue (Bloebaum et al., 1997; Engh et al., 1993; Pidhorz et al., 1993), it is unclear how much bony ingrowth is necessary to achieve a stable interface (Clarke et al., 2000). Stress shielding may occur with certain designs, especially with more distal fixation (Kang et al., 2000; Peterson et al., 1979).

As one would expect, loose uncemented prostheses are subject to increased wear. There are occasional reports of debonding or degradation of the porous or textured surface (Agins et al., 1988; Jacobs et al., 2009). This can result in implant loosening as well as third-body wear (Kleinhans et al., 2009). Furthermore, screw holes, if present, may act as a portal for migration of wear debris to the bone interface (Wasielewski et al., 1997).

Several strategies have been undertaken to enhance the biologic fixation of orthopaedic implants. The bioactivities of ceramics have made them good candidates for coatings. Hydroxyapatite (HAp) and hydroxyapaptite-tricalcium phosphate (HAp-TCP) coatings can be applied to the surface of an implant to stimulate osteogenesis, facilitating osteointegration, and resulting in a mechanical stable interface (Akizuki et al., 2003; Tonino et al., 2001). Another approach is to use porous tantalum for the fixation surface. Reflecting its high porosity and interconnectivity, the rate of ingrowth was shown to be accelerated in an animal model (Bobyn *et al.*, 1999). Early results in patients regarding implant stability and bony apposition have been favorable (Simon and Bellemans, 2009).

12.2.4 Manufacturing factors

Manufacturing processes are directly related to material choice and implant design.

Polyethylene

Much has been published concerning the manufacturing of polyethylene. Sterilization methods have been shown to affect the material properties of high molecular weight polyethylene. Polyethylene that was gamma sterilized in air was shown to have significantly higher wear rates than that sterilized in ethylene oxide (Sutula *et al.*, 1995; Williams *et al.*, 1998). Subsurface oxidation, reduced ductility and reduced strength have been observed in polyethylene gamma sterilized in air (Bargmann *et al.*, 1999; Currier *et al.*, 2007; Sutula *et al.*, 1995). Subsurface damage has been associated with delamination (Medel *et al.*, 2011; Watanabe *et al.*, 2002). To address this, gamma irradiation in an inert gas (such as argon or nitrogen) was introduced. This was found to significantly reduce the wear rate of polyethylene components (Faris *et al.*, 2006). Irradiation is associated with the formation of free radicals (Premnath *et al.*, 1996). The development of free radicals may continue to occur after irradiation and a long shelf life may have a negative impact on the material (Bargmann *et al.*, 1999; Premnath *et al.*, 1996; Simon and Bellemans, 2009; Sutula *et al.*, 1995; Wasielewski *et al.*, 1997; Williams *et al.*, 1998). One approach to reduce the production of free radicals is to add a free-radical scavenger, such as vitamin E, to the polyethylene (Crowninshield and Muratoglu, 2008; Oral *et al.*, 2005; Tomita *et al.*, 1999). The wear rates of other non-irradiation methods of sterilization (e.g. ethylene oxide and gas plasma) have also been studied and may show improved material properties depending on the type of polyethylene studied (Sutula *et al.*, 1995; Sychterz *et al.*, 2004; Willie *et al.*, 2004).

The process used to shape polyethylene into components has been shown to have a significant effect on wear. The three methods of consolidation that have been used primarily in the manufacture of medical implants are direct molding, ram-extrusion and sheet molding (Poggie *et al.*, 1998). Ram-extruded polyethylene was used with several implant designs during the 1980s and 1990s. Reports of significant wear with implants utilizing this type of polyethylene started to appear in the medical literature in the early 1990s (Collier *et al.*, 1992; Cook and Thomas, 1991; Tsao *et al.*, 1993). Since then, several studies have substantiated that implants made from compression molded stock have superior wear performance compared with ram-extruded stock (Berzins et al., 2002; Faris et al., 2006; Meding et al., 2011).

Most polyethylene components have been made using one of two methods: machine milling or heat pressing. In 1991, Bloebaum et al. (1991) observed severe delamination in retrieved polyethylene tibial inserts that had been manufactured using heat-pressed polyethylene. They suggested that this may be a consequence of changes in the crystallinity of the polyethylene surfaces as well as increases in the microhardness of the surface. In a series of 487 patients with a porous-coated anatomic total knee prosthesis with a heat-pressed polyethylene tibial tray, Tsao et al. (1993) reported a significant level of wear in 7% of patients implanted. Hirakawa et al. (1994) noted significantly larger wear particles with heat-pressed implants. However, Engh et al. (1992b) suggested that it is likely that heat-pressing alone does not lead to increased wear but that it is a combination of variables that contribute to accelerated wear such as the thinness of the polyethylene component, screw holes, incongruous surfaces, and third-body wear, as well as the heat-pressed polyethylene.

Other factors regarding the wear of polyethylene may include the use of specific additives such as calcium stearate, as well as the type of resin, lot-to-lot variability, the method of final geometry shaping and shelf life (Berzins et al., 2002; Meding et al., 2011; Pienkowski et al., 1996; Poggie et al., 1998; Premnath et al., 1996).

Metals

Concerns regarding the potential effects of manufacturing processes regarding metal implants were stimulated recently by reports of pseudotumors around metal-on-metal implants. In a meta-analysis of wear of metal-on-metal implants, Kretzer at al.(2009) evaluated several factors including manufacturing method, clearance, head size and carbon content. They concluded that an increase in head size and a smaller clearance reduces running-in wear; low surface roughness and low deviation on roundness reduce wear; the influence of alloy carbon content is unclear; manufacturing process (wrought vs. cast) had no effect; and heat treatment processes increased wear.

12.3 Surgical factors

If we accept that loose implants accelerate wear, any surgical factors that contribute to early loosening would then promote wear. Eftekhar et al. (1976) proposed that there were three factors that produce early loosening of a hip replacement: error in operative technique in preparation of bone;

error in technique in insertion of cement; faulty selection of the design of the implant (small femoral head, thin plastic socket). These three factors can also be extrapolated to implants with uncemented fixation. While the last factor relates to the implant design choice, there remain intraoperative decisions relating to component selection and implant fixation.

12.3.1 Bone resection and component position

Malpositioned and malaligned components have been observed with all types of arthroplasty procedures and generally have poor long-term outcomes (Fehring, 2000; Franta *et al.*, 2007; Parvizi *et al.*, 2006; van Riet *et al.*, 2009). These may be a consequence of malrotation (internal or external), malalignment with the mechanical or anatomical axis of the joint (off-axis; varus/valgus), malposition regarding the joint line as is seen with over- or under-resection, and malposition regarding anterior–posterior placement or posterior slope.

Soft-tissue balance (laxity vs. over constraint) of ligaments and tendons can also have an impact on the outcome and wear of components (Lewallen *et al.*, 1984; Swank *et al.*, 2007). The soft-tissue imbalance is frequently noted with pre-operative deformity that may be corrected during surgery (Krackow *et al.*, 1991). While pre-operative deformity and constraint may prevent the proper placement of components, post-operative laxity or over-constraint may affect the range of motion of the affected joint (Favorito *et al.*, 2002).

The consequences of malposition or malalignment include improper tracking, unbalanced loading, edge loading, impingement, subluxation and dislocation. This has been observed in simulator tests as well as clinically (Heegaard *et al.*, 2001; Moskal and Capps, 2010; Romero *et al.*, 2002).

Computer navigation has been introduced to arthroplasty procedures to improve alignment. Laboratory and clinical studies have demonstrated that results following computer alignment are more reproducible, with fewer outliers (Chin *et al.*, 2005; Haaker *et al.*, 2007; Krackow *et al.*, 2003). On the other hand, computer navigation adds another level of complexity to the surgical procedure and is associated with a significant learning curve (Hungerford, 2005). Bonutti *et al.*(2008) found a higher complication rate and a longer operative time with computer-assisted total knee arthroplasty. Also, differences in the reference systems between different navigation systems can have a significant impact on the results (Mihalko *et al.*, 2009).

Minimally invasive surgical approaches to total joint arthroplasty were introduced in order to improve recovery time. Minimally invasive procedures are associated with smaller incision sizes, minimal or no incision of muscles and tendons, and minimal dislocation or subluxation of the joint during surgery (Kolisek *et al.*, 2008; Mont *et al.*, 2010). However, issues regarding malalignment and other complications as well as longer surgical times may have an impact on wear and the long-term outcome (Khanna et al., 2009; Kolisek et al., 2008). Computer navigation may lead to improved results for alignment following minimally invasive surgery (Dutton and Yeo, 2009; Pagnano et al., 2009). Improved integration of these technologies is worthy of further exploration.

12.3.2 Implant fixation

Total joint implants are most frequently designed for fixation with bone cement (PMMA) or for biologic fixation. The long-term outcome of each has been variable and dependent on implant design, materials, surgical technique and host factors such as bone quality. Based on past results, hybrid fixation – where one component is cemented and the other is uncemented – is also frequently used.

Experience has proven that the long-term survival of cemented implants is highly dependent on good cement technique. Contemporary cement techniques may involve preparation of the bone bed with use of pulsatile lavage and/or a medullary brush, cement plugs or cement centralizers, centrifugation, vacuum mixing, retrograde filling of the prepared cavity, pressurization during application (cement gun), and topical agents including epinephrine and thrombin. Inadequate mixing of the bone cement (powder and monomer) can result if unpolymerized powder, bubbles (voids) within the cement mantle or inadequate penetration. In a study of autopsy specimens, while debonding was the most frequent observation (82%), other cement technique related findings were also noted: thin cement mantle (74%); stem–bone contact (48%); soft tissue at the stem interface (44%); no cement–bone interdigitation (30%); a gap at the stem interface (28%); and voids in the cement (22%) (Bishop et al., 2009). Cement mantle thickness has been shown to affect strains observed in the cement mantle (Fisher et al., 1997) and uneven distribution of cement may affect the loading of the implant and lead to fracture of the cement mantle.

The fixation success of biologic ingrowth prostheses is also highly technique dependent. While small gaps can be bridged by new bone (Onsten, 1995), larger interface distances may become filled by fibrous tissue, significantly impacting the initial stability of the implant (Jasty et al., 2007). In addition, small adjustments with cement to correct less than 1 mm over-resection and minor surface preparation irregularities are possible, although transitioning to cement fixation may become necessary.

12.3.3 Surgical decision making

As suggested by Eftekhar *et al.*, (1976) selection of the type and size of the implant is ultimately the responsibility of the surgeon. Decisions regarding type include not only implant design and manufacturer, but also type of fixation and articulating couple. This is particularly apropos to wear with the recent debate regarding the use of metal-on-metal implants.

A surgeon's overall experience, as well as experience with a particular design, may also have an impact on alignment of an implant. While instrumentation and computer navigation may facilitate the proper placement of prosthetic components, they do not replace the input and impact of the surgeon. Implant sizing may also influence the tracking and wear behavior of prostheses. Mismatched sizes are sometimes used and this may prevent proper articulation of the components.

12.3.4 Other surgical factors

Particles of bone cement, bone and metal (during cutting) may have been created during the surgical procedure. If they migrate between the articulating surfaces they will act as third bodies and may initiate abrasive wear of one or more of the components. This underscores the importance of thorough debridement of the prosthetic surfaces following implantation. Another source of iatrogenic damage takes place if the surface of the prosthesis is scratched during implantation. This compromise in the integrity of the articulating surface can act as a source of wear debris as well as a point of initiation for abrasive or adhesive wear.

12.4 Patient factors

A number of patient-related factors can have a profound effect on the surgical procedure as well as the long-term outcome. Factors that may impact implant wear are:

- activity level
- age
- anatomy
- body mass
- bone quality
- comorbidities
- cultural demands
- deformity
- falls
- gait

- general health
- patient expectations
- gender
- post-operative complications
- pre-operative diagnosis
- prior surgery
- race and ethnicity
- service – length of implantation

Historically, poorer survivorship rates have been reported in patients with higher levels of activity, higher body mass index (BMI), lower age and with specific pathologies (Bordini et al., 2007; Wright and Goodman, 2000). As one would expect, these factors are interrelated. For example, younger patients are associated with greater activity level and certain diseases are more prevalent in younger patients. Younger patients may also be associated with longer times of implantation. A higher BMI is associated with lower activity level (McClung et al., 2000). It is also important to appreciate that the patient's anatomy and health are not static but ever-changing.

12.4.1 Body mass index

There are mixed results reported for total joint arthroplasty in obese patients (Foran et al., 2004; Stukenborg-Colsman et al., 2005). Berend et al. (2004) reported that elevated BMI (> 33.7) when combined with varus tibial component alignment was associated with a 168-fold increase in failure, although no knees were revised specifically for polyethylene wear. Several authors have reported decreased activity with obesity and this is likely to mitigate the wear behavior of the components (Foran et al., 2004; McClung et al., 2000; Wright and Goodman, 2000).

12.4.2 Use

Wear rates have been shown to change during the service life of the implant. There is an initial 'bedding-in' period followed by a more steady-state period (Walker et al., 1996; Wroblewski et al., 1996). While there is a relationship between wear rate and length of implantation (Engh et al., 1992b; Lavernia et al., 2001), we generally agree with Schmalzreid et al. (2000) that 'wear is a function of use'. Use is influenced by activity level, joint load and loading cycles (McClung et al., 2000; Tsao et al., 2008). The activity level of a patient encompasses their activities of daily living, work-related activities, the level and frequency of exercise, the level of sports activity (occasional, recreational, professional, low-impact vs. high impact) and cultural practices (kneeling for prayer, for example). The magnitude of the load, range of motion and the interrelationship between the two during activity influence the mechanical conditions to which implants are subjected. It is generally accepted that the more physical activity that a person engages in, the more the implant is likely to wear (Lavernia et al., 2001; Wright and Goodman, 2000).

Patient expectations may also influence activity level positively or negatively. Patient motivation can determine how rapidly they return to their routine activities. However, there is an increased risk of falls with the elderly and post-operative complications (Kearns et al., 2008; Swinkels et al., 2009). In addition, sports activities with high contact or a high incidence of falling (skiing, snowboarding) are not recommended.

12.4.3 Anatomy

Anatomic diversity is determined by gender, age, disease, deformity, activity, ethnicity, gait and health. Variations in anatomy are not limited to size and morphometry, but also include differences in limb alignment and rotational angles. Regarding orthopaedic implants, musculoskeletal anatomy can affect implant selection, surgical approach, and alignment and position. The implant size selected is based upon the patient's anatomy and deformity (Low et al., 2000; Tsao et al., 2008). There is a limit to off-the-shelf sizes of implants. Although customized implants can be manufactured, they are not tested in the same way as the off-the-shelf sizes and their wear characteristics are unknown. In addition, soft-tissue diversity (origins, insertions, laxity, constraint) may also influence surgical approach, implant placement and function.

12.4.4 Pre-operative diagnosis, deformity and general health

Historically, specific diseases have lower survival rates than that reported for osteoarthritis. This may be a consequence of bone quality (e.g. osteoporosis), deformity (e.g. congenital hip dysplasia) or disease progression (e.g. rheumatoid arthritis). Pre-operative ligamentous laxity or contractures (Robbins et al., 2001) and limb length discrepancies (Berend et al., 2010) can influence component placement and it may not be possible to correctly balance the soft-tissue structures during surgery. Prior surgery on the affected limb can alter the anatomy and bone quality as well as create scar tissue, thereby having an effect on the surgical exposure, implant positioning and subsequent wound healing.

Post-operatively, the patient's overall health and the presence of comorbidities can have an impact on the healing and remodeling that occurs following orthopaedic surgery. In addition to diseases (e.g.

osteoporosis, rheumatoid arthritis, diabetes), comorbidities may include obesity, trauma, tumors and infection. There is also an increased risk of infection for patients with bacterial infections related to dental procedures (LaPorte et al., 1999; Waldman et al., 1997). Smoking has been shown to impair bone healing and osteogenesis in both dental and orthopaedic applications (Esposito et al., 1998; Lavernia et al., 1999).

12.4.5 Bone quality

The quality of host bone can have a significant effect on the outcome of the orthopaedic procedure. This may reflect disease, age, use or disuse, or prior surgery. Osteopetrotic and osteoporotic bone can both affect the seating of an implant, as can screw fixation (Matsuno and Katayama, 1997; Zardiackas et al., 1989).

12.4.6 Gender

More women than men undergo total joint arthroplasty. It has been suggested that women present with higher morbidity than men. However, outcomes for both patient groups are similar. If the sex of the patient did have an impact on wear, it is more likely to be a result of differences in pre-operative diagnosis, activity type and activity level, BMI and anatomy.

12.4.7 Age

Historically, younger patients have experienced lower joint survivorship than older patients. The primary reason for this was thought to be increased mechanical demands associated with activity. As improvements in implant design and surgical technique have led to improved longevity of orthopaedic implants, prostheses are being implanted into relatively younger patients. It is difficult to analyze the effect of age due to the many confounding variables that may be present. For example, on the one hand, the patient may have significant morbidity associated with their degenerative disease (such as with congenital hip dysplasia or juvenile arthritis) but, on the other, the osteogenic and healing capacity may be greater in younger patients.

12.5 Interactions between different factors

While specific factors that are associated with increasing wear rates have been discussed, in reality, wear usually occurs under conditions where several of these factors interact and thereby instigate a cyclic amplification of wear leading to the ultimate failure of the surgical procedure. The medical literature contains numerous case reports illustrating this point. For example, an acetabular cup can be placed into too much anteversion, causing frequent subluxation. This places high stresses on the rim of the cup, which fractures. There is now metal-on-metal impingement of a femoral head on the metal backing of the cup. The debris incites osteolysis and loss of fixation with instability. More wear is generated, and so on. In general, poor surgical technique such as with a poorly balanced total knee replacement or an unstable fracture fixation construct will exhibit increased wear as a component of potential catastrophic failure accelerating the overall clinical failure.

12.6 Conclusion

Wear, and its subsequent effects, can compromise the long-term survivorship of orthopaedic implants. Based upon laboratory tests and analysis of retrieved implants, factors have been identified that may contribute to different wear processes. These factors may be related to the specific implant (materials, design, manufacturing), surgical technique and decision making, or type of patient. Over the past few decades, new materials, designs and manufacturing processes have been introduced that have improved the wear properties of many orthopaedic implants. The development of improved instrumentation and surgeon education (fellowships, courses) has also had an impact on the reproducibility of these surgical procedures. Patient factors are the least controllable. While certain patient aspects such as weight and activity (types and level) are modifiable, others are not (e.g. age, anatomy, gender). Advancements in the treatment of diseases such as osteoporosis may ultimately reduce or at least delay the need for implant itself.

There have been concerns regarding component wear since the advent of orthopaedic implants. The biological response to wear debris has been shown to adversely affect the interface between the implant and host tissue. The future depends on continuing efforts to produce materials and designs that minimize implant wear as well as the development of treatment strategies to reduce the chronic inflammatory response to wear debris.

12.7 References

Agins, H. J., Alcock, N. W., Bansal, M., Salvati, E. A., Wilson, P. D. J., Pellicci, P. M. and Bullough, P. G. 1988. Metallic wear in failed titanium-alloy total hip replacements. A histological and quantitative analysis. *J Bone Joint Surg Am*, 70, 347–56.

Akizuki, S., Takizawa, T. and Horiuchi, H. 2003. Fixation of a hydroxyapatite-tricalcium phosphate-coated cementless knee prosthesis. Clinical and radiographic evaluation seven years after surgery. *J Bone Joint Surg Br*, 85, 1123–7.

Amstutz, H. C. 1969. Polymers as bearing materials for total hip replacement: a friction and wear analysis. *J Biomed Mater Res*, 3, 547–68.

Au, A., Ha, J., Hernandez, M., Polotsky, A., Hungerford, D. S. and Frondoza, C. G. 2006. Nickel and vanadium metal ions induce apoptosis of T-lymphocyte Jurkat cells. *J Biomed Mater Res A*, 79, 512–21.

Bargmann, L. S., Bargmann, B. C., Collier, J. P., Currier, B. H. and Mayor, M. B. 1999. Current sterilization and packaging methods for polyethylene. *Clin Orthop Relat Res*, 369, 49–58.

Barrack, R. L., Folgueras, A., Munn, B., Tvetden, D. and Sharkey, P. 1997. Pelvic lysis and polyethylene wear at 5-8 years in an uncemented total hip. *Clin Orthop Relat Res*, 335, 211–7.

Bartel, D. L., Bicknell, V. L. and Wright, T. M. 1986. The effect of conformity, thickness, and material on stresses in ultra-high molecular weight components for total joint replacement. *J Bone Joint Surg Am*, 68, 1041–51.

Bauer, T. W. and Schils, J. 1999. The pathology of total joint arthroplasty.II. Mechanisms of implant failure. *Skeletal Radiol*, 28, 483–97.

Beaule, P. E., Harvey, N., Zaragoza, E., Le Duff, M. J. and Dorey, F. J. 2007. The femoral head/neck offset and hip resurfacing. *J Bone Joint Surg Br*, 89, 9–15.

Bellare, A. and Kurtz, S. M. 2009. High pressure crystallized UHMWPEs. In Kurtz, S. M. (ed.) *UHMWPE*. Oxford, Academic Press.

Berend, K. R., Sporer, S. M., Sierra, R. J., Glassman, A. H. and Morris, M. J. 2010. Achieving stability and lower-limb length in total hip arthroplasty. *J Bone Joint Surg Am*, 92, 2737–52.

Berend, M. E., Ritter, M. A., Meding, J. B., Faris, P. M., Keating, E. M., Redelman, R., Faris, G. W. and Davis, K. E. 2004. Tibial component failure mechanisms in total knee arthroplasty. *Clin Orthop Relat Res*, 428, 26–34.

Berzins, A., Jacobs, J. J., Berger, R., Ed, C., Natarajan, R., Andriacchi, T. and Galante, J. O. 2002. Surface damage in machined ram-extruded and net-shape molded retrieved polyethylene tibial inserts of total knee replacements. *J Bone Joint Surg Am*, 84A, 1534–40.

Billi, F., Sangiorgio, S. N., Aust, S. and Ebramzadeh, E. 2010. Material and surface factors influencing backside fretting wear in total knee replacement tibial components. *J Biomechanics*, 43, 1310–5.

Bishop, N. E., Schoenwald, M., Schultz, P., Puschel, K. and Morlock, M. M. 2009. The condition of the cement mantle in femoral hip prosthesis implantations – a post mortem retrieval study. *Hip Int*, 19, 87–95.

Black, J. 1992. *Biological Performance of Materials*. New York, Marcel Dekker.

Bloebaum, R. D., Nelson, K., Dorr, L. D., Hofmann, A. A. and Lyman, D. J. 1991. Investigation of early surface delamination observed in retrieved heat-pressed tibial inserts. *Clin Orthop Relat Res*, 269, 120–7.

Bloebaum, R. D., Mihalopoulus, N. L., Jensen, J. W. and Dorr, L. D. 1997. Postmortem analysis of bone growth into porous-coated acetabular components. *J Bone Joint Surg Am*, 79, 1013–22.

Bobyn, J. D., Toh, K. K., Hacking, S. A., Tanzer, M. and Krygier, J. J. 1999. Tissue response to porous tantalum acetabular cups: a canine model. *J Arthroplasty*, 14, 347–54.

Bolland, B. J., Culliford, D. J., Langton, D. J., Millington, J. P., Arden, N. K. and Latham, J. M. 2011. High failure rates with a large-diameter hybrid metal-on-metal total hip replacement: clinical, radiological and retrieval analysis. *J Bone Joint Surg Br*, 93, 608–15.

Bonutti, P. M., Dethmers, D., Ulrich, S. D., Seyler, T. M. and Mont, M. A. 2008. Computer navigation-assisted versus minimally invasive TKA: benefits and drawbacks. *Clin Orthop Relat Res*, 466, 2756–62.

Bordini, B., Stea, S., De Clerico, M., Strazzari, S., Sasdelli, A. and Toni, A. 2007. Factors affecting aseptic loosening of 4750 total hip arthroplasties: multivariate survival analysis. *BMC Musculoskelet Disord*, 8, 69.

Boutin, P., Christel, P., Dorlot, J. M., Meunier, A., De Roquancourt, A., Blanquaert, D., Herman, S., Sedel, L. and Witvoet, J. 1988. The use of dense alumina–alumina ceramic combination in total hip replacement. *J Biomed Mater Res*, 22, 1203–32.

Burke, D. W., O'connor, D. O., Zalenski, E. B., Jasty, M. and Harris, W. H. 1991. Micromotion of cemented and uncemented femoral components. *J Bone Joint Surg Br*, 73, 33–7.

Caicedo, M. S., Pennekamp, P. H., McAllister, K., Jacobs, J. J. and Hallab, N. J. 2010. Soluble ions more than particulate cobalt-alloy implant debris induce monocyte costimulatory molecule expression and release of proinflammatory cytokines critical to metal-induced lymphocyte reactivity. *J Biomed Mater Res A*, 93, 1312–21.

Callaghan, J. J., O'rourke, M. R., Goetz, D. D., Schmalzried, T. P., Campbell, P. A. and Johnston, R. C. 2002. Tibial post impingement in posterior-stabilized total knee arthroplasty. *Clin Orthop Relat Res*, 404, 83–8.

Callaghan, J. J., Bracha, P., Liu, S. S., Piyaworakhun, S., Goetz, D. D. and Johnston, R. C. 2009. Survivorship of a Charnley total hip arthroplasty. A concise follow-up, at a minimum of thirty-five years, of previous reports. *J Bone Joint Surg Am*, 91, 2617–21.

Campbell, P., Takamura, K., Lundergan, W., Esposito, C. and Amstutz, H. C. 2009. Cement technique changes improved hip resurfacing longevity–implant retrieval findings. *Bull NYU Hosp Joint Dis*, 67, 146–53.

Campbell, P., Ebramzadeh, E., Nelson, S., Takamura, K., De Smet, K. and Amstutz, H. C. 2010. Histological features of pseudotumor-like tissues from metal-on-metal hips. *Clin Orthop Relat Res*, 468, 2321–7.

Caton, J. and Prudhon, J. L. 2011. Over 25 years survival after Charnley's total hip arthroplasty. *Int Orthop*, 35, 185–8.

Champion, J. A., Walker, A. and Mitragotri, S. 2008. Role of particle size in phagocytosis of polymeric microspheres. *Pharm Res*, 25, 1815–21.

Charnley, J. 1961. Arthroplasty of the hip. A new operation. *Lancet*, 1, 1129–32.

Charnley, J. 1972. The long-term results of low-friction arthroplasty of the hip performed as a primary intervention. *J Bone Joint Surg Br*, 54, 61–76.

Charnley, J. and Halley, D. K. 1975. Rate of wear in total hip replacement. *Clin Orthop Relat Res*, 112, 170–9.

Chin, K. R., Dalury, D. F., Zurakowski, D. and Scott, R. D. 2002. Intraoperative measurements of male and female distal femurs during primary total knee arthroplasty. *J Knee Surg*, 15, 213–7.

Chin, P. L., Yang, K. Y., Yeo, S. J. and Lo, N. N. 2005. Randomized control trial comparing radiographic total knee arthroplasty implant placement using computer navigation versus conventional technique. *J Arthroplasty*, 20, 618–26.

Chmell, M. J., Poss, R., Thomas, W. H. and Sledge, C. B. 1996. Early failure of Hylamer acetabular inserts due to eccentric wear. *J Arthroplasty*, 11, 351–3.
Cinotti, G., Lucioli, N., Malagoli, A., Calderoli, C. and Cassese, F. 2011. Do large femoral heads reduce the risks of impingement in total hip arthroplasty with optimal and non-optimal cup positioning? *Int Orthop*, 35, 317–23.
Clarke, I. C., Good, V., Williams, P., Schroeder, D., Anissian, L., Stark, A., Oonishi, H., Schuldies, J. and Gustafson, G. 2000. Ultra-low wear rates for rigid-on-rigid bearings in total hip replacements. *Proc Inst Mech Eng H*, 214, 331–47.
Collier, J. P., Surprenant, V. A., Jensen, R. E. and Mayor, M. B. 1991. Corrosion at the interface of cobalt-alloy heads on titanium-alloy stems. *Clin Orthop Relat Res*, 271, 305–12.
Collier, J. P., Mayor, M. B., Jensen, R. E., Surprenant, V. A., Surprenant, H. P., McNamar, J. L. and Belec, L. 1992. Mechanisms of failure of modular prostheses. *Clin Orthop Relat Res*, 285, 129–39.
Collier, M. B., Jewett, B. A. and Engh, C. A., JR. 2003. Clinical assessment of tibial polyethylene thickness: comparison of radiographic measurements with as-implanted and as-retrieved thicknesses. *J Arthroplasty*, 18, 860–6.
Conditt, M. A., Ismaily, S. K., Alexander, J. W. and Noble, P. C. 2004a. Backside wear of modular ultra-high molecular weight polyethylene tibial inserts. *J Bone Joint Surg Am*, 86A, 1031–7.
Conditt, M. A., Stein, J. A. and Noble, P. C. 2004b. Factors affecting the severity of backside wear of modular tibial inserts. *J Bone Joint Surg Am*, 86A, 305–11.
Conditt, M. A., Thompson, M. T., Usrey, M. M., Ismaily, S. K. and Noble, P. C. 2005. Backside wear of polyethylene tibial inserts: mechanism and magnitude of material loss. *J Bone Joint Surg Am*, 87, 326–31.
Cook, S. D. and Thomas, K. A. 1991. Fatigue failure of noncemented porous-coated implants. A retrieval study. *J Bone Joint Surg Br*, 73, 20–4.
Cook, S. D., Barrack, R. L., Baffes, G. C., Clemow, A. J., Serekian, P., Dong, N. and Kester, M. A. 1994. Wear and corrosion of modular interfaces in total hip replacements. *Clin Orthop Relat Res*, 298, 80–8.
Cooke, C. C., Hozack, W., Lavernia, C., Sharkey, P., Shastri, S. and Rothman, R. H. 2003. Early failure mechanisms of constrained tripolar acetabular sockets used in revision total hip arthroplasty. *J Arthroplasty*, 18, 827–33.
Counsell, A., Heasley, R., Arumilli, B. and Paul, A. 2008. A groin mass caused by metal particle debris after hip resurfacing. *Acta Orthop Belg*, 74, 870–4.
Crowninshield, R. D. and Muratoglu, O. K. 2008. How have new sterilization techniques and new forms of polyethylene influenced wear in total joint replacement? *J Am Acad Orthop Surg*, 16, Suppl 1, S80–5.
Currier, B. H., Currier, J. H., Mayor, M. B., Lyford, K. A., Van Citters, D. W. and Collier, J. P. 2007. In vivo oxidation of gamma-barrier-sterilized ultra-high-molecular-weight polyethylene bearings. *J Arthroplasty*, 22, 721–31.
Currier, J. H., Bill, M. A. and Mayor, M. B. 2005. Analysis of wear asymmetry in a series of 94 retrieved polyethylene tibial bearings. *J Biomechanics*, 38, 367–75.
D'Lima, D. D., Chen, P. C. and Colwell, C. W., JR. 2001. Polyethylene contact stresses, articular congruity, and knee alignment. *Clin Orthop Relat Res*, 392, 232–8.
Davis, J. R. 2003. *Handbook of Materials for Medical Devices*. Materials Park, OH, ASM International.

Dolan, M. M., Kelly, N. H., Nguyen, J. T., Wright, T. M. and Haas, S. B. 2011. Implant design influences tibial post wear damage in posterior-stabilized knees. *Clin Orthop Relat Res*, 469, 160–7.

Dutton, A. Q. and Yeo, S. J. 2009. Computer-assisted minimally invasive total knee arthroplasty compared with standard total knee arthroplasty. Surgical technique. *J Bone Joint Surg Am*, 91, Suppl 2 Pt 1, 116–30.

Ebramzadeh, E., Campbell, P. A., Takamura, K. M., Lu, Z., Sangiorgio, S. N., Kalma, J. J., De Smet, K. A. and Amstutz, H. C. 2011. Failure modes of 433 metal-on-metal hip implants: how, why, and wear. *Orthop Clin North Am*, 42, 241–50.

Eftekhar, N. S., Kiernan, H. A., Jr. and Stinchfield, F. E. 1976. Systemic and local complications following low-friction arthroplasty of the hip joint. A study of 800 consecutive operations. *Arch Surg*, 111, 150–5.

ElMaraghy, A. and Devereaux, M. 2008. Medial wear of the polyethylene component associated with heterotopic ossification after reverse shoulder arthroplasty. *Can J Surg*, 51, E103–4.

Engh, C. A., O'connor, D., Jasty, M., McGovern, T. F., Bobyn, J. D. and Harris, W. H. 1992a. Quantification of implant micromotion, strain shielding, and bone resorption with porous-coated anatomic medullary locking femoral prostheses. *Clin Orthop Relat Res*, 285, 13–29.

Engh, C. A., Zettl-Schaffer, K. F., Kukita, Y., Sweet, D., Jasty, M. and Bragdon, C. 1993. Histological and radiographic assessment of well functioning porous-coated acetabular components. A human postmortem retrieval study. *J Bone Joint Surg Am*, 75, 814–24.

Engh, G. A. and Ammeen, D. J. 2004. Epidemiology of osteolysis: backside implant wear. *Instr Course Lect*, 53, 243–9.

Engh, G. A., Dwyer, K. A. and Hanes, C. K. 1992b. Polyethylene wear of metal-backed tibial components in total and unicompartmental knee prostheses. *J Bone Joint Surg Br*, 74, 9–17.

Esposito, M., Hirsch, J. M., Lekholm, U. and Thomsen, P. 1998. Biological factors contributing to failures of osseointegrated oral implants. (II). Etiopathogenesis. *Eur J Oral Sci*, 106, 721–64.

Ezzet, K. A. 1996. Early failure of Hylamer acetabular inserts due to eccentric wear. *J Arthroplasty*, 11, 761–2.

Faris, P. M., Ritter, M. A., Pierce, A. L., Davis, K. E. and Faris, G. W. 2006. Polyethylene sterilization and production affects wear in total hip arthroplasties. *Clin Orthop Relat Res*, 453, 305–8.

Favorito, P. J., Mihalko, W. M. and Krackow, K. A. 2002. Total knee arthroplasty in the valgus knee. *J Am Acad Orthop Surg*, 10, 16–24.

Fehring, T. K. 2000. Rotational malalignment of the femoral component in total knee arthroplasty. *Clin Orthop Relat Res*, 380, 72–9.

Fehring, T. K., Murphy, J. A., Hayes, T. D., Roberts, D. W., Pomeroy, D. L. and Griffin, W. L. 2004. Factors influencing wear and osteolysis in press-fit condylar modular total knee replacements. *Clin Orthop Relat Res*, 428, 40–50.

Firkins, P. J., Tipper, J. L., Ingham, E., Stone, M. H., Farrar, R. and Fisher, J. 2001. A novel low wearing differential hardness, ceramic-on-metal hip joint prosthesis. *J Biomechanics*, 34, 1291–8.

Fisher, D. A., Tsang, A. C., Paydar, N., Milionis, S. and Turner, C. H. 1997.

Cement-mantle thickness affects cement strains in total hip replacement. *J Biomechanics*, 30, 1173–7.

Foran, J. R., Mont, M. A., Rajadhyaksha, A. D., Jones, L. C., Etienne, G. and Hungerford, D. S. 2004. Total knee arthroplasty in obese patients: a comparison with a matched control group. *J Arthroplasty*, 19, 817–24.

Franta, A. K., Lenters, T. R., Mounce, D., Neradilek, B. and Matsen, F. A., 3rd 2007. The complex characteristics of 282 unsatisfactory shoulder arthroplasties. *J Shoulder Elbow Surg*, 16, 555–62.

Freeman, M. A., Swanson, S. A. and Heath, J. C. 1969. The production characterization and biological significance of the wear particles produced in vitro from cobalt–chromium–molybdenum total joint-replacement prostheses. *Br J Surg*, 56, 701.

Fujishiro, T., Moojen, D. J., Kobayashi, N., Dhert, W. J. and Bauer, T. W. 2011. Perivascular and diffuse lymphocytic inflammation are not specific for failed metal-on-metal hip implants. *Clin Orthop Relat Res*, 469, 1127–33.

Garcia-Rey, E. and Garcia-Cimbrelo, E. 2008. Clinical and radiographic results and wear performance in different generations of a cementless porous-coated acetabular cup. *Int Orthop*, 32, 181–7.

Gelb, H., Schumacher, H. R., Cuckler, J., Ducheyne, P. and Baker, D. G. 1994. In vivo inflammatory response to polymethylmethacrylate particulate debris: effect of size, morphology, and surface area. *J Orthop Res*, 12, 83–92.

Gilbert, J. L., Buckley, C. A., Jacobs, J. J., Bertin, K. C. and Zernich, M. R. 1994. Intergranular corrosion-fatigue failure of cobalt-alloy femoral stems. A failure analysis of two implants. *J Bone Joint Surg Am*, 76, 110–5.

Goldberg, J. R., Gilbert, J. L., Jacobs, J. J., Bauer, T. W., Paprosky, W. and Leurgans, S. 2002. A multicenter retrieval study of the taper interfaces of modular hip prostheses. *Clin Orthop Relat Res*, 40, 49–61.

Goldring, S. R., Schiller, A. L., Roelke, M., Rourke, C. M., O'neill, D. A. and Harris, W. H. 1983. The synovial-like membrane at the bone–cement interface in loose total hip replacements and its proposed role in bone lysis. *J Bone Joint Surg Am*, 65, 575–84.

Goldring, S. R., Jasty, M., Roelke, M. S., Rourke, C. M., Bringhurst, F. R. and Harris, W. H. 1986. Formation of a synovial-like membrane at the bone–cement interface. Its role in bone resorption and implant loosening after total hip replacement. *Arthritis Rheum*, 29, 836–42.

Goldsmith, A. A., Dowson, D., Isaac, G. H. and Lancaster, J. G. 2000. A comparative joint simulator study of the wear of metal-on-metal and alternative material combinations in hip replacements. *Proc Inst Mech Eng H*, 214, 39–47.

Gonzalez Della Valle, A., Ruzo, P. S., Li, S., Pellicci, P., Sculco, T. P. and Salvati, E. A. 2001. Dislodgment of polyethylene liners in first and second-generation Harris–Galante acetabular components. A report of eighteen cases. *J Bone Joint Surg Am*, 83A, 553–9.

Goodman, S. B. 2007. Wear particles, periprosthetic osteolysis and the immune system. *Biomaterials*, 28, 5044–8.

Goodman, S. B., Schatzker, J., Sumner-Smith, G., Fornasier, V. L., Goften, N. and Hunt, C. 1985. The effect of polymethylmethacrylate on bone: an experimental study. *Arch Orthop Trauma Surg*, 104, 150–4.

Goodman, S. B., Gomez Barrena, E., Takagi, M. and Konttinen, Y. T. 2009.

Biocompatibility of total joint replacements: A review. *J Biomed Mater Res A*, 90, 603–18.

Haaker, R. G., Tiedjen, K., Ottersbach, A., Rubenthaler, F., Stockheim, M. and Stiehl, J. B. 2007. Comparison of conventional versus computer-navigated acetabular component insertion. *J Arthroplasty*, 22, 151–9.

Hallab, N. J. and Jacobs, J. J. 2009. Biologic effects of implant debris. *Bull NYU Hosp Joint Dis*, 67, 182–8.

Hallab, N. J., Jacobs, J. J. and Katz, J. L. 2004. Orthopedic applications. In: Ratner, B. D., Hoffman, A. S., Schoen, F. J. and Lemons, J. E. (eds) *Biomaterials Science: An Introduction to Materials in Medicine*. New York, Elsevier.

Hannouche, D., Nich, C., Bizot, P., Meunier, A., Nizard, R. and Sedel, L. 2003. Fractures of ceramic bearings: history and present status. *Clin Orthop Relat Res*, 417, 19–26.

Harman, M., Affatato, S., Spinelli, M., Zavalloni, M., Stea, S. and Toni, A. 2010. Polyethylene insert damage in unicondylar knee replacement: a comparison of *in vivo* function and *in vitro* simulation. *Proc Inst Mech Eng H*, 224, 823–30.

Harman, M. K., Banks, S. A. and Hodge, W. A. 2007. Backside damage corresponding to articular damage in retrieved tibial polyethylene inserts. *Clin Orthop Relat Res*, 458, 137–44.

Harris, W. H. 1984. Advances in total hip arthroplasty. The metal-backed acetabular component. *Clin Orthop Relat Res*, 183, 4–11.

Harris, W. H., Schiller, A. L., Scholler, J. M., Freiberg, R. A. and Scott, R. 1976. Extensive localized bone resorption in the femur following total hip replacement. *J Bone Joint Surg Am*, 58, 612–8.

Hart, A. J., Ilo, K., Underwood, R., Cann, P., Henckel, J., Lewis, A., Cobb, J. and Skinner, J. 2011. The relationship between the angle of version and rate of wear of retrieved metal-on-metal resurfacings: a prospective, CT-based study. *J Bone Joint Surg Br*, 93, 315–20.

Heegaard, J. H., Leyvraz, P. F. and Hovey, C. B. 2001. A computer model to simulate patellar biomechanics following total knee replacement: the effects of femoral component alignment. *Clin Biomech*, 16, 415–23.

Hertel, R. and Ballmer, F. T. 2003. Observations on retrieved glenoid components. *J Arthroplasty*, 18, 361–6.

Hirakawa, K., Bauer, T. W., Yamaguchi, M., Stulberg, B. N. and Wilde, A. H. 1999. Relationship between wear debris particles and polyethylene surface damage in primary total knee arthroplasty. *J Arthroplasty*, 14, 165–71.

Hoeltzel, D. A., Walt, M. J., Kyle, R. F. and Simon, F. D. 1989. The effects of femoral head size on the deformation of ultrahigh molecular weight polyethylene acetabular cups. *J Biomechanics*, 22, 1163–73.

Hood, R. W., Wright, T. M. and Burstein, A. H. 1983. Retrieval analysis of total knee prostheses: a method and its application to 48 total condylar prostheses. *J Biomed Mater Res*, 17, 829–42.

Hopkins, A. R., Hansen, U. N., Amis, A. A., Knight, L., Taylor, M., Levy, O. and Copeland, S. A. 2007. Wear in the prosthetic shoulder: association with design parameters. *J Biomech Eng*, 129, 223–30.

Horowitz, S. M., Frondoza, C. G. and Lennox, D. W. 1988. Effects of polymethylmethacrylate exposure upon macrophages. *J Orthop Res*, 6, 827–32.

Hosman, A. H., Van der Mei, H. C., Bulstra, S. K., Busscher, H. J. and Neut, D.

2010. Effects of metal-on-metal wear on the host immune system and infection in hip arthroplasty. *Acta Orthop*, 81, 526–34.

Huber, M., Reinisch, G., Zenz, P., Zweymuller, K. and Lintner, F. 2010. Postmortem study of femoral osteolysis associated with metal-on-metal articulation in total hip replacement: an analysis of nine cases. *J Bone Joint Surg Am*, 92, 1720–31.

Hungerford, D. S. 2005. Computer-assisted surgery: still just 'boy toys' for the passionate few. Counterpoint. *Orthopedics*, 28, 941.

Ianuzzi, A., Kurtz, S. M., Kane, W., Shah, P., Siskey, R., Van ooij, A., Bindal, R., Ross, R., Lanman, T., Buttner-Janz, K. and Isaza, J. 2010. In vivo deformation, surface damage, and biostability of retrieved Dynesys systems. *Spine (Phila Pa 1976)*, 35, E1310–6.

Isaac, G. H., Wroblewski, B. M., Atkinson, J. R. and Dowson, D. 1992. A tribological study of retrieved hip prostheses. *Clin Orthop Relat Res*, 276, 115–25.

Ishikawa, Y., Muramatsu, N., Ohshima, H. and Kondo, T. 1991. Effect of particle size on phagocytosis of latex particles by guinea-pig polymorphonuclear leucocytes. *J Biomater Sci Polym Ed*, 2, 53–60.

Jacobs, J. J., Shanbhag, A., Glant, T. T., Black, J. and Galante, J. O. 1994. Wear debris in total joint replacements. *J Am Acad Orthop Surg*, 2, 212–20.

Jacobs, M. A., Bhargava, T., Lathroum, J. M. and Hungerford, M. W. 2009. Debonding of the acetabular porous coating in hip resurfacing arthroplasty. A report of two cases. *J Bone Joint Surg Am*, 91, 961–4.

Jasty, M., Jiranek, W. and Harris, W. H. 1992. Acrylic fragmentation in total hip replacements and its biological consequences. *Clin Orthop Relat Res*, 285, 116–128.

Jasty, M., Kienapfel, H. and Griss, P. 2007. Fixation by ingrowth. In Callaghan, J. J., Rosenberg, A. G. and Rubash, H. E. (eds) *The Adult Hip*. Philadelphia, PA, Lipincott Williams and Wilkins.

Jayabalan, P., Furman, B. D., Cottrell, J. M. and Wright, T. M. 2007. Backside wear in modern total knee designs. *HSS J*, 3, 30–4.

Jerosch, J. and Moursi, M. G. 2008. Foreign body reaction due to polyethylene's wear after implantation of an interspinal segment. *Arch Orthop Trauma Surg*, 128, 1–4.

Jones, L. C. and Hungerford, D. S. 1987. Cement Disease. *Clin Orthop Relat Res*, 225, 192–206.

Jones, L. C., Frondoza, C. G. and Hungerfrod, D. S. 1999. Immunohistochemical evaluation of interface membranes from failed cemented and uncemented acetabular components. *J Biomed Mater Res*, 48, 889–98.

Jones, L. C., Frondoza, C. and Hungerford, D. S. 2001. Effect of PMMA particles and movement on an implant interface in a canine model. *J Bone Joint Surg Br*, 83, 448–58.

Jung, Y. L. and Kim, S. Y. 2010. Alumina-on-polyethylene bearing surfaces in total hip arthroplasty. *Open Orthop J*, 4, 56–60.

Kang, J. S., Dorr, L. D. and Wan, Z. 2000. The effect of diaphyseal biologic fixation on clinical results and fixation of the APR-II stem. *J Arthroplasty*, 15, 730–5.

Kearns, R. J., O'Connor, D. P. and Brinker, M. R. 2008. Management of falls after total knee arthroplasty. *Orthopedics*, 31, 225.

Khan, W. S., Agarwal, M., Malik, A. A., Cox, A. G., Denton, J. and Holt, E. M. 2008. Chromium, cobalt and titanium metallosis involving a Nottingham shoulder replacement. *J Bone Joint Surg Br*, 90, 502–5.

Khanna, A., Gougoulias, N., Longo, U. G. and Maffulli, N. 2009. Minimally invasive total knee arthroplasty: a systematic review. *Orthop Clin North Am*, 40, 479–89.

Kim, H. D., Kim, K. S., Ki, S. C. and Choi, Y. S. 2007. Electron microprobe analysis and tissue reaction around titanium alloy spinal implants. *Asian Spine J*, 1, 1–7.

Kim, J. M., Mudgal, C. S., Konopka, J. F. and Jupiter, J. B. 2011. Complications of total elbow arthroplasty. *J Am Acad Orthop Surg*, 19, 328–39.

Kim, Y. H., Oh, S. H., Kim, J. S. and Koo, K. H. 2003. Contemporary total hip arthroplasty with and without cement in patients with osteonecrosis of the femoral head. *J Bone Joint Surg Am*, 85A, 675–81.

Kleinhans, J. A., Jakubowitz, E., Seeger, J. B., Heisel, C. and Kretzer, J. P. 2009. Macroscopic third-body wear caused by porous metal surface fragments in total hip arthroplasty. *Orthopedics*, 32, 364.

Kligman, M., Furman, B. D., Padgett, D. E. and Wright, T. M. 2007. Impingement contributes to backside wear and screw-metallic shell fretting in modular acetabular cups. *J Arthroplasty*, 22, 258–64.

Kolisek, F. R., Seyler, T. M., Ulrich, S. D., Marker, D. R., Jessup, N. M. and Mont, M. A. 2008. A comparison of the minimally invasive dual-incision versus posterolateral approach in total hip arthroplasty. *Surg Technol Int*, 17, 253–8.

Krackow, K. A., Jones, M. M., Teeny, S. M. and Hungerford, D. S. 1991. Primary total knee arthroplasty in patients with fixed valgus deformity. *Clin Orthop Relat Res*, 273, 9–18.

Krackow, K. A., Phillips, M. J., Bayers-Thering, M., Serpe, L. and Mihalko, W. M. 2003. Computer-assisted total knee arthroplasty: navigation in TKA. *Orthopedics*, 26, 1017–23.

Kretzer, J. P., Kleinhans, J. A., Jakubowitz, E., Thomsen, M. and Heisel, C. 2009. A meta-analysis of design- and manufacturing-related parameters influencing the wear behavior of metal-on-metal hip joint replacements. *J Orthop Res*, 27, 1473–80.

Krieg, A. H., Speth, B. M. and Ochsner, P. E. 2009. Backside volumetric change in the polyethylene of uncemented acetabular components. *J Bone Joint Surg Br*, 91, 1037–43.

Kurtz, S. M. and Devine, J. N. 2007. PEEK biomaterials in trauma, orthopedic, and spinal implants. *Biomaterials*, 28, 4845–69.

Kurtz, S. M., Ochoa, J. A., White, C. V., Srivastav, S. and Cournoyer, J. 1998. Backside nonconformity and locking restraints affect liner/shell load transfer mechanisms and relative motion in modular acetabular components for total hip replacement. *J Biomechanics*, 31, 431–7.

Kurtz, S. M., Muratoglu, O. K., Evans, M. and Edidin, A. A. 1999. Advances in the processing, sterilization, and crosslinking of ultra-high molecular weight polyethylene for total joint arthroplasty. *Biomaterials*, 20, 1659–88.

Kurtz, S. M., Peloza, J., Siskey, R. and Villarraga, M. L. 2005. Analysis of a retrieved polyethylene total disc replacement component. *Spine J*, 5, 344–50.

Kurtz, S. M., Van Ooij, A., Ross, R., De Waal Malefijt, J., Peloza, J., Ciccarelli, L.

and Villarraga, M. L. 2007. Polyethylene wear and rim fracture in total disc arthroplasty. *Spine J*, 7, 12–21.

Kuzyk, P. R., Saccone, M., Sprague, S., Simunovic, N., Bhandari, M. and Schemitsch, E. H. 2011. Cross-linked versus conventional polyethylene for total hip replacement: a meta-analysis of randomised controlled trials. *J Bone Joint Surg Br*, 93, 593–600.

LaPorte, D. M., Waldman, B. J., Mont, M. A. and Hungerford, D. S. 1999. Infections associated with dental procedures in total hip arthroplasty. *J Bone Joint Surg Br*, 81, 56–9.

Lavernia, C. J., Sierra, R. J. and Gomez-Marin, O. 1999. Smoking and joint replacement: resource consumption and short-term outcome. *Clin Orthop Relat Res*, 367, 172–80.

Lavernia, C. J., Sierra, R. J., Hungerford, D. S. and Krackow, K. 2001. Activity level and wear in total knee arthroplasty: a study of autopsy retrieved specimens. *J Arthroplasty*, 16, 446–53.

Lee, P. C., Shih, C. H., Chen, W. J., Tu, Y. K. and Tai, C. L. 1999. Early polyethylene wear and osteolysis in cementless total hip arthroplasty: the influence of femoral head size and polyethylene thickness. *J Arthroplasty*, 14, 976–81.

Lennox, D. W., Schofield, B. H., McDonald, D. F. and Riley, L. H. J. 1987. A histologic comparison of aseptic loosening of cemented, press-fit, and biologic ingrowth prostheses. *Clin Orthop Relat Res*, 225, 171–191.

Lewallen, D. G., Bryan, R. S. and Peterson, L. F. 1984. Polycentric total knee arthroplasty. A ten-year follow-up study. *J Bone Joint Surg Am*, 66, 1211–8.

Lewis, J. L., Askew, M. J. and Jaycox, D. P. 1982. A comparative evaluation of tibial component designs of total knee prostheses. *J Bone Joint Surg Am*, 64, 129–35.

Li, G., Papannagari, R., Most, E., Park, S. E., Johnson, T., Tanamal, L. and Rubash, H. E. 2005. Anterior tibial post impingement in a posterior stabilized total knee arthroplasty. *J Orthop Res*, 23, 536–41.

Li, S., Scuderi, G., Furman, B. D., Bhattacharyya, S., Schmieg, J. J. and Insall, J. N. 2002. Assessment of backside wear from the analysis of 55 retrieved tibial inserts. *Clin Orthop Relat Res*, 404, 75–82.

Liu, C., Green, S. M., Watkins, N. D., Gregg, P. J. and McCaskie, A. W. 2001. Some failure modes of four clinical bone cements. *Proc Inst Mech Eng H*, 215, 359–66.

Lombardi, A. V., Jr., Skeels, M. D., Berend, K. R., Adams, J. B. and Franchi, O. J. 2011. Do large heads enhance stability and restore native anatomy in primary total hip arthroplasty? *Clin Orthop Relat Res*, 469, 1547–53.

Low, F. H., Khoo, L. P., Chua, C. K. and Lo, N. N. 2000. Kinematic analysis of total knee prosthesis designed for Asian population. *Crit Rev Biomed Eng*, 28, 33–40.

MacDonald, D., Sakona, A., Ianuzzi, A., Rimnac, C. M. and Kurtz, S. M. 2011. Do first-generation highly crosslinked polyethylenes oxidize in vivo? *Clin Orthop Rel Res*, 469, 2278–85.

Manson, T. T., Kelly, N. H., Lipman, J. D., Wright, T. M. and Westrich, G. H. 2010. Unicondylar knee retrieval analysis. *J Arthroplasty*, 25, 108–11.

Mathieu, G., Roue, J., Poignard, A. and Hernigou, P. 2008. Metal/alumine metallosis on tibial osteotomy. A case report. *Rev Chir Orthop Reparatrice Appar Mot*, 94, 297–300.

Matsen, F. A., 3rd, Bicknell, R. T. and Lippitt, S. B. 2007. Shoulder arthroplasty: the socket perspective. *J Shoulder Elbow Surg*, 16, S241–7.

Matsen, F. A., 3rd, Clinton, J., Lynch, J., Bertelsen, A. and Richardson, M. L. 2008. Glenoid component failure in total shoulder arthroplasty. *J Bone Joint Surg Am*, 90, 885–96.

Matsuno, T. and Katayama, N. 1997. Osteopetrosis and total hip arthroplasty. Report of two cases. *Int Orthop*, 21, 409–11.

Matthies, A., Underwood, R., Cann, P., Ilo, K., Nawaz, Z., Skinner, J. and Hart, A. J. 2011. Retrieval analysis of 240 metal-on-metal hip components, comparing modular total hip replacement with hip resurfacing. *J Bone Joint Surg Br*, 93, 307–14.

McClung, C. D., Zahiri, C. A., Higa, J. K., Amstutz, H. C. and Schmalzried, T. P. 2000. Relationship between body mass index and activity in hip or knee arthroplasty patients. *J Orthop Res*, 18, 35–9.

McGovern, T. E., Black, J., Jacobs, J. J., Graham, R. M. and Laberge, M. 1996. In vivo wear of Ti6A14V femoral heads: a retrieval study. *J Biomed Mater Res*, 32, 447–57.

McKellop, H., Clarke, I., Markolf, K. and Amstutz, H. 1981. Friction and wear properties of polymer, metal, and ceramic prosthetic joint materials evaluated on a multichannel screening device. *J Biomed Mater Res*, 15, 619–53.

McKellop, H., Park, S. H., Chiesa, R., Doorn, P., Lu, B., Normand, P., Grigoris, P. and Amstutz, H. 1996. In vivo wear of three types of metal on metal hip prostheses during two decades of use. *Clin Orthop Relat Res*, 329, S128–40.

McKellop, H., Shen, F. W., Dimaio, W. and Lancaster, J. G. 1999a. Wear of gamma-crosslinked polyethylene acetabular cups against roughened femoral balls. *Clin Orthop Relat Res*, 369, 73–82.

McKellop, H., Shen, F. W., Lu, B., Campbell, P. and Salovey, R. 1999b. Development of an extremely wear-resistant ultra high molecular weight polyethylene for total hip replacements. *J Orthop Res*, 17, 157–67.

McKellop, H. A. and Rostlund, T. V. 1990. The wear behavior of ion-implanted Ti-6A1-4V against UHMW polyethylene. *J Biomed Mater Res*, 24, 1413–25.

McKellop, H. A., Campbell, P., Park, S. H., Schmalzried, T. P., Grigoris, P., Amstutz, H. C. and Sarmiento, A. 1995. The origin of submicron polyethylene wear debris in total hip arthroplasty. *Clin Orthop Relat Res* 311, 3–20.

McNamara, J. L., Collier, J. P., Mayor, M. B. and Jensen, R. E. 1994. A comparison of contact pressures in tibial and patellar total knee components before and after service in vivo. *Clin Orthop Relat Res*, 299, 104–13.

Medel, F. J., Kurtz, S. M., Parvizi, J., Klein, G. R., Kraay, M. J. and Rimnac, C. M. 2011. In vivo oxidation contributes to delamination but not pitting in polyethylene components for total knee arthroplasty. *J Arthroplasty*, 26, 802–10.

Meding, J. B., Keating, E. M. and Davis, K. E. 2011. Acetabular UHMWPE survival and wear changes with different manufacturing techniques. *Clin Orthop Relat Res*, 469, 405–11.

Mihalko, W. M., Kammerzell, S. and Saleh, K. J. 2009. Acetabular orientation with different pelvic registration landmarks. *Orthopedics*, 32, 11–3.

Mont, M. A., Zywiel, M. G., McGrath, M. S. and Bonutti, P. M. 2010. Scientific evidence for minimally invasive total knee arthroplasty. *Instr Course Lect*, 59, 73–82.

Moskal, J. T. and Capps, S. G. 2010. Improving the accuracy of acetabular component orientation: avoiding malposition. *J Am Acad Orthop Surg*, 18, 286–96.

Muratoglu, O. K., Bragdon, C. R., O'Connor, D. O., Perinchief, R. S., Jasty, M. and Harris, W. H. 2002. Aggressive wear testing of a cross-linked polyethylene in total knee arthroplasty. *Clin Orthop Relat Res*, 404, 89–95.

Murtagh, R. D., Quencer, R. M., Cohen, D. S., Yue, J. J. and Sklar, E. L. 2009. Normal and abnormal imaging findings in lumbar total disk replacement: devices and complications. *Radiographics*, 29, 105–18.

Nam, D., Kepler, C. K., Neviaser, A. S., Jones, K. J., Wright, T. M., Craig, E. V. and Warren, R. F. 2010a. Reverse total shoulder arthroplasty: current concepts, results, and component wear analysis. *J Bone Joint Surg Am*, 92, Suppl 2, 23–35.

Nam, D., Kepler, C. K., Nho, S. J., Craig, E. V., Warren, R. F. and Wright, T. M. 2010b. Observations on retrieved humeral polyethylene components from reverse total shoulder arthroplasty. *J Shoulder Elbow Surg*, 19, 1003–12.

Nasser, S., Campbell, P. A., Kilgus, D., Kossovsky, N. and Amstutz, H. C. 1990. Cementless total joint arthroplasty prostheses with titanium-alloy articular surfaces. A human retrieval analysis. *Clin Orthop Relat Res*, 261, 171–85.

Nho, S. J., Nam, D., Ala, O. L., Craig, E. V., Warren, R. F. and Wright, T. M. 2009. Observations on retrieved glenoid components from total shoulder arthroplasty. *J Shoulder Elbow Surg*, 18, 371–8.

Noble, P. C., Conditt, M. A., Thompson, M. T., Stein, J. A., Kreuzer, S., Parsley, B. S. and Mathis, K. B. 2003. Extraarticular abrasive wear in cemented and cementless total knee arthroplasty. *Clin Orthop Relat Res*, 416, 120–8.

Okamoto, T., Inao, S., Gotoh, E. and Ando, M. 1997. Primary Charnley total hip arthroplasty for congenital dysplasia: effect of improved techniques of cementing. *J Bone Joint Surg Br*, 79, 83–6.

Ong, A., Wong, K. L., Lai, M., Garino, J. P. and Steinberg, M. E. 2002. Early failure of precoated femoral components in primary total hip arthroplasty. *J Bone Joint Surg Am*, 84A, 786–92.

Onsten, I. 1995. Appositional bone bridging of primary gaps in the dome area of uncemented, porous acetabular components. *J Arthroplasty*, 10, 702–6.

Onsten, I., CArlsson, A. S. and Besjakov, J. 1998. Wear in uncemented porous and cemented polyethylene sockets: a randomised, radiostereometric study. *J Bone Joint Surg Br*, 80, 345–50.

Oral, E., Greenbaum, E. S., Malhi, A. S., Harris, W. H. and Muratoglu, O. K. 2005. Characterization of irradiated blends of alpha-tocopherol and UHMWPE. *Biomaterials*, 26, 6657–63.

Ozeki, K., Masuzawa, T. and Hirakuri, K. K. 2010. The wear properties and adhesion strength of the diamond-like carbon film coated on SUS, Ti and Ni-Ti with plasma pre-treatment. *Biomed Mater Eng*, 20, 21–35.

Pagnano, M. W., Argenson, J. N., Parratte, S., Scuderi, G. R. and Booth, R. E., Jr. 2009. Minimally invasive total knee arthroplasty meets computer navigation. *J Bone Joint Surg Am*, 91, Suppl 5, 56–8.

Parvizi, J., Kim, K. I., Goldberg, G., Mallo, G. and Hozack, W. J. 2006. Recurrent instability after total hip arthroplasty: beware of subtle component malpositioning. *Clin Orthop Relat Res*, 447, 60–5.

Peterson, L. F., Fitzgerald, R. H., Jr. and Johnson, E. W., Jr. 1979. Total joint arthroplasty. The knee. *Mayo Clin Proc*, 54, 564–9.

Pidhorz, L. E., Urban, R. M., Jacobs, J. J., Sumner, D. R. and Galante, J. O. 1993. Histological study of the porous coating of the uncemented acetabulum. Apropos of 11 implants removed at autopsy. *Chirurgie*, 119, 334–9.

Pienkowski, D., Hoglin, D. P., Jacob, R. J., Saum, K. A., Nicholls, P. J. and Kaufer, H. 1996. Shape and size of virgin ultrahigh molecular weight GUR 4150 HP polyethylene powder. *J Biomed Mater Res*, 33, 65–71.

Pitzen, T., Kettler, A., Drumm, J., Nabhan, A., STeudel, W. I., Claes, L. and Wilke, H. J. 2007. Cervical spine disc prosthesis: radiographic, biomechanical and morphological post mortal findings 12 weeks after implantation. A retrieval example. *Eur Spine J*, 16, 1015–20.

Plante-Bordeneuve, P. and Freeman, M. A. 1993. Tibial high-density polyethylene wear in conforming tibiofemoral prostheses. *J Bone Joint Surg Br*, 75, 630–6.

Poggie, R. A., Takeuchi, M., Averill, R. and Nasser, S. 1998. Accelerated aging and associated changes in ultra-high molecular weight polyethylene (UHMWPE) materials following irradiation and aging. In Gsell, R. A., Stein, H. L. and Ploskonka, K. J. (eds) *Characterization and Properties of Ultra-High Molecular Weight Polyethylene*. Philadelphia, PA, ASTM International.

Popoola, O. O., Yao, J. Q., Johnson, T. S. and Blanchard, C. R. 2010. Wear, delamination, and fatigue resistance of melt-annealed highly crosslinked UHMWPE cruciate-retaining knee inserts under activities of daily living. *J Orthop Res*, 28, 1120–6.

Premnath, V., Harris, W. H., Jasty, M. and Merrill, E. W. 1996. Gamma sterilization of UHMWPE articular implants: an analysis of the oxidation problem. Ultra high molecular weight poly. *Biomaterials*, 17, 1741–53.

Pruitt, L. A. 2005. Deformation, yielding, fracture and fatigue behavior of conventional and highly cross-linked ultra high molecular weight polyethylene. *Biomaterials*, 26, 905–15.

Que, L. and Topoleski, L. D. 1999. Surface roughness quantification of CoCrMo implant alloys. *J Biomed Mater Res*, 48, 705–11.

Ries, M. D., Guiney, W., Jr. and Lynch, F. 1994. Osteolysis associated with cemented total knee arthroplasty. A case report. *J Arthroplasty*, 9, 555–8.

Robbins, G. M., Masri, B. A., Garbuz, D. S. and Duncan, C. P. 2001. Preoperative planning to prevent instability in total knee arthroplasty. *Orthop Clin North Am*, 32, 611–26.

Romero, J., Duronio, J. F., Sohrabi, A., Alexander, N., MacWilliams, B. A., Jones, L. C. and Hungerford, D. S. 2002. Varus and valgus flexion laxity of total knee alignment methods in loaded cadaveric knees. *Clin Orthop Relat Res*, 394, 243–53.

Sathasivam, S. and Walker, P. S. 1994. Optimization of the bearing surface geometry of total knees. *J Biomechanics*, 27, 255–64.

Scarlat, M. M. and Matsen, F. A., 3rd 2001. Observations on retrieved polyethylene glenoid components. *J Arthroplasty*, 16, 795–801.

Schmalzried, T. P. and Harris, W. H. 1993. Hybrid total hip replacement. A 6.5-year follow-up study. *J Bone Joint Surg Br*, 75, 608–15.

Schmalzried, T. P., Jasty, M., Rosenberg, A. and Harris, W. H. 1993. Histologic identification of polyethylene wear debris using Oil Red O stain. *J Appl Biomater*, 4, 119–25.

Schmalzried, T. P., Shepherd, E. F., Dorey, F. J., Jackson, W. O., Dela Rosa, M., Fa'Vae, F., McKellop, H. A., McClung, C. D., Martell, J., Moreland, J. R. and Amstutz, H. C. 2000. The John Charnley Award. Wear is a function of use, not time. *Clin Orthop Relat Res*. 381, 36–46.

Schmiedberg, S. K., Jones, L. C., Chang, D. H., Hungerford, D. S. and Frondoza, C. G. 2007. Extraction and characterization of metallic wear debris from total joint arthroplasty. *Biomed Sci Instrum*, 43, 104–109.

Schroder, D. T., Kelly, N. H., Wright, T. M. and Parks, M. L. 2011. Retrieved highly crosslinked UHMWPE acetabular liners have similar wear damage as conventional UHMWPE. *Clin Orthop Relat Res*, 469, 387–94.

Scotchford, C. A., Garle, M. J., Batchelor, J., Bradley, J. and Grant, D. M. 2003. Use of a novel carbon fibre composite material for the femoral stem component of a THR system: in vitro biological assessment. *Biomaterials*, 24, 4871–9.

Shahgaldi, B. F. and Compson, J. 2000. Wear and corrosion of sliding counterparts of stainless-steel hip screw-plates. *Injury*, 31, 85–92.

Shahgaldi, B. F., Heatley, F. W., Dewar, A. and Corrin, B. 1995. In vivo corrosion of cobalt-chromium and titanium wear particles. *J Bone Joint Surg Br*, 77, 962–6.

Shiers, L. G. 1959. Hinge arthroplasty of right knee. *Proc R Soc Med*. 52, 577.

Sieber, H. P., Rieker, C. B. and Kottig, P. 1999. Analysis of 118 second-generation metal-on-metal retrieved hip implants. *J Bone Joint Surg Br*, 81, 46–50.

Simon, J. P. and Bellemans, J. 2009. Clinical and radiological evaluation of modular trabecular metal acetabular cups. Short-term results in 64 hips. *Acta Orthop Belg*, 75, 623–30.

Smith, S. L. and Unsworth, A. 2001. An in vitro wear study of alumina-alumina total hip prostheses. *Proc Inst Mech Eng H*, 215, 443–6.

Smith, S. W., Estok, D. M., 2nd and Harris, W. H. 1998. Total hip arthroplasty with use of second-generation cementing techniques. An eighteen-year-average follow-up study. *J Bone Joint Surg Am*, 80, 1632–40.

Sobieraj, M. C. and Rimnac, C. M. 2009. Ultra high molecular weight polyethylene: mechanics, morphology, and clinical behavior. *J Mech Behav Biomed Mater*, 2, 433–443.

Stern, S. H., Wills, R. D. and Gilbert, J. L. 1997. The effect of tibial stem design on component micromotion in knee arthroplasty. *Clin Orthop Relat Res*, 345, 44–52.

Stoller, A. P., Johnson, T. S., Popoola, O. O., Humphrey, S. M. and Blanchard, C. R. 2011. Highly crosslinked polyethylene in posterior-stabilized total knee arthroplasty: in vitro performance evaluation of wear, delamination, and tibial post durability. *J Arthroplasty*, 26, 483–91.

Stukenborg-Colsman, C., Ostermeier, S. and Windhagen, H. 2005. What effect does of obesity have on the outcome of total hip and knee arthroplasty. Review of the literature. *Orthopäde*, 34, 664–7.

Stulberg, S. D., Stulberg, B. N., Hamati, Y. and Tsao, A. 1988. Failure mechanisms of metal-backed patellar components. *Clin Orthop Relat Res*, 236, 88–105.

Sutula, L. C., Collier, J. P., Saum, K. A., Currier, B. H., Currier, J. H., Sanford, W.

M., Mayor, M. B., Wooding, R. E., Sperling, D. K., Williams, I. R. *et al.* 1995. The Otto Aufranc Award. Impact of gamma sterilization on clinical performance of polyethylene in the hip. *Clin Orthop Relat Res*, 319, 28–40.

Swank, M., Romanowski, J. R., Korbee, L. L. and Bignozzi, S. 2007. Ligament balancing in computer-assisted total knee arthroplasty: improved clinical results with a spring-loaded tensioning device. *Proc Inst Mech Eng H*, 221, 755–61.

Swinkels, A., Newman, J. H. and Allain, T. J. 2009. A prospective observational study of falling before and after knee replacement surgery. *Age Ageing*, 38, 175–81.

Sychterz, C. J., Engh, C. A., JR., Swope, S. W., McNulty, D. E. and Engh, C. A. 1999. Analysis of prosthetic femoral heads retrieved at autopsy. *Clin Orthop Relat Res*, 358, 223–34.

Sychterz, C. J., Orishimo, K. F. and Engh, C. A. 2004. Sterilization and polyethylene wear: clinical studies to support laboratory data. *J Bone Joint Surg Am*, 86A, 1017–22.

Taki, N., Goldberg, V. M., Kraay, M. J. and Rimnac, C. M. 2004. Backside wear of Miller-Galante I and Insall-Burstein II tibial inserts. *Clin Orthop Relat Res*, 428, 198–206.

Tomita, N., Kitakura, T., Onmori, N., Ikada, Y. and Aoyama, E. 1999. Prevention of fatigue cracks in ultrahigh molecular weight polyethylene joint components by the addition of vitamin E. *J Biomed Mater Res*, 48, 474–8.

Tonino, A., Oosterbos, C., Rahmy, A., Therin, M. and Doyle, C. 2001. Hydroxyapatite-coated acetabular components. Histological and histomorphometric analysis of six cups retrieved at autopsy between three and seven years after successful implantation. *J Bone Joint Surg Am*, 83A, 817–25.

Tower, S. S., Currier, J. H., Currier, B. H., Lyford, K. A., Van Citters, D. W. and Mayor, M. B. 2007. Rim cracking of the cross-linked longevity polyethylene acetabular liner after total hip arthroplasty. *J Bone Joint Surg Am*, 89, 2212–7.

Triclot, P. 2011. Metal-on-metal: history, state of the art (2010). *Int Orthop*, 35, 201–6.

Tsao, A., Mintz, L., McRae, C. R., Stulberg, S. D. and Wright, T. 1993. Failure of the porous-coated anatomic prosthesis in total knee arthroplasty due to severe polyethylene wear. *J Bone Joint Surg Am*, 75, 19–26.

Tsao, A., Jones, L. and Lewallen, D. 2008. What patient and surgical factors contribute to implant wear and osteolysis in total joint arthroplasty? *J Am Acad Orthop Surg*, 16, S7–S13.

Uehara, K., Kadoya, Y., Kobayashi, A., Ohashi, H. and Yamano, Y. 2002. Anthropometry of the proximal tibia to design a total knee prosthesis for the Japanese population. *J Arthroplasty*, 17, 1028–32.

Usrey, M. M., Noble, P. C., Rudner, L. J., Conditt, M. A., Birman, M. V., Santore, R. F. and Mathis, K. B. 2006. Does neck/liner impingement increase wear of ultrahigh-molecular-weight polyethylene liners? *J Arthroplasty*, 21, 65–71.

van Riet, R. P., Morrey, B. F. and O'Driscoll, S. W. 2009. The Pritchard ERS total elbow prosthesis: lessons to be learned from failure. *J Shoulder Elbow Surg*, 18, 791–5.

Vertullo, C. J., Easley, M. E., Scott, W. N. and Insall, J. N. 2001. Mobile bearings in primary knee arthroplasty. *J Am Acad Orthop Surg*, 9, 355–64.

Villarraga, M. L., Cripton, P. A., Teti, S. D., Steffey, D. L., Krisnamuthy, S., Albert, T., Hilibrand, A. and Vaccaro, A. 2006. Wear and corrosion in retrieved thoracolumbar posterior internal fixation. *Spine (Phila Pa 1976)*, 31, 2454–62.

Waldman, B. J., Mont, M. A. and Hungerford, D. S. 1997. Total knee arthroplasty infections associated with dental procedures. *Clin Orthop Relat Res*, 343, 164–72.

Walker, P. S., Blunn, G. W. and Lilley, P. A. 1996. Wear testing of materials and surfaces for total knee replacement. *J Biomed Mater Res*, 33, 159–75.

Wang, J. C., Yu, W. D., Sandhu, H. S., Betts, F., Bhuta, S. and Delamarter, R. B. 1999. Metal debris from titanium spinal implants. *Spine (Phila Pa 1976)*, 24, 899–903.

Wasielewski, R. C., Galante, J. O., Leighty, R. M., Natarajan, R. N. and Rosenberg, A. G. 1994. Wear patterns on retrieved polyethylene tibial inserts and their relationship to technical considerations during total knee arthroplasty. *Clin Orthop Relat Res*, 299, 31–43.

Wasielewski, R. C., Parks, N., Williams, I., Surprenant, H., Collier, J. P. and Engh, G. 1997. Tibial insert undersurface as a contributing source of polyethylene wear debris. *Clin Orthop Relat Res*, 345, 53–9.

Watanabe, E., Suzuki, M., Nagata, K., Kaneeda, T., Harada, Y., Utsumi, M., Mori, A. and Moriya, H. 2002. Oxidation-induced dynamic changes in morphology reflected on freeze-fractured surface of gamma-irradiated ultra-high molecular weight polyethylene components. *J Biomed Mater Res*, 62, 540–9.

Weber, A. B. and Morris, H. G. 1996. Thickness of tibial inserts in total knee arthroplasty. *J Arthroplasty*, 11, 856–8.

Willert, H. G., Buchhorn, G. H., Gobel, D., Koster, G., Schaffner, S., Schenk, R. and Semlitsch, M. 1996. Wear behavior and histopathology of classic cemented metal on metal hip endoprostheses. *Clin Orthop Relat Res*, 329, S160–86.

Williams, I. R., Mayor, M. B. and Collier, J. P. 1998. The impact of sterilization method on wear in knee arthroplasty. *Clin Orthop Relat Res*, 356, 170–80.

Williams, S., Leslie, I., Isaac, G., Jin, Z., Ingham, E. and Fisher, J. 2008. Tribology and wear of metal-on-metal hip prostheses: influence of cup angle and head position. *J Bone Joint Surg Am*, 90, Suppl 3, 111–7.

Williams, V. G., 2nd, Whiteside, L. A., White, S. E. and McCarthy, D. S. 1997. Fixation of ultrahigh-molecular-weight polyethylene liners to metal-backed acetabular cups. *J Arthroplasty*, 12, 25–31.

Willie, B. M., Ashrafi, S., Alajbegovic, S., Burnett, T. and Bloebaum, R. D. 2004. Quantifying the effect of resin type and sterilization method on the degradation of ultrahigh molecular weight polyethylene after 4 years of real-time shelf aging. *J Biomed Mater Res A*, 69, 477–89.

Willis-Owen, C. A., Keene, G. C. and Oakeshott, R. D. 2011. Early metallosis-related failure after total knee replacement: a report of 15 cases. *J Bone Joint Surg Br*, 93, 205–9.

Wright, T. M. and Goodman, S. B. (eds) 1996. *Implant Wear: The Future of Total Joint Replacement*. Rosemont, Il, American Academy of Orthopaedic Surgeons.

Wright, T. M. and Goodman, S. B. 2000. *Implant Wear in Total Joint Replacement*. Rosemont, IL, American Academy of Orthopaedic Surgeons.

Wright, T. M., Rimnac, C. M., Stulberg, S. D., Mintz, L., Tsao, A. K., Klein, R. W.

and McCrae, C. 1992. Wear of polyethylene in total joint replacements. Observations from retrieved PCA knee implants. *Clin Orthop Relat Res*, 276, 126–34.

Wroblewski, B. M., Siney, P. D., Dowson, D. and Collins, S. N. 1996. Prospective clinical and joint simulator studies of a new total hip arthroplasty using alumina ceramic heads and cross-linked polyethylene cups. *J Bone Joint Surg Br*, 78, 280–5.

Wrona, M., Mayor, M. B., Collier, J. P. and Jensen, R. E. 1994. The correlation between fusion defects and damage in tibial polyethylene bearings. *Clin Orthop Relat Res*, 299, 92–103.

Yamaguchi, M., Bauer, T. W. and Hashimoto, Y. 1999. Deformation of the acetabular polyethylene liner and the backside gap. *J Arthroplasty*, 14, 464–9.

Zardiackas, L. D., Black, R. J., Hughes, J. L. Reeves, R. B. and Jun, J. N. 1989. Metallurgical evaluation of retrieved implants and correlation of failures to patient record data. *Orthopedics*, 12, 85–92.

13
Diagnosis and surveillance of orthopaedic implants

S. AFFATATO, D. BRANDO, Istituto Ortopedico Rizzoli, Italy and
D. TIGANI, Santa Maria alle Scotte Hospital, Italy

Abstract: The number of patients who undergo total joint arthroplasty, and consequently revision, has been increasing in recent years. The increase is due to an ageing population, with whom arthritic diseases are more associated, and also because this surgery can offer a better quality of life for young people. In order to achieve the best outcome from the substitution of a joint with a prosthesis it is important for the surgeon to make a correct diagnosis, and so choose the most suitable prosthesis, time and type of surgery for the patient. Wear and infections are the primary causes of failure in implants. Their presence can be monitored by means of radiography and microbiological analyses, but there are now other and more specific techniques that guarantee greater accuracy. Several types of hip and knee prostheses are commercially available, differing from each other in design, materials, bone setting mechanism and degree of invasiveness. Choosing the correct option increases implant lifetime and stability. The establishment of registries means that prosthetic devices can be monitored and patients traced in case of adverse events. The first regional registry in Italy was activated at the Rizzoli Orthopaedic Institute in 1990. It collects data relating to hip, knee and shoulder prostheses implanted in Emilia Romagna and reports on the clinical condition of patients, surgical procedures and the type and fixation of implants for both primary and revision prostheses. Managing such a registry is costly, but it means that fewer revisions are necessary, resulting in savings overall.

Key words: diagnosis, radiography, hip prosthesis, knee prosthesis, surveillance, registry.

13.1 The importance of a correct diagnosis

Total joint replacement (TJR), a surgical treatment performed to solve disabling joint pathologies, consists of replacing a damaged joint with an artificial joint or prosthesis (Corten *et al.*, 2011; Hohler, 2008). The goals of

TJR are to relieve pain, to restore movement of the joint combined with good stability and to correct deformity if present. Current joint replacements, if properly implanted, achieve high success rates in meeting these goals according to both short- and long-term follow-up studies. TJR can be used for any joint of the body but hips and knees are most commonly replaced. The number of TJRs performed has increased in recent years and will continue to increase in the future because of an ageing population, linked to the occurrence of arthrosis, and use of the technique to solve disabilities in younger patients (Kurtz et al., 2007). The increase in primary joint replacements also leads to an increased number of revisions as patients survive longer than the life expectation of prostheses. Revision surgery is a more difficult procedure, with higher morbidity and mortality, than the primary operations (Engelbrecht et al., 1990). Reducing the number of primary and revision surgeries will lead to important cost savings.

Making a correct initial diagnosis is of fundamental importance in ensuring a positive outcome for joint replacement surgery (Muller et al., 2008). A surgeon must know what is affecting the patient or the causes of failure in order to plan the correct solution to the problem. A correct diagnosis includes complete characterization of the disease, knowledge of the degree of progression and impairment of the structures, and chances of recovery. In order to give a proper prognosis, an expert surgeon will need to consider the patient history and conduct physical examinations using modern technology.

TJR is generally appropriate for individuals with a painful disabling joint deterioration that is no longer responsive to conservative treatment. Following these criteria, neither limited but pain-free joint motion nor roentgenographic evidence of severe joint disease without significant clinical symptoms is an indication for joint replacement. Although there are indications for TJR in younger people, especially those with multiple joint involvements from a systemic disorder such as rheumatoid arthritis, lupus erithematosus or emophilia, the procedure is normally reserved for older individuals. Historically, patients between 60 and 75 years of age were considered the most suitable for joint replacement, but over recent decades this age range has expanded. With continual improvements in quality of life and an ageing population, many older individuals are becoming candidates for surgery. Advanced age is not a contraindication for surgery. What is important from this perspective are the characteristic of the patients, so that outcome appears to correlate more to co-morbidities than to age alone. The disorders most commonly treated by joint arthroplasty are summarized in Table 13.1.

Table 13.1 Joints disorders in which arthroplasty may be indicated

Primary joint disorder	Secondary joint disorder
Inflammatory disorders	
Degenerative joint disease	Primary osteoarthritis
	Secondary osteoarthritis
Osteonecrosis	
Sequelae of paediatric disease	

13.1.1 Inflammatory arthritis

Inflammatory arthritis is a term used to describe the occurrence of joint destruction in the presence of systemic diseases involving the immune system. Some of the more common diseases associated with inflammatory arthritis include rheumatoid arthritis (RA), ankylosing spondylitis, psoriatric arthritis and systemic lupus erythematosus. Among these, RA is by far the most common subgroup among older patients who require TJR. RA is a chronic inflammatory disease that causes progressive disability with a relatively constant incidence in North America and northern Europe. It is estimated at 20 to 50 cases per 100,000 people with a prevalence of 0.5–1.1% (Tobon *et al.*, 2010); however, this can reach 5–7% in some groups (e.g. some native American-Indian populations) (Peschken *et al.*, 2010).

The pathology of RA is characterized by infiltration of the synovium with mononuclear phagocytes, lymphocytes, plasma cells and polymorphonuclear leukocytes. As the disease progresses, the synovium becomes progressively hypertrophic and begins to erode the joint space. Structural damage of the articular surface is characterized by cartilage loss and erosion of the periarticular bone.

No single diagnostic test definitively confirms the diagnosis of RA. However, several tests can provide objective data that increase diagnostic certainty and allow disease progression to be followed. Rheumatoid factors are found in the serum of about 85% of patients with RA and in about 5% of healthy normal individuals. The detection of these factors is of clinical value because their presence tends to correlate with the severe and unremitted disease. RA is a primarily clinical diagnosis. Patients commonly present with pain and stiffness in multiple joints. In most patients, symptoms emerge over weeks to months, starting with one joint and often accompanied by prodromal symptoms of anorexia, weakness or fatigue. Rheumatoid joints typically are boggy, tender to the touch and warm. RA is diagnosed formally using seven American Rheumatism Association criteria (Arnett *et al.*, 1988; Saraux *et al.*, 2001), as reported in Table 13.2.

In the Norwegian Arthroplasty Register (NAR, 2010), in 2009, the rate of RA patients in total joint arthroplasty databases ranged from 1.8% for hip

Table 13.2 Criteria for diagnosis of rheumatoid arthritis according to the American Rheumatism Association

Sign or symptom	Definition
Morning stiffness	Stiffness in or around the affected joints for at least one hour after initiating movement
Arthritis of three or more joint areas	Three or more of the following joints noted to be fluid-filled or have soft tissue swelling: wrist, PIP, MCP, elbow, knee, ankle, MTP
Hand joint involvement	Wrist, MCP or PIP joints among the symptomatic joints observed
Symmetric arthritis	Right and left joints involved for one or more of the following: wrist, PIP, MCP, elbow, knee, ankle, MTP[1]
Rheumatoid nodules	Subcutaneous nodules in region surrounding joints, extensor surfaces, or bony prominescences
Serum rheumatoid factor positive	Positive results using any laboratory test that has a positive predictive value of 95% or more, i.e. positive in no more than 5% of patients without rheumatoid arthritis
Radiographic changes	Hand and wrist films show typical changes of erosion or loss density adjacent to affected joints

Note: PIP, proximal interphalangeal; MCP, metacarpophalangeal; MTP, metatarsophalangeal.
[1]PIP, MCO and MTP joints need not be absolutely symmetrical.

arthroplasty to 4.3% for total knee arthroplasty. RA is more predominant for the upper arm, rising to 16% for shoulder, 35% for elbow and 92% for finger prostheses. The incidence of ankle prostheses in 2009 was about 27%.

Juvenile rheumatoid arthritis

Juvenile rheumatoid arthritis (JRA) may develop at any age during childhood. The disease is associated with growth disturbance from the effects of inflammation on epiphyseal growth, resulting in overgrowth or undergrowth of bones. Destructive disabling arthritis occurs in as many as 50% of those with consistent positive rheumatoid factor and in 10–15% of negative rheumatoid factor patients.

Seronegative spondyloarthropathies

The seronegative spondyloarthropathies are a series of rheumatic disorders that affect the spine and peripheral joint of the lower extremity. Most of these disorders show an increased prevalence among individuals who have the human lymphocyte antigen HLA-B27 gene. Ankilosing spondylitis, Reiter's syndrome and psoriasis arthritis are the most common diagnostic entities within this category.

Ankilosing spondylitis is the prototypical disease of the spondyloarthropathies, a group of disorders characterized by:

- involvement of the sacroiliac joints;
- peripheral arthropathy;
- absence of rheumatoid factor;
- enthesopathy;
- a tendency towards familial aggregation;
- association with HLA-B27 ranging from about 60% in psoriatic and enteropathic spondylitis to more than 95% in ankylosing spondylitis, depending on ethnic group.

Ankylosing spondylitis occurs more commonly in men than in women (2.7:1). Women tend to have more peripheral joint involvement; men have more severe spinal disease. Peripheral joint involvement, particularly in the lower limbs, occurs at some stage in about 20–30% of patients; the incidence increases with the severity of the disease. Inflammatory disease of the hip and shoulder may produce progressive disability. End-stage hip disease requiring total hip replacement (often bilateral) occurs within 15–20 years of disease onset in about 20% of patients with juvenile-onset ankylosing spondylitis (age at onset 10–16 years) and in about 10% of those in whom onset is in the late teens; it is rare for onset to occur in adulthood (Brophy and Calin, 2001; Brown *et al.*, 1997; Calin and Taurog, 1998; Calin *et al.*, 1999; Khan, 2001).

Reiter's syndrome

Reiter's syndrome is the development of arthritis involving a small number of joints, frequently accompanied by infections of the eyes, mucous membranes, and the genitourinary or gastrointestinal tracts. Arthritis usually appears some weeks after urethritis or diarrhea and involves a few joints in an asymmetric pattern. Knees, ankles and wrists are most commonly involved.

Systemic lupus erythematosus

Systemic lupus erythematosus (SLE) is an autoimmune rheumatic disease that predominantly affects young women. It involves many organs and systems, resulting in vasculitis, renal and central nervous system involvement, arthritis, and mucocutaneous, peritoneal or pleuropericardial disorders. One of the most frequently presenting manifestations of SLE is arthritis. The distribution of affected joints is not dissimilar to that of RA, but SLE-associated arthritis does not cause joint deformity. A small number of patients with SLE need total joint replacement. Information concerning

500 patients was collected in a cohort series of SLE at University College of London Hospital from 1978 to 2008. Nineteen were found to have at least one TJR in most cases because of avascular necrosis (AVN) or concomitant RA (Mourao et al., 2009). The hip was the most commonly replaced joint (20/46, 43.5%), followed by the knee (15/46, 32.6%), elbow (5/46, 10.9%), shoulder (4/46, 8.7%), metacarpophalangeal joint (1/46, 2.2%) and metatarsophalangeal joint (1/46, 2.2%). One patient was submitted for six TJRs during the course of his life.

3.1.2 Osteoarthritis

Osteoarthritis is the most common diagnosis among patients selected to undergo TJR and certainly the most common cause of musculoskeletal pain and disability. Osteoarthritis is classified as either primary or secondary. Primary or idiopathic refers to the development of osteoarthritis in the absence of a causative factor, while secondary refers to the development of osteoarthritis as a direct consequence of a certain event or condition. Osteoarthritis is a very common disease; most individuals beyond the age of 50 years have some degree of osteoarthritis, although it may be asymptomatic. A radiograph of a patient with a bilateral osteoarthritis is shown in Fig. 13.1(a) and a radiograph of a bilateral staged uncemented total hip arthroplasty is shown in Fig. 13.1(b).

Osteoarthritis is a disorder that affects an entire joint, involving cartilage, bone synovium and capsule; however, the principal target tissue is the cartilage. The focal area of damage, identified by fibrillation and loss of volume, can be evident by gross observation or artroscopically at an early

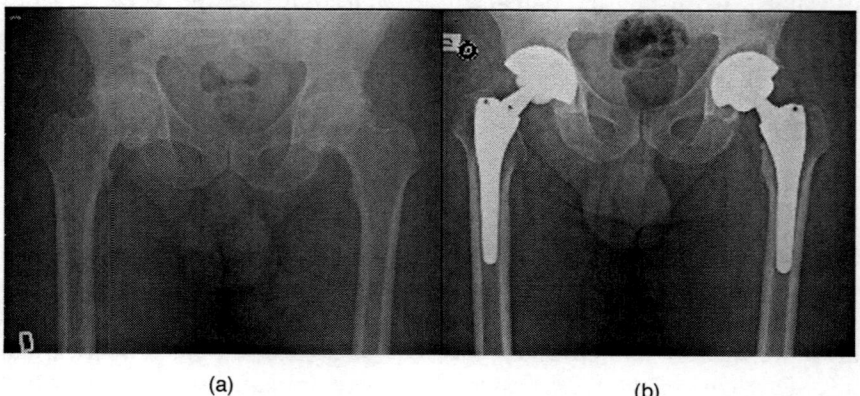

(a)   (b)

13.1 (a) Anteroposterior radiograph of the pelvis of a 67 year old man with bilateral osteoarthritis of the hip. (b) Radiograph of bilateral staged uncemented total hip arthroplasty.

stage (Schurman and Smith, 2004). Initially, there is loss of proteoglycan from the matrix of the articular cartilage. This results in the structure of this tissue becoming less resilient and is accompanied by vertical splitting or fibrillation of the articular cartilage. Cartilage is lost as the disease advances, ultimately resulting in the subchondral bone becoming the articulating joint surface. There is an increase in vascularity and activity of the subcondral bone, with areas of relative sclerosis and porosis secondary to its remodeling. It is often possible to find change in the joint margin, including outgrowths of cartilage as well as ostheophyte. Extensive thickening of the capsule is common and synovitis may be present at any stage. Remodeling of the subchondral bone can dramatically alter the anatomy of the affected joint.

It is not possible to detect early cartilage abnormalities radiographically, but they are detectable with magnetic resonance imaging. X-ray findings that can diagnose osteoarthritis include: joint space narrowing secondary to deterioration and loss of cartilage; osteophytes, which typically develop as a reparative response by remaining cartilage; and increased density of the subchondral bone, where it is possible to see some cysts filled by fluid extruded from the joint. Some degrees of deformity and subluxation can be evident in all affected joints according to the severity of the disease.

The causes of osteoarthritis are not completely understood. It is thought to be a disease associated with increased joint loading, for example in long-term impact exercise or obesity. However, the risk varies from individual to individual and some forms of osteoarthritis, the so-called idiopathic osteoarthritis, do not seem to be load related. There is increasing evidence that some individuals develop osteoarthritis as a result of hereditary factors. A radiograph showing moderate degrees of deformity and degenerative arthritis in a right knee is shown in Fig. 13.2. Figure 13.3 shows a radiograph of 75 year old woman with total hip arthroplasty, total knee arthroplasty and mild valgus deformity with degenerative change of the tibio-femoral joint. Recent studies have identified a few consistent osteoarthritis susceptibility genes (FRZB, GDF5 and DIO2) that are thought to have functions in the process of endochondral ossification (Bos et al., 2008).

Sequelae of pediatric disease

Among the childhood conditions that may lead to a need for future intervention, developmental dysplasia of the hip (DDH) is certainly the most problematic and redoubtable. DDH is an important cause of childhood disability. Developments in ultrasound imaging have lent DDH a greater prominence in recent years; in several European countries all newborn infants routinely undergo ultrasonography. One consequence of

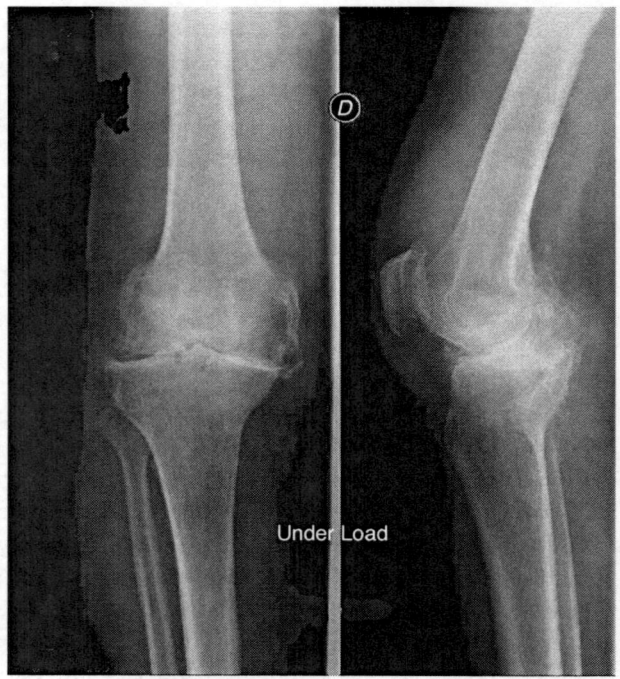

13.2 Radiograph showing moderate deformity and degenerative arthritis of a right knee.

routine ultrasonographic screening has been a pronounced increase in treatment of neonates, which arises from clinical uncertainty about the management of ultrasonography findings.

The underlying aetiology is likely to be multi-factorial. DDH is predominantly a female condition (5:1). It is more common in the left hip because this is the adducted hip lying against the sacrum in the most commonly occurring intrauterine position. The disease is bilateral in 20% of patients. There is a geographical predilection. It is common in native American Indians (1 in 20) and rare in sub-Saharan Africans, supporting postnatal influences such as swaddling as a causative factor.

The important effort directed at diagnostic neonatal screening will certainly reduce the incidence of sequelae in adults as early detection and appropriate management can prevent or delay the necessity for total hip replacement. In the last century, according to the Norwegian Arthroplasty Register, this disorder underlay up to 9% of all primary hip replacements and up to 29% of those in people aged 60 years and younger (Furnes *et al.*, 2001).

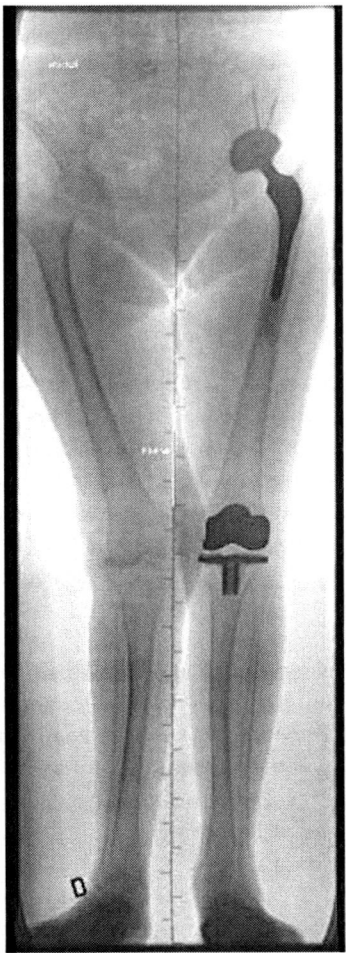

13.3 A long-standing X-ray of a 75 year old woman with total hip arthroplasty, total knee arthroplasty and mild valgus deformity with degenerative change of the tibio-femoral joint.

13.1.3 Slipped capital femoral epiphysis

Slipped capital femoral epiphysis (SCFE) is a disorder in which there is displacement of the capital femoral epiphysis from the metaphysic through the physeal plate due to an alteration of the proximal femoral growth plate. It occurs in the pediatric population at a rate of 1 in 1200 (Jerre *et al.*, 1996). Physiolysis occurs through a widened hypertrophic zone, which is weakened because of abnormalities in chondrocyte maturation and enchondral ossification (Ippolito *et al.*, 1981). The etiology has not been established, but endocrine abnormalities and increased weight are both associated with an increased risk of an SCFE (Loder, 1996). The incidence of degenerative joint disease in patients with known, or radiographic signs attributed to old, SCFE varies greatly among different series: from 5% to 40% (Johnston and Larson, 1969; Stulberg *et al.*, 1975).

Other less frequent disorders that may necessitate total hip arthroplasty in adults are Legg–Calvé–Perthes disease, developmental *coxa vara* and sequelae of septic arthritis.

13.1.4 Osteonecrosis

Osteonecrosis refers to bone death. The most frequent site of osteonecrosis is that of the femoral head, where the death of osteocytes following structural changes can lead to femoral head collapse and secondary hip joint osteoarthritis. Many patients with osteonecrosis of the femoral head will eventually undergo total hip arthroplasty. Most series estimate that approximately 10% (range 8–12%) of total hip arthroplasties performed in the USA are for cases involving osteonecrosis of the femoral head (Mankin; 1992; Ortiguera *et al.*, 1999).

Osteonecrosis primarily affects the epiphysis of long bones such as the femur head followed by the proximal humerus and the distal femur. A number of medical conditions have been associated with osteonecrosis. It is difficult to assess the frequency of each cause, because the reporting center data vary widely. It is possible, however, to distinguish in a general way between traumatic and non-traumatic causes of the condition.

Osteonecrosis of the femoral head as a consequence of trauma usually involves dislocation of the hip or fracture of the femoral neck. The incidence after dislocation is reported to be 10–25% depending on the severity of injury and associated femoral head or acetabular fractures (Antapur *et al.*, 2011). For patients with no traumatic osteonecrosis, several etiologic associations have been proposed: dysbarism, corticosteroids, alcoholism and hemoglobinopaties remain the most common causes of osteonecrosis (see Table 13.3).

13.1.5 Fractures

In the acute setting, TJR is identified as an acceptable option for a few indications, excluding hip fractures where the use of TJR is the indication of choice in elderly patients. Hip fractures are extremely common in all age groups but particularly affect the elderly. It is estimated that 500,000 hip fractures will occur annually in the USA by 2040. The majority of these, approximately 95–97%, occur in the older adult population. The cause is usually due to a combination of baseline osteoporosis and minor trauma

Table 13.3 Causes of osteonecrosis

Definite factors	Probable factors
Major trauma fractures	Corticosteroids
Disorders	Alcohol
Dislocations	Lipid disturbance
Caisson disease (deep sea divers)	Connective tissue disease
Sickle cell disease	Smoking
Post-irradiation	High dosage blood clotting disorders
Lupus	Clotting
Chemotherapy	Pancreatitis
Arterial disease	Kidney disease
Gaucher's disease	

such as falls. A fracture of the cervical aspect of a right femur is shown in Fig. 13.4(a) and a hybrid total hip arthroplasty is shown in Fig. 13.4(b).

The rationale for treating displaced hip fractures with hip arthroplasty is as follows. Fractures are connected with a significant risk of disruption to the ascending cervical branches that ascend the femoral neck and provide the majority of the vascular supply to the femoral head. This disruption in vascular supply to the femoral head results in osteonecrosis.

Total hip arthroplasty as the primary operative procedure in elderly patients with a displaced hip fracture is becoming increasingly popular. Numerous reports have shown better functional and quality of life outcomes when compared with other types of treatment (Ravikumar and Marsh, 2000; Rogmark *et al.*, 2002; Tidermark *et al.*, 2003). There are increasing reports of the use of total hip arthroplasty as a primary procedure for a

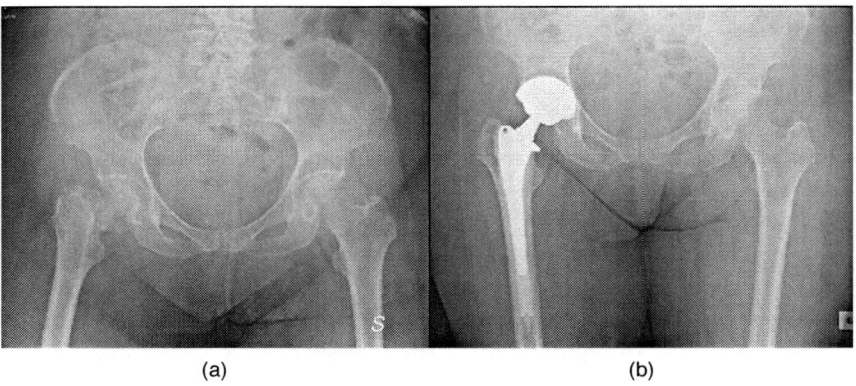

(a)   (b)

13.4 (a) Fracture of the cervical aspect of the right femur in a 75 year old woman. She was treated with an uncemented acetabular component and a cemented femoral component. (b) Hybrid total hip arthroplasty.

fractured neck of the femur in healthy elderly patients. There is now significant evidence that older patients treated with hip arthroplasty have a better functional outcome and quality of life and fewer complications when compared with those undergoing internal fixation. The potential advantages of total hip arthroplasty must be considered against an increased initial cost and possibly a higher risk of dislocation and infection when compared with internal fixation.

There is some debate concerning the use of hemiarthroplasty and total hip arthroplasty in elderly patients. Tidermark *et al.* (2003), comparing these procedures, concluded that the total hip arthroplasty group had better results and better functional outcomes, with no increase in complication rates. Bipolar hemiarthroplasty is generally recommended in older patients who are less active and have a shorter life expectancy (Antapur *et al.*, 2011) for fractures and some proximal humeral fractures. A fracture through the neck of a left femur is shown in Fig. 13.5(a) and anteroposterior and lateral radiographs of the patient treated with a total cementless arthroplasty are shown in Figs 13.5(b) and (c).

13.1.6 Proximal humeral arthroplasty for acute fractures

Proximal humeral replacement can be a useful surgical technique for acute displaced fractures of the proximal humerus. The indications for the use of a prosthesis are as follows (Neer, 2006).

- Four-part fractures and fracture dislocation. This refers to a fracture involving four distinct fragments, including a humeral head fragment, a great tuberosity, a lesser tuberosity fragment and a humeral shaft fragment.
- Head-splitting fractures. This is where a segment of the humeral head is fractured and subluxes or dislocates, while the articular surface of the unfractured part of the humeral head remains attached to the shaft.
- Impression fractures involving more than 40% of the reticular surface.
- Selected three-part fractures in older patients with osteoporosis.

13.1.7 Reasons for revision

The complexity and variety of phenomena leading to revision range from the very simple to the very complicated (Fevang *et al.*, 2010). A common and obvious cause of hip implant failure is that the operated limb was fixed so that it was too long or too short. Very often, a hip prosthesis is unstable and may dislocate, and the reasons for dislocation can vary (e.g. weak muscles, improper positioning of the hip or knee components, or broken or worn out parts). Particle debris generated from the worn surface can induce

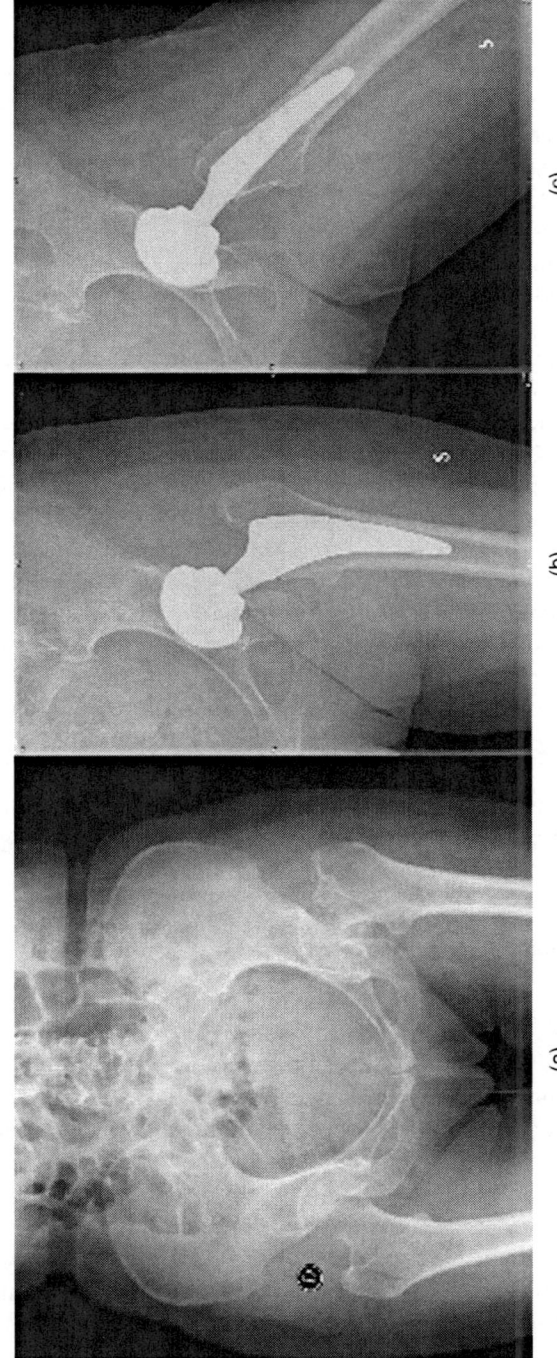

13.5 (a) Fracture through the neck of the left femur in a 61 year old woman, then treated with a total cementless arthroplasty. (b) Anteroposterior radiograph. (c) Lateral radiograph.

a localized inflammatory reaction, with consequent periprosthetic bone loss, component loosening and pain.

Another important reason for revision is prosthetic infection. This can occur due to organisms introduced during surgery (if it occurs within 12 months of surgery) or can be hematogenously acquired (if it occurs 12 months or more after surgery) (Matthews *et al.*, 2009). The primary cause for joint infection is a previous joint arthroplasty; indeed, people undergoing prosthesis revision have a greater risk of infection than those who undergo primary joint replacement. Advanced age, obesity, poor nutrition, skin disease and pre-existing joint disease are other risk factors for infection.

Very often, a minutely detailed interview and examination of the patient, together with an X-ray, allow proper diagnosis. Particular diagnostic tests and non-orthopaedic specialist advice will be necessary when the diagnosis is more complicated. It has been found that surgeons who perform more joint arthroplasties per year are more likely to have an excellent outcome than surgeons who performed fewer procedures (Moran *et al.*, 2010). This could well be due to the fact that surgeons who perform more procedures gain more practice, and usually have the support of a more sophisticated and experienced rehabilitation staff. Additionally, they may be used to recognizing indications and factors in choosing appropriate patients for surgery.

Before surgery, subjecting the patient to an infiltrative therapy with hyaluronic acid may be useful; this therapy can allow quite a long period of remission of painful symptoms (Hunter *et al.*, 2010). However, surgery should be avoided while symptoms can be managed by other treatment modalities. Weight management and exercise are important though often neglected conservative treatments for delaying surgery.

13.2 Predictive and detection methods

The most common reasons for revision in hip and knee prostheses are aseptic loosening and infection. The revision procedure is very costly and complicated. Knowledge of the mechanisms of defect formation allows primary and secondary prevention. Primary prevention, through the choice of prosthetic model according to surgical technique and proper indications, provides for the conservation of bone stock, while secondary prevention provides early revision of those implants that are doomed to failure.

Plain serial radiographs are usually used to determine clinical wear and for measuring the degree of penetration of the femoral head in the acetabular socket of a hip prosthesis (Sutherland, 1988). In the past, this technique was manual, so it was very imprecise and useless in short-term follow-up. Radiographs are also used to assess the amount of bone loss owing to osteolysis, though it is often underestimated. The major drawback of conventional radiography is the fact that it returns two-dimensional (2D) images rather than allowing a 3D view of the joint. Furthermore, chronic infection can lead to bone loss and loosening of the prosthesis, visible in a radiograph, but these are not specific signs of infection so other tests are necessary.

The most accurate method for assessing wear in a hip prosthesis is radiostereometric analysis (RSA) (Kadar *et al.*, 2011). RSA allows measurements of the bone–implant relative movement repeated over the course of routine monitoring of patients. Small tantalum markers are inserted in the prosthetic components and the bone; these are then monitored with great accuracy using a double standard radiographic exposure of the joint in question. Early identification of movement reveals likely failure of the prosthesis in advance. The use of tantalum, however, limits this technique to a small number of patients. Some computer-assisted methods can also be used. They are less accurate than RSA but applicable to a larger number of patients, using edge detection on a standard plan radiograph.

Computer tomography (CT) is more accurate than standard radiographs in detecting osteolysis, if beam-hardening artefacts are minimized with the use of a multi-detector helical CT (Kitamura *et al.*, 2005). This technique improves penetration of the radiographic beam, resulting in better quality images and increasing the effectiveness of the ionising radiation. Post-processing software may improve the obtained results. The formation of artefacts is due to the attenuation of the radiographic beam through the overlap of the high attenuation coefficient of metal and the lower one of the surrounding soft tissues.

Magnetic resonance imaging (MRI) has a higher soft tissue contrast than either radiography or CT and so can be used to detect early-stage osteolysis occurring in the synovial soft tissue (Potter *et al.*, 2005). Painful and symptomatic arthroplasty can be studied with this technique, permitting estimation of the intracapsular synovial load and bone loss. In the past, the main problem encountered with MRI was the formation of artefacts due to the overlap of very easily magnetized ferromagnetic metallic components and poorly magnetized soft tissue, leading to image distortion and frequency shift. Better results are obtained with components made of oxide zirconia because of its lower magnetic moment. Several methods can help reduce the formation of artefacts – the use of wide receiver sampling bandwidth, increasing the signal-to-noise ratio, following determinate protocols and taking advantage of commercially available software.

Diagnosing infection requires the conjunction of clinical, histological and microbiological tests (Moran *et al.*, 2010). A blood test might indicate the presence of infection after the early post-operative period, but positive results can be indicative of infection in another part of the body. When possible, a biopsy or aspiration should be performed for microbiological and histological analysis before subjecting the patient to antibiotics. Periprosthetic biopsy under fluorescence helps to sample the area in which there is a higher density of infectious micro-organisms. If a revision of the prosthesis is necessary, a preliminary biopsy and microbiological test can help in confirming the diagnosis and selection of an appropriate surgical strategy.

Sometimes, the difficulty in making a proper diagnosis is due to the fact that single surgeons face only a few complex cases. The creation of specialist centers where the collaboration of experts is possible will allow delays to be avoided and pathology to be properly managed (Thomas and Sethares, 2008).

13.3 Choice of prosthesis

13.3.1 Hip prostheses

Hip replacement surgery typically consists of dissection of the diseased femoral head and removing the diseased cartilage that covers the bottom of the acetabulum. A new artificial socket is then placed in the acetabulum and a new femoral head is secured to the femur using an intramedullary taproot. There are several kinds of hip prostheses, which differ in the type of material used, the bone setting mechanism and design. The surgeon, based on clinical and radiographic examination, will determine the need for intervention on the basis of the disease, age and patient expectations. However, three major classes of hip prostheses can be identified – the resurfacing prosthesis, the short-stem prosthesis and the long-stem prosthesis (from least to most invasive). A minimally invasive prosthesis is implanted to find good bone at the next reoperation and to make revision surgery easier. In a revision, the same type of prosthesis cannot usually be reimplanted but a more invasive implant should be chosen. So, in young patients, at the first implant, it would be better to use the least invasive prosthesis available. The choice of less invasive implants should be well balanced and carefully considered depending on the patient, because the less invasive the prosthesis, the less it grips to the bone. Not all patients are suitable for all prostheses.

The least invasive hip prosthesis is the resurfacing prosthesis, which preserves the femoral head of the patient rather than replacing it, covering it with a metal cup (Vail, 2011). The use of this kind of prosthesis is contraindicating in some forms of joint disease and in the case of old patients.

In the short-stem implant, the femoral head of the patient is sacrificed (Zeh *et al.*, 2011). The prosthesis grips the socket on the femoral neck and the metaphysis of the femur. The advantage of this prosthesis is that it can usually be revised with a classical prosthesis, without the need for a revision prosthesis. However, it is important that the patient has a well-preserved femoral neck and good quality bone. Typically, a classical prosthesis must be replaced with a revision prosthesis (i.e. one that is 'long' enough to engage the distal femur (Sathappan et al., 2009)). Therefore, this is a good solution in those patients, even young people, who display one or more contraindications to the use of less invasive implants. Prostheses are modular (consisting of several assembled parts), so that wear or breakage of a component does not involve the replacement of the entire implant, except in rare cases (Barrack, 1994).

The choice of materials plays a crucial role (Dearnley, 1999). Factors to consider are not only the age of the patient, but also many other aspects such as sex, weight, allergies, occupation, activities and, of course, basic pathology. The classical hip prosthesis has a cobalt–chromium head with a cup of high molecular weight polyethylene. This combination of metal-on-polyethylene exposes the patient to almost no risk of allergic sensitization or breakage of the implant. However, for younger patients a better solution might be a ceramic-on-polyethylene, which reduces the risk of allergic sensitization and has better wear resistance and thus longer life. The ceramic-on-ceramic coupling has an excellent wear resistance but there is a small risk of rupture, which does not suggest its suitability for patients who are very athletic or very heavy. The metal-on-metal coupling has an excellent resistance to wear, but has a small risk of sensitization to metal ions, which could cause the system to fail.

Primary stability, which allows the patient to place load on the limb immediately, is now achieved by cementing the prosthesis to the bone of the patient or using a mechanism called press-fit (Wixson et al., 1991). The use of cement gives a stable anchorage of the prosthesis by filling the space between the stem and the femoral canal. The cement is a polymethylmethacrylate-based material charged with radio opaque substances (DiMaio, 2002). The bone cement can adapt the prosthesis to the bone host by changing the size, shape and volume of the gap and allowing a distribution of mechanical stress by means of its elastic modulus. The use of bone cement has some major disadvantages; for example, volumetric shrinkage following the polymerization reaction and the inflammatory response evoked by the reaction of cement particles in contact with the surrounding tissues.

The press-fit technique consists of using a pressure mechanism to carefully prepare a chamber in the patient's bone into which the prosthesis fits well (Gebert et al., 2009). This is the technique of choice in young patients because, in the event of further surgery to replace an old and worn prosthesis, removing it will be easier and tissues will be better preserved and so the implant of a new prosthesis will be simpler and less invasive. In the case of uncemented prostheses, problems that arise are mainly related to lack of mechanical primary anchoring and significant differences between the bone and implant that can lead to harmful effects such as loosening, bone necrosis and bone resorption.

13.3.2 Knee prostheses

The unicompartmental knee is the ideal solution for a knee presenting damage limited to one compartment (more often the medial one) (Griffin *et al.*, 2007). This prosthesis allows much of the natural joint to be retained, thereby reducing the invasiveness of the surgical procedure. It is a resurfacing prosthesis because it covers the damaged femoral condyle with a metal component and the tibial plateau with a polyethylene component fixed with bone cement. It is used in mono-compartmental arthritis with integral or poorly damaged patello-femoral joint and integrity of the anterior cruciate ligament. The prosthetic knee replacement is applicable for both primary and secondary knee arthritis, when the symptoms are no longer controllable by medication and physiotherapy. It is contraindicated in cases of obesity, osteoporosis, instability and severe axial deviation.

A total prosthesis should be considered only when all other treatment options have been exhausted and only if the patient is fully aware that he cannot return to activities of high physical effort. A total knee prosthesis is indicated when the knee is affected by a degenerative process overall, involving more than one compartment. In these cases, partial replacement would inevitably lead to failure. The prosthesis consists of a metal tibial and femoral component, fixed to the bone through the use of acrylic cement (Thongtrangan *et al.*, 2003). Unlike the hip, the use of porous components without cement is less common. A polyethylene insert, fixed or rotating depending on the prosthetic model, is assembled on the tibial component allowing for sliding and rolling movement. In the mobile-bearing knee prosthesis, the polyethylene insert can rotate inside the metal tibial tray, so that the articulating tibial geometry can more highly conform to the femoral condylar geometry, with a reduction of contact stress and polyethylene wear (Callaghan *et al.*, 2001). Compared with fixed-bearing designs, mobile-bearing knee implants require more support from soft tissues and the ligaments surrounding the knee. If the soft tissues are not strong enough, a mobile-bearing knee prosthesis is more likely to dislocate.

Several type of knee prostheses are available, differing from each other in design and degree of stability (Morgan *et al.*, 2005). A prosthesis that preserves the posterior cruciate ligament is appropriate for patients with limited arthritis and intact cruciate ligaments. Prostheses with back stability are more stable and can also be used in more advanced arthritic knees with damage and injury to the cruciate ligaments. There are some constraint designs used in cases of prosthetic reimplantation, for failure of a previous installation or whenever major losses of bone or a large ligamentous laxity require prosthesis of greater stability. Constraint condylar prostheses, which have greater stability, are used in cases of significant ligamentous injuries or in cases of serious joint instability. They have a bond 'hinge' associated with femoral intramedullary rods and/or longer tibial.

Young or relatively young patients may benefit from high-flexion prosthesis designs (Endres and Wilke, 2011). The high-flexion designs are characterized by the ability of the system to perform deep flexion, comparable to those of a normal knee, without causing serious overloading of the articular surfaces. In this way, even those with active lifestyles can limit the prosthetic implant wear, with the theoretical expectation of increased longevity of their implants.

13.4 Patient education

Patient education plays an important role in successful joint arthroplasties, both pre- and post-operatively (Hawker, 2006). Very often, patients who undergo an arthroplasty are not fully prepared psychologically or organizationally and this affects their post-operative functional recovery. It has been demonstrated that proper pre-surgical preparation can have a positive effect in decreasing the level of pre-surgical anxiety and improving patient autonomy immediately after the operation (Thomas and Sethares, 2008). In spite of this, it is necessary that information is given to the patient in understandable language, meeting the patient's expectations (Lieberman et al., 2003). Patient education is important to ensure that the patient arrives at the operation in a healthy state. In this context, the physician has the unenviable task of correcting poor conditions, such as excess weight, diabetes, and cardiovascular and vascular disease. Any excess of weight is absolutely contraindicated for the possible anaesthesia complications and for the accentuated overload on the joint. It is also necessary to clear up any outbreak of infections (dental abscess, cystitis) that could affect the success of the implant. It is important to keep muscles toned using joint and muscle exercises to facilitate recovery after surgery. The patient must be aware that there are generic and specific risks related to surgery, varying according to age and general and local conditions. These include risk of infection and thromboembolism. Post-operatively, it is necessary to prepare the patient for any special needs (such as prolonged use of crutches, the need for a brace or a cast) or special modifications to the home, to the point of removing anything that could hinder or make paths insecure (such as carpets and floor wax). Patients must also be trained in management of the new implanted prosthesis, for example on how to move the limb (up and down stairs, staying in bed, staying sitting). Leading an active life and avoiding carrying excessive loads and gaining weight will help to preserve the prosthesis.

In order to diagnose problems early, the patient would have to submit to periodical clinical and radiographic controls, even if, often, when the patient contacts the physician, the bone situation is already compromised. If the patient does not comply with the recommendations, the implanted prosthesis will incur early wear, raising the risk of a new intervention.

13.5 Surveillance

Because of the ageing population, the number of joint replacement surgeries has been increasing in recent years (Lawrence et al., 2008). Consequently, the number of revision surgeries is also growing, as the life expectancy of patients is longer than that of prostheses (Kurtz et al., 2007). As a result, there is an increase in health expenses and it is necessary to reduce the number of revisions in order to diminish these costs (Persson et al., 1999). It is therefore important to know how individual prostheses behave in certain clinical conditions. At present, there is a large number of prosthetic models on the market and little scientific evidence of good methodological quality to support the use of most of them (Malchau et al., 2002). In these conditions, it is difficult to monitor the use of prosthetic devices and ensure the traceability of the patients in case of adverse events.

In many countries, a registry for post-marketing surveillance has been established in order to collect specific data on the performance of joint prostheses (Kolling et al., 2007). Registers can be set up at international, national or regional level but also at local level, such as at a hospital. They are useful for different purposes, the first of which is quality control (Ahn et al., 2009). In fact, through them, it is possible to evaluate the effectiveness of an implant in terms of its lifetime and performance for the treatment of specific cases. In this way, the registry can inform surgeons of the better types of prostheses and surgical techniques. Consequently, healthcare resources will be properly used.

Registers are an important tool for research. They allow the identification of patients with a certain condition or outcome for large prospective observational studies. The systematic collection of essential information on the surgery and the definition of a single endpoint, the failure of the system and its replacement, make it possible to monitor the device over time after its commercial introduction (Graves et al., 2004). Registries have the ability to identify defective prostheses early, to implement procedures for the identification and recall of patients at risk, and to subject such patients to appropriate monitoring strategies and analysis. Without a register, it is not easy to identify people who received failed prostheses; hospitals would need to scan all the clinical folders of patients who underwent joint replacement in the period of use of the prosthesis.

Before implementing a register, it is important that all users agree on its purpose and on the type of data to be reported, so as not to have too much useless information that makes compilation and research difficult. The following data are usually recorded: patient details; type of prosthesis; type of surgery; side; diagnosis; details of the components used. Errors of coding and transcription must be avoided through coding fields in user-friendly software. Moreover, all patients have to be included in the registry. This can be ensured, for example, by comparing registry data with other databases. Moreover, the system should be able to detect lack of information and check if the entered values are acceptable. Indeed, in spite of data analysis, missing data can lead to erroneous conclusions if its absence is not random. This involves a reduction of the number of cases in the study, because it is necessary to ignore cases with missing data.

The first national arthroplasty registers to be implemented were the Swedish Arthroplasty Registers (Böhler and Labek, 2009), composed of the knee register created in 1975 and the hip register created in 1979. These registers have proven to be effective in evaluating the behavior of joint prostheses and treatments. On this model, new national registries have been set up over the years. Important contributions have been provided by the Danish (Lucht, 2000), Finnish (Puolakka et al., 2001), Canadian (Bohm et al., 2010) and Norwegian (Havelin et al., 2000) registers.

In Italy, the first regional registry was set up in the Emilia Romagna region in 1990 (Stea et al., 2009): the Register of Orthopaedic Prosthetic Implants (RIPO) was initiated at the Rizzoli Orthopaedic Institute. Orthopaedic units in the region began to use it in January 2000 and involvement was very high (97.3% in 2009), unlike previous attempts that failed because of low participation of physicians. RIPO is partially financed by the Regional Health of the Emilia Romagna and is coordinated by the Regional Orthopaedic Commission. RIPO also collaborates with the Department of Health of the Emilia-Romagna and with the Regional Health Agency to conduct analysis about the cost-effectiveness of hip prostheses. By 31 December 2009, the register had collected data concerning nearly 56,000 total hip replacements, 21,700 hemiarthoplasties, 8,900 revisions, 40,000 knee replacements and 3,500 knee revisions (Servizio Sanitario Regionale, 2009). More than 100 types of hip prostheses and 70 knee prostheses have been considered. Since 2008, RIPO included shoulder prostheses: between 1 July 2008 and 31 December 2009, the register collected data on nearly 300 total shoulder replacements, 170 hemiarthoplasties and 50 revisions.

The main information collated in the RIPO multi-centric databases is clinical condition of patients, surgical procedures, and type and fixation of the implant for both primary and revision prostheses. Revision is defined as the failure endpoint of the prosthesis. Surgeons have to report patient information in a specific form, together with the label of each component of the prosthesis implanted. The data are then entered in the database by means of specific procedures for assuring data quality, which is one of the fundamental problems related to database management. As a consequence, related costs are also an issue, even though, till now, this cost has been covered by funds from the Rizzoli Institute and public grants. These high management costs are compensated by the cost savings resulting from a consequent smaller number of revisions.

13.6 References

Ahn, H., Court-Brown, C. M., McQueen, M. M. and Schemitsch, E. H. (2009) The use of hospital registries in orthopaedic surgery. *J Bone Joint Surg Am*, 91, Suppl 3, 68–72.

Antapur, P., Mahomed, N. and Gandhi, R. (2011) Fractures in the elderly: when is hip replacement a necessity? *Clin Interv Aging*, 6, 1–7.

Arnett, F. C., Edworthy, S. M., Bloch, D. A., McShane, D. J., Fries, J. F., Cooper, N. S., Healey, L. A., Kaplan, S. R., Liang, M. H., Luthra, H. S. *et al.* (1988) The American Rheumatism Association 1987 revised criteria for the classification of rheumatoid arthritis. *Arthr Rheum*, 31, 315–24.

Barrack, R. L. (1994) Modularity of Prosthetic Implants. *J Am Acad Orthop Surg*, 2, 16–25.

Böhler, N. and Labek, G. (2009) Current status of arthroplasty registers in Europe. *Euro Instruct Lect*, 9, 3–10.

Bohm, E. R., Dunbar, M. J. and Bourne, R. (2010) The Canadian Joint Replacement Registry – what have we learned? *Acta Orthop*, 81, 119–21.

Bos, S. D., Slagboom, P. E. and Meulenbelt, I. (2008) New insights into osteoarthritis: early developmental features of an ageing-related disease. *Curr Opin Rheumatol*, 20, 553–9.

Brophy, S. and Calin, A. (2001) Ankylosing spondylitis: interaction between genes, joints, age at onset, and disease expression. *J Rheumatology*, 28, 2283–8.

Brown, M. A., Kennedy, L. G., MacGregor, A. J., Darke, C., Duncan, E., Shatford, J. L., Taylor, A., Calin, A. and Wordsworth, P. (1997) Susceptibility to ankylosing spondylitis in twins: the role of genes, HLA, and the environment. *Arthr Rheum*, 40, 1823–8.

Calin, A. and Taurog, J. (1998) *The Spondylarthritides*. Oxford, Oxford University Press.

Calin, A., Brophy, S. and Blake, D. (1999) Impact of sex on inheritance of ankylosing spondylitis: a cohort study. *Lancet*, 354, 1687–90.

Callaghan, J. J., Insall, J. N., Greenwald, A. S., Dennis, D. A., Komistek, R. D., Murray, D. W., Bourne, R. B., Rorabeck, C. H. and Dorr, L. D. (2001) Mobile-bearing knee replacement: concepts and results. *Instr Course Lect*, 50, 431–49.

Corten, K., Ganz, R., Simon, J. P. and Leunig, M. (2011) Hip resurfacing arthroplasty: current status and future perspectives. *Eur Cell Mater*, 21, 243–58.

Dearnley, P. A. (1999) A review of metallic, ceramic and surface-treated metals used for bearing surfaces in human joint replacements. *Proc Inst Mech Eng H*, 213, 107–35.

DiMaio, F. R. (2002) The science of bone cement: a historical review. *Orthopedics*, 25, 1399–407; quiz 1408–9.

Endres, S. and Wilke, A. (2011) High flexion total knee arthroplasty – mid-term follow up of 5 years. *Open Orthop J*, 5, 138–42.

Engelbrecht, D. J., Weber, F. A., Sweet, M. B. and Jakim, I. (1990) Long-term results of revision total hip arthroplasty. *J Bone Joint Surg Br*, 72, 41–5.

Fevang, B. T., Lie, S. A., Havelin, L. I., Engesaeter, L. B. and Furnes, O. (2010) Improved results of primary total hip replacement. *Acta Orthop*, 81, 649–59.

Furnes, O., Lie, S. A., Espehaug, B., Vollset, S. E., Engesaeter, L. B. and Havelin, L. I. (2001) Hip disease and the prognosis of total hip replacements. A review of 53,698 primary total hip replacements reported to the Norwegian Arthroplasty Register 1987–99. *J Bone Joint Surg Br*, 83, 579–86.

Gebert, A., Peters, J., Bishop, N. E., Westphal, F. and Morlock, M. M. (2009) Influence of press-fit parameters on the primary stability of uncemented femoral resurfacing implants. *Med Eng Phys*, 31, 160–4.

Graves, S. E., Davidson, D., Ingerson, L., Ryan, P., Griffith, E. C., McDermott, B. F., McElroy, H. J. and Pratt, N. L. (2004) The Australian Orthopaedic Association National Joint Replacement Registry. *Med J Aust*, 180, S31–4.

Griffin, T., Rowden, N., Morgan, D., Atkinson, R., Woodruff, P. and Maddern, G. (2007) Unicompartmental knee arthroplasty for the treatment of unicompartmental osteoarthritis: a systematic study. *ANZ J Surg*, 77, 214–21.

Havelin, L. I., Engesaeter, L. B., Espehaug, B., Furnes, O., Lie, S. A. and Vollset, S. E. (2000) The Norwegian Arthroplasty Register: 11 years and 73,000 arthroplasties. *Acta Orthop Scand*, 71, 337–53.

Hawker, G. A. (2006) Who, when, and why total joint replacement surgery? The patient's perspective. *Curr Opin Rheumatol*, 18, 526–30.

Hohler, S. E. (2008) Total knee arthroplasty: past successes and current improvements. *AORN J*, 87, 143–58; quiz 159–62.

Hunter, D. J., Neogi, T. and Hochberg, M. C. (2010) Quality of osteoarthritis management and the need for reform in the US. *Arthr Care Res (Hoboken)*, 63, 31–8.

Ippolito, E., Mickelson, M. R. and Ponseti, I. V. (1981) A histochemical study of slipped capital femoral epiphysis. *J Bone Joint Surg Am*, 63, 1109–13.

Jerre, R., Karlsson, J. and Henrikson, B. (1996) The incidence of physiolysis of the hip: a population-based study of 175 patients. *Acta Orthop Scand*, 67, 53–6.

Johnston, R. C. and Larson, C. B. (1969) Results of treatment of hip disorders with cup arthroplasty. *J Bone Joint Surg Am*, 51, 1461–79.

Kadar, T., Hallan, G., Aamodt, A., Indrekvam, K., Badawy, M., Skredderstuen, A., Havelin, L. I., Stokke, T., Haugan, K., Espehaug, B. and Furnes, O. (2011) Wear and migration of highly cross-linked and conventional cemented polyethylene cups with cobalt chrome or Oxinium femoral heads: A randomized radiostereometric study of 150 patients. *J Orthop Res*, 29, 1222–9.

Khan, M. A. (2001) Spondyloarthropathies. *Curr Opin Rheumatol*, 13, 245–90.

Kitamura, N., Leung, S. B. and Engh, C. A., Sr. (2005) Characteristics of pelvic osteolysis on computed tomography after total hip arthroplasty. *Clin Orthop Relat Res*, 441, 291–7.

Kolling, C., Simmen, B. R., Labek, G. and Goldhahn, J. (2007) Key factors for a successful National Arthroplasty Register. *J Bone Joint Surg Br*, 89, 1567–73.

Kurtz, S., Ong, K., Lau, E., Mowat, F. and Halpern, M. (2007) Projections of primary and revision hip and knee arthroplasty in the United States from 2005 to 2030. *J Bone Joint Surg Am*, 89, 780–5.

Lawrence, R. C., Felson, D. T., Helmick, C. G., Arnold, L. M., Choi, H., Deyo, R. A., Gabriel, S., Hirsch, R., Hochberg, M. C., Hunder, G. G., Jordan, J. M., Katz, J. N., Kremers, H. M. and Wolfe, F. (2008) Estimates of the prevalence of arthritis and other rheumatic conditions in the United States. Part II. *Arthr Rheum*, 58, 26–35.

Lieberman, J. R., Thomas, B. J., Finerman, G. A. and Dorey, F. (2003) Patients' reasons for undergoing total hip arthroplasty can change over time. *J Arthroplasty*, 18, 63–8.

Loder, R. T. (1996) The demographics of slipped capital femoral epiphysis. An international multicenter study. *Clin Orthop Relat Res*, 322, 8–27.

Lucht, U. (2000) The Danish Hip Arthroplasty Register. *Acta Orthop Scand*, 71, 433–9.

Malchau, H., Herberts, P., Eisler, T., Garellick, G. and Soderman, P. (2002) The Swedish Total Hip Replacement Register. *J Bone Joint Surg Am*, 84A, Suppl 2, 2–20.

Mankin, H. J. (1992) Nontraumatic necrosis of bone (osteonecrosis). *N Engl J Med*, 326, 1473–9.

Matthews, P. C., Berendt, A. R., McNally, M. A. and Byren, I. (2009) Diagnosis and management of prosthetic joint infection. *BMJ*, 338, 1378–83.

Moran, E., Byren, I. and Atkins, B. L. (2010) The diagnosis and management of prosthetic joint infections. *J Antimicrob Chemother*, 65, Suppl 3, 45–54.

Morgan, H., Battista, V. and Leopold, S. S. (2005) Constraint in primary total knee arthroplasty. *J Am Acad Orthop Surg*, 13, 515–24.

Mourao, A. F., Amaral, M., Caetano-Lopes, J. and Isenberg, D. (2009) An analysis of joint replacement in patients with systemic lupus erythematosus. *Lupus*, 18, 1298–302.

Muller, M., Morawietz, L., Hasart, O., Strube, P., Perka, C. and Tohtz, S. (2008) Diagnosis of periprosthetic infection following total hip arthroplasty-evaluation of the diagnostic values of pre- and intraoperative parameters and the associated strategy to preoperatively select patients with a high probability of joint infection. *J Orthop Surg Res*, 3 (31), 1–8.

NAR (Norwegian Arthroplasty Register) (2010) Hauteland University Hospital, Bergen, Norway.

Neer, C. S., 2nd (2006) Displaced proximal humeral fractures: part I. Classification and evaluation. 1970. *Clin Orthop Relat Res*, 442, 77–82.

Ortiguera, C. J., Pulliam, I. T. and Cabanela, M. E. (1999) Total hip arthroplasty for osteonecrosis: matched-pair analysis of 188 hips with long-term follow-up. *J Arthroplasty*, 14, 21–8.

Persson, U., Persson, M. and Malchau, H. (1999) The economics of preventing revisions in total hip replacement. *Acta Orthop Scand*, 70, 163–9.

Peschken, C. A., Hitchon, C. A., Robinson, D. B., Smolik, I., Barnabe, C. R., Prematilake, S. and El-Gabalawy, H. S. (2010) Rheumatoid arthritis in a north american native population: longitudinal followup and comparison with a white population. *J Rheumatology*, 37, 1589–95.

Potter, H. G., Foo, L. F. and Nestor, B. J. (2005) What is the role of magnetic resonance imaging in the evaluation of total hip arthroplasty? *HSS J*, 1, 89–93.

Puolakka, T. J., Pajamaki, K. J., Halonen, P. J., Pulkkinen, P. O., Paavolainen, P. and Nevalainen, J. K. (2001) The Finnish Arthroplasty Register: report of the hip register. *Acta Orthop Scand*, 72, 433–41.

Ravikumar, K. J. and Marsh, G. (2000) Internal fixation versus hemiarthroplasty versus total hip arthroplasty for displaced subcapital fractures of femur – 13 year results of a prospective randomised study. *Injury*, 31, 793–7.

Rogmark, C., Carlsson, A., Johnell, O. and Sernbo, I. (2002) A prospective randomised trial of internal fixation versus arthroplasty for displaced fractures of the neck of the femur. Functional outcome for 450 patients at two years. *J Bone Joint Surg Br*, 84, 183–8.

Saraux, A., Berthelot, J. M., Chales, G., Le Henaff, C., Thorel, J. B., Hoang, S., Valls, I., Devauchelle, V., Martin, A., Baron, D., Pennec, Y., Botton, E., Mary, J. Y., Le Goff, P. and Youinou, P. (2001) Ability of the American College of Rheumatology 1987 criteria to predict rheumatoid arthritis in patients with early arthritis and classification of these patients two years later. *Arthr Rheum*, 44, 2485–91.

Sathappan, S., Pang, H.-N., Manoj, A., Ashwin, T. and Satku, K. (2009) Does stress shielding occur with the use of long-stem prosthesis in total knee arthroplasty? *Knee Surg Sports Traumatol Arthrose*, 17, 179–83.

Schurman, D. J. and Smith, R. L. (2004) Osteoarthritis: current treatment and future prospects for surgical, medical, and biologic intervention. *Clin Orthop Relat Res*, 427, S183–9.

Servizio Sanitario Regionale, E.-R. (2009) *Annual Report 2009 Regione Emilia Romagna. Dati Complessivi Interventi di Protesi d'anca, di Ginocchio e di Spalla in Emilia Romagna* 2000–2009.

Stea, S., Bordini, B., De Clerico, M., Petropulacos, K. and Toni, A. (2009) First hip arthroplasty register in Italy: 55,000 cases and 7 year follow-up. *Int Orthop*, 33, 339–46.

Stulberg S. D., Cordell, L. D., Harris, W. H., Ramsey, P. L., and MacEwen, G. D. (1975) Unrecognized childhood hip disease: a major cause of idiopathic osteoarthritis of the hip. *The Hip: Proceedings of the Third Open Scientific Meeting of the Hip Society*. St Louis, CV Mosby, pp. 212–28.

Sutherland, C. J. (1988) Radiographic evaluation of acetabular bone stock in failed total hip arthroplasty. *J Arthroplasty*, 3, 73–9.

Thomas, K. M. and Sethares, K. A. (2008) An investigation of the effects of preoperative interdisciplinary patient education on understanding postoperative expectations following a total joint arthroplasty. *Orthop Nurs*, 27, 374–81.

Thongtrangan, I., Yoon, P. and Saleh, K. J. (2003) Principles of revision total knee arthroplasty. *Sem Arthroplasty*, 14, 142–7.

Tidermark, J., Ponzer, S., Svensson, O., Soderqvist, A. and Tornkvist, H. (2003) Internal fixation compared with total hip replacement for displaced femoral neck fractures in the elderly. A randomised, controlled trial. *J Bone Joint Surg Br*, 85, 380–8.

Tobon, G., Youinou, P. and Saraux, A. (2010) The environment, geo-epidemiology, and autoimmune disease: Rheumatoid arthritis. *Autoimmun Rev*, 9, A288–92.

Vail, T. P. (2011) Hip resurfacing. *J Am Acad Orthop Surg*, 19, 236–44.

Wixson, R. L., Stulberg, S. D. and Mehlhoff, M. (1991) Total hip replacement with cemented, uncemented, and hybrid prostheses. A comparison of clinical and radiographic results at two to four years. *J Bone Joint Surg Am*, 73, 257–70.

Zeh, A., Weise, A., Vasarhelyi, A., Bach, A. G. and Wohlrab, D. (2011) Medium-term results of the Mayo short-stem hip prosthesis after avascular necrosis of the femoral head. *Z Orthop Unfall*, 149, 200–5.

14
Failure analysis of orthopaedic implants

D. W. VAN CITTERS, Dartmouth College, USA

Abstract: It is generally accepted that failure of total joint arthroplasty can be broadly attributed to patient factors, procedure factors or device factors. Whereas patient and procedure factors account for many revisions in any year, the majority of revisions are due to prosthesis failure. Because manufacturers do not proactively seek to evaluate retrieved devices, which could demonstrate long-term problems, it is imperative that retrieval centers exist to identify industry-wide problems that may impact thousands of patients. This chapter examines the history of retrieval laboratories, the typical failure modes of implants and the tools used to evaluate retrieved devices.

Key words: retrieval analysis, historical failure modes, modern analysis techniques.

14.1 Introduction

Total joint arthroplasty is often cited as one of the most successful and financially valuable elective surgeries available to patients. While the procedure itself is technically demanding and requires a skilled surgical team, worldwide outcomes are outstanding. This is particularly remarkable given how recently the modern total joint device was developed. In fewer than 50 years, devices and techniques have evolved that will accommodate most patients with debilitating joint disease or injury, returning them to activities of daily living in relatively short periods of time. Patients who, prior to surgery, might not have been capable of walking without pain are routinely returned to the tennis courts, the golf course or the ski slopes.

Due in part to these highly favorable published outcomes, the pool of candidates eligible for total joint arthroplasty is growing. As the number of total knee and hip arthroplasties performed annually increases (Kurtz et al., 2005), data show that an increasing number of patients aged under 65 are receiving artificial joints (Kurtz et al., 2009a). This younger and more active population will expect their prosthetic joints to accommodate an active lifestyle without multiple revisions, necessitating an implant designed to withstand a high number of cycles at high stress.

Unfortunately, this specification for implant longevity often is not met. Nearly 80,000 total joints are revised every year in the USA (Kurtz et al., 2009b). As a percentage of total joint procedures performed, historical data as well as extrapolations suggest that approximately 10% of today's procedures can be classified as revision procedures, though this value is country-dependent (Falbrede et al., 2011). Joint replacement surgery is inherently risky, carrying the potential for adverse events secondary to general anesthesia, infection and bleeding. Moreover, patients undergoing a revision joint surgery have aged since their primary surgery – they develop more scar tissue, they have less bone stock for the surgeon to work with and they tend to recover more slowly. For these reasons and many others, revision surgery is inherently risky and expensive. A better understanding of arthroplasty failures would therefore allow developers and surgeons to optimize materials, designs and procedures to minimize failures, decrease overall healthcare costs and improve patient outcomes.

The focus of this chapter is the detection and analysis of the variety of failure modes of joint prostheses. By its nature, failure analysis is a complex science informed by obfuscated clues, 'red herrings' and a biological system that, firstly, is unique to each individual and, secondly, can chemically and mechanically adapt to its surroundings. As such, the reader is cautioned that individual devices can have discrete failure modes associated with them (e.g. fracture, wear-through, or malalignment), but classes of devices and materials might also have less obvious, global failure modes that only become apparent through studying large numbers of retrievals and performing statistical analysis.

14.2 Implant retrieval laboratories

The orthopaedic industry is driven by rapid technological changes geared toward product differentiation in the marketplace. These rapid technological changes have led to significant technical problems with medical devices in the past (e.g. Poly II, a carbon-fiber reinforced polyethylene that shed fibers due to wear *in vivo*; corrosion from mixed modular interfaces, poor metallurgy and poorly maintained tolerances; thin bearings subject to rapid fatigue; and gamma sterilization in air resulting in oxidative degradation and fatigue failure of polyethylene). Orthopaedic manufacturers are required to file medical device reports (MDRs) for all retrieved devices that are known to them, acknowledging poor clinical outcomes. However, manufacturers do not proactively seek to evaluate retrieved devices, which could demonstrate long-term problems. There is no perceived financial incentive for a company to look for long-term performance problems when the results of such a study could not only hurt competitive market position but, in today's climate of litigation, could also represent significant legal liability. As a result, unforeseen detrimental impacts are discovered sometime later, after broad use and a significant period of application.

Retrieval laboratories with no proprietary affiliation with orthopaedic device brands, designs, manufacturing techniques or materials are rare in the field of orthopaedic research. They are nonetheless critical to identifying industry-wide predictors of failure, whether these are material related or design related. Often administered through academic institutions with federal grants or research contracts from collections of industry representatives, such laboratories have been responsible for changing the design, fabrication and implantation of devices over the last three decades.

Pioneering work by Hood and colleagues at the Hospital for Special Surgery in New York provided retrieval laboratories with a common nomenclature for feature identification, and later researchers began to identify techniques and trends that continue to be used and standardized across institutions. International standards organizations also recognize the importance of retrieval analysis, publishing standards such as ASTM F561 (ASTM, 2003b) and ISO 12891-(1-4) (ISO, 2011).

Because many failures would not happen in the absence of mechanical input from the user, patient history is an important factor in failure analysis. As such, compliance with ethical principles of human subjects research is of paramount importance. Before starting a new study center at an institution, the researcher is cautioned to seek approval from an appropriate institutional review board for retrieval studies.

14.3 Failure modes

It is generally accepted that failure of total joint arthroplasty can be broadly attributed to factors relating to the patient, the procedure or the device (Morrey, 1993). Whereas patient and procedure factors account for many revisions in any year, the majority of revisions are due to prosthesis failure (Sharkey et al., 2002) (Fig. 14.1).

Historically, mechanical failure of polymer bearings occurred through contact fatigue modes such as cracking, spalling and delamination (Kennedy et al., 2003) (see Fig. 14.1(a)). One would not predict such failures based on the mechanical properties of virgin polyethylene, and retrieval studies in the 1980s and 1990s focused on determining the conditions that led to material degradation. In the mid-1990s, scientists determined that sterilization using gamma irradiation allowed for subsequent oxidation of the material, thereby changing the mechanical

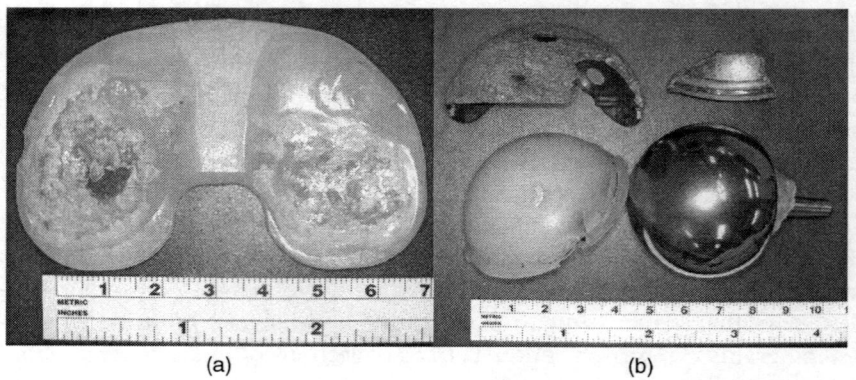

14.1 Over half of all orthopaedic retrievals are related to device failure. (a) A severely delaminated total knee arthroplasty after 186 months *in vivo*. (b) A hip arthroplasty showing cracking of the metallic acetabular shell, thinning of the polymer bearing and scratching of the TiN coating on the femoral head.

character of the finished product (Collier *et al.*, 1996; Currier *et al.*, 1997; Sutula *et al.*, 1995b; Williams *et al.*, 1998).

During radiation sterilization, gamma radiation from a cobalt-60 source disrupts all biological activity. Simultaneously, the radiation causes chain scission and hydrogen separation from the carbon backbone of the polymer chain. Free radicals created within the material seek a lower energy state through recombining in their original conformation, combining with each other or remaining in a high-energy state until they combine with other chemical species found in the polymer bulk. Oxygen is one such active species that, in a poorly understood process, catalyzes a self-perpetuating reaction of chain scission and further oxidation (Daly and Yin, 1998). This is evidenced by the accumulation of carbonyl species (aldehydes, acids and ketones) within the material. Although free radicals are created uniformly through the material, it is thought that oxidation only occurs in amorphous regions, owing to an inability of oxygen to diffuse through the crystalline lattice (Goldman *et al.*, 1997; Kurtz *et al.*, 1999; Nevoralova *et al.*, 2005).

Less well understood is the profile of oxidation with depth. In materials retrieved from patients or materials exposed to air on the shelf, the maximum carbonyl concentration is found 1–2 mm below the exposed surface (Fig. 14.2). Originally it was thought that the radiation dose varied through the depth of the polymer, resulting in an increased free radical population below the surface (Blanchet and Burroughs, 2001). However, later studies determined that bulk-irradiated polyethylene could be cut to expose new surfaces, and the same characteristic oxidation profile would appear (Van Citters, 2003). Researchers are further perplexed in that retrieved devices show that oxidation is not uniform around the free

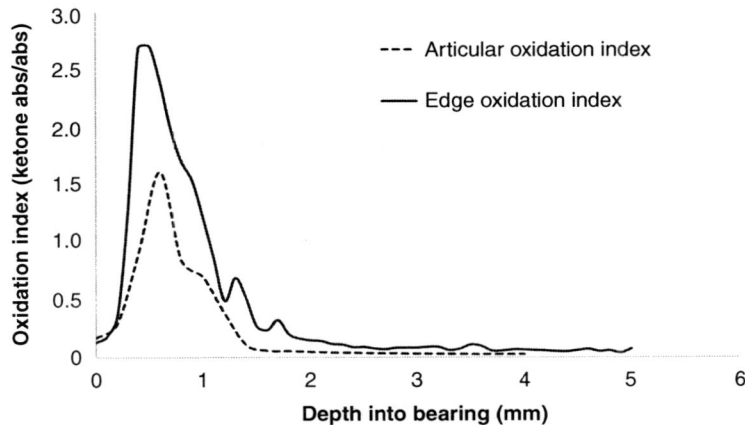

14.2 Typical oxidation profile of polyethylene showing a subsurface peak in the oxidation index. Different regions can have different oxidation maxima.

surfaces. In some cases, regions near the edge of a tibial insert or the flange of an acetabular cup oxidize faster than the articular surfaces (Currier *et al.*, 2007) (Fig. 14.3).

Oxidation is detectable as more than just double-bonded oxygen species within the polymer bulk. Because the mechanical properties of polyethylene change with oxidation, any freshly cut surfaces will show the appearance of 'white bands' below the exposed surface (Fig. 14.3). The white band is the result of localized brittle failure during sectioning and is often the locus of failure in retrieved devices.

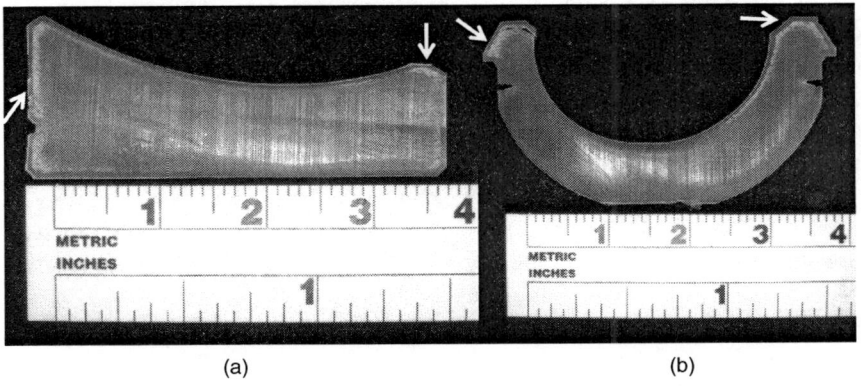

14.3 Thin cross-sections of (a) knee and (b) hip (R) bearings show subsurface white bands. Oxidation is typically higher in areas exposed to body fluids. This is indicated by more pronounced whitening (indicated by arrows).

The maximum oxidation level of a component exposed to atmospheric oxygen will increase exponentially with time (Sutula *et al.*, 1995a). This degradation will render an orthopaedic bearing useless after as few as 5 years due to loss of toughness (Sutula *et al.*, 1995a). Therefore, to avoid shelf oxidation of orthopaedic bearings, all US manufacturers have discontinued radiation sterilization in the presence of oxygen.

14.3.1 Osteolysis

Concerns surrounding wear of an orthopaedic device are not limited to volume loss or wear-through of the polymer bearing. The fate of the polymer wear debris has become an increasingly important concern in orthopaedic science. Previous researchers have found that wear particles generated by total knee devices are generally sub-micron in dimensions and of polymer origin (Harris, 1994; Schmalzried *et al.*, 1994). These particles differ greatly in size from those found in the hip, and tend to be smaller and more biologically active (Schmalzried *et al.*, 1994).

Polyethylene, at the macro-scale, is quiescent in the body. Hence, it is used for a range of medical applications beyond bearings for the knee and the hip. However, as a piece of polyethylene is decreased in size, the cellular self-defense mechanism of the human body begins to take over. Throughout the body exist phagocytic cells whose purpose is to rid the body of old blood cells, cellular debris and micro-organisms. The cells operate through binding to, and subsequently engulfing, the invader or dead tissue. Because this recognition and interaction occur on the cellular level, the most inflammatory particles will be cellular or sub-cellular in size. In early studies, researchers determined that polyethylene particles must be in the 'phagocytosable size range of 0.3 to 10 microns to be biologically active' (Green *et al.*, 1998). Later studies have shown that particle sizes in the range of 0.1 to 1 microns are the most biologically active (Ingham and Fisher, 2005).

If a wear particle is 'biologically active,' it stimulates a cascade of events that will ultimately lead to a loss of bone stock and implant loosening. In addition to phagocytosing the particle, a macrophage will send a variety of signals to other cells in and around the joint space. These signals include proteolytic enzymes, inflammatory mediators and osteolytic mediators (Green *et al.*, 1998; Ingham and Fisher, 2005). Osteoclasts are either recruited by or differentiated from the macrophages and begin to break down the bone in the vicinity of the total joint device. For the patient, this translates to potential pain, swelling and implant loosening. In some cases, osteolysis is pain free and the loss of bone stock continues asymptomatically (Fig. 14.4). This clinical condition of bone resorption as a result of biological activity of wear debris is known as osteolysis. It is unclear

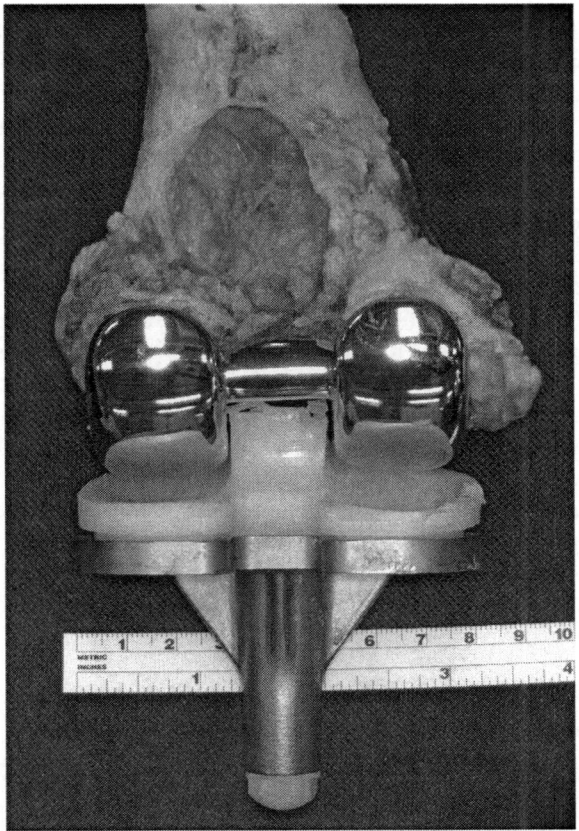

14.4 Loss of bone stock near an implant is indicative of osteolysis secondary to polyethylene wear.

whether certain patient groups are more or less susceptible to this activity; it has been proposed that a host-related factor is responsible for the magnitude of cytokine response (Wilkinson et al., 2003).

Detailed retrieval analyses have not led to specific characteristics of the orthopaedic components that can be positively attributed to an increased incidence of osteolysis (Atwood et al., 2005; Currier et al., 2005b). Therefore research has been extended into the analysis of the debris and the patient. Of particular importance would be a study of the osteolytic cysts. The cyst must contain the material causing the osteolysis, and documentation of the characteristics should provide insight into the size, shape and volumetric concentration of particles.

To examine *in vivo* wear particle production, tissue can be analyzed through optical microscopy, using birefringence to identify polymer particles. However, the sub-micron nature of the particles often requires the use of shorter wavelength radiation for detection. Tissue digestion followed by subsequent filtration and electron microscope imaging has been recently employed for particle characterization. Digestion and filtration techniques vary widely, and there exists a wealth of literature supporting acid digestion, base digestion, and enzymatic digestion. Each technique has benefits and drawbacks, but they all appear to produce evidence of the mechanism of wear or damage to the articulating surfaces.

While a detailed discussion of debris analysis techniques is beyond the scope of this chapter, the retrieval scientist is nonetheless urged to understand the nature and activity of wear debris related to a metal on polymer sliding contact. This is particularly important because newer cross-linked and remelted materials have demonstrated lower linear wear rates both in the laboratory and in clinical use. These wear rates come at the cost of an increased proportion of debris in the sizes considered to be biologically active (Ingham and Fisher, 2005). Moreover, studies have shown that the overall functional activity of this smaller volume but more active debris is essentially equivalent to the larger volume of debris produced by conventional polymer bearings (Endo et al., 2002).

14.3.2 Total hip arthroplasty failure

In most contemporary hip bearings, manufacturers have tried to eliminate the residual free radicals that result from ionizing radiation. After the polymer is irradiated, it is heated above its crystalline melt temperature and subsequently cooled under controlled conditions. Not only does this remelting process quench most of the residual free radicals, but the polymer is further cross-linked as the free radicals annihilate each other. These 'first-generation' cross-linked polymers are known to have lower wear rates in laboratory tests and have therefore been seen as beneficial in a multi-directional sliding environment such as the human hip (McKellop et al., 1999b).

In the hope of capitalizing on the lower linear wear rate associated with the level of cross-linking, manufacturers have subjected polyethylene to radiation doses approaching four times those used in conventional gamma-inert or gamma-vacuum devices. Conventional polyethylene devices may see doses in the 25–40 kGy range, while cross-linked materials have been dosed from 50 to 100 kGy (Collier et al., 2003).

Wear rate reductions of up to 90% have been reported in the literature for materials cross-linked in this way (McKellop et al., 1999a). However, increased cross-linking and wear resistance come at the cost of reduced mechanical properties, particularly fracture toughness. A number of studies have been published showing *in vivo* fracture of the polymer components of total hip devices (Furmanski et al., 2009; Tower et al., 2006). The fractured

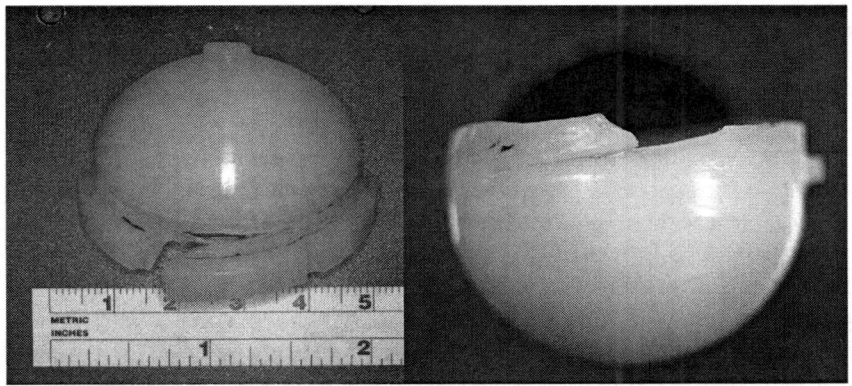

14.5 Devices placed in challenging mechanical loading scenarios are susceptible to cracking and fatigue failure. (a) A vertically oriented cup that failed after 3 months. (b) A bearing loaded extensively on the edge due to patient anatomy that failed after 24 months.

devices all appear to show damage secondary to fatigue loading of the polymer, oftentimes in areas of very high stress (Fig. 14.5). These would include locations of thin polyethylene, sharp corners causing stress concentrations or locking mechanisms designed to restrict movement of the polymer bearing in the metal shell.

In an effort to decrease wear rates, improve surgeon choice during surgery, minimize fracture and more closely mimic natural biomechanics, the orthopaedic industry has provided alternative bearing couples to the market. Specifically, hard-on-hard bearings in the form of ceramic-on-ceramic (CoC) or metal-on-metal (MoM) couples have enjoyed a resurgence in recent years. While osteolysis and wear-through of these bearings are rare, additional failure modes have been introduced.

Historically, early ceramic bearings failed through fracture or chipping, adding very hard third-body debris to the joint space (Boutin, 1972; Knahr *et al.*, 1987). Newer alumina ceramics and recently introduced zirconia–alumina ceramic composites have addressed many of these issues, allowing for CoC bearing couples with very low revision rates (D'Antonio *et al.*, 2005; Lusty *et al.*, 2007; Murphy *et al.*, 2006) and seldom-reported mechanical failure (Huet *et al.*, 2011). Retrieved devices still show evidence of metal transfer and worn 'stripes' of the alumina heads (Fig. 14.6). The literature also reports a varying incidence of audible squeaking between 1% and 20% (Capello *et al.*, 2008; Mesko *et al.*, 2009; Walter *et al.*, 2008). While this does not necessarily represent a clinical complication, it can be categorized as a tribological failure and a potential social concern for the joint recipient.

A recent study of never implanted CoC devices has shown that the squeaking phenomenon can be reproduced in the laboratory, in the absence of metallic components such as the acetabular shell or the femoral stem (Currier *et al.*, 2010a). Audible squeaks have similar frequency characteristics to clinically recorded squeaks, demonstrating that the driving force behind the vibration is likely related to a stick–slip phenomenon in the CoC contact. It is apparent from studies such as this that failure analysis should focus on patient factors, lubrication and loading of affected devices (Currier *et al.*, 2010a).

MoM hip arthroplasty is a second alternative bearing couple that has been in use since the early days of arthroplasty. Early success with devices such as the McKee Farrar and the Ring prostheses demonstrated that a cobalt-on-cobalt articulation is possible. Because squeaking and fracture are two potential failure modes of the otherwise low-wear CoC bearing couple, there has been renewed interest in MoM. Wear simulator studies and early clinical results pointed toward good outcomes, but current clinical results are unexpected. It has become apparent through retrieval analysis that surgeon placement of the device, material selection, design and patient sensitivity can all impact the outcomes of arthroplasty surgery. As with other orthopaedic failures, none of these factors were predicted during the device design and preliminary testing phases.

Given the potentially traumatic outcomes associated with metal sensitivity or metallosis, the causes of failure for these devices are being actively researched. Techniques such as the Hood scoring technique (Hood *et al.*, 1983) are proving inadequate for device analysis. As such, it is important for retrieval laboratories to establish common methods and

14.6 Metal transfer and stripe wear are typically found in retrieved ceramic bearings. The metal transfer stands proud of the substrate, while stripe wear is characterized as a roughening through material loss. The rough area (shown in the micrograph) allows pencil to be rubbed onto the ceramic for better visualization.

terminologies for assessing MoM devices. For instance, laboratories are working on standardization of biochemical techniques for ion assessment, optical and profilometry techniques for surface analysis, and coordinate measurement techniques for wear analysis.

14.3.3 Total knee arthroplasty failure

In knee bearings, the most common alternative to gamma in air treatment involves sterilizing the bearing using a radiation source in an inert or vacuum environment. Although free radicals are still created in this method, the exclusion of oxygen precludes shelf oxidation (Greer *et al.*, 1999; Lu *et al.*, 2003). This method has a mechanical benefit in that irradiation causes hydrogen separation from the carbon backbones and, through recombination, the polyethylene acquires a low level of cross-linking.

In vivo, several studies have documented the benefit of gamma sterilization in a vacuum relative to gas plasma sterilization, reporting up to 50% wear reduction with irradiated materials (Sychterz *et al.*, 2004). Components that are sterilized in this fashion have residual free radicals. While shelf oxidation in the package is eliminated, retrieved devices have shown that oxidation occurs in the body (Currier *et al.*, 2007). Therefore, gamma vacuum or gamma inert sterilized devices may still be susceptible to mechanical failure subsequent to polyethylene oxidation *in vivo* (Currier *et al.*, 2007; Muratoglu *et al.*, 2004).

While current polymer treatments might eliminate or delay fatigue failure secondary to oxidative embrittlement, wear at articular and non-articular modular interfaces is important to analyze. An important design objective of modular knee arthroplasty devices is to allow intraoperative flexibility and ease of bearing replacement. The intent has been to securely lock the insert onto the metal tray such that relative motion of the components *in vivo* is prevented. However, despite the robustness of the insert-to-tray locking mechanism or its design, it is not practical in engineering terms to entirely eliminate relative motion at the interface between the components under *in vivo* loads. The metal tray and the ultra-high molecular weight polyethylene (UHMWPE) insert have very large differences in material properties that will govern relative motion under load. For example, the modulus of elasticity is approximately 0.7 GPa for UHMWPE and 116 GPa for titanium. This indicates that, under a given load, the deformation of UHMWPE will be 100 times greater than that of titanium, and there is a high likelihood of relative motion between two materials in contact. Since the majority of tibial trays in modular fixed-bearing knee devices have historically been titanium with an unpolished modular interface surface, the relative motion of the insert will be against a relatively abrasive surface.

It is therefore not surprising that studies of knee devices have documented

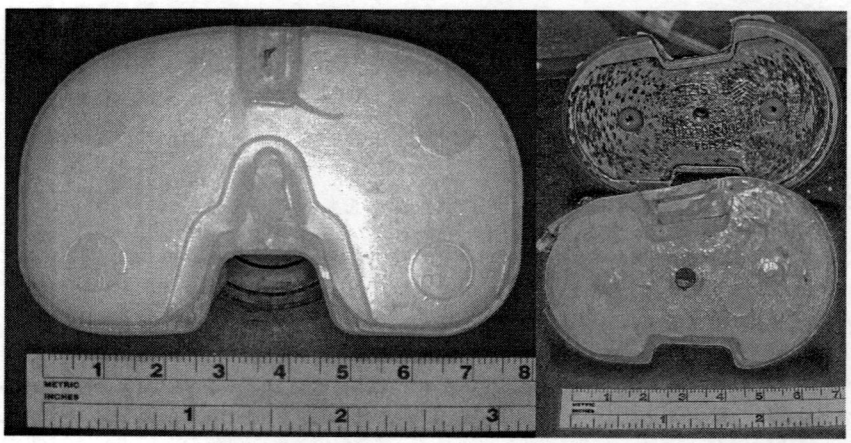

14.7 Backside wear of devices typically results from abrasive motion against a rough titanium alloy tibial tray.

that modular knees designed as fixed bearings are in fact not 'fixed' in place, but move and experience abrasive wear. Engh *et al.* (2001) performed an important *in vitro* study measuring multi-directional motion of tibial inserts in tray locking mechanisms with clinically relevant loads. This motion is sufficient to liberate debris in the biologically active range, and results in visible abrasion and burnishing (Muratoglu *et al.*, 2003; Schmalzried *et al.*, 1994; Wasielewski *et al.*, 1997). Studies of retrievals from several centers have documented marked wear of UHMWPE due to relative motion (Fig. 14.7) (Conditt *et al.*, 2004a; Mayor *et al.*, 2005; Noble *et al.*, 2003). Although this relative displacement is often termed 'micromotion', it is clear that the impact of this motion can be the degradation of locking mechanisms and the release of a significant amount of wear debris (Conditt *et al.*, 2004b; Engh *et al.*, 1992, 2001; Parks *et al.*, 1998; Rao *et al.*, 2002).

Growing concern over wear-related osteolysis has led a number of retrieval centers to invest time and resources into documenting *in vivo* changes of failed devices. Publications related to a number of these studies have employed the terms 'damage' and 'wear' to describe changes, but they cannot be used interchangeably. Historically, the two could have been synonymous given the gross failure modes of cracking and delamination leading to material loss. Visual assessment of these phenomena would enable a researcher to identify the poor appearance of a device. However, in cases where adhesive/abrasive wear is occurring, visual surface changes might not be as evident. Atwood *et al.* (2008) and Currier *et al.* (2011), through investigations of low contact stress rotating platform bearings, have documented that there is no correlation between damage and wear. A

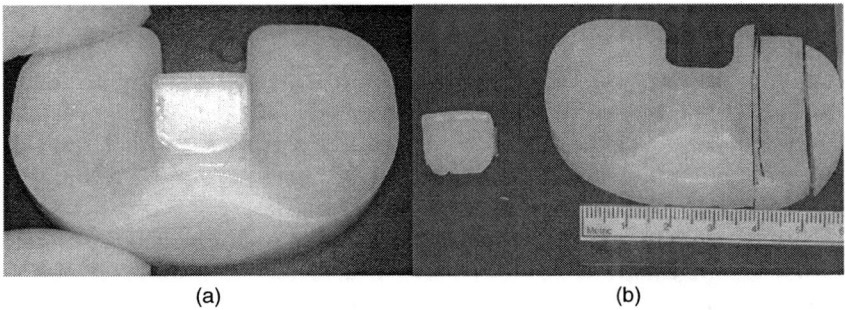

(a)   (b)

14.8 Anterior impingement of the femoral component on the tibial bearing results in a 'bowtie' appearance in posterior-stabilized devices (a). In some cases, this can result in separation of the tibial post from the remainder of the tibial insert (b).

damaged appearance can be identified after short durations *in vivo* and is likely impacted by third-body debris (Atwood *et al.*, 2006).

Another location of damage and potential failure in total knee arthroplasty is the tibial eminence on posterior-stabilized knee inserts. Posterior-stabilized knee bearings with a post-and-cam mechanism are designed to facilitate 'roll-back' through contact of the femoral component cam and the posterior aspect of the post. The anterior facet and the top of the post are generally not designed to incur significant contact under normal knee articulation. Posterior-stabilized knee inserts retrieved from clinical service provide important insight into whether the tibio-femoral contacts are, in fact, performing as designed. Evidence of significant impingement on the front and top of the post would indicate knee alignment or kinematics different from those intended. Failures have been reported in the literature; anterior impingement or the 'bowtie' effect (Fig. 14.8) is commonly documented and in one study was reported in 100% of retrieved tibial inserts (Banks *et al.*, 2002; Hendel *et al.*, 2003; Orozco and Hozack, 2008; Puloski *et al.*, 2001; Silva *et al.*, 2003).

Post fracture, while rare in the literature, nonetheless occurs and is attributed to impingement, high stresses in a specific biomechanical environment, or wear (Chiu *et al.*, 2004; Hendel *et al.*, 2003). Notably, three recent cases of fracture of highly cross-linked UHMWPE have been reported, and concerns surround the suitability of materials with lower toughness for application in a posterior-stabilized total knee (Huot *et al.*, 2010; Jung *et al.*, 2008; Medel *et al.*, 2007).

14.3.4 Other joints

Total joint arthroplasty for smaller joints in the body, including shoulder, spine, ankle and elbow, is becoming increasingly prevalent. While each of these joints can be characterized by a unique environment with respect to range of motion and loading, failures can be characterized by techniques similar to those used in total hip and knee prostheses.

Shoulder arthroplasty, for instance, does not enjoy the same success rate as total hip or total knee arthroplasty. In a review, Bohsali *et al.* (2006) document failure rates of over 14% in studies reporting results at more than 2 years. While the majority of shoulder failures are attributed to loosening of the glenoid component, gross mechanical failure of the polymer component of the joint and wear-related osteolysis have also been extensively documented (Scarlat and Matsen, 2001).

Total ankle arthroplasty is growing as an alternative to ankle fusion around the world due to the potential for increased range of motion after surgery. Failures of total ankle prostheses are typically secondary to loosening or instability and, according to large joint registry datasets, 5 year survival rates do not exceed 90% (Skytta *et al.*, 2010). Failure analysis studies of these devices are not as common in the literature as other arthroplasty devices, although features similar to those found in total hips and knees have been identified in retrieved ankles (Vaupel *et al.*, 2009). Affatato and colleagues were able to take such studies further by demonstrating the ability to reproduce these features in a laboratory setting (Affatato *et al.*, 2007).

Total disc arthroplasty is a relatively new procedure in which the native tissue is replaced by a bearing construct most typically using a cobalt counterface and a polymer bearing surface. Similar to artificial knees and hips, failures reported in the literature for artificial discs are most commonly documented as mechanical fatigue failure secondary to radiation-induced oxidation (Kurtz *et al.*, 2007). Few long-term outcomes have been reported and it is unknown whether a solution to the fatigue failure problem will allow wear-related phenomena to manifest in patients. Specifically, Grupp and colleagues have shown that wear particles from artificial disc constructs are biologically active and may lead to osteolysis (Grupp *et al.*, 2009). Alternative bearing materials such as carbon fiber reinforced polyaryletheretherketone might lead to improved outcomes, though the tribological behavior of these bearings needs additional research (Grupp *et al.*, 2010; Langohr *et al.*, 2011; Scholes and Unsworth, 2010).

14.4 Analysis techniques

Tools for failure analysis of total joint arthroplasty range in size, cost, complexity and utility. Often, the most valuable tool is a large database and a systematic method to characterize and store data related to device characteristics. While case reports and identification of trends are of great importance to the field, some of the strongest publications are those in which statistical significance is achieved through analysis of larger numbers (e.g. more than 100) of retrieved devices. Larger numbers of failed devices allow for control of patient factors or device design factors. This is particularly important when assessing tribological failure of a device or a material since low wear rates in orthopaedics can be masked by manufacturing tolerances or variations in patient behavior or measurement techniques.

Analysis techniques can be broadly grouped into surface characterization, mechanical characterization and chemical characterization. While these techniques are not exhaustive, they have proven useful to past generations of retrieval laboratories in identifying the root cause of orthopaedic failures.

14.4.1 Surface characterization

The first two pieces of equipment used by any retrieval laboratory are a camera and a microscope. Levels of sophistication can vary greatly for these, but studies at Dartmouth College have found that macro-photographs of all received devices, followed by careful micrographs of salient features can provide a great deal of evidence of a failure mode. Such photographs can help identify tribological failures such as contact fatigue failure, pitting or scratching. Alone, or in conjunction with scanning electron microscopy, fatigue failures and locations of crack initiation can also be identified.

Notably, lighting of components for photography can be very difficult. Imaging polyethylene, due to its white color and semi-translucent character, often requires reflected light from low angles, polarized light, transmitted light or multiple light sources to bring out burnishing marks, shadows from scratches or pits, or subsurface cracks that might not have propagated to the surface. Likewise, lighting of metallic components, particularly highly polished articular surfaces, might require a ring light, diffusers or oblique lighting to best document a feature. Digital image processing techniques such as high dynamic range can be employed to more faithfully represent surface appearances visible to the eye.

Digital images also lend themselves well to either qualitative or quantitative analysis. Qualitative analysis was first used by Hood *et al.* (1983) to triage failed artificial joints and the technique continues to be used

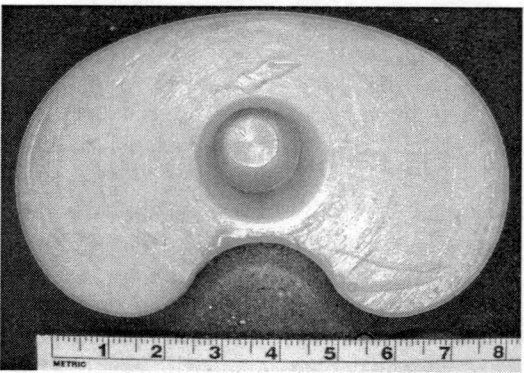

14.9 The damaged appearance of the rotating platform knee bearing does not indicate material removal in this device after 2 months of service.

today. As articular materials and failure modes change, updates to the Hood scoring system have been made and are continually reported to the literature (e.g. Collier *et al.*, 2008; Currier *et al.*, 2005b, 2010b). There is room in the literature for a new nomenclature and ranking system for metal and ceramic components as the Hood system was developed primarily for polymer articular surfaces. Recently, there have been reports that the clinical damage ranking system might not be predictive of tribological failure or material removal in polymer components. For instance, Atwood *et al.* (2008) note that a damaged appearance of a device did not correlate with material removal (Fig. 14.9). Therefore, non-destructive measurement of material dimensions is merited.

Surface measurements can range in scale from using a dial indicator for discrete dimensional analysis (indicating wear, creep or deformation) to profilometry (to identify changes in surface roughness, scratches or microscopic features identifying contact conditions) to coordinate measurement machines (to identify global changes in device geometry).

Occasionally, destructive testing is necessary for imaging. This is particularly true if a device needs metallurgical or microstructural analysis. For instance, in the late 1980s and early 1990s, many corrosion-related failures in femoral head–neck junctions were attributed to mixed metals and a galvanic effect (Collier *et al.*, 1992). However, a subset of these devices was identified as being metallurgically deficient. Careful metallurgy showed grain boundary attack secondary to growth of carbides in the cobalt alloy (Gilbert *et al.*, 1993). More recently, while corrosion and fatigue failure in tapered interfaces of modular hip stems might be attributed to poor choice of materials, metallurgy and microscopic analysis has shown failures secondary to fretting and the presence of a crevice (Fraitzl *et al.*, 2011; Rodrigues *et al.*, 2009).

14.4.2 Chemical analysis

Beyond visual analysis, chemical techniques have also been used for failure analysis of total joints. One of the most valuable techniques developed over the last two decades is Fourier transform infrared spectroscopy (FTIR). This technique allows a variety of features to be determined from analysis of polymer components. For instance, one can identify the original degree of irradiation if the device was cross-linked or sterilized using a gamma or electron beam source (ASTM, 2004). Similarly, the crystallinity of the polymer can be estimated (Nagy and Li, 1990). Perhaps most importantly, chemical changes in the bearing material can be deduced, including the degree of absorbed species and the oxidation of the material (ASTM, 2001). Because oxidation of a barrier-packaged material can occur in the body during service, or on the shelf after retrieval, care must be taken to minimize or account for shelf-ageing. This has recently become even more important given the indication that cross-linked and stabilized materials can oxidize both in the body and on the shelf after retrieval.

Numerous other chemical techniques can be used to identify chemical changes in a failed device, for example:

- differential scanning calorimetry, useful for determination of crystallinity and crystal size distribution;
- gel permeation chromatography, employed to determine molecular weight and molecular weight distribution, though difficult for cross-linked materials;
- mass spectrometry, detection of chemical species present in a material or tissue;
- densitometry, an older method for determining degree of oxidation and/or crystallinity.

14.4.3 Mechanical testing

Mechanical properties of materials have the potential to change with time, sometimes dramatically. The result can be a change in wear rate, accelerated contact fatigue failure, or gross mechanical failure of the device. To fully analyze materials that have been explanted from the body, the retrieval scientist has a number of standardized tests at their disposal. For polymers, mechanical testing can be performed by:

- dynamic mechanical analysis – identification of changes to a material's viscoelastic properties;

- small punch testing – standardized technique used to test small, thin polymer specimens (ASTM, 2002);
- tensile testing – standardized technique to test larger polymer specimens (ASTM, 2003a);
- durometer/hardness testing – alternative method to examine mechanical properties.

For metals and ceramics, mechanical testing includes microhardness, hardness and scratch testing.

14.5 Importance of validation

While identification of failures and hypothesizing their cause is the primary function of a retrieval laboratory, it is important to note that few of these failures, if any, were predicted by the original manufacturer of an orthopaedic device. Despite thorough scientific and clinical testing required by entities such as the US Food and Drug Administration (FDA) and conformity standards established by ASTM International, the International Organization for Standardization (ISO) and the European Union (e.g. the CE mark), sometimes alarming failure rates exist.

In vitro validation of failure modalities therefore serves dual purposes. Firstly, creation of a controlled mechanical, chemical or tribological environment allows verification of the hypotheses formed during observation and analysis of the original failure. Being able to recreate the failure and observe it or document its progression provides valuable information for surgeons, manufacturers and patients with respect to predictions for future failure.

The second, and perhaps equally valuable, aspect of *in vitro* validation is the ability to test new designs against older designs that failed. Tribotesting of prostheses in particular has benefitted from *in vitro* validation of failure modes. For instance, the best-known failure prediction devices include hip, knee, ankle and shoulder simulators. Each of these has been developed to provide insight into failure modes before any clinical use. Examples of other successful testing modalities include the following:

- performing tests on devices using microseparation in a total hip simulator to better identify wear behavior (Bowsher *et al*., 2008; Leslie *et al*., 2009);
- performing tests on devices using edge loading in compression to better identify susceptibility to fatigue failure of locking mechanisms (Anglin *et al*., 2000; Saleh *et al*., 2008);
- artificial ageing of new materials to provide insight into predicting long-term chemical and mechanical behavior of devices (Collier *et al*., 2003; Currier *et al*., 2005a; Edidin *et al*., 2002).

14.6 Conclusion

The near-constant introduction of 'improved materials' for joint arthroplasty has led to marketing of new materials without a proven *in vivo* track record. Often, there is sparse basic science that has been published to allow prediction or explanation of the mechanical properties of the material, and predictions of *in vivo* performance often are based on phenomenological experimental techniques that may or may not be clinically relevant. Nonetheless, devices manufactured through novel methods gain FDA approval and are implanted in humans every day. These devices also comprise a growing portion of the revision load. Whereas oxidation-related contact fatigue was originally responsible for a large number of bearing failures, today's failures are related to less predictable phenomena such as the reduced mechanical properties of highly cross-linked materials, wear-particle-induced osteolysis, metal sensitivity of a patient or tribocorrosion of a construct (Hirakawa *et al.*, 2004).

Despite this incomplete understanding of the material behavior of contemporary UHMWPE treatments and hard-on-hard bearings, 'next-generation' cross-linked polyethylenes are beginning to appear before the FDA for approval. These polymers have novel treatments that attempt to decrease the oxidation susceptibility of irradiated and cross-linked polyethylene while at the same time preserving the fracture toughness of non-irradiated polyethylene. Examples include materials that incorporate antioxidants such as alpha tocopherol to halt oxidation, those that are annealed through mechanical deformation rather than heat and those that are chemically cross-linked (Muratoglu, 2005).

Characterization and test techniques must therefore be constantly adapted and developed to help explain the current range of failures and to predict the engineering limits of such candidate materials before they are incorporated into orthopaedic devices. Steps taken during processing and subsequent treatment provide thermal and mechanical energy that may alter the structure of the polyethylene. These structural changes, in turn, may affect the mechanical properties and material behavior of the polymer in ways that can significantly impact the long-term success of an orthopaedic device.

14.7 References

Affatato, S., Leardini, A., Leardini, W., Giannini, S. and Viceconti, M. 2007. Meniscal wear at a three-component total ankle prosthesis by a knee joint simulator. *J Biomech*, 40, 1871–6, S0021-9290(06)00302-2 [pii], DOI 10.1016/j.jbiomech.2006.08.002.

Anglin, C., Wyss, U. P. and Pichora, D. R. 2000. Mechanical testing of shoulder prostheses and recommendations for glenoid design. *J Shoulder Elbow Surg*, 9, 323–31, S1058-2746(00)15673-3 [pii], DOI 10.1067/mse.2000.105451.

ASTM. 2001. *F2102-01 Standard Guide for Evaluating the Extent of Oxidation in Ultra High Molecular Weight Polyethylene Fabricated Forms Intended for Surgical Implants*. Philadelphia, PA, ASTM.

ASTM. 2002. *F2183-02 Standard Test Method for Small Punch Testing of Ultra-High Molecular Weight Polyethylene Used in Surgical Implants*. Philadelphia, PA, ASTM.

ASTM. 2003a. *D638-03 Standard Test Method for Tensile Properties of Plastics*. Philadelphia, PA, ASTM.

ASTM. 2003b. *F561-97 Practice for Retrieval and Analysis of Implanted Medical Devices, and Associated Tissues*. Philadelphia, PA, ASTM.

ASTM. 2004. *F2381-04 Standard Test Method for Evaluating Trans Vinylene Yield in Irradiated Ultra High Molecular Weight Polyethylene Fabricated Forms Intended for Surgical Implants by Infrared Spectroscopy*. Philadelphia, PA, ASTM.

Atwood, S. A., Kennedy, F. E., Currier, J. H., Van Citters, D. W. and Collier, J. P. 2005 In-vitro study of backside wear mechanisms on mobile platform knee bearings. *Proceedings of World Tribology Congress III*, 2005. Washington, DC, ASME International, Vol. 2, pp. 633–4.

Atwood, S. A., Kennedy, F. E., Currier, J. H., Van Citters, D. W. and Collier, J. P. 2006. In-vitro study of backside wear mechanisms on mobile knee bearing components. *ASME J Tribology*, 128, 275–81.

Atwood, S. A., Currier, J. H., Mayor, M. B., Collier, J. P., Van Citters, D. W. and Kennedy, F. E. 2008. Clinical wear measurement on low contact stress rotating platform knee bearings. *J Arthroplasty*, 23, 431–40, S0883-5403(07)00342-7 [pii], DOI 10.1016/j.arth.2007.06.005.

Banks, S. A., Harman, M. K. and Hodge, W. A. 2002. Mechanism of anterior impingement damage in total knee arthroplasty. *J Bone Joint Surg Am*, 84A, Suppl 2, 37–42.

Blanchet, T. A. and Burroughs, B. 2001. Numerical oxidation model for gamma radiation-sterilized UHMWPE: Consideration of dose-depth profile. *J Biomed Mater Res*, 58, 684–93.

Bohsali, K. I., Wirth, M. A. and Rockwood, C. A., Jr. 2006. Complications of total shoulder arthroplasty. *J Bone Joint Surg Am*, 88, 2279–92, 88/10/2279 [pii], DOI 10.2106/JBJS.F.00125.

Boutin, P. 1972. Total hip arthroplasty made of dense ceramics – fritted alumina. *Rev Chir Orthop Repara Appar Mot*, 58, 229–46.

Bowsher, J. G., Williams, P. A., Clarke, I. C., Green, D. D. and Donaldson, T. K. 2008. 'Severe' wear challenge to 36 mm mechanically enhanced highly crosslinked polyethylene hip liners. *J Biomed Mater Res B Appl Biomater*, 86, 253–63, DOI 10.1002/jbm.b.31013.

Capello, W. N., D'Antonio, J. A., Feinberg, J. R., Manley, M. T. and Naughton, M. 2008. Ceramic-on-ceramic total hip arthroplasty: update. *J Arthroplasty*, 23, 39–43.

Chiu, Y. S., Chen, W. M., Huang, C. K., Chiang, C. C. and Chen, T. H. 2004. Fracture of the polyethylene tibial post in a NexGen posterior-stabilized knee prosthesis. *J Arthroplasty*, 19, 1045–9, S0883540304003122 [pii].

Collier, J. P., Surprenant, V. A., Jensen, R. E., Mayor, M. B. and Surprenant, H. P.

1992. Corrosion between the components of modular femoral hip prostheses. *J Bone Joint Surg Br*, 74, 511–7.

Collier, J. P., Sutula, L. C., Currier, B. H., Currier, J. H., Wooding, R. E., Williams, I. R., Farber, K. B. and Mayor, M. B. 1996. Overview of polyethylene as a bearing material: comparison of sterilization methods. *Clin Orthop Relat Res*, 333, 76–86.

Collier, J. P., Currier, B. H., Kennedy, F. E., Currier, J. H., Timmins, G. S., Jackson, S. K. and Brewer, R. L. 2003. Comparison of cross-linked polyethylene materials for orthopaedic applications. *Clin Orthop Relat Res*, 414, 289–304.

Collier, J. P., Mayor, M. B., Lyford, K. A., Hughlock, M. K. and Van Citters, D. W. 2008. How retrieval analysis provides insight into the development of the 30-year knee. *2008 Annual Meeting of the American Academy of Orthopaedic Surgeons, San Francisco, CA*, Poster P154, p. 214.

Conditt, M. A., Ismaily, S. K., Alexander, J. W. and Noble, P. C. 2004a. Backside wear of modular ultra-high molecular weight polyethylene tibial inserts. *J Bone Joint Surg Am*, 86A, 1031–7.

Conditt, M. A., Stein, J. A. and Noble, P. C. 2004b. Factors affecting the severity of backside wear of modular tibial inserts. *J Bone Joint Surg Am*, 86A, 305–11.

Currier, B. H., Currier, J. H., Collier, J. P., Mayor, M. B. and Scott, R. D. 1997. Shelf life and in vivo duration. Impacts on performance of tibial bearings. *Clin Orthop Relat Res*, 342, 111–22.

Currier, B. H., Currier, J. H., Collier, J. P., Mayor, M. B., Lyford, K. A. and Van Citters, D. W. 2007. In vivo oxidation of gamma-barrier sterilized UHMWPE bearings. *J Arthroplasty*, 22, 721–31.

Currier, J. H., Currier, B. H., Rice, P. J., Van Citters, D. W. and Collier, J. P. 2005a. A clinically relevant method for accelerated aging of UHMWPE. *51st Annual Meeting of the Orthopedic Research Society, Washington, DC*, Poster 1665, p.110.

Currier, J. H., Rice, P. J., Lyford, K. A., Van Citters, D. W. and Mayor, M. B. 2005b Clinical damage from post impingement on retrieved PS knee inserts. *51st Annual Meeting of the Orthopedic Research Society, Washington, DC*, Poster 1212, p. 88.

Currier, J. H., Aanderson, D. E. and Van Citters, D. W. 2010a. A proposed mechanism for squeaking of ceramic-on-ceramic hips. *Wear*, 269, 782–789, DOI 10.1016/j.wear.2010.08.006.

Currier, J. H., Van Citters, D. W., Reinitz, S. R., Carlson, E. M., Currier, B. H. and Collier, J. P. 2010b. Ceramic hips: an investigation of the mechanism of squeaking. *2010 Annual Meeting of the American Academy of Orthopaedic Surgeons, New Orleans, LA*, Poster P042, p. 235.

Currier, J. H., Mayor, M. B., Collier, J. P., Currier, B. H. and Van Citters, D. W. 2011. Wear rate in a series of retrieved RP knee bearings. *J ASTM Int*, 8, DOI 10.1520/JAI103166.

D'Antonio, J., Capello, W., Manley, M., Naughton, M. and Sutton, K. 2005. Alumina ceramic bearings for total hip arthroplasty: five-year results of a prospective randomized study. *Clin Orthop Relat Res*, 436, 164–71.

Daly, B. M. and Yin, J. 1998. Subsurface oxidation of polyethylene. *J Biomed Mater Res*, 42, 523–9.

Edidin, A. A., Herr, M. P., Villarraga, M. L., Muth, J., Yau, S. S. and Kurtz, S. M.

2002. Accelerated aging studies of UHMWPE. I. Effect of resin, processing, and radiation environment on resistance to mechanical degradation. *J Biomed Mater Res*, 61, 312–322.

Endo, M., Tipper, J. L., Barton, D. C., Stone, M. H., Ingham, E. and Fisher, J. 2002. Comparison of wear, wear debris and functional biological activity of moderately crosslinked and non-crosslinked polyethylenes in hip prostheses. *Proc Inst Mech Eng H*, 216, 111–22.

Engh, G. A., Dwyer, K. A. and Hanes, C. K. 1992. Polyethylene wear of metal-backed tibial components in total and unicompartmental knee prostheses. *J Bone Joint Surg Br*, 74, 9–17.

Engh, G. A., Lounici, S., Rao, A. R. and Collier, M. B. 2001. In vivo deterioration of tibial baseplate locking mechanisms in contemporary modular total knee components. *J Bone Joint Surg Am*, 83A, 1660–5.

Falbrede, I., Widmer, M., Kurtz, S., Schneidmüller, D., Dudda, M. and Röder, C. 2011. Verwendungsraten von Prothesen der unteren Extremität in Deutschland und der Schweiz. *Der Orthopäde*, 40, 793–801, DOI 10.1007/s00132-011-1787-5.

Fraitzl, C. R., Moya, L. E., Castellani, L., Wright, T. M. and Buly, R. L. 2011. Corrosion at the stem-sleeve interface of a modular titanium alloy femoral component as a reason for impaired disengagement. *J Arthroplasty*, 26, 113–9, S0883-5403(09)00515-4 [pii], DOI 10.1016/j.arth.2009.10.018.

Furmanski, J., Anderson, M., Bal, S., Greenwald, A. S., Halley, D., Penenberg, B., Ries, M. and Pruitt, L. 2009. Clinical fracture of cross-linked UHMWPE acetabular liners. *Biomaterials*, 30, 5572–82, S0142-9612(09)00718-2 [pii], DOI 10.1016/j.biomaterials.2009.07.013.

Gilbert, J. L., Buckley, C. A. and Jacobs, J. J. 1993. In vivo corrosion of modular hip prosthesis components in mixed and similar metal combinations. The effect of crevice, stress, motion, and alloy coupling. *J Biomed Mater Res*, 27, 1533–44, DOI 10.1002/jbm.820271210.

Goldman, M., Lee, M., Gronsky, R. and Pruitt, L. 1997. Oxidation of ultrahigh molecular weight polyethylene characterized by Fourier transform infrared spectrometry. *J Biomed Mater Res*, 37, 43–50.

Green, T. R., Fisher, J., Stone, M., Wroblewski, B. M. and Ingham, E. 1998. Polyethylene particles of a 'critical size' are necessary for the induction of cytokines by macrophages in vitro. *Biomaterials*, 19, 2297–302.

Greer, K. W., Hamilton, J. V., Schmidt, M. B. and Urian, C. 1999. The effects of accelerated shelf aging on the stability of gamma vacuum sterilized UHMWPE. *Trans Soc Biomater*, XXII.

Grupp, T. M., Yue, J. J., Garcia, R., Jr., Basson, J., Schwiesau, J., Fritz, B. and Blomer, W. 2009. Biotribological evaluation of artificial disc arthroplasty devices: influence of loading and kinematic patterns during in vitro wear simulation. *Eur Spine J*, 18, 98–108, DOI 10.1007/s00586-008-0840-5.

Grupp, T. M., Meisel, H. J., Cotton, J. A., Schwiesau, J., Fritz, B., Blomer, W. and Jansson, V. 2010. Alternative bearing materials for intervertebral disc arthroplasty. *Biomaterials*, 31, 523–31, S0142-9612(09)00996-X [pii], DOI 10.1016/j.biomaterials.2009.09.064.

Harris, W. H. 1994. Osteolysis and particle disease in hip replacement. A review. *Acta Orthop Scand*, 65, 113–23.

Hendel, D., Garti, A. and Weisbort, M. 2003. Fracture of the central polyethylene tibial spine in posterior stabilized total knee arthroplasty. *J Arthroplasty*, 18, 672–4, S088354030300192X [pii].

Hirakawa, K., Jacobs, J. J., Urban, R. and Saito, T. 2004. Mechanisms of failure of total hip replacements: lessons learned from retrieval studies. *Clin Orthop*, 420, 10–7.

Hood, R. W., Wright, T. M. and Burstein, A. H. 1983. Retrieval analysis of total knee prostheses: a method and its application to 48 total condylar prostheses. *J Biomed Mater Res*, 17, 829–42.

Huet, R., Sakona, A. and Kurtz, S. M. 2011. Strength and reliability of alumina ceramic femoral heads: Review of design, testing, and retrieval analysis. *J Mech Behav Biomed Mater*, 4, 476–83, S1751-6161(10)00185-2 [pii], DOI 10.1016/j.jmbbm.2010.12.010.

Huot, J. C., Van Citters, D. W., Currier, J. H., Currier, B. H., Mayor, M. B. and Collier, J. P. 2010. Evaluating the suitability of highly cross-linked and remelted materials for use in posterior stabilized knees. *J Biomed Mater Res Appl Biomater*, 95B, 298–307, DOI 10.1002/Jbm.B.31714.

Ingham, E. and Fisher, J. 2005. The role of macrophages in osteolysis of total joint replacement. Biomaterials, 26, 1271–86.

ISO. 2011. *ISO 12891: Retrieval and analysis of surgical implants.* Geneva, ISO.

Jung, K. A., Lee, S. C., Hwang, S. H. and Kim, S. M. 2008. Fracture of a second-generation highly cross-linked UHMWPE tibial post in a posterior-stabilized scorpio knee system. *Orthopedics*, 31, 1137–9, orthopedics.32904 [pii].

Kennedy, F. E., Currier, B. H., Van Citters, D. W., Currier, J. H. and Collier, J. P. 2003. Oxidation of ultra-high molecular weight polyethylene and its influence on contact fatigue and pitting of knee bearings. *Tribology Trans*, 46, 111–8.

Knahr, K., Bohler, M., Frank, P., Plenk, H. and Salzer, M. 1987. Survival analysis of an uncemented ceramic acetabular component in total hip-replacement. *Archi Orthop Trauma Surg*, 106, 297–300.

Kurtz, S., Mowat, F., Ong, K., Chan, N., Lau, E. and Halpern, M. 2005. Prevalence of primary and Revision total hip and knee arthroplasty in the United States from 1990 through 2002. *J Bone Joint Surg Am*, 87, 1487–97.

Kurtz, S., Lau, E., Ong, K., Zhao, K., Kelly, M. and Bozic, K. 2009a. Future young patient demand for primary and revision joint replacement: national projections from 2010 to 2030. *Clin Orthop Relat Res*, 467, 2606–12, DOI 10.1007/s11999-009-0834-6.

Kurtz, S. M., Pruitt, L. A., Crane, D. J. and Edidin, A. A. 1999. Evolution of morphology in UHMWPE following accelerated aging: the effect of heating rates. *J Biomed Mater Res*, 46, 112–20.

Kurtz, S. M., van Ooij, A., Ross, R., de Waal Malefijt, J., Peloza, J., Ciccarelli, L. and Villarraga, M. L. 2007. Polyethylene wear and rim fracture in total disc arthroplasty. *Spine J*, 7, 12–21, S1529-9430(06)00289-0 [pii], DOI 10.1016/j.spinee.2006.05.012.

Kurtz, S. M., Ong, K. L., Schmier, J., Zhao, K., Mowat, F. and Lau, E. 2009b. Primary and revision arthroplasty surgery caseloads in the United States from 1990 to 2004. *J Arthroplasty*, 24, 195–203, DOI 10.1016/j.arth.2007.11.015.

Langohr, G. D. G., Gawel, H. A. and Medley, J. B. 2011. Wear performance of all-polymer PEEK articulations for a cervical total level arthroplasty system. *Proc. IMechE Part J: J Eng Tribol*, 225, 449–513.

Leslie, I. J., Williams, S., Isaac, G., Ingham, E. and Fisher, J. 2009. High cup angle and microseparation increase the wear of hip surface replacements. *Clin Orthop Relat Res*, 467, 2259–65, DOI 10.1007/s11999-009-0830-x.

Lu, S., Orr, J. F. and Buchanan, F. J. 2003. The influence of inert packaging on the shelf ageing of gamma-irradiation sterilised ultra-high molecular weight polyethylene. *Biomaterials*, 24, 139–45.

Lusty, P. J., Watson, A., Tuke, M. A., Walter, W. L., Walter, W. K. and Zicat, B. 2007. Wear and acetabular component orientation in third generation alumina-on-alumina ceramic bearings: an analysis of 33 retrievals [corrected]. *J Bone Joint Surg Br*, 89, 1158–64.

Mayor, M. B., Currier, J. H., Collier, J. P., Shields, W. H. and Atwood, S. A. 2005. Measurement of backside wear in retrieved PFC polyethylene tibial bearings. *Podium Presentation 72nd Annual Meeting of the American Academy of Orthopaedic Surgeons, Washington, DC, February* 23–27, 2005.

McKellop, H., Shen, F. W., DiMaio, W. and Lancaster, J. G. 1999a. Wear of gamma-crosslinked polyethylene acetabular cups against roughened femoral balls. *Clin Orthop Relat Res*, 369, 73–82.

McKellop, H., Shen, F. W., Lu, B., Campbell, P. and Salovey, R. 1999b. Development of an extremely wear-resistant ultra high molecular weight polythylene for total hip replacements. *J Orthop Res*, 17, 157–67.

Medel, F. J., Pena, P., Cegonino, J., Gomez-Barrena, E. and Puertolas, J. A. 2007. Comparative fatigue behavior and toughness of remelted and annealed highly crosslinked polyethylenes. *J Biomed Mater Res B Appl Biomater*, 83, 380–90, DOI 10.1002/jbm.b.30807.

Mesko, J. W., D'Antonio, J., Capello, W. and Naughton, M. 2009. 3rd Generation alumina-alumina total hip arthroplasty: Has it met expectations? *2009 American Academy of Orthopaedic Surgeons Annual Meeting, Las Vegas, NV*, Poster P077, p. 225.

Morrey, B. F. (ed.) 1993. *Biological, Material, and Mechanical Considerations of Joint Replacement*, New York, NY, Raven Press.

Muratoglu, O. K., Ruberti, J., Melotti, S., Spiegelberg, S. H., Greenbaum, E. S. and Harris, W. H. 2003. Optical analysis of surface changes on early retrievals of highly cross-linked and conventional polyethylene tibial inserts. *J Arthroplasty*, 18, 42–7.

Muratoglu, O. K., Bhattacharyya, S., Wannomae, K. K., Freiberg, A. A. and Harris, W. H. 2004. Oxygen concentration in synovial fluid and potential for in vivo oxidation of UHMWPE with residual free radicals. *Transactions of the 50th Annual Meeting of the Orthopedic Research Society, San Francisco, CA*, Poster 1475, p. 95.

Muratoglu, O. K. 2005. Improving the wear resistance of ultra high molecular-weight polyethylene. *Proceedings of the World Tribology Congress*, 2005. *Washington, DC*, p. 54.

Murphy, S. B., Ecker, T. M. and Tannast, M. 2006. Two-to 9-year clinical results of alumina ceramic-on-ceramic THA. *Clin Orthop Relat Res*, 453, 97–102.

Nagy, E. and Li, S. 1990. A Fourier transform infrared technique fo the evaluation of polyethylene orthopaedic bearing materials. *16th Annual Meeting of the Society for Biomaterials, Charleston, SC, Mt Laurel, NJ, Society for Biomaterials*, p. 109.

Nevoralova, M., Baldrian, J., Pospisil, J., Chodak, I. and Horak, Z. 2005. Structure modification of UHMWPE used for total joint replacements. *J Biomed Mater Res B Appl Biomater*, 74B, 800–7.
Noble, P. C., Conditt, M. A., Thompson, M. T., Stein, J. A., Kreuzer, S., Parsley, B. S. and Mathis, K. B. 2003. Extraarticular abrasive wear in cemented and cementless total knee arthroplasty. *Clin Orthop*, 416, 120–8.
Orozco, F. and Hozack, W. J. 2008. Outcomes of posterior stabilized total knee arthroplasty. *Curr Orthop Prac*, 19, 160–4.
Parks, N. L., Engh, G. A., Topoleski, L. D. and Emperado, J. 1998. The Coventry Award. Modular tibial insert micromotion. A concern with contemporary knee implants. *Clin Orthop Relat Res*, 356, 10–5.
Puloski, S. K., McCalden, R. W., MacDonald, S. J., Rorabeck, C. H. and Bourne, R. B. 2001. Tibial post wear in posterior stabilized total knee arthroplasty. An unrecognized source of polyethylene debris. *J Bone Joint Surg Am*, 83A, 390–7.
Rao, A. R., Engh, G. A., Collier, M. B. and Lounici, S. 2002. Tibial interface wear in retrieved total knee components and correlations with modular insert motion. *J Bone Joint Surg Am*, 84A, 1849–55.
Rodrigues, D. C., Urban, R. M., Jacobs, J. J. and Gilbert, J. L. 2009. In vivo severe corrosion and hydrogen embrittlement of retrieved modular body titanium alloy hip-implants. *J Biomed Mater Res B Appl Biomater*, 88, 206–19, DOI 10.1002/jbm.b.31171.
Saleh, K. J., Bear, B., Bostrom, M., Wright, T. and Sculco, T. P. 2008. Initial stability of press-fit acetabular components: an in vitro biomechanical study. *Am J Orthop (Belle Mead NJ)*, 37, 519–22.
Scarlat, M. M. and Matsen, F. A., 3rd 2001. Observations on retrieved polyethylene glenoid components. *J Arthroplasty*, 16, 795–801, S0883-5403(01)81342-5 [pii], DOI 10.1054/arth.2001.23725.
Schmalzried, T. P., Jasty, M., Rosenberg, A. and Harris, W. H. 1994. Polyethylene wear debris and tissue reactions in knee as compared to hip replacement prostheses. *J Appl Biomater*, 5, 185–90.
Scholes, S. C. and Unsworth, A. 2010. The wear performance of PEEK-OPTIMA based self-mating couples. *Wear*, 268, 380–7, DOI 10.1016/j.wear.2009.08.023.
Sharkey, P. F., Hozack, W. J., Rothman, R. H., Shastri, S. and Jacoby, S. M. 2002. Insall Award paper. Why are total knee arthroplasties failing today? *Clin Orthop Relat Res*, 404, 7–13.
Silva, M., Kabbash, C. A., Tiberi, J. V., 3rd, Park, S. H., Reilly, D. T., Mahoney, O. M. and Schmalzried, T. P. 2003. Surface damage on open box posterior-stabilized polyethylene tibial inserts. *Clin Orthop*, 416, 135–44.
Skytta, E. T., Koivu, H., Eskelinen, A., Ikavalko, M., Paavolainen, P. and Remes, V. 2010. Total ankle replacement: a population-based study of 515 cases from the Finnish Arthroplasty Register. *Acta Orthop*, 81, 114–8, DOI 10.3109/17453671003685459.
Sutula, L. C., Collier, J. P., Saum, K., Currier, B. H., Currier, J. H., Sanford, W. M., Mayor, M. B., Wooding, R. E., Sperling, D. K., Williams, I. R., Kasprzak, D. J. and Surprenant, V. A. 1995a. Impact of gamma sterilization on clinical performance of polyethylene in the hip. *Clin Orthop Relat Res*, 319, 28–40.
Sutula, L. C., Collier, J. P., Saum, K. A., Currier, B. H., Currier, J. H., Sanford, W. M., Mayor, M. B., Wooding, R. E., Sperling, D. K. and Williams, I. R. 1995b.

The Otto Aufranc Award. Impact of gamma sterilization on clinical performance of polyethylene in the hip. *Clin Orthop*, 319, 28–40.

Sychterz, C. J., Orishimo, K. F. and Engh, C. A. 2004. Sterilization and polyethylene wear: clinical studies to support laboratory data. *J Bone Joint Surg Am*, 86, 1017–22.

Tower, S., Lyford, K. A., Mayor, M. B., Van Citters, D. W. and Currier, B. H. 2006. Acetabular rim cracking in crosslinked longevity polyethylene. *2006 Annual Meeting of the American Academy of Orthopaedic Surgeons, Chicago, IL*, Paper 323, p. 485.

Van Citters, D. W. 2003. *Fatigue Failure of UHMWPE: The Development and Application of Novel Methods and Devices*. Master of Science Thesis, Dartmouth College, NH.

Vaupel, Z., Baker, E. A., Baker, K. C., Kurdziel, M. D. and Fortin, P. T. 2009. Analysis of retrieved agility total ankle arthroplasty systems. *Foot Ankle Int*, 30, 815–23, 50029028 [pii], DOI 10.3113/FAI.2009.0815.

Walter, W. L., Waters, T. S., Gillies, M., Donohoo, S., Kurtz, S. M., Ranawat, A. S., Hozack, W. J. and Tuke, M. A. 2008. Squeaking hips. *J Bone Joint Surg Am*, 90, Suppl 4, 102–11.

Wasielewski, R. C., Parks, N., Williams, I., Surprenant, H., Collier, J. P. and Engh, G. 1997. Tibial insert undersurface as a contributing source of polyethylene wear debris. *Clin Orthop Relat Res*, 345, 53–9.

Wilkinson, J. M., Wilson, A. G., Stockley, I., Scott, I. R., Macdonald, D. A., Hamer, A. J., Duff, G. W. and Eastell, R. 2003. Variation in the TNF gene promoter and risk of osteolysis after total hip arthroplasty. *J Bone Miner Res*, 18, 1995–2001, DOI 10.1359/jbmr.2003.18.11.1995.

Williams, I. R., Mayor, M. B. and Collier, J. P. 1998. The impact of sterilization method on wear in knee arthroplasty. *Clin Orthop Relat Res*, 356, 170–180.

15
Wear prediction of orthopaedic implants

F. LIU and J. FISHER, University of Leeds, UK and
Z. JIN, University of Leeds, UK and Xi'an Jiaotong
University, People's Republic of China

Abstract: Computational wear modelling is an efficient simulation tool for the wear assessment of artificial joints, which can be developed to investigate wear mechanisms, provide guidance for further experimental tests and optimise implant design. This chapter outlines such a tool, based on current developments in the wear modelling of artificial joints. Wear modelling consists of the development of wear equations, determination of wear factors/coefficients, contact modelling and numerical calculations of wear. In addition to the conventional Archard wear law, which is suitable for metallic/ceramic bearings, a contact-area-dependent new wear law is described for the polyethylene bearings widely used in hip, knee and spinal disc replacements. The wear predictions are illustrated with examples of metal-on-polyethylene and metal-on-metal hip joint replacements. Using such modelling, wear mechanisms can be highlighted and better understood. For example, the effect of bearing geometry design and the long-term wear performance of artificial hip joints demonstrate the efficiency and potential of wear modelling to complement or provide an alternative to experimental simulations.

Key words: artificial joints, computational modelling, wear prediction.

15.1 Introduction

As already discussed in preceding chapters, implant wear can cause adverse tissue reactions that may lead to implant failure. For patients with artificial joints, wear debris generated at the bearing surfaces can induce osteolysis and consequent loosening of the artificial joint fixation. Wear is a major factor that limits the long-term clinical performance of an implant. Implant design should therefore consider not only improvements in biomechanical functions but also long-term wear performance.

Studies of wear performance play a crucial role in implant design.

Historically, the wear simulation of artificial joints has been largely carried out using experimental methods (e.g. using a simple tribometer such as a pin-on-plate tetster for material selection and ranking) or more sophisticated joint simulators for considering both implant materials and design geometry. With advances in modern computing technology, compuational wear modelling has been increasingly developed and used. Wear prediction using computer modelling techniques can be powerful for parametric analyses or providing guidance for further laboratory experimental tests. It is also necessary in situations where experimental measurements are difficult, such as the evaluation of contact stresses at articulating bearing surfaces, or for longer term wear predictions. Computational simulation provides an efficient tool with which to understand wear mechanisms; implant designs can then be optimised to minimise wear and hence improve longevity of the implant. The main purpose of this chapter is to outline such a tool. The focus is on the development of computational wear models for artificial joints, the underlying fundamental mechanisms and practical applications and implementations to help improve implant design through better wear performance.

This chapter is mainly concerned with the computational wear modelling of artificial hip joints. Both metal-on-metal (MoM) and metal-on-polyethylene (MoP) bearings are considered as examples. The methodologies described can be readily extended to other joints such as knee, spinal disc and ankle replacements. The chapter covers the conventional Archard wear law, largely developed for metallic bearing surfaces, and a new wear law specifically for ultra-high molecular weight polyethylene (UHMWPE) bearings. The model formulation deals with surface wear occurring during sliding of articulating bearing surfaces under physiological conditions. This type of wear accounts for the majority of the wear encountered in artificial joint replacements under normal walking conditions.

15.2 Overall wear modelling

Wear is considered to be progressive material loss resulting from the relative motion of articulating bearing surfaces. Many factors are involved in wear generation, including bearing materials, geometries, loading/motion and other environmental variables such as lubrication. Wear modelling can be started with the formulation of a wear model, usually expressed by an empirical equation since direct wear modelling from first principle is still quite challenging. The wear equation is generally derived from wear tests, linking the wear data with some input variables such as material properties and operational conditions of load and motion. The wear process is so complicated that it is difficult to develop a universal wear law or equation that can model all practical situations. For different wear models, a wear parameter is invariably introduced in the wear equation to cover the effect of other factors that are not explicitly expressed. As wear usually occurs within the contact area, a contact model is required in wear modelling. The major wear mechanisms of artificial joints using different biomaterials such as metal, ceramic and polyethylene can be computationally modelled using specific wear models. A typical wear model for artificial joints can be considered to include the following major components, which will be addressed separately in this chapter:

- development of wear models
- determination of wear parameters
- contact modelling
- numerical calculation of wear.

15.3 Wear models

The term wear model can be used in a variety of contexts, for example as a description of a wear process or a representative laboratory wear simulation with a set of specific materials, geometry and operating conditions. Wear is not an intrinsic material property but is closely related to both the material property and environmental conditions such as the surface contact stress, surface roughness and lubrication of the articulating bearing surfaces. In a wear formulation, wear (volumetric or linear) is usually expressed as a function of well-controlled operational conditions such as loads and motion, and a wear factor (dimensional) or a coefficient (dimensionless) is generally incorporated.

The wear model mostly considered for artificial joints is the classical Archard wear law, given by (Archard, 1953):

$$V = KFL \qquad [15.1]$$

where V is the volumetric wear, F is the normal load, L is the sliding distance and K is a dimensional constant known as the wear factor in orthopaedic biotribology (Maxian *et al.*, 1996). This equation is derived from the experimental observation that the wear volume is proportional to the normal load applied and the sliding distance associated with the load, commonly observed for metallic bearing surfaces. Asperities on the metallic bearing surfaces in contact are usually deformed plastically and the real contact area is directly proportional to the load (Archard, 1953); hence the wear is linearly related to the load. The wear factor K, usually quoted in units of $mm^3 \, N^{-1} \, m^{-1}$, represents the wear volume per unit sliding distance per unit normal load, and can be seen as a specific wear rate. This factor is used to reflect the effects of bearing material combinations and other variables such as surface roughness, lubrication, etc. Given a laboratory wear test with specific load and sliding motion and the volumetric wear measured, the wear factor can be calculated using equation 15.1. For wear prediction of artificial joints, selection of the wear factor is vital; it is generally chosen from a representative experimental wear test such as the pin-on-plate wear test (Kang *et al.*, 2008a) or calibrated from a simulator test (Liu *et al.*, 2008). However, it should be noted that the latter approach does not give an independent prediction.

To numerically calculate wear on bearing surfaces, a linear wear depth equation is required. This can be derived by dividing both sides of equation (15.1) by the contact area A in association with the load F:

$$\delta = KpL \qquad [15.2]$$

where δ is the linear wear depth and p is the contact pressure associated with the load F. The volumetric or linear wear equations can be considered locally for each point on the bearing surface. The contact pressure of the points on the bearing surfaces can be determined from a contact model of the articulating bearing surfaces (contact models will be discussed in Section 15.5). The distributed wear depth at each point generates the worn bearing surface, while the overall wear volume can be obtained by integration of the wear depths over the bearing surface. The worn bearing surface geometry needs to be incorporated in the contact model during the progressive wear calculation in order to take into account the effect of the bearing surface geometry change on the contact mechanics.

For UHMWPE bearing surfaces, a new wear law has been developed (Liu *et al.*, 2011) that is based on the hypothesis that the volumetric wear V of the polyethylene bearing surface is explicitly proportional to the real contact area A and the sliding distance L under a certain range of contact pressure. This is given by:

$$V = CAL \qquad [15.3]$$

where C is a dimensionless constant referred to as the wear coefficient. Correspondingly, a wear depth equation can also be derived as:

$$\delta = CL \qquad [15.4]$$

For the polymeric bearing materials used in artificial joints, due to the relatively low elastic modulus of the material, the deformation of the asperity contacts is largely elastic and hence the contact area of the bearing surface is not linearly proportional to the load applied and a weak relationship between volumetric wear and load is expected. This also leads to the conclusion that the real area of contact in these soft-on-hard contacts is similar to the apparent area of contact, which can be determined from the contact models to be discussed in Section 15.5. Use of Archard's law for a polyethylene bearing indicates that the wear factor K is a strong function of nominal contact pressure (Barbour et al., 1997). Use of the new wear law results in the wear coefficient C being largely constant within the pressure range for artificial joint bearings (Liu et al., 2011). Since the contact pressure varies considerably on the worn bearing surface as well as during wear simulation, the use of the wear factor as a function of contact pressure may be difficult to implement and may lead to larger numerical errors. Use of the new wear equation and the wear coefficient can be numerically more accurate and more physically sound.

It has been recognised that, for polyethylene, multi-directional sliding motion causes significantly more wear than uni-directional sliding (Wang, 2001). This is defined as the cross-shear effect of polyethylene and can be explicitly incorporated in the wear coefficient. The wear coefficient is a function of the cross-shear ratio, a parameter used for quantifying the multi-directional motion. The cross-shear ratio can be numerically determined for each point on the bearing surface using the frictional work and the principal molecular orientation of the polyethylene bearing surface; this will be described in detail in Section 15.4.

15.4 Determination of wear factors and coefficients

As already mentioned, wear factors are used in association with the Archard wear equation. For a computational wear formulation of artificial joints, the wear factors are considered to be constant and are selected from a wide range of data from the literature (Goreham-Voss et al., 2010). The wear factor values are adjusted in the computational wear formulation using a trial-and-error approach, by matching the computed volumetric wear with that of either simulator results or clinical measurements. The computational prediction with the wear factor thus obtained is therefore not generic and not independent, but is relevant to the specific set of conditions in a specific application.

For UHMWPE bearings, the major factor that can significantly affect the wear rate is the cross-shear effect resulting from the multi-directional sliding motion of polyethylene surfaces. The cross-shear motion refers to a counterface motion that is transverse to the direction of strain hardening of the polyethylene surface. With a linear tracking motion, molecules of the UHMWPE surface are stretched along the sliding direction, leading to significant strain hardening and increase in wear resistance. With multi-directional motion, surface molecules align preferentially in the principal direction of sliding, resulting in strengthening of wear resistance in this particular direction and weakening in the transverse direction. This weakening is known as orientation softening, which increases surface wear

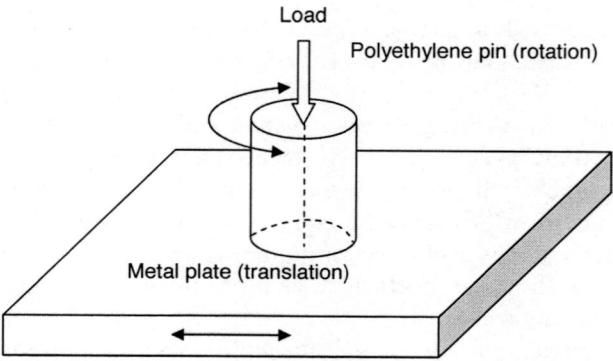

15.1 Schematic pin-on-plate wear test with reciprocal rotation of the polyethylene pin, reciprocal translation of the metal plate and the loading force applied along the symmetrical axis of the pin.

generation (Wang, 2001). The principal direction of sliding is also considered as the principal molecular orientation (PMO) of the polyethylene in the computational wear calculation.

Cross-shear can be quantified using the ratio of frictional work in the direction perpendicular to the PMO to the total frictional work. This is defined as the cross-shear ratio (CSR), given by:

$$\mathrm{CSR} = \sum W_{ti} \Big/ \sum (W_{ti} + W_{pi}) \qquad [15.5]$$

where W_{ti} and W_{pi} are the frictional work components perpendicular to and along the PMO direction respectively. Details of the determination of the PMO and calculation of the CSR can be found in the work of Kang *et al.*, (2008a).

A multi-directional pin-on-plate wear test was used to obtain the wear factors or coefficients for the computational wear model of UHMWPE bearings (Fig. 15.1). In the pin-on-plate wear test, a polyethylene pin with a small bearing surface of a few millimetres in diameter represents a small fraction of the total polyethylene bearing surface. Multi-directional sliding of the polyethylene bearing can be achieved by rotating the polyethylene pin against a translating metal plate under lubricated conditions similarly to simulator testing. Different cross-shear motions can be obtained by combining different rotation angles of the pins and translation lengths of the plates during tests (Kang *et al.*, 2008a). The test is subjected to a practical range of contact pressures likely to be experienced in artificial hip and knee joints. Wear factors or coefficients as a function of the CSR can be determined based on wear data from multi-directional pin-on-plate testing.

For MoM bearings, it is generally accepted that wear is lubrication dependent. Incorporation of lubrication into the wear equation was attempted by Harun *et al.* (2009), but such approaches are still limited. The common approach to wear modelling is largely based on a calibration procedure, i.e. adjusting the wear factor to match the volumetric wear from simulator testing and then extending to a longer term prediction. A similar approach was developed for ceramic-on-ceramic (CoC) bearings by Sari-ali (2009).

15.5 Contact models

Contact mechanics are modelled with finite-element (FE) methods to obtain the contact pressure distribution or contact area on the unworn or worn articulating surfaces throughout the whole formulation process. Using FE methods, complicated geometries and boundary conditions (including implant fixation and support for the bearing components) can be incorporated. A contact model with smooth bearing surfaces without incorporation of surface roughness and under dry contact conditions can be utilised to obtain the contact pressure distribution on bearing surfaces. Such an approach is considered to be valid because the pressure distribution under lubricated contacts is close to that of dry contacts. Also, asperities can be expected to be fully deformed in the case of polyethylene. The smooth surface assumption has a small effect on the overall pressure prediction. Numerically, quasi-static contact analyses can be considered based on discretised time instants over a motion/loading cycle instead of a full transient simulation. The static analyses are able to provide fast convergence for the contact solution without losing accuracy in calculating contact pressure. FE contact modelling is widely available in many commercial FE software packages; with this software, material properties of the bearings (such as the plastic deformation of UHMWPE) can be readily incorporated using true stress–strain data.

15.6 Numerical calculation of wear

To solve equations 15.1–15.4, a continuously varying motion/loading cycle of a joint activity is temporally divided into small time intervals. Spatially, the bearing surface can be discretised into the mesh of a FE contact model. For each point on the bearing surface, variables such as the increment of sliding distance and direction and the contact pressure can be numerically averaged and considered to be constant within each of the discretised time intervals.

The wear depth equations for Archard's wear model and the new wear model for polyethylene can be expressed over one motion cycle, respectively, by:

$$\delta = \sum_{i=1}^{n} Kp_i \Delta L_i \qquad [15.6]$$

and

$$\delta = \sum_{i=1}^{n} C(\text{CSR}) \Delta L_i \qquad [15.7]$$

where δ is the wear depth at a certain point, n is the total number of time intervals discretised over a motion cycle, p_i and s_i denote the instantaneous contact pressure and sliding distance respectively and C is the wear coefficient for the polyethylene bearing as a function of CSR as determined from equation 15.5.

For wear calculation using equations 15.6 and 15.7, FE contact models are required to obtain the values of the contact pressure and the contact area for each point on the bearing surface. The FE contact model can be solved using the quasi-static solution at each of the discretised time instants over a motion cycle. For each point on the bearing surface, a tangential plane to the surface at the point in consideration needs to be determined first; the sliding increment of the distance and direction at that point is then calculated on the tangential plane. The individual tangential plane at each point can be numerically determined by using the coordinates of the point and the transformation of the relative motions of the articulating bearings. Geometry update due to wear is usually only required in the FE contact model at a certain time interval, such as 250,000 motion cycles for a representative hip joint model. Therefore, the linear wear depth is multiplied to obtain the wear for the time interval within the corresponding geometry update. The geometry update is considered for the FE contact model by modifying the coordinates of the FE node points on the bearing surface. The FE mesh is also updated with respect to the modified coordinates. The contact pressure, the PMO direction and the CSR are accordingly calculated after each geometry modification. The calculated linear wear depths can be converted to the volumetric wear for the bearing surface. A flowchart of wear modelling is shown in Fig. 15.2.

15.7 Applications

15.7.1 Metal-on-UHMWPE bearings

The use of the Archard wear equation for UHMWPE hip joints results in the wear factor being a strong function of contact pressure and hence gives a wide range of wear factor values. This has been further complicated by

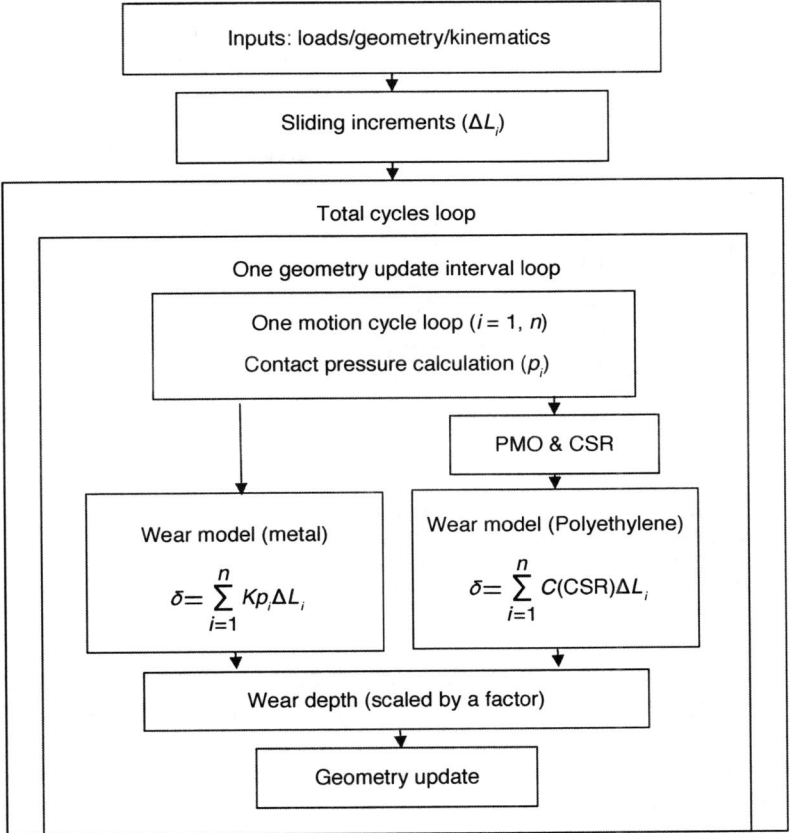

15.2 Wear modelling flowchart.

incorporating the cross-shear effect into the wear factor (Kang *et al.*, 2009), the curve-fitted wear factor K being a function of both the CSR and the contact pressure p as follows:

$$K(\text{CSR}, p) = e^{(-13.1 + 0.19 \ln(\text{CSR}) - 0.29p)} \quad [15.8]$$

Use of the alternative wear equation leads to a relatively constant wear coefficient over the contact pressure range considered for UHMWPE hip joints and hence the wear coefficient C is a function of the CSR only:

$$C = (32.0 + 0.3) \times 10^{-9} \text{ when CSR} < 0.04 \quad [15.9a]$$

$$C = (1.9 + 1.6) \times 10^{-9} \text{ when } 0.04 < \text{CSR} < 0.5 \quad [15.9b]$$

The volumetric wear rates predicted for UHMWPE hip joint bearings with

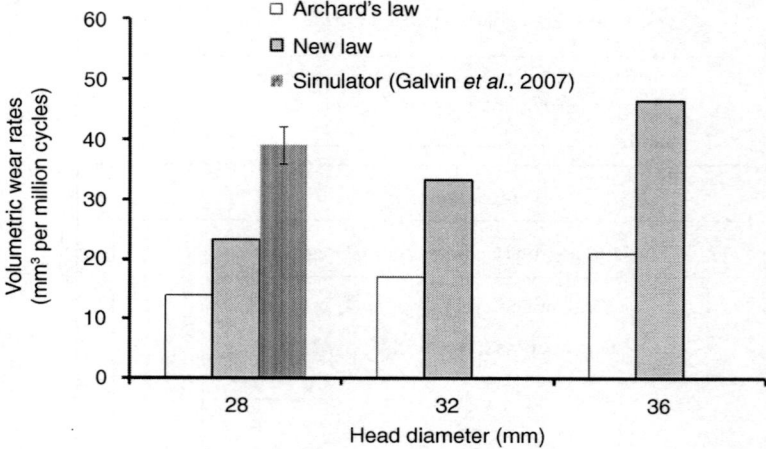

15.3 Comparison of wear rates predicted for UHMWPE hip joint bearings with different femoral head diameters (28–36 mm) using Archard's wear law and the new wear law (under simulated gait conditions used in the simulator) and a typical simulator test (Galvin *et al.*, 2007).

different femoral head sizes using Archard's law, the new wear law and a typical simulator test are compared in Fig. 15.3. The prediction using the new wear law agrees more closely with simulator testing (as shown in Fig. 15.3) and with clinical wear measurements (Livermore *et al.*, 1990). Volumetric wear increases for larger bearings (Fig. 15.4(a)) as a result of both larger sliding distance and contact area associated with larger head sizes. The normalised wear in Fig. 15.4(b) (volumetric wear values in Fig. 15.4(a) divided by femoral head diameter), however, illustrates the difference in wear as a result of contact area only for polyethylene hip joint bearings with different head sizes.

15.7.2 Metal-on-metal bearings

Artificial hip joints consisting of a metallic femoral head articulating against a metallic acetabular cup are used as low-wear bearings and alternatives to conventional UHMWPE bearings (Fisher *et al.*, 2006). One type of MoM bearing is the resurfacing hip joint replacement. This type of bearing is designed for long-term use, particularly for younger, more active and high-demand patients. Simulator wear testing of artificial hip joints is generally carried out for 5–10 million cycles, representing clinical follow-up of 3–5 years. Resurfacing joints are expected to function for up to 50 years, equivalent to 50–100 million cycles. Such long-term use is, however,

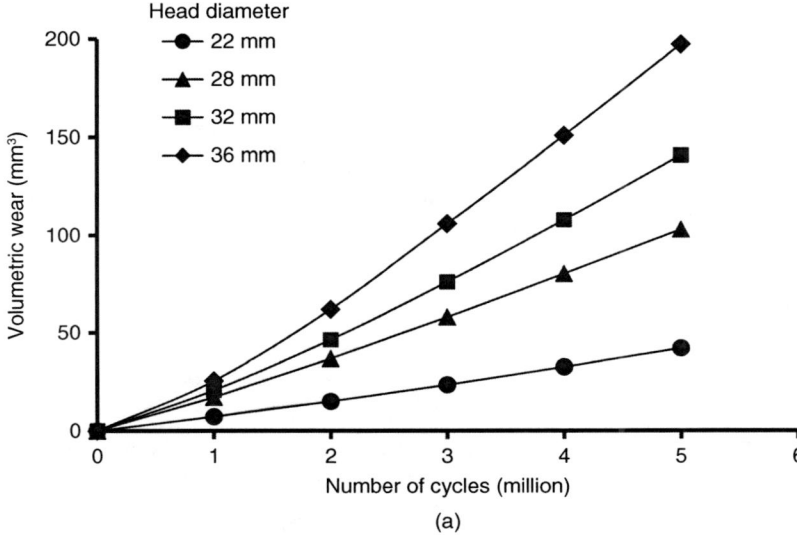

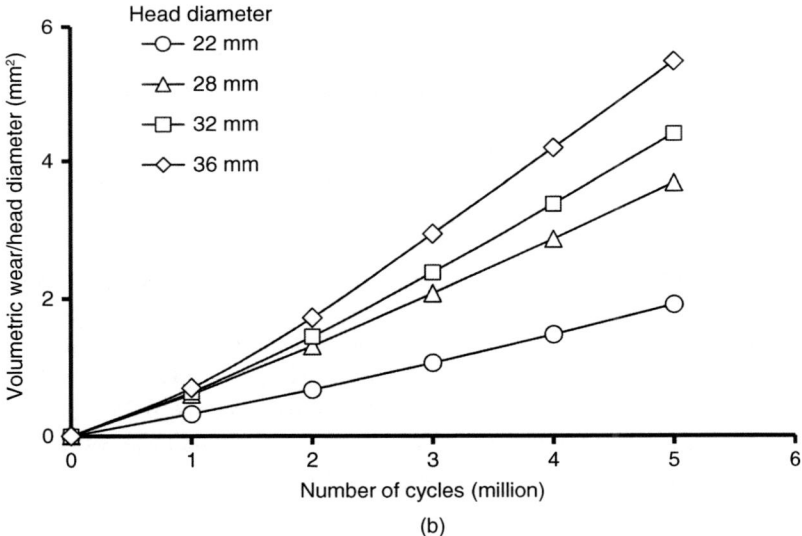

15.4 (a) Comparison of volumetric wear over the simulation cycles computationally predicted for UHMWPE hip joint bearings with different femoral head diameters (22–36 mm) using the new wear law (under simulated gait conditions used in the simulator). (b) Comparison of normalised wear (volumetric wear in Fig. 15.4(a) divided by femoral head diameter) over the simulation cycles for UHMWPE hip joint bearings (under the simulated gait conditions).

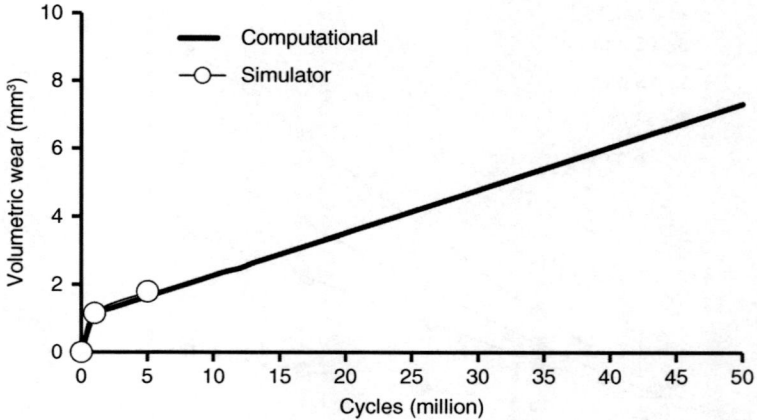

15.5 Computational prediction of volumetric wear for MoM hip resurfacing bearing (head diameter 55 mm) over 50 million cycles (under simulator testing conditions) compared with the simulator testing result of 5 million cycles (Liu *et al.*, 2008).

extremely difficult to simulate experimentally and computational models are more suitable for long-term simulations (Liu *et al.*, 2008).

The wear of the MoM resurfacing bearings has been modelled with Archard's law using different wear factors for running-in and steady-state phases. A FE contact model created using a commercial FE package (ABAQUS version 6.5-1, ABAQUS Inc., Rhode Island, USA) was used to obtain contact pressures on both the cup and head bearing surfaces. Wear factors of 1.13×10^{-8} and 1.20×10^{-9} mm^3 N^{-1} m^{-1} were computationally calibrated to match the simulator volumetric wear results, and these were used for the running-in and steady-state wear phases in the modelling, respectively. The computationally predicted worn areas on the bearing surfaces agreed well with those of simulator testing results at 15 million cycles (Liu *et al.*, 2008). The results of volumetric wear and linear wear depth distributions on the bearings of the simulation extended to 50 million cycles are shown in Figs 15.5 and 15.6, respectively.

15.8 Future trends

Determination of wear factors/coefficients is key to computational wear predictions. Pin-on-plate wear tests are generally adopted, but the test should be designed to incorporate all the major variables inherent in artificial joints. Currently, constant loads are used in the majority of pin-on-plate tests, which may be a limiting factor that leads to the wear rate being underestimated for UHMWPE hip joints (Liu *et al.*, 2011). The role of dynamic loading related to the fatigue wear of polyethylene bearing surfaces

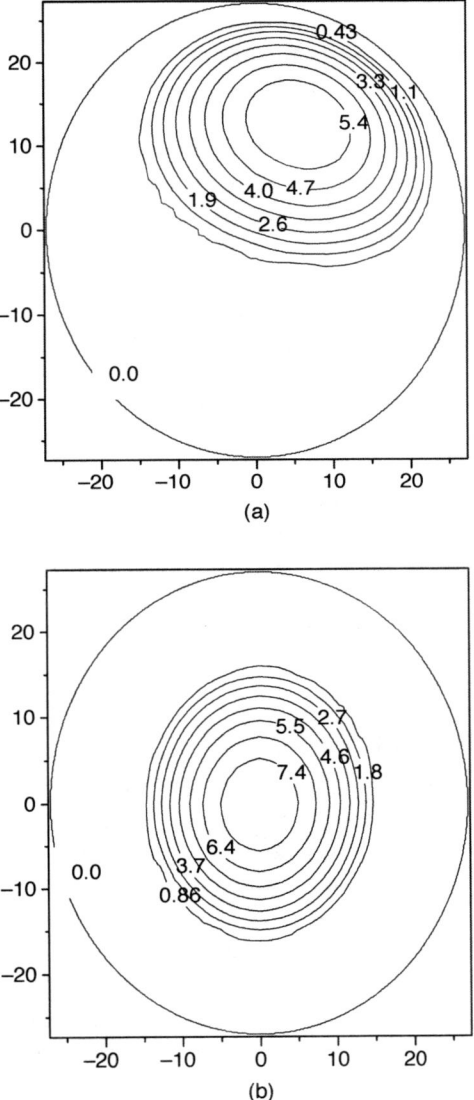

15.6 Corresponding computational predictions of the distributed linear wear depths (μm) on (a) the cup and (b) head bearing surfaces for metal hip resurfacing bearings after 50 million cycles (under simulator testing conditions). The plots show a projection viewed from the centre of the spherical bearing surface to the pole (bearing geometry unit, mm), the maximum linear wear depths being 6.0 and 8.0 μm for the cup and head bearing respectively.

may need further attention in terms of pin-on-plate wear tests. On the other hand, due to large differences in both bearing geometry design and operational conditions of different artificial joints, pin-on-plate wear tests need to be specifically designed to replicate different mechanisms.

Particularly for conventional UHMWPE bearings, other factors that may affect surface deformation and lead to differences in UHMWPE wear predictions should also be considered in future modelling work. For example, the effect of polyethylene creep (known to increase the surface worn area), material properties (e.g. Young's modulus) and heat effects generated during bearing contact may all be important.

The conventional Archard wear equation is generally used as a starting point in modelling the wear of hard-on-hard bearings such as MoM hip joints. An important characteristic of these bearings is lubrication, which can vary between mixed and fluid film regimes. It may be possible to incorporate the lubrication effect into wear modelling via the use of the lambda ratio to characterise lubrication regimes. However, further development of lubrication-dependent wear models is required.

The methodology outlined in this chapter can be extended to other joint designs and material applications. Particular interests may include metal-on-ceramic bearings, polyether ether ketone (PEEK) and cervical spinal disc replacements.

15.9 Further information

For polyethylene artificial bearings, Kang et al. (2008a, 2008b) have reported calculations of the cross-shear and principal molecular orientation for simulation either with a pin-on-plate tester or a full joint simulator. For MoM bearings, Harun et al. (2009) described an approach using the wear factor as a function of a lambda ratio determined to quantify the fluid film lubrication; in this way the effect of lubrication on wear was numerically incorported and analysed. In an attempt to model the wear of CoC total hip joints, Sari-ali (2009) obtained wear factors for ceramic bearings based on experimental simulator wear tests. These data can be used further in the prediction of wear of ceramic total hip joints.

15.10 Acknowledgments

This work was partially funded through WELMEC, a Centre of Excellence in Medical Engineering funded by the Wellcome Trust and EPSRC, under grant number WT 088908/Z/09/Z and additionally supported by the National Institute for Health Research (NIHR) as part of a collaboration with the Leeds Musculoskeletal Biomedical Research Unit (LMBRU). Professor John Fisher is a NIHR senior investigator.

15.11 References

Archard JF (1953) Contact and rubbing of flat surfaces. *J Appl Phys*, 24, 981–8, DOI 10.1063/1.1721448.

Barbour PS, Barton DC and Fisher J (1997) The influence of stress conditions on the wear of UHMWPE for total joint replacements. *J Mater Sci Mater Med*, 8, 603–11, DOI 10.1023/A:1018515318630.

Fisher J, Jin Z, Tipper J, Stone M and Ingham E (2006) Presidential Guest Lecture: Tribology of alternative bearings. *Clin Orthop Relat Res*, 453, 25–34, DOI 10.1097/01.blo.0000238871.07604.49.

Galvin AL, Tipper JL, Jennings LM, Stone MH, Jin ZM, Ingham E and Fisher J (2007) Wear and biological activity of highly crosslinked polyethylene in the hip under low serum protein concentrations. *Proc IMechE H J Eng Med*, 221, 1–10, DOI 10.1243/09544119JEIM99.

Goreham-Voss CM, Hyde PJ, Hall RM, Fisher J and Brown TD (2010) Cross-shear implementation in sliding-distance-coupled finite element analysis of wear in metal-on-polyethylene total joint arthroplasty: Intervertebral total disc replacement as an illustrative application. *J Biomechanics*, 43, 1674–81, DOI 10.1016/j.jbiomech.2010.03.003.

Harun MN, Wang FC, Jin ZM and Fisher J (2009) Long-term contact-coupled wear prediction for metal-on-metal total hip joint replacement. *Proc IMechE J: J Eng Tribol*, 223, 993–1001, DOI 10.1243/13506501JET592.

Kang L, Galvin AL, Brown TD, Jin Z and Fisher J (2008a) Quantification of the effect of cross-shear on the wear of conventional and highly cross-linked UHMWPE. *J Biomechanics*, 41, 340–6, DOI 10.1016/j.jbiomech.2007.09.005.

Kang L, Galvin AL, Brown TD, Fisher J and Jin ZM (2008b) Wear simulation of ultra-high molecular weight polyethylene hip implants by incorporating the effects of cross-shear and contact pressure. *Proc IMechE H J Eng Med*, 222, 1049–64, DOI 10.1243/09544119JEIM431.

Kang L, Galvin AL, Fisher J and Jin Z (2009) Enhanced computational prediction of polyethylene wear in hip joints by incorporating cross-shear and contact pressure in additional to load and sliding distance: Effect of head diameter. *J Biomechanics*, 42, 912–8, DOI 10.1016/j.jbiomech.2009.01.005.

Liu F, Leslie L, Williams S, Fisher J and Jin Z (2008) Development of computational wear simulation of metal-on-metal hip resurfacing replacements. *J Biomechanics*, 41, 686–94, DOI 10.1016/j.jbiomech.2007.09.020.

Liu F, Galvin A, Jin Z and Fisher J (2011) A new formulation for the prediction of polyethylene wear in artificial hip joints. *Proc IMechE H J Eng Med*, 225, 6–24, DOI 10.1243/09544119JEIM819.

Livermore J, Ilstrup D and Morrey B (1990) Effect of femoral head size on wear of the polyethylene acetabular component. *J Bone Joint Surg Am*, 72A, 518–28.

Maxian TA, Brown TD, Pedersen DR and Callaghan JJ (1996) The Frank Stinchfield Award. 3-Dimensional sliding/contact computational simulation of total hip wear. *Clin Orthop Relat Res*, 333, 41–50.

Sari-ali E (2009) *Experimental and Computational Simulation of Micro-separation and its Effect on Ceramic-on-Ceramic Total Hip Prostheses*. PhD Thesis, University of Leeds, UK.

Wang A (2001) A unified theory of wear for ultra-high molecular weight polyethylene in multi-directional sliding. *Wear*, 248, 38–47, DOI 10.1016/S0043-1648(00)00522-6.

Index

α-tocopherol, 226
abduction–adduction rotation, 59–60, 61
abrasive wear, 5–7, 312
  hip implants, 7
  illustration, 6
acetabulum, 95
acquired immunity, 317
adhesive wear, 7–9, 312
  hip implants, 9
  illustration, 7
AISI 316L stainless steel, 188–9
alpha alloys, 135
alternative wear equation, 411
alumina, 137, 197–8, 227, 281–3
  Biolox, Biolox forte, ZTA, and Biolox delta SEM analysis, 282
  Biolox and Biolox forte fluorescence spectra, 283
  first-generation, 281
  orthopaedic ceramic materials characteristics, 281
alumina–zirconia micro-composite, 286
American Rheumatism Association, 353
amorphous diamond, 202
ankylosing spondylitis, 355
anterior cruciate ligament, 118–19
anterior–posterior translation, 61–3
Archard model, 8–9
Archard wear law, 405, 409–10
ArCom XL, 169
arthroplasty, 227
articular capsule, 118
articulations, 320–4
  ceramics, 323–4
  metal-on-metal, 323
  metal-on-polyethylene, 321–3
artificial cartilage, 223

aseptic loosening, 27–8, 33, 34, 35, 37, 42
aseptic lymphocytic vasculitis-associated lesion (ALVAL), 31–2, 35
asperity aspect ratio, 239
asperity shape ratio, 239
ASTM F138, 73
ASTM F561, 379

β-stabilising agents, 249
beta alloys, 135
bioactive ceramics, 204–6
bioactive glasses, 204–6
bioinert material, 318
biologic ingrowth prostheses, 325–6
biological fixation, 155, 157, 315
biologically active particle, 382
Biolox, 281
Biolox delta, 73, 137, 199, 286, 293
Biolox forte, 281
biomimetic coating, 206
biotribocorrosion
  corrosion and wear interactions, 258–60
    biotribocorrosion events sequence, 259
    wear-accelerated corrosion schematic, 260
  measuring corrosion–wear interactions, 260–2
    surface layers removal and regrowth measurement, 261
  orthopaedic implants tribological contacts, 257–8
    contacts types and interfacing materials illustration, 258
  surface phenomena, 257–62
bipolar hemiarthroplasty, 362

Index

bisphosphonates (BPs), 42, 44
bone bonding
  bioactive ceramics and glasses coatings, 204–6
  porous coatings, 194–6
bone cement, 106–7, 146–7, 186
  see also polymethylmethacrylate (PMMA)
bone multicellular units (BMUs), 31
bone resorption, 34
bone tumours, 105
bone–cement interface, 107
bones, 115–20
  knee joint, 119
  left femur, 116
  right tibia, 117
'bowtie' effect, 389

calcium phosphate, 204
calf bone *see* fibula
carbide–metal matrix, 264
cement fixation, 315
cemented acetabular components, 153–4
  total hip arthroplasty with cemented 'all-polyethylene' acetabular cup, 154
cemented femoral components, 158–9
  Exeter stem with distal centraliser, 159
cemented total hip arthroplasty, 106
cementless acetabular components, 154–7
  mechanical and biological fixation, 155
  revision stemmed cup and severe bone loss requires additional fixation, 156
cementless femoral components, 159–65
  curved anatomical stems, 164
  cylindrical stems, 162
  double-wedge femoral stem, 161
  full-modular stems, 163
  non-neck and neck-preserving short femoral stem, 165
  single-wedge femoral stem, 160
  stems with more than one plane taper, 162
cementless total hip arthroplasty, 106, 108
ceramic joints
  ceramic components wear, 288–93
    microseparation phenomenon schematic, 292
    total hip replacements, 289–91
    total knee replacements, 291–3
  ceramic technology developments, 280–8
    alumina, 281–3
    Biolox forte and Biolox delta, 280
    zirconia, 283–5
    zirconia-toughened alumina, 285–7
  wear phenomena, 278–93
ceramic-on-ceramic (CoC), 73, 74, 76, 79, 83, 108, 137
ceramic-on-ceramic coupling, 367, 385–6
ceramic-on-metal (CoM), 73, 74, 138
ceramic-on-polyethylene (CoP), 79
ceramic-on-polyethylene coupling, 367
ceramics, 137–42, 279
  evolution and internal/surface treatment *in vivo*, 196–206
    average physical properties used in hip and knee implants, 198
    bearing surface, 197–9
    bioactive and glasses coatings to improve bone bonding, 204–6
    coatings to improve wear resistance, 199–204
  hip arthroplasty, 138–40
  knee arthroplasty, 140–2
    first-generation ceramic components, 140
    Multigen Plus TKR symmetric femoral component made with Biolox Delta ceramic, 141
    second-generation femoral ceramic components, 141
  oxidised zirconium femoral head component, 139
  zirconia, ZTA and femoral head components, 138
CeramTec, 293
cerivastatin, 45
chemical analysis, 393
chemical solution deposition *see* sol-gel
chemical vapour deposition (CVD), 199
chromium oxide, 254
cobalt alloys, 190
cobalt-based alloys, 36
cobalt–chromium alloy, 134, 187
CoCrMo alloys, 247
commercially pure titanium (CPTi), 189
computational simulation, 404
computer-aided design (CAD) software, 239
computer navigation, 328

computer tomography (CT), 365
constrained condylar knee, 127–8
constraint condylar prostheses, 369
contact conditions
  hip and knee implant lubrication, 71–80
    hip prostheses, 73–6
    knee prostheses, 77–80
    mechanical properties of orthopaedic prosthesis materials, 72
coordinate measuring machines (CMMs), 20
Corail *see* titanium alloy stem
corrosion, 249–53
corrosive wear, 11–12, 312
corundum, 281
crevice corrosion, 256
cross-shear motion, 407
cross-shear ratio, 408
cruciate-retaining prostheses, 127, 148
curved anatomic stems, 163
  illustration, 164
cutting, 6
cyclic loading, 267

3D Knee, 150
debris analysis techniques, 384
delamination, 16–17, 222, 231–6
  orthopaedic implants, 17
  UHMWPE tibial insert delamination schematic, 235
  UHMWPE tibial insert surface changes, 233
  UHMWPE tibial insert worn surface, 234
delayed type hypersensitivity *see* Type IV hypersensitivity
densitometry, 393
depassivation rate, 259
destructive testing, 392
developmental coxa vara, 360
developmental dysplasia of hip (DDH), 357–8
diagnosis
  importance, 351–64
    acute fractures proximal humeral arthroplasty, 362
    fracture radiographs in different angles, 363
    fractures, 360–2
    inflammatory arthritis, 353–6
    osteoarthritis, 356–8

    osteonecrosis, 360
    osteonecrosis causes, 361
    revision reasons, 363–4
    slipped capital femoral epiphysis, 359–60
  orthopaedic implants, 351–72
    patient education, 369–70
    predictive and detection methods, 364–6
diamond, 200
diamond-like carbon film, 321
Diamond Rota Gliding knee, 203
differential scanning calorimetry, 393
diffusion bonding, 195
digital imaging, 391
DLC coating, 199, 200–1, 203
DLC-PDMS-h, 203–4
DLC polymer hybrid (DLC-p-h), 203
DLC-PTFE-h, 203–4
double-wedge femoral stem, 160
  illustration, 161
doxycycline (DOX), 46
durometer testing, 394
dynamic mechanical analysis, 393

E-Poly, 169
elasto-plastic contact analysis, 236
elasto-plastic material model, 237
elastohydrodynamic lubrication (EHL), 57, 72–3, 74, 75, 77–8
electrochemical impedance spectroscopy, 262
electrochemical testing, 260
electron beam deposition, 196
electrophoretic deposition, 205–6
endothelial cells, 38
Epoch hip stem system, 185
erosive wear, 9–10, 312
  hip implants, 10
  illustration, 10
erythromycin (EM), 46
etanecerp, 45
ethylene oxide (EtO), 180–1
external collateral ligament, 118

failure, 313, 315–17
failure analysis
  failure modes, 379–90
    osteolysis, 382–4
    other joints, 390
    total hip arthroplasty failure, 384–7
    total knee arthroplasty failure, 387–9

techniques, 391–4
  chemical analysis, 393
  damaged platform knee bearing, 392
  mechanical testing, 393–4
  surface characterisation, 391–3
failure modes, 379–90
  orthopaedic retrievals from device failures, 380
  osteolysis, 382–4
    bone stock loss photo, 383
  other joints, 390
  polyethylene oxidation profile, 381
  total hip arthroplasty failure, 384–7
    devices from mechanical loading tests, 385
    metal transfer and stripe wear, 386
  total knee arthroplasty failure, 387–9
    backside wear from abrasive motion, 388
    femoral component impingement, 389
  white bands in knee, hip and bearings, 381
fatigue wear, 12–13, 312
  hip implants, 14
  illustration, 13
femoral anteversion, 302
femoral condyles, 115–16
femoral lateralisation, 300
femoral stem, 257
femur, 95, 115
fibroblasts, 38
fibula, 118
fibular collateral ligament see external collateral ligament
filtered pulsed arc discharge (FPAD), 203
finite-element analysis, 304
finite-element method, 409
finite-element model, 236, 409
fixation method, 324–6
  biologic ingrowth prostheses, 325–6
  cement, 324–5
flash temperature, 8
flexion balance, 305
flexion–extension rotation, 59–60, 61, 62–3
Food and Drug Administration (FDA), 289
four-part fractures, 362
Fourier transform infrared spectroscopy, 393

fovea capitis, 95
fracture dislocation, 362
fractures, 360–2
  femur cervical fracture and hybrid total hip arthroplasty, 361
  fractures radiographs in different angles, 362
fragmentation, 6
free radicals, 380
fretting corrosion, 11–12, 267–72
  cemented and uncemented interface stem fixation, 270–2
  cemented implants, 270–2
  retrieved femoral stem SEM images, 271
  uncemented implants, 270
  modular implants neck–head junction, 268–70
    alloy surface alterations, 269
fretting wear, 13–15
  hip implants, 15
  illustration, 14
frustrated phagocytosis, 313
fully conforming MB, 151

gait analysis, 58
gait cycle, 59, 63
galling, 8
galvanic corrosion, 256–7
gel permeation chromatography, 393
gene therapy, 47
genu recurvatum, 120
geometry update, 410
ginglymus, 118
granulation tissue, 31
guided motion, 149

hard-on-hard bearing surfaces, 108
hard-on-hard hip prostheses, 223
hardness testing see durometer testing
Harris–Galante acetabular components, 303
head-splitting fractures, 362
heat pressing, 327
high-density polyethylene (HDPE), 180
high-purity alumina, 281
highly cross-linked polyethylene, 180–3, 321–2
hinge joint see ginglymus
hip abduction, 98–9
  illustration, 99
hip adduction, 99
  illustration, 100

hip and knee implants
  future trends, 86
  implications, 80–6
  joint biomechanics, 56–86
  kinematics, 57–64
  kinetics and joint force, 64–71
  lubrication and contact conditions, 71–80
  materials, 178–206
    ceramic evolution and internal/surface treatment *in vivo*, 196–206
    metal evolution and internal/surface treatment *in vivo*, 187–96
    polymer evolution and internal/surface treatment, 179–86
hip and knee joints
  implant wear, 56–86
    future trends, 86
    implications, 80–6
    kinematics, 57–64
    kinetics and joint force, 64–71
    lubrication and contact conditions, 71–80
hip arthroplasty, 299–303
  materials, 134–47
    cement, 146–7
    ceramics, 137–42
    metals and alloys, 134–7
    polyethylene, 142–3
    trabecular metal technology (TMT)/non-TMT, 143–6
hip extension, 98
  illustration, 99
hip external rotation, 99–101
  illustration, 101
hip flexion, 98
hip internal rotation, 99–101
  illustration, 100
hip joint, 93–110
  anatomy, 93–8
    biomechanics, 101–4
    coxal bone, 94
    femur, 96
    future trends, 109–110
    hip joint, 97
    kinematics, 98–101
    pelvis, 94
hip pain, 105
hip prostheses, 73–6, 80–4
  designs and bearing surface, 105–9
  components of a standard total hip arthroplasty, 106
  future trends, 109–10
  resurfacing prosthesis, 110
  hip joint anatomy, 93–110
  minimum, centre and average thickness of lubricant film, 75
  predicted variation of maximum contact pressure in MoP, 82
  total hip replacement history and indication, 104–5
Holm, R., 4
Hood scoring technique, 386
hybrid fixation, 329
hydrogenated tetrahedral amorphous carbon (ta-C:H), 202
hydroxyapatite, 184–5, 204–5, 325
hydroxyapatite-tricalcium phosphate, 325
Hylamer, 321

idiopathic osteoarthritis *see* primary osteoarthritis
ilium, 95
implant sizing, 330
implant wear
  surgical techniques influence, 298–305
    hip arthroplasty, 299–303
    knee arthroplasty, 303–5
impression fractures, 362
in vitro measurements, 19–21
in vivo measurements, 18–19
inert oxide ceramics, 197
infiltrative therapy, 364
inflammasome, 30
inflammatory arthritis, 353–6
  juvenile rheumatoid arthritis, 354
  Reiter's syndrome, 355
  rheumatoid arthritis, 354
  seronegative spondyloarthropathies, 354–5
  systemic lupus erythematosus, 355–6
inflammatory reaction
  particulate materials, 28–32
    particle characteristics, 28, 30
    tissue response, 30–2
innate immunity, 316–17
Insall–Burstein Modular, 149
Insall–Burstein prosthesis, 149
insert-to-tray locking mechanism, 387
Interax Integrated Secure Asymmetric prosthesis, 151
intercondyloid fossa, 97
internal collateral ligament, 118

Index

internal–external rotation, 59–60, 61, 62–3
ion beam assisted deposition (IBAD), 199
ion beam mixing, 205
ion beam sputter deposition (IBSD), 199
ion implantation, 192, 205
ischium, 95
ISO 14242-1: 2002, 19, 75, 83
ISO 14242-2: 2000, 19, 20
ISO 14243-1: 2009, 19
ISO 14243-2: 2009, 19
ISO 14243-3: 2004, 61, 69–70
isostatic pressing, 321

joint biomechanics
  hip, 101–4
    anteversion angle, 104
    illustration, 102
    inclination angle, 103
  implant wear, 56–86
    future trends, 86
    hip and knee joints kinematics, 57–64
    hip and knee lubrication and contact conditions, 71–80
    implications, 80–6
    kinetics and joint force, 64–71
  knee, 123–4
    anatomical and the mechanical axis, 124
    patella function to improve extensor lever arm, 125
joint force, 64–71
  hip, 67–8
    joint contact force components and resultant, 67
    peak force as multiple of body weight for variety of daily activities, 68
  knee, 68–71
    joint contact force, 69
    peak force as multiple of body weight for variety of daily activities, 70
  model for musculoskeletal analysis of lower limb loads, 66
joint kinematics, 57–64
  hip, 59–61, 98–101
    paths traced on acetabular cup, 62
    rotations during normal gait, 60
    typical rotations during normal walking, running and stair climbing, 61
  human walking cycle, 59
  knee, 61–4, 120–3
    amount of knee rotation, 122
    range of knee extension and flexion, 121
    typical motions of contact paths on medial and lateral condyles, 65
    typical rotations during normal walking, running and stair climbing, 64
    typical rotations during walking cycle, 63
joint kinetics, 64–71
  model for musculoskeletal analysis of lower limb loads, 66
joint replacement surgery, 378
joint simulator tests, 290
juvenile rheumatoid arthritis, 354

kinetic barriers, 250
knee arthroplasty, 303–5
  materials, 134–47
    cement, 146–7
    ceramics, 137–42
    metals and alloys, 134–7
    polyethylene, 142–3
    trabecular metal technology (TMT)/non-TMT, 143–6
knee extension, 120, 121, 122
knee flexion, 120, 121–2
knee flexors, 122–3
knee internal rotation, 121
knee joint
  anatomy, 115–29
  biomechanics, 123–4
  bones and ligaments, 115–20
  future trends, 129
  kinematics, 120–3
knee prostheses, 77–80, 84–6, 115–29
  design and bearing surfaces, 126–9
  components of a standard total knee arthroplasty, 126
  unicompartmental knee arthroplasty, 128
  future trends, 129
  loads and velocity used in elastohydrodynamic analysis of MoP, 77
  total knee replacement history and indications, 124–6

transient plots of minimum thickness of synovial lubricant film, 78

lateral collateral ligament *see* external collateral ligament
lattice system, 201
Legg–Calvé–Perthes disease, 360
ligamentous balancing, 304–5
ligamentous contraction, 332
ligamentous laxity, 332
ligaments, 115–20
  tendons around the knee, 120
ligamentum teres, 95, 97
linea aspera, 95
linear low density polyethylene (LLDPE), 180
lip failure, 182
longevity, 182
Low Contact Stress knee system, 150
low-density polyethylene (LDPE), 180
lubricants, 313
lubrication
  hip and knee implant contact conditions, 71–80
  hip prostheses, 73–6
  knee prostheses, 77–80
  mechanical properties of orthopaedic prothesis materials, 72
lymphocyte transformation test (LTT), 37
lymphocytes, 35–7

machine milling, 327
macroscopic contact analysis, 236–42
  PFC type UHMWPE knee joint FEM, 236
  PFC type UHMWPE tibial insert contour plots, 238
magnesia partially stabilised zirconia (Mg-PSZ), 284
magnetic resonance imaging (MRI), 365
Marathon®, 182
mass spectrometry, 393
maximum plastic strain, 232
McKee Farrar prostheses, 386
mean prosthetic offset, 301
mechanical testing, 393–4
medial collateral ligament *see* internal collateral ligament
Medial Pivot knee, 149–50
medialisation, 299
Medially Based Kinematics knee, 151

medical device reports, 378
menisci, 120
metal, 327
  evolution and internal/surface treatment *in vivo*, 187–96
    average physical properties used in hip and knee implants, 187
    cobalt alloys, 190
    material treatment to improve mechanical properties, 192–4
    porous coatings to improve bone bonding, 194–6
    stainless steel, 188–9
    titanium alloys, 189–90
metal joints
  articulating interface tribocorrosion, 262–6
    metal-on-metal implants, 264–6
    metal-on-polyethylene implants, 263–4
  biotribocorrosion surface phenomena, 257–62
    interactions between corrosion and wear, 258–60
    measuring corrosion–wear interactions, 260–2
    orthopaedic implants tribological contacts, 257–8
  electrochemical aspects of corrosion, 249–53
    human blood serum composition, 252
    human body corrosive environment, 251–3
    metal oxidation, 249–51
    physiological solutions composition, 252
    polarisation curve schematic, 251
  fretting corrosion, 267–72
    cemented and uncemented interface stem fixation, 270–2
    modular implants neck–head junction, 268–70
  implant alloys passivity and corrosion, 253–7
    biomolecules interaction, 255
    ion release, 255–6
    orthopaedic implants corrosion mechanisms, 256–7
    passive layers, 253–4
  orthopaedic implants alloys, 246–9
    chemical composition, 247–8
    common alloys composition, 247

joint replacement materials
    properties, 248
    mechanical properties, 248–9
    wear phenomena, 246–272
metal-on-metal bearings, 412–14
    linear wear depth computational
        prediction, 415
    volumetric wear computational
        prediction, 414
metal-on-metal coupling, 367, 386
metal-on-metal (MoM), 35, 42, 73,
    74–6, 77, 82–3, 167
metal-on-polyethylene (MoP), 80, 81,
    84, 108
metal-on-UHMWPE bearings, 410–12
    volumetric and normalised wear vs
        simulation cycles, 413
    wear rates predictions, 412
metal particle, 28, 30
2-methacryloyloxyethyl
    phosphorylcholine (MPC), 226
micro-focus X-ray CT apparatus, 230
micromotion, 388
microscopic contact analysis, 239–42
    contact analysis 3D FEM, 240
    UHMWPE contour plots, 241
Miller–Galante total knee, 148, 228
minimally invasive procedures, 328–9
mobile-bearing knee designs, 323
mobile-bearing knee prosthesis, 368
mobile bearing knees, 150–1
modular implants, 319
monocytes/macrophages, 33–5
Morich particles, 263
Morse cone, 268
mould arthroplasty, 320
multi-axial joint kinematics, 242
multi-directional wear test, 225
multi-variate analysis, 303

nanocrystalline microstructure, 266
nitriding, 192–3
nitrogen ion implantation, 321
non-neck-preserving stems, 164
    illustration, 165
non-steroidal anti-inflammatory drugs
    (NSAIDs), 42
Norwegian Arthroplasty Register,
    353–4, 358
nuclear factor κB ligand *see* RANKL

obturator foramen, 95
OP-1, 47

Optetrak Posterior-Stabilized knee, 149
optimisation, 66
orientation softening, 407
orthopaedic implant, 377–95
    corrosion mechanisms, 256–7
        crevice corrosion, 256
        other mechanisms, 256–7
        pitting corrosion, 256
    diagnosis and surveillance, 351–72
        importance of correct diagnosis,
            351–64
        joint disorders for arthroplasty, 353
        patient education, 369–70
        predictive and detection methods,
            364–6
        surveillance, 370–2
    factors contributing to wear, 310–34
    failure, 313, 315–17
    failure analysis, 377–95
        failure modes, 379–90
        failure techniques, 391–4
        validation importance, 394
    interactions between different factors,
        333–4
    materials and design, 133–70, 318–27
        articulations, 320–4
        considerations, 320–6
        existing hip and knee joint
            arthroplasty registers, 170
        fixation method, 324–6
        future trends, 168–9
        general design considerations,
            319–20
        general material considerations,
            318–19
        knee and hip arthroplasty, 134–47
        manufacturing factors, 326–7
        material and design considerations,
            320–6
        structure, 320
        total hip arthroplasty history,
            151–68
        total knee arthroplasty evolution,
            147–51
    patient factors, 330–3
        age, 333
        anatomy, 332
        body mass index, 331
        bone quality, 333
        gender, 333
        preoperative diagnosis, deformity
            and general health, 332–3
        use, 331–2

prothesis choices, 366–9
　hip prostheses, 366–8
　knee prostheses, 368–9
retrieval laboratories, 378–9
surgical factors, 327–30
　bone resection and component position, 328–9
　implant fixation, 329
　other factors, 330
　surgical decision making, 330
wear, 3–22, 311–13
　future trends, 22
　history, 3–5
　in vitro measurements, 19–21
　in vivo measurements, 18–19
　mechanisms, 5–17
　mechanisms importance and evaluation, 17–18
　socio-economic impact, 21
　types, 314–15
wear biology, 27–48
　cellular/molecular response, 32–40
　inflammatory reaction to particulate materials, 28–32
　osteolytic areas along the stem of a Co–Cr hip prosthesis, 29
　therapeutic targets, 40–8
wear prediction, 403–16
　applications, 410–14
　contact models, 409
　future trends, 414–16
　numerical calculation of wear, 409–10
　overall wear modelling, 404–5
　wear factors and coefficients determination, 407–9
　wear models, 405–7
osteoarthritis, 356–8
　moderate deformity and degenerative arthritis radiograph, 358
　paediatric disease sequelae, 357–8
　pelvis and THA radiographs, 356
　THA, TKA and valgus deformation X-ray image, 359
osteoblasts/osteocytes, 38–9
osteoclasts, 39–40
　role of the RANK/RANKL/OPG system in wear particle-induced osteolysis, 41
osteolysis, 30–1, 42, 303
osteonecrosis, 105, 126, 360
osteophytes, 357

osteoprotegerin (OPG), 34, 38, 39, 45, 47
oxidation–reduction reaction, 249
oxidised zirconium, 137–8
OXINIUM, 73
oxynitriding, 193

pamidronate, 44
parathyroid hormone (PTH), 47–8
partially conforming MB, 150–1
particulate materials
　inflammatory reaction, 28–32
　　particle characteristics, 28, 30
　　tissue response, 30–2
passive layers, 253–4
　metals and alloys layers illustration, 254
　potentiodynamic polarisation curves, 253
patella, 118, 123
patello-femoral joint, 118
pathogen-associated molecular patterns (PAMPs), 37
PEEK–HA composites, 184
peripheral blood mononuclear cells (PBMCs), 37
periprosthetic biopsy, 366
periprosthetic infection, 317
periprosthetic osteolysis, 27–8
phagocytic response, 316–17
photo-induced polymerisation technique, 226
physical vapour deposition (PVD), 199
physiolysis, 359
pin-on-plate wear test, 406, 408
pitting, 240
pitting corrosion, 11, 256
plasma electrolytic oxidation, 192
plasma spraying, 195–6
plastic deformation, 7–8
Plexiglas, 185
plowing, 6
polished stem, 272
polyaromatic polymers, 184
poly(aryl-ether-ether-ketone) (PEEK), 179, 184–5
polycarbonate tumbling, 322
polycrystalline diamond compact surface, 321
polyethylene, 142–3, 326–7, 382
　creep, 416
　cross-linking, 225
　wear, 299

polymer
 evolution and internal/surface treatment, 179–86
  average physical properties used in hip and knee implants, 179
  poly(aryl-ether-ether-ketone) (PEEK), 184–5
  poly(methylmethacrylate) (PMMA), 185–6
  UHMWPE and highly cross-linked polyethylene, 180–3
polymeric brush treatment, 226
polymethylmethacrylate (PMMA), 106–7, 146, 147, 185–6, 312, 315, 324
polytetrafluoroethylene (PTFE) cups, 222
porous-coated anatomical knee, 148
porous coatings, 194–6
post-marketing surveillance, 370
posterior cruciate ligament, 119
posterior-cruciate-retaining prosthesis, 304
posterior-cruciate-substituting prosthesis, 304
posterior-stabilised knee bearings, 389
posterior-stabilized MB, 151
posterior-stabilized prostheses, 127
Press-Fit Condylar type total knee system, 228, 322
press-fit mechanism, 368
primary osteoarthritis, 105, 126, 356
prosthetic infection, 364
proximal humeral arthroplasty, 362
pseudotumour, 317
pubis, 95

quasi-static contact analysis, 409

radiation sterilisation, 181, 380
radiostereometric analysis (RSA), 19, 365
Raman spectroscopy, 287
RANK/RANKL/OPG, 34, 39, 40, 42
RANKL, 34, 38–9, 39–40
reduction, 66
Register of Orthopaedic Prosthetic Implants (RIPO), 371
registers, 370
Reiter's syndrome, 355
resurfacing hip prostheses, 165–8
 failure modes of resurfacing arthroplastics, 168
 Paltrinieri–Trentani, 166

resurfacing prosthesis, 366
retrieved artificial knee joints, 227–31
 M–G I type knee joint components, 228
 PFC type knee joint components, 228
 PFC type UHMWPE tibial insert X-ray CT image, 231
 UHMWPE tibial inserts micrographs, 229
revision, 372
revision surgery, 352, 378
rheumatoid arthritis, 105
rim cracking, 182
ring-on-disk tests, 284
Ring prostheses, 386
Rotaglide Total Knee System, 151

S-ROM super cup, 156
secondary osteoarthritis, 105, 126, 356
selective cyclo-oxygenase inhibitors, 42
Self Aligning MB, 150
septic arthritis, 105, 360
serial radiographs, 364
seronegative spondyloarthropathies, 354–5
shoulder arthroplasty, 390
silicon nitride, 138
single-wedge femoral stem illustration, 160
sintering, 195
SL Plus, 194
slipped capital femoral epiphysis, 359–60
small punch testing, 394
smoking, 332–3
soft-tissue balance, 328
sol-gel, 205
squeaking phenomenon, 384, 386
stainless steel, 135, 247
316L stainless steel, 255
stem–cement interface, 107, 270–1
stents, 246
stick–slip phenomenon, 386
stress corrosion, 12
stress shielding, 316
Stribeck analysis, 223
'stripe' wear, 291
surface characterisation, 391–3
surgical techniques
 hip arthroplasty, 299–303
  acetabular side, 299–300
  femoral side, 300–3
 influence on implant wear, 298–305

knee arthroplasty, 303–5
surveillance
   orthopaedic implants, 351–72
      patient education, 369–70
      predictive and detection methods, 364–6
      prosthesis choices, 366–9
Swedish Arthroplasty Registers, 371
synovial fluid, 98, 313
systemic lupus erythematosus, 355–6

TACK MB, 150–1
tantalum, 144, 325–6, 368
Teflon, 321
tensile testing, 394
thermal spraying, 195
third-generation alumina, 281
three-body abrasion, 263
three-body wear, 311–12
three-part fractures, 362
Ti-based alloys, 247
tibia, 116–17
tibial collateral ligament *see* internal collateral ligament
TiN coating, 199–200
titanium, 135–7
   names and properties of prosthetic biomaterials, 136
titanium alloy, 135–7, 187, 189–90
   names and properties of prosthetic biomaterials, 136
titanium alloy stem, 194
titanium-based alloys, 36
total ankle arthroplasty, 390
total condylar prosthesis, 148–9
total disc arthroplasty, 390
total hip arthroplasty, 28, 31, 151–68, 178–9, 183, 300, 362
   acetabular components, 153–7
   femoral components, 157–65
   resection – reconstruction of hip joint, 152
   resurfacing hip prostheses, 165–8
total hip replacement, 30, 36, 104–5, 278, 289–3, 302
   retrieved alumina hip stripe wear, 291
   volumetric wear data, 290
total joint arthroplasty, 377
total joint replacement, 310, 351–2
total knee arthroplasty (TKA), 35, 147–51, 183, 291, 293
   anatomical approach, 147–8

modern cruciate-retaining knee prosthesis, 149
   functional design, 148–50
   mobile bearing (MB) knees, 150–1
total knee replacement, 124–6
Total Rotating Knee (TRK), 151
Trabecular Metal™, 196
trabecular metal technology (TMT), 143–6
   acetabular polyethylene component, 145
   TM modular augments, 145
transfer film, 312
triaxial electrogoniometers, 58
tribocorrosion
   articulating interface, 262–6
      typical surface, friction and wear parameters of implants articulation, 262
   metal-on-metal implants, 264–6
      tribochemical reaction layer photos, 265
   metal-on-polyethylene implants, 263–4
tricalciumphosphate (TCP), 204–5
two-body wear, 311
Two Radii Area Contact (TRAC), 151
Type IV hypersensitivity, 317

ultra-high molecular weight polyethylene (UHMWPE), 17, 20, 31, 35, 42, 57, 73, 74, 77, 80, 85, 134, 137, 139, 140, 179, 180–3, 298, 387
ultra-high molecular weight polyethylene (UHMWPE) joints
   knee joints wear phenomena, 227–42
      delamination mechanism study, 231–6
      femoral component and tibial insert analysis, 236–9
      retrieved joints wear characteristics, 227–31
      surface asperities and tibial insert analysis, 239–42
   UHMWPE-on-hard lubrication modes in artificial joints, 223–5
      knee prostheses fluid film formation evaluation, 224
   wear phenomena, 221–42
   wear reduction methods improvement, 225–7
      articulation mating material improvement, 227

MPC grafting treatment wear
  properties improvement, 227
 polyethylene cross-linking, 225
 polymeric brush treatment, 226
 vitamin E addition, 226
ultrasonographic screening, 358
uncemented prosthesis, 315
uni-variate analysis, 303
unicompartmental knee, 368
unicompartmental knee replacement, 128–9

valgus angle, 103
validation importance, 394
Variall, 194
varus angle, 103
Versys *see* Epoch hip stem system
vibration, 14
vitamin E, 226, 326
volumetric wear, 18

wear, 311–13
 cellular/molecular response, 32–40
  endothelial cells, 38
  fibroblasts, 38
  lymphocytes, 35–7
  monocytes/macrophages, 33–5
  osteoblasts/osteocytes, 38–9
  osteoclasts, 39–40
 future trends, 22, 86
 hip and knee implant lubrication and contact conditions, 71–80
 hip and knee joint kinematics, 57–64
 history, 3–5
 implications, 80–6
  hip prostheses, 80–4
  knee prostheses, 84–6
 in vitro measurements, 19–21
 in vivo measurements, 18–19
 inflammatory reaction to particulate materials, 28–32
 joint biomechanics, 56–86
 kinetics and joint force, 64–71
 mechanisms, 5–17
  abrasive, 5–7
  adhesive, 7–9
  corrosive, 11–12
  delamination, 16–17
  erosive, 9–10
  fretting, 13–15
  importance and evaluation, 17–18
 orthopaedic implants, 3–22, 27–48

 osteolytic areas along the stem of a Co–Cr hip prosthesis, 29
 socio-economic impact, 21
 therapeutic targets, 40–8
  biologic treatments for particle-induced osteolysis, 43
wear-accelerated corrosion, 257, 259
wear debris, 316, 403
wear equation, 404
wear phenomenon
 ceramic joints, 278–93
  ceramic components wear, 288–93
  ceramic technology developments, 280–8
 importance in artificial joints, 222–3
 metal joints, 246–272
  articulation interface tribocorrosion, 262–6
  biotribocorrosion surface phenomena, 257–62
  electrochemical aspects of corrosion, 249–53
  fretting corrosion, 267–72
  implant alloys passivity and corrosion, 253–7
  orthopaedic implants alloys, 246–9
 UHMWPE knee joints, 227–42
  delamination mechanism study, 231–6
  femoral component and tibial insert analysis, 236–9
  retrieved artificial knee joints, 227–31
  surface asperities and tibial insert analysis, 239–42
  ultra-high molecular weight polyethylene (UHMWPE) joints, 221–42
  knee joints, 227–42
wear prediction
 applications, 410–14
  metal-on-metal bearings, 412–14
  metal-on-UHMWPE bearings, 410–12
 contact models, 409
 numerical calculation of wear, 409–10
  wear modelling flowchart, 411
 orthopaedic implants, 403–16
  future trends, 414–16
 overall wear modelling, 404–5
 wear factors and coefficients determination, 407–9

pin-on-plate wear test schematic, 408
wear models, 405–7
wear resistance, 199–204
wearing-in period, 312
welding wear, 8
Wolff's law, 316

X3 polyethylene, 169
X-ray fluoroscopy, 58

yttria-stabilised tetragonal zirconia polycrystals (Y-TZP), 284

Zimmer, 194
zirconia, 137, 198, 283–5
Y-TZP-based ceramics phase conversion toughening mechanism, 284
ZTA and Biolox phase conversion toughening mechanism, 285
zirconia-toughended alumina, 285–7
  Biolox delta micro-Raman spectra data, 288
  Biolox delta strontium aluminate platelets, 287
zirconia-toughened alumina (ZTA), 137, 198–9
zoledronic acid, 45
Zweymuller implant, 194
Zweymuller threaded cup, 156